Management of Sexual Dysfunction in Men and Women

Larry I. Lipshultz
Alexander W. Pastuszak
Andrew T. Goldstein
Annamaria Giraldi
Michael A. Perelman
Editors

Management of Sexual Dysfunction in Men and Women

An Interdisciplinary Approach

Springer

Editors
Larry I. Lipshultz
Baylor College of Medicine
Chief, Division of Male Reproductive Medicine and Surgery
Center for Reproductive Medicine
Scott Department of Urology
Houston, TX, USA

Andrew T. Goldstein
The Center for Vulvovaginal Disorders
Department of Obstetrics and Gynecology
George Washington University
School of Medicine and Health Sciences
Washington, DC, USA

Michael A. Perelman
Clinical Professor of Psychiatry, Reproductive Medicine and Urology
Weill Medical College Cornell University
New York, NY, USA

Co-Director, Human Sexuality Program
The New York Presbyterian Hospital
New York, NY, USA

Founder, MAP Education and Research Fund
New York, NY, USA

Alexander W. Pastuszak
Baylor College of Medicine
Assistant Professor
Division of Male Reproductive Medicine and Surgery
Center for Reproductive Medicine
Scott Department of Urology
Houston, TX, USA

Annamaria Giraldi
Sexological Clinic
Psychiatric Center Copenhagen
Institute of Clinical Medicine
University of Copenhagen
Copenhagen, Denmark

ISBN 978-1-4939-3099-9 ISBN 978-1-4939-3100-2 (eBook)
DOI 10.1007/978-1-4939-3100-2

Library of Congress Control Number: 2015957426

Springer New York Heidelberg Dordrecht London

Printed on acid-free paper
Springer Science+Business Media LLC New York is part of Springer Science+Business Media (www.springer.com)

Preface

Understanding both the physical and psychosocial-behavioral and cultural basis of sexual and reproductive health is essential in instituting effective treatments for men, women, and couples with sexual dysfunctions. The mental and physical aspects of sexual function are intricately interrelated, with established relationships between depression and sexual function in both males and females and links between sexual dysfunction and hormonal dysregulation and fertility in both sexes as well. In addition, a genetic basis for many conditions affecting sexual function is becoming apparent, which will inevitably lead to the rapid expansion of the diagnostic and potentially the therapeutic approaches used to evaluate and treat these patients. The evaluation and management of sexual dysfunction in the male, the female, and the couple is clinically complicated and does not fit into routine conceptualization of gender-specific diseases.

Integrating the individual approaches of urology, gynecology, psychiatry, and psychology, this book is truly transdisciplinary and unique among textbooks addressing sexual dysfunction.

The text provides a comprehensive, state-of-the-art review of the intersection of male and female reproductive and sexual health and will serve as a valuable resource for clinicians and researchers with an interest in abnormalities of sexual function. The book comprehensively discusses the evaluation and management of physical, genetic, and psychological causes of male and female sexual dysfunction. Examined in detail, one finds medical and surgical therapies in both the male and female, specifically focusing on erectile, ejaculatory, and orgasmic disorders in the male, arousal and orgasmic disorders in the female, and an integrated medico-psychosocial approach to the couple. Lifestyle modification through diet and exercise, resulting in optimization of anthropomorphic characteristics, is also reviewed. This approach highlights a holistic view of these disorders that goes beyond the typical focus on obvious pathophysiologic disorders of the genital system.

We believe the text will serve as a resource for physicians, mental health professionals, and researchers interested in sexual medicine, providing a concise and comprehensive overview of the field. Written by experts in their specialties, the text is divided into three sections: sexual dysfunction in the male, in the female, and in the couple. Many of the chapters are complemented by unique commentaries written by mental health professionals, giving an in-depth interdisciplinary approach to the subject of the chapter.

We hope this book will become a unique reference for all healthcare professionals interested in better understanding and treating human sexual dysfunction. Furthermore, it is anticipated that this comprehensive edition will help guide patient management and stimulate novel research efforts to further enhance progress in the field of human sexuality.

Houston, TX, USA — Larry I. Lipshultz
Houston, TX, USA — Alexander W. Pastuszak
Washington, DC, USA — Andrew T. Goldstein
Copenhagen, Denmark — Annamaria Giraldi
New York, NY, USA — Michael A. Perelman

Contents

Part II Sexual Dysfunction in the Female

Contributors

List of Editors

Annamaria Giraldi, M.D., Ph.D., F.E.C.S.M. Sexological Clinic, Psychiatric Center Copenhagen, Institute of Clinical Medicine, University of Copenhagen, Copenhagen, Denmark

Andrew T. Goldstein, M.D., FACOG, IF Director, The Center for Vulvovaginal Disorders, The George Washington University School of Medicine, Washington, DC, USA

Larry I. Lipshultz, M.D., Ph.D. Baylor College of Medicine, Division of Male Reproductive Medicine and Surgery, Center for Reproductive Medicine, Scott Department of Urology, Houston, TX, USA

Alexander W. Pastuszak, M.D., Ph.D. Baylor College of Medicine, Division of Male Reproductive Medicine and Surgery, Center for Reproductive Medicine, Scott Department of Urology, Houston, TX, USA

Michael A. Perelman, Ph.D. Psychiatry, Reproductive Medicine and Urology, Weill Medical College Cornell University, New York, NY, USA

Co-Director, Human Sexuality Program, The New York Presbyterian Hospital, New York, NY, USA

Founder, MAP Education and Research Fund, New York, NY, USA

List of Authors

Stanley E. Althof, Ph.D. Case Western Reserve University School of Medicine, Cleveland, OH, USA

Center for Marital and Sexual Health of South Florida, West Palm Beach, FL, USA

Phil Bach, M.D. Division of Urology, Faculty of Medicine and Dentistry, University of Alberta, Edmonton, AB, Canada

Natan Bar-Chama, M.D. Department of Urology, Mount Sinai School of Medicine, New York, NY, USA

Richard Balon, M.D. Department of Psychiatry, Detroit, MI, USA

Boback M. Berookhim, M.D., M.B.A. Department of Urology, Lenox Hill Hospital, New York, NY, USA

Johannes Bitzer, M.D. Department Obstetrics and Gynecology, University Hospital Basel, Switzerland

Yitzchak M. Binik, Ph.D. Department of Psychology, McGill University, Montreal, QC, Canada

Marianne Brandon, Ph.D. Wellminds Wellbodies, LLC, Annapolis, MD, USA

Robert E. Brannigan, M.D. Department of Urology, Northwestern University, Feinberg School of Medicine, Chicago, IL, USA

Claudia Brown, M.Sc., P.T. Faculty of Medicine, School of Physical and Occupational Therapy, McGill University, Montreal, QC, Canada

Physiotherapie Polyclinique Cabrini, UroSanté, Montreal, QC, Canada

Arthur L. Burnett, M.D. Brady Urological Institute, Johns Hopkins School of Medicine, Baltimore, MD, USA

John E. Buster, M.D. Division of Reproductive Endocrinology and Infertility, Women and Infants Hospital, Providence, RI, USA

Rafael Carrion, M.D. Department of Urology, University of South Florida, Tampa, FL, USA

F. Andrew Celigoj, M.D. Department of Urology, University of Virginia, Charlottesville, VA, USA

Shahin T. Chandrasoma, M.D. Skyline Urology, Los Angeles, CA, USA

Seth D. Cohen, M.D., M.P.H. Advanced Urological Care, New York, NY, USA

R. Matthew Coward, M.D. Department of Urology, University of North Carolina, Chapel Hill, NC, USA

Emma Dargie, M.Sc. Department of Psychology, Queen's University, Kingston, ON, Canada

James M. Dupree, M.D., M.P.H. Department of Urology, University of Michigan Medical Center, Ann Arbor, MI, USA

Alyssa Dweck, M.S., M.D., F.A.C.O.G., C.S.T. Mount Kisco Medical Group, Northern Westchester Hospital, Mt Kisco, NY, USA

Mt. Sinai School of Medicine, New York, NY, USA

Michael L. Eisenberg, M.D. Department of Urology, Stanford University School of Medicine, Palo Alto, CA, USA

William Fisher, Ph.D. Department of Psychology, University of Western Ontario, London, Ontario, Canada

Department of Obstetrics and Gynaecology, University of Western Ontario, London, Ontario, Canada

Martin K. Gelbard, M.D. Clinical Faculty, Skyline Urology, University of California, Los Angeles, Burbank, CA, USA

Irwin Goldstein, M.D. San Diego Sexual Medicine, San Diego, CA, USA

Juan Ramon Flores Gonzalez, M.D. Department of Surgery, University of Texas Medical School at Houston, Houston, TX, USA

Alessandra Graziottin, M.D. Center of Gynecology and Medical Sexology, H. San Raffaele Resnati, Milan, Italy

Graziottin Foundation for the Cure and Care of Pain in Women, Milan, Italy

Elizabeth Grill, Psy.D. The Ronald O. Perelman and Claudia Cohen Center for Reproductive Medicine, Weill Cornell Medical College, New York, NY, USA

Ethan D. Grober, M.Ed., M.D. Division of Urology, Department of Surgery, Mount Sinai and Women's College Hospital, University of Toronto, Toronto, ON, Canada

Steven R. Hahn, M.D., F.A.C.P. Albert Einstein College of Medicine, Bronx, NY, USA

Tariq S. Hakky, M.D. Advanced Urology, Snellville, GA, USA

Kathryn S.K. Hall, Ph.D. HallWatter Institute, Princeton, NJ, USA

T. Mike Hsieh, M.D. Department of Urology, University of California, San Diego, San Diego, CA, USA

Brett A. Johnson, M.D. Department of Urology, University of Wisconsin-Madison, Madison, WI, USA

Rose Khavari, M.D. Houston Methodist Center for Restorative Pelvic Medicine, Houston Methodist Hospital Department of Urology, Houston, TX, USA

Mohit Khera, M.D., M.B.A. Scott Department of Urology, Baylor College of Medicine, Houston, TX, USA

Jason R. Kovac, M.D., Ph.D. Urology of Indiana, Carmel, IN, USA

Yonah Krakowsky, B.Sc., M.D. Division of Urology, Department of Surgery, University of Toronto, Toronto, ON, Canada

Jill M. Krapf, M.D. Department of Obstetrics and Gynecology, George Washington University School of Medicine, Washington, DC, USA

Michael Krychman, M.D., C.M. Southern California Center for Sexual Health and Survivorship Medicine, Newport Beach, CA, USA

University of California Irvine, Irvine, CA, USA

Gavin M. Langille, M.D., F.R.C.S.C. Dalhousie University, Saint John, NB, Canada

Brian V. Le, M.D. Department of Urology, University of Wisconsin School of Medicine and Public Health, Madison, WI, USA

Stephen B. Levine, M.D. Case Western Reserve University School of Medicine, Beachwood, OH, USA

Center for Marital and Sexual Health, Beachwood, OH, USA

Kirk C. Lo, M.D., F.R.C.S.C. Division of Urology, Department of Surgery, Mount Sinai Hospital, Faculty of Medicine, Institute of Medical Science, University of Toronto, Toronto, ON, Canada

Monika Ewa Lukasiewicz, M.D. Department of Obstetrics and Gynecology, The Medical Center of Postgraduate Education, Bielanski Hospital, Warsaw, Poland

Marita P. McCabe, Ph.D. Institute for Health and Ageing, Australian Catholic University, Melbourne, Australia

Barry McCarthy, Ph.D. Department of Psychology, American University, Washington, DC, USA

Rachel Needle, Psy.D. Center for Marital and Sexual Health of South Florida, West Palm Beach, FL, USA

Advanced Mental Health Training Institute, West Palm Beach, FL, USA

Nova Southeastern University, West Palm Beach, FL, USA

Christian J. Nelson, Ph.D. Memorial Sloan Kettering Cancer Center, New York, NY, USA

Michael Pan, M.D. Scott Department of Urology, Baylor College of Medicine, Houston, TX, USA

Sharon J. Parish, M.D. Weill Cornell Medical College, New York, NY, USA

Westchester Division, New York Presbyterian Hospital, White Plains, NY, USA

Nishant Patel, M.D. Department of Urology, University of California, San Diego, San Diego, CA, USA

Samara Perez, Ph.D. (c). Department of Psychology, McGill University and Jewish General Hospital, Montreal, QC, USA

William D. Petok, Ph.D. Independent Practice, Severna Park, MD, USA

Caroline F. Pukall, Ph.D. Department of Psychology, Queen's University, Kingston, ON, Canada

Eusebio Rubio-Aurioles, M.D., Ph.D. Asociación Mexicana para la Salud Sexual, A.C. Profesor de posgrado, Departamento de Psiquiatría y Salud Mental, Facultad de Medicina, Universidad Nacional Autónoma de México, Mexico City, Mexico

Mary K. Samplaski, M.D. Department of Surgery, Institute of Urology, University of Southern California, Los Angeles, CA, USA

Glenn L. Schattman, M.D. The Ronald O. Perelman and Claudia Cohen Center for Reproductive Medicine, Weill Cornell Medical College, New York, NY, USA

Jason M. Scovell Center for Reproductive Medicine, Scott Department of Urology, Baylor College of Medicine, Houston, TX, USA

Ryan P. Smith, M.D. Department of Urology, University of Virginia, Charlottesville, VA, USA

Amy Stein, DPT, BCB-PMD, IF Beyond Basics Physical Therapy, LLC, New York, NY, USA

Matthew D. Timberlake, M.D. Department of Urology, University of Virginia, Charlottesville, VA, USA

Lana M. Wald, M.A. Department of Psychology, American University, Washington, DC, USA

Marcel Waldinger, M.D., Ph.D. Division Pharmacology, Department of Pharmaceutical Sciences, Faculty of BetaSciences, Utrecht University, Utrecht, The Netherlands

Practice for Psychiatry and Neurosexology, Amstelveen, The Netherlands

Daniel N. Watter, Ed.D. The Society for Sex Therapy and Research (SSTAR), Morris Psychological Group, P.A., Parsippany, NJ, USA

Daniel H. Williams IV, M.D. Department of Urology, University of Wisconsin School of Medicine and Public Health, Madison, WI, USA

Terri L. Woodard, M.D. Department of Gynecologic Oncology and Reproductive Medicine, MD Anderson, Houston, TX, USA

Christopher Yang, M.D. North Austin Urology, Austin, TX, USA

Jonathan Zurawin, M.D. Baylor College of Medicine, Houston, TX, USA

Introduction: Advocating for a Transdisciplinary Approach to the Management of Sexual Disorders

1

Michael A. Perelman

Two concepts were particularly important to me in developing this textbook: (1) a desire to cultivate a transdisciplinary sexual medicine perspective for the reader that emphasized integrating counseling with current and future medical/surgical approaches for the treatment of male and female sexual disorders and (2) emphasizing the need and benefit for the reader to use a biopsychosocial-behavioral and cultural lens when contemplating sexual response and sexual dysfunction.

When asked to coedit this volume, I was concerned about the need for yet another edited text about sexual disorders and their treatments. It was agreed that if we were to write a text for a truly multidisciplinary clinical audience, our editorial and author group would need to be diverse in terms of both gender and professions of origin. Through editorial discussions, a concept emerged of a book whose chapters would be written primarily by sexual medicine physicians and typically with additional commentary from those with a mental health background—often sex therapists. We believed such a dialectic would provide a unique contribution to the literature as well as support the emerging viewpoint that sexual medicine should share a transdisciplinary perspective which has characterized the most recent advances in many areas of medicine [1]. Such an approach goes beyond the multidisciplinary view, previously held by others as well as ourselves. Instead, transdisciplinarity speaks to the need for healthcare practitioners to exchange information in a manner that each contributing discipline and specialty begins to alter its own practices to share an integrated knowledge and achieve common scientific and clinical goals [2].

We hope the reader will develop insights and wisdom that transcends the information explicitly contained in the chapters and commentaries offered within this volume. Why and how? The dialogue between the mental health authors and the medical/surgical authors was often an implicit one. The reason for this was twofold. First, some of the commentaries were written to express the viewpoint of the mental health author in response to their perception of a physician's/surgeon's general approach to sexual problems today. These authors spoke about their view of the generic trends, rather than addressing a specific chapter author's writing. Other commentaries were written to directly complement a specific chapter and commented on the work of a given author. Obtaining a thorough understanding of sexual medicine requires an understanding of the mind/body issues inherent within human experience in general and sex in

M.A. Perelman, Ph.D. (✉)
Psychiatry, Reproductive Medicine and Urology, Weill Medical College Cornell University, 70 East 77th Street, New York, NY 10075, USA

Co-Director, Human Sexuality Program, The New York Presbyterian Hospital, New York, NY, USA

Founder, MAP Education and Research Fund, New York, NY, USA
e-mail: perelman@earthlink.net

L.I. Lipshultz et al. (eds.), *Management of Sexual Dysfunction in Men and Women*, DOI 10.1007/978-1-4939-3100-2_1

particular. The purpose of this book was to evoke a dialogue within the mind of the reader about a more comprehensive perspective on how to view patient's sexual disorders and concerns. In other words, the book is designed to teach an integrated treatment approach; yet our ultimate goal was to nurture for at least some of you a transdisciplinary perspective for the future of sexual medicine.

Of course, there is no reason to believe a single pathogenetic pathway to sexual disorders exists. Clarity of understanding requires that the clinician and researcher alike maintain a biopsychosocial-behavioral and cultural view of sexual response and dysfunction. Besides the obvious common sense appeal of such models, there is an ever-expanding body of empirically based quantitative and qualitative evidence supporting a multidimensional conceptualization, especially in the areas of treatment optimization, treatment adherence, and continuation of recommended therapies [3–26].

The reader may choose from a number of multidimensional models, but sexual medicine and sex therapy have recently been most influenced by various "dual-control models" [27–36]. Earlier, Helen S. Kaplan brought to sex therapy and to sexual medicine the principles of multideterminism and multilevel causality [32, 37]. However, in her last book *The Sexual Desire Disorders*, published in 1995, Kaplan foreshadowed the important work of Bancroft and colleagues [27] when she both described and illustrated dual-control elements of human sexual motivation and identified sexual "inciters" and "suppressors" to sexual desire dysregulation [31, 38]. She attributed her conceptualization to Kupferman [39] who had noted earlier that "all examples of physiological motivational control seem to involve dual effects—inhibitory and excitatory—which function together to adjust the system" (p. 751). Kaplan felt that control of sexual motivation was no exception and also operated on such a "dual steering" principle (Fig. 1.1).

The seminal works of Bancroft and colleagues are the best known and researched of the various dual-control models [27]. Bancroft's 1999 manuscript [27] and subsequent work with his Kinsey Institute colleagues (Graham, Heiman, Janssen, Sanders, etc.) have provided outstanding, erudite articulation of their dual-control theory, psychometrics, and comprehensive research for over 15 years

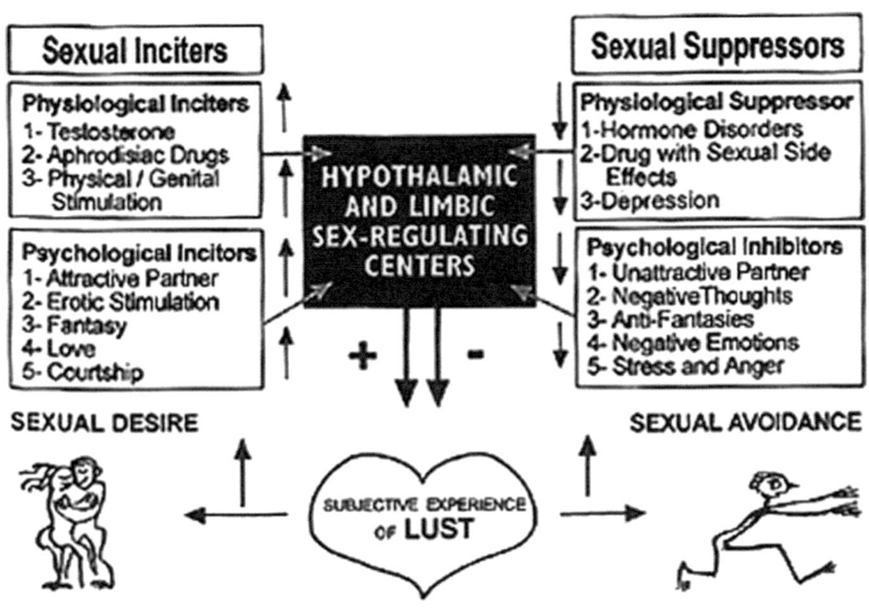

Fig. 1.1 Helen S. Kaplan's (1995) Dual-control elements of human sexual motivation: a psychosomatic model. With permission from Kaplan HS, The Sexual Desire Disorders. Dysfunctional Regulation of Sexual Motivation. Brunner-Routledge (Taylor and Frances, London, 1995: p. 15

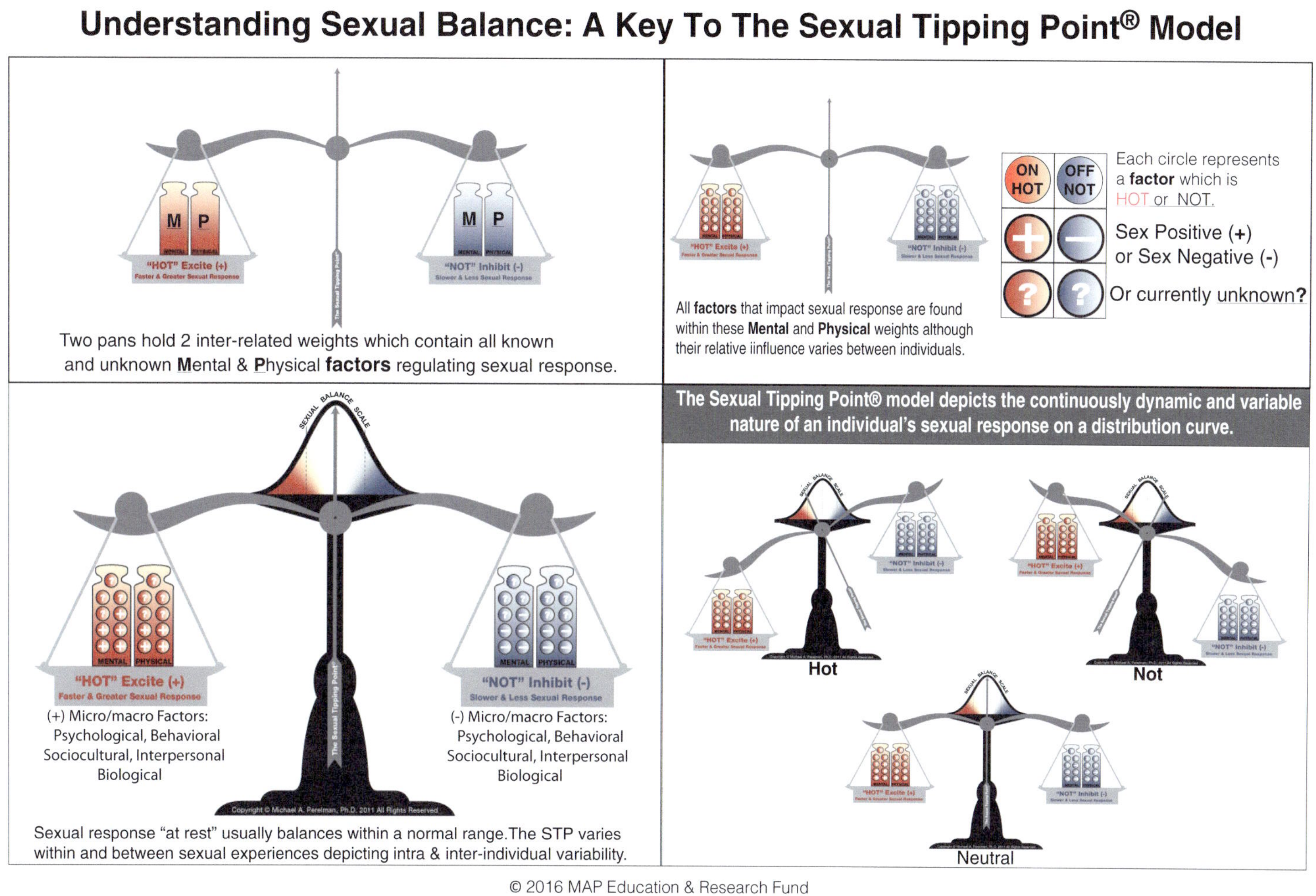

Fig. 1.2 A sequential key to the STP model. mapedfund.org provides a video explanation of the STP model as well as continuously updated images and other resources which are all available for free download by healthcare professionals

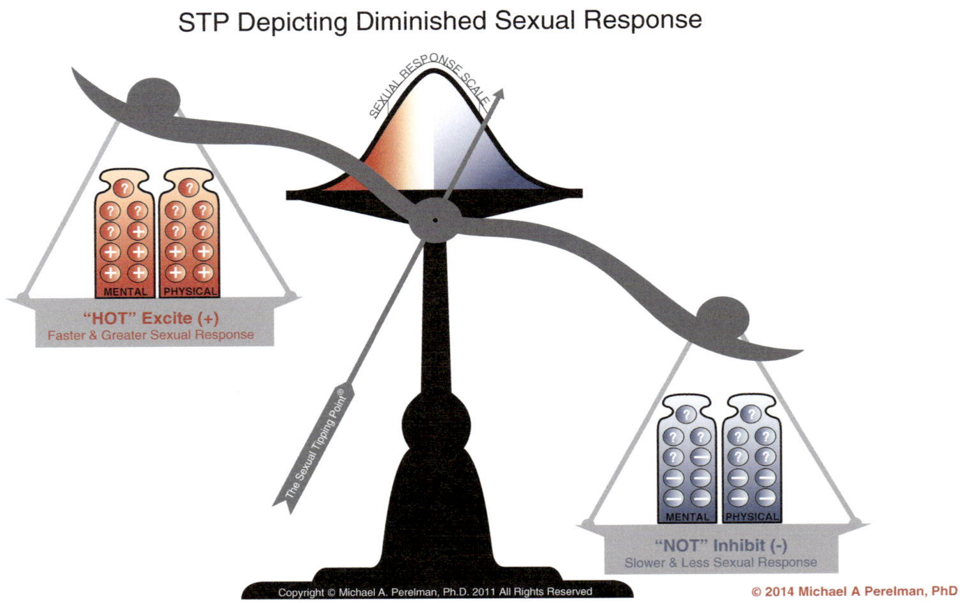

Fig. 1.3 STP illustrates diminished response. mapedfund.org provides a video explanation of the STP model as well as continuously updated images and other resources which are all available for free download by healthcare professionals

[40–42]. In short, they postulate and attempt to demonstrate "that sexual response and associated arousal occurs in a particular individual, in a particular situation, and is ultimately determined by the balance between two systems in that individual's brain, the sexual activation or excitation system and the sexual inhibition system, each of which has a neurobiological substrate" [27, p. 15].

Yet, from our perspective when contemplating the clinical need for understanding etiology, diagnosis, and treatment, we find the Sexual Tipping Point ® (STP) dual-control model particularly useful in its ability to illustrate both intra- and interindividual variability that characterizes sexual response and its disorders for both men and women (Fig. 1.2) [13].[1]

The Sexual Tipping Point® model easily illuminates the mind/body concept that mental factors can "turn you on" as well as "turn you off"; and the same is true of the physical factors. The Sexual Tipping Point® is the characteristic threshold for an expression of a given sexual response. Therefore, an individual's Sexual Tipping Point® represents the cumulative impact of the interaction of their constitutionally established capacity to express a sexual response which is elicited by different types of stimulation as dynamically impacted by various psychosocial-behavioral and cultural factors. An individual's threshold will vary somewhat from one sexual experience to another, based on the proportional effect of all the different factors that determine that tipping point at a particular moment in time. For instance, an individual suffering from a diminished sexual response (desire, arousal, orgasm) is illustrated by the cartoon in Fig. 1.3.

Besides illustrating all etiological permutations, including normal sexual balance, the Sexual Tipping Point® concept is particularly useful for modeling treatment and can easily be used to explain risks and benefits for patients with sexual disorders. The STP model can be used to teach patients where different treatment

[1] The STP model is a registered trademark of the MAP Education and Research Fund, a 501(c)(3) public charity. STP illustrations are available free from mapedfund.org.

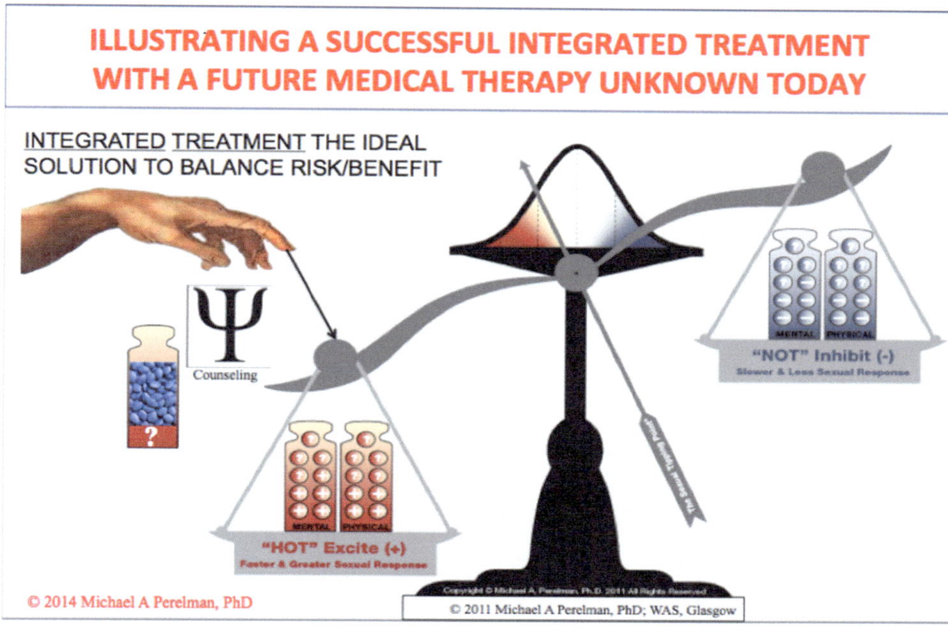

Fig. 1.4 STP depicts integrated treatment with a future medical therapy unknown today. mapedfund.org provides a video explanation of the STP model as well as continuously updated images and other resources which are all available for free download by healthcare professionals

targets should be focused, depending on diagnosis of their etiological determinants. Typically expressed erroneous binary beliefs can be politely disabused, and the patient can be reassured that "no it is not all in your head" nor "all a physical problem." Reciprocally, their partner can be assured it is "not all their fault!" Teaching the STP model to the patient and partner can reduce patient and partner despair and anger, while providing hope through a simple explanation of how the problem's causes can be diagnosed, parsed, and "fixed." In fact, the Sexual Tipping Point® also allows for modeling of a variety of future treatments, including medical or surgical interventions not yet discovered or proven such as novel pharmacotherapy, genetic engineering, or nanotechnology [35] (Perelman, 2011b). This is illustrated in Fig. 1.4.

Indeed, all the biopsychosocial-behavioral and cultural models of sexual dysfunction provide a compelling argument for sexual medicine treatments that integrate sex counseling and medical and/or surgical treatments [43]. Our work is not just to alleviate our patient's sexual symptom but when possible to improve their intimate relational lives. Restoration of lasting and satisfying sexual function requires a multifactorial understanding of all of the forces that created the problem, whether a solo physician or multidisciplinary team approach is applied. The healthcare professional that can accomplish an integrated treatment will offer the most optimized approach and the most elegant solution [43].[2] Treatment formats vary according to the preference and expertise of healthcare providers and tend to incorporate three processes: (a) the clinician's interest, training, and competence; (b) the biopsychosocial-behavioral and cultural severity of the sexual dysfunction; and (c) patient preference as to which healthcare professional

[2] Telemedicine through today's Internet technologies offers the opportunity for inexpensive video conferencing of diverse experts across geographic boundaries, which will perhaps increase the productive interaction between disciplines. Such technology offers the potential of multispecialty referral or consultation being available for the patient or partner when required, independent of geography.

they first choose to consult. Perelman [44] recommended that the degree of medical and psychosocial complexity determines whether a healthcare provider would work alone or as part of a multidisciplinary team. For instance, a physician working alone would assess all needed physical findings (examination, laboratory testing, etc.), as well as diagnose the patient as suffering from mild, moderate, or severe psychosocial obstacles to successful restoration of sexual function and satisfaction. In addition to the physical factors, the physician would attempt to identify the cognitive, behavioral, relational, and contextual cultural factors predisposing, precipitating, and maintaining the patient's sexual dysfunction. The physician would either continue treatment or make a referral(s) on the basis of perceived complexity and the actual progress obtained [5, 43].

Each clinician needs to carefully evaluate his or her own competencies and interests when considering treatments for sexual dysfunction. Having a multidimensional understanding of sexual dysfunction does not mandate a multidisciplinary approach. Solo practitioners may question whether to collaborate with a multidisciplinary team or to provide an integrated treatment themselves. Regardless of which healthcare professional the patient consults first, he or she is entitled to receive optimized care. For many patients, neither sex therapy alone nor medical/surgical interventions alone are sufficient to facilitate lasting improvement and satisfaction for a patient or partner with sexual dysfunction. For those patients who have sexual dysfunction based on deep-seated psychosocial and emotional issues, the use of a simple single-agent pharmacologic therapeutic will not be sufficient. Furthermore, a patient who has physical issues related to age, illness, and so forth is extremely unlikely to be fully restored (versus helped to adapt) by sex counseling exclusively. Indeed, some primary care physicians as well as many specialists will not have the expertise to adequately diagnose psychological obstacles to success, independent of their willingness to treat these factors. Alternatively, most mental health practitioners are neither capable nor licensed to provide medical care to the full extent needed by the patient. And as in all areas of healthcare, professionals should appropriately refer their patients for adjunctive consultation as needed.

We hope medical research will one day bring us more and better treatments to help ameliorate the biological factors that underlie some people's failure to function sexually in ways they would prefer. We believe the multidisciplinary perspective that emerged from an emphasis on the empirical success of combination treatments will be replaced by an integrated approach to sexual issues and dysfunctions by clinicians who will consult to these patients in the future. As that transdisciplinary view becomes more prevalent, we hope it will become the teaching model for all healthcare practitioners early in their training. In other words, we hope our readers will advance sexual medicine with an enlightened appreciation of etiology, diagnosis, and treatment based on a biopsychosocial-behavioral and cultural model. It is our hope that such sophistication will lead to an improved personalized sexual medicine benefitting both patient and practitioner alike. Our aspiration is for all healthcare practitioners to maintain a patient-centered holistic view of healing that integrates a variety of treatment approaches as needed whether for sexual dysfunction or any sexual concern. We hope this book provides a window on how this can be accomplished both now and in the future.

References

1. Perelman MA. Advocating for a transdisciplinary perspective in sexual medicine. Curr Sex Health Rep. 2015;7(1):1–2.
2. Rosenfield PL. The potential of transdisciplinary research for sustaining and extending linkages between the health and social sciences. Soc Sci Med. 1992;35(11):1343–57.
3. Abdo C, Afif-Abdo J, Otani F, Machado A. Sexual satisfaction among patients with erectile dysfunction treated with counseling, sildenafil, or both. J Sex Med. 2008;5(7):1720–6. doi:10.1111/j.1743-6109.2008.00841.x.
4. Althof SE. Sexual therapy in the age of pharmacotherapy. Annu Rev Sex Res. 2006;17:116–32. New York: Taylor and Francis.

5. Althof SE, Needle RB. Psychological factors associated with male sexual dysfunction: screening and treatment for the urologist [Review]. Urol Clin N Am. 2011;38(2):141–6. doi:10.1016/j.ucl.2011.02.003.
6. Aubin S, Heiman J, Berger R, Murallo A, Yung-Wen L. Comparing Sildenafil alone vs. Sildenafil plus brief couple sex therapy on erectile dysfunction and couples' sexual and marital quality of life: a pilot study. J Sex Marital Ther. 2009;35(2):122–43.
7. Bach A, Barlow D, Wincze J. The enhancing effects of manualized treatment for erectile dysfunction among men using sildenafil: a preliminary investigation. Behav Ther. 2004;35:55–73.
8. Banner L, Anderson R. Integrated sildenafil and cognitive-behavior sex therapy for psychogenic erectile dysfunction: a pilot study. J Sex Med. 2007;4(4 Pt 2):1117–25.
9. Brock G, Carrier S, Casey R, et al. Can an educational program optimize PDE5i therapy? A study of canadian primary care practices. J Sex Med. 2007;4(5): 1404–13.
10. Mahmoud A, Drake RJ, Lewis SW, Hayhurst KP, Barnes TRE. The ANNSERS (antipsychotic non-neurological side effects rating scale): validation of sexual side-effect measurement. Ther Adv Psychopharmacol. 2011;1(4):97–100.
11. McCabe M, Price E, Piterman L, Lording D. Evaluation of an internet-based psychological intervention for the treatment of erectile dysfunction. Int J Impot Res. 2008. doi:10.1038/ijir.2008.3.
12. Perelman M. Abstract #121: The sexual tipping point: a model to conceptualize etiology and combination treatment of female and male sexual dysfunction. J Sex Med. 2006;3 Suppl 1:52.
13. Perelman MA. The Sexual Tipping Point™: a model to conceptualize etiology, diagnosis and combination treatment of female and male sexual dysfunction. J Sex Med. 2006;3 Suppl 1:52.
14. Perelman M. Post-prostatectomy orgasmic response. J Sex Med. 2008;5(1):248–9.
15. Perelman MA. The history of sexual medicine. In: Tolman D, Diamond L, editors. APA handbook of sexuality and psychology. Washington, DC: American Psychiatric Association; 2013. p. 137–79.
16. Perelman M. Sexual balance: the universal versatility of the sexual tipping point model. Paper presented at the world meeting on sexual medicine: the 18th scientific meeting of the sexual medicine society of North America (SMSNA) and the 15th world meeting of the international society for sexual medicine (ISSM); 2012.
17. Phelps J, Jain A, Monga M. The PsychoedPlusMed approach to erectile dysfunction treatment: the impact of combining a psychoeducational intervention with sildenafil. J Sex Marital Ther. 2004;30(5):305–14.
18. Rosen R. Medical and psychological interventions for erectile dysfunction: toward a combined treatment approach. In: Leiblum S, Rosen R, editors. Principles and practice of sex therapy. 3rd ed. New York: Guilford Press; 2000. p. 276–304.
19. Rosen L, Rosen R. Fifty years of female sexual dysfunction research and concepts: from Kinsey to the present. In: Goldstein I, Meston C, Davis S, Traish A, editors. Women's sexual function and dysfunction: study, diagnosis and treatment. London: Taylor and Francis; 2006.
20. Rosen R, Brown C, Heiman J, et al. The female sexual function index (FSFI): a multidimensional self-report instrument for the assessment of female sexual function. J Sex Marital Ther. 2000;26(2):191–208.
21. Titta M, Tavolini I, Moro F, Cisternino A, Bassi P. Sexual counseling improved erectile rehabilitation after non-nerve-sparing radical retropubic prostatectomy or cystectomy – results of a randomized prospective study. J Sex Med. 2006;3(2):267–73.
22. Goldstein A, Pukall C, Goldstein I, editors. Female sexual pain disorders: evaluation and management. Oxford: Blackwell Publishing; 2009.
23. Brotto L, Basson R, Luria M. A mindfulness-based group psychoeducational intervention targeting sexual arousal disorder in women. J Sex Med. 2008;5: 1646–59.
24. Brotto L, Heiman J, Goff B, Greer B, Lentz G, Swisher E, Van Blaricom A. A psychoeducational intervention for sexual dysfunction in women with gynecologic cancer. Arch Sex Behav. 2008;37(2):317–29. doi:10.1007/s10508-007-9196-x.
25. Brotto L, Woo J. Cognitive-behavioral and mindfulness-based therapy for low sexual desire. In: Leiblum S, editor. Treating sexual desire disorders: a clinical casebook. New York: Guilford Press; 2010.
26. Brotto L, Heiman J. Mindfulness in sex therapy: applications for women with sexual difficulties following gynaecologic cancer. Leading comment. Sex Relat Ther. 2007;22(1):3–11.
27. Bancroft J, Graham CA, Janssen E, Sanders SA. The dual control model: current status and future directions. J Sex Res. 2009;46(2/3):121–42. doi:10.1080/00224490902747222.
28. Bancroft J, Janssen E. The dual control model of male sexual response: a theoretical approach to centrally mediated erectile dysfunction. Neurosci Biobehav Rev. 2000;24(5):571–9.
29. Basson R. The female sexual response: a different model. J Sex Marital Ther. 2000;26:51–65.
30. Basson B. Sexual desire and arousal disorders in women. N Engl J Med. 2006;354:1497–506.
31. Kaplan H. The sexual desire disorders: dysfunctional regulation of sexual motivation. New York: Brunner/Mazel, Inc; 1995.
32. Kaplan H. The new sex therapy. New York: Brunner/Mazel; 1974.
33. Metz ME, McCarthy BW. The "Good-Enough Sex" model for couple sexual satisfaction. Sex Relat Ther. 2007;22(3):351–62.
34. Perelman M. The sexual tipping point: a mind/body model for sexual medicine. J Sex Med. 2009;6(3):629–32. doi:10.1111/j.1743-6109.2008.01177.x.
35. Perelman M. The sexual tipping point: a mind/body model for the past, present and future. J Sex Med. 2011;8 Suppl 3:87.
36. Pfaus J. Pathways of sexual desire. J Sex Med. 2009; 6(6):1506–33.doi:10.1111/j.1743-6109.2009.01309.x.

37. Perelman M. Delayed ejaculation and other diminished ejaculatory disorders (DED). In: Binik Y, Hall K, editors. Principles and practice of sexual therapy. 5th ed. New York: Guilford; 2014.
38. Perelman MA. Helen Singer Kaplan's legacy and the future of sexual medicine. J Sex Med. 2012;9 Suppl 4:227.
39. Kupferman I. Hypothalamus and limbic system motivation. In: Kandel ER, Schwartz JH, Jessell TM, editors. Principle of neural science. 3rd ed. New York: Elsevier; 1991.
40. Bancroft J. Central inhibition of sexual response in the male: a theoretical perspective. Neurosci Biobehav Rev. 1999;23(6):763–84.
41. Graham C, Sanders S, Milhausen R. The sexual excitation/sexual inhibition inventory for women: psychometric properties. Arch Sex Behav. 2006;35(4):397–409. doi:10.1007/s10508-006-9041-7.
42. Janssen E, Vorst H, Finn P, Bancroft J. The sexual inhibition (SIS) and sexual excitation (SES) scales: I. Measuring sexual inhibition and excitation proneness in men. J Sex Res. 2002;39(2):114–26.
43. Perelman M. Integrated sex therapy: a psychosocial-cultural perspective integrating behavioral, cognitive, and medical approaches. In: Carson C, Kirby R, Goldstein I, Wyllie M, editors. Textbook of erectile dysfunction. 2nd ed. London: Informa Healthcare; 2008. p. 298–305.
44. Perelman MA. Psychosocial evaluation and combination treatment of men with erectile dysfunction [Review]. Urol Clin N Am 2005;32(4):431–45, vi. doi:10.1016/j.ucl.2005.08.010.

Additional Reading

Barlow D. Causes of sexual dysfunction: the role of anxiety and cognitive interference. J Consult Clin Psychol. 1986;54(2):140–8.

Bella A, Perelman M, Brant W, Lue T. Peyronie's disease (CME). J Sex Med. 2007;4(6):1527–38.

Hatzichristou D, Moysidis K, Apostolidis A, Bekos A, Tzortzis V, Hatzimouratidis K, Ioannidis E. Sildenafil failures may be due to inadequate patient instructions and follow-up: a study on 100 non-responders. Eur Urol 2005;47(4):518–22; discussion 522–13.

Jemtå L, Fugl-Meyer K, Öberg K. On intimacy, sexual activities and exposure to sexual abuse among children and adolescents with mobility impairment. Acta Paediatr. 2008;97:641–5.

McCarthy B. Integrating Viagra into cognitive-behavioral couple's sex therapy. J Sex Educ Ther. 1998;23:302–8.

Perelman M. Sex coaching for physicians: combination treatment for patient and partner. Int J Impot Res. 2003;15 Suppl 5:S67–74.

Perelman M. A new combination treatment for premature ejaculation: a sex therapist's perspective. J Sex Med. 2006;3(6):1004–12. doi:10.1111/j.1743-6109.2006.00238.x.

Perelman M. Clinical application of CNS-acting agents in FSD. J Sex Med. 2007;4 Suppl 4:280–90. doi:10.1111/j.1743-6109.2007.00611.x.

Perelman M. Guest editorial: female sexual dysfunction and the central nervous system. J Sex Med. 2007; 4(s4):257–9.

2 Why Is Sex Important?

Stephen B. Levine

2.1 Introduction

As the reader begins this book devoted to the modern treatment of sexual problems, it is useful to state the obvious. The primary purpose of clinical medicine is to assist patients with their limitations to physical and mental health. To this end, healthcare professionals are continuously educated about disorders and their therapies. Since 1970, this traditional focus on disease has been applied to sexual dysfunction, a term that artfully dodges the idea that many sexual problems are diseases. For several decades the scope of urology and gynecology has expanded to include sexual dysfunctions. A less than obvious benefit of the focus on diseases and their response to treatments is a clearer understanding of the processes that maintain health. For example, as clinical research recognized disease-inducing forms of immunological incompetence, the complex overlapping systems that preserve our health from pathogens were clarified. Similarly, as interventions for sexual dysfunction have evolved, knowledge has accumulated about sexual health. But sexual health, per se, is rarely the subject of sexual medicine articles. These articles assume sexual health equates with arousal or orgasmic functionality and suggest methods for restoring these capacities.

This chapter explores subtle, private aspects of sexual health. In doing so, it will define the lurking sources of disappointment that our patients are likely to feel when they request our assistance. In addition, the examination of sexual health and sexual distress will provide clinicians with some concepts concerning the psychological pathogenesis of many problems.

Sexual problems, theories of their cause, and treatment approaches date back to the earliest of medical writings [1]. Today, the sexual problems that attract clinical attention involve two broad categories: (1) *sexual identity* (transpositions of gender identity, variations in orientation, paraphilic patterns of arousal within and outside of a sexual addiction pattern) and (2) *sexual dysfunction* (symptoms include deficient sexual desire, incapacities in maintaining sexual arousal, anorgasmia, orgasm without pleasure, ejaculatory latency extremes, painful intercourse, and unwanted sexual arousal). Urologists, gynecologists, psychologists, psychiatrists, relationship therapists, sex therapists, and physical therapists each stake out their territories within this expanding array.

S.B. Levine, M.D. (✉)
Case Western Reserve University School of Medicine, Beachwood, OH, USA

Center for Marital and Sexual Health, Beachwood, OH, USA
e-mail: sbl2@case.edu

L.I. Lipshultz et al. (eds.), *Management of Sexual Dysfunction in Men and Women*, DOI 10.1007/978-1-4939-3100-2_2

2.2 The First Principle of Clinical Sexuality

All sexual behavior—solitary or partnered, normal or dysfunctional, morally acceptable or socially disapproved of—is ultimately constructed from four general sources: biology, psychology, interpersonal relationships, and culture [2]. This principle is a humbling reminder not to oversimplify the determinants of sexual phenomena in our rush to find solutions to patients' problems. Despite knowledge of this principle, all healthcare professionals are forced by their education, knowledge, and skill set to oversimplify this ordinary complexity in their everyday work. An elegant model that schematically illustrates the interaction of these four major determinants exists [3].

2.3 The Two Systems of Adult Nurturance in Sexual Relationships

Adult sexual relationships are well known to have the potential to stabilize and enrich individuals and make them happy with their interpersonal status. *Psychological intimacy* and *partner sexual behavior* are the two behavioral systems that nurture adults. Partner sexual behavior can exist without psychological intimacy just as psychological intimacy can occur without partner sexual behavior. When they are successfully integrated, however, a positive feedback between them creates a greater degree of mutual nurturance and results in maximization of sexual functional capacities. Psychological intimacy motivates partner sexual behavior, and sexual behaviors create a new degree of psychological intimacy. In sexual health, the two systems function as one.

2.4 Three Paths to the Creation of Psychological Intimacy

2.4.1 Conversation

The usual way to attain psychological intimacy is through conversion [4]. One person speaks; the other person listens. In order to achieve a moment of psychological intimacy, the speaker has to meet three requirements. The speaker must talk about his or her inner subjective psychological self. The speaker must be able to trust in the safety of sharing this with the listener. The speaker must possess the language skills to express in words his or her thoughts, feelings, perceptions, and history. Psychological intimacy will not occur, however, unless the listener is able to evidence the following characteristics: The listener must provide undivided, uninterrupted attention to the speaker. The listener's comments must be noncritical and reflect an accurate comprehension of what is being said and felt by the speaker. The listener needs to construe the opportunity to listen as a privilege to learn about the inner experiences of the speaker. Much conversation, even between established lovers, does not create psychological intimacy.

Psychological intimacy is a transformative moment of connection that occurs simultaneously in both the speaker and the listener. It is a bonding process that creates or reinforces the sense of belonging to one another. There are two basic forms of psychological intimacy. The first is the *two-way psychological intimacy* that ideally recurs in a couple's life. Each member of the couple, of course, takes a turn being a speaker and a listener to potentially re-create moments of connection. In *one-way psychological intimacy*, however, a particular person is almost always the speaker and the other person is predominantly the listener. Physicians and mental health professionals create a one-way psychological intimacy with patients, as do parents with their young children. Psychological intimacies are part of the landscape of numerous kinds of relationships, ranging from friendship to sibling bonds to lawyer-client relationships. Unlike this wide array of psychological intimacies, psychological intimacy within a sexual relationship possesses a special power to repeatedly ease the way to sexual behavior.

These bonding moments of connection have profound consequences for the speaker. The moments strengthen the bond to the listener, causing pleasing thoughts such as "I am accepted." "I feel more stable." "I am happier." "I feel healthier." These moments erase loneliness, create optimism, and cause the speaker to look forward to the next opportunity for connection. After repeated moments of psychological intimacy, the speaker generates interest in sexual behavior with the listener. Psychological intimacy can be a powerful erotic stimulus. In certain contexts it is the most reliable and safest known aphrodisiac.

Moments of psychological intimacy have positive consequences for the listener as well. The listener gains a deeper understanding of the speaker and experiences pleasure in being of value to the speaker. The listener demonstrates an increased willingness to think about his or her own subjective self and comes to realize how important he or she is to the speaker. These subjective experiences reaffirm the bond to the speaker.

Psychological intimacy is not confined to the adult-adult relationship. Parents ideally maintain it with their children; friendships among any age group exist because of the individuals' capacities to share aspects of themselves. The skill of psychotherapists is their ability to create and maintain psychological intimacy in order to promote psychological growth. Psychological intimacy creates a rarely discussed erotic stimulus in many relationships that are not intended to be sexual. As such, people have to carefully manage themselves so as not to complicate their lives.

2.4.2 Shared Intense Experiences

A second way of creating psychological intimacy, shared intense emotional experiences, does not require much conversation. An intense bond can readily be established or reestablished, for example, by enduring a frightening febrile illness in an infant, caring for a dying friend together, being together in combat, or being on an athletic team.

2.4.3 Sexual Behavior

The third way of attaining psychological intimacy is through sexual behaviors. It, too, is a largely nonverbal shared emotional experience. Many aspects of sex create private emotion. The sight of the partner's naked body is a powerful experience of knowing the person, particularly early in the relationship. To this is added the perception of what the naked person feels about his or her naked body. One learns of the partner's interest in and attitude toward specific sexual behaviors. Each person witnesses the other in arousal, a pleasurable knowledge that is augmented by facilitating, listening to, and watching the partner's orgasm. These intensely private subjective experiences create the sense of knowing the partner in a way that others could not. This is a privilege. In these ways, sex creates a profound degree of connection.

The unmodified word "intimacy" is used to describe shared conversations about private experiences, nonverbal emotional experiences, and sexual pleasure. All avenues of attaining psychological intimacies promote the sense of loving and being loved.

2.5 What Is Learned Over Time Through Sex

Over time, individuals discover their partners' range of sexual comfort. They witness the changing nature of this comfort. They come to discern their own and their partner's variations in desire, arousal, and orgasm. They appreciate some of their partner's motivations for sexual behaviors. Over months, years, or decades, sexual behavior may deepen the couple's bond such that each has a rich, nuanced conviction of the sensual capacities of the other and how best to relate to them [5].

2.6 What Accounts for the Pleasures of Sex?

The pleasures of sex are physical and psychological. Sex can create novel delicious sensations and pleasant emotions before, during, and after orgasm. A person experiences the sense of power in giving the partner pleasure. The ability to give and to receive pleasure increases interest in the other, adds to the knowledge of the other, and creates the sense of being intertwined with the other. These are the means of creating a sense of oneness. The seamless interplay of physical and psychological pleasure during sex attenuates the sense of time as the individuals transport one another into the realm of sensation. The psychological pleasures of sex also involve personal meanings. These meanings, however, are often either closely held privacies from the partner or indescribable. "I feel it, but I can't describe it. It just is!" "I love you!" is the occasional summary of this complexity.

2.7 Why Is Sex Important?

Sexual behavior stabilizes our sexual identity. Sex allows us to feel that we are confident as a man or woman. It helps us to clarify and stabilize our identity as a heterosexual, homosexual, or bisexual person. It clarifies the nature of our intentions as consisting of peaceable mutuality or varieties of sadomasochism or fetishism.

Sex is the vehicle for early romantic attachment at every stage in life—among the never attached, divorced, widowed, and those having affairs. It can facilitate the vital process of creating an entity from two individuals. Romance conveys the hidden quest for a safe, secure, comforting lasting unity. It is typically accompanied by an intense erotic desire for each other.

In established relationships, sexual behavior reinforces the sense that one is loved and capable of loving. It strengthens the sense of oneness enabling individuals to feel themselves to be an integral part of another. Sex has the capacities to erase the ordinary angers of everyday life, to elevate one's mood, and to increase resiliency for tomorrow. It improves our capacity to withstand extra relationship temptation. And, of course, it is vital to our reproductive ambitions.

Sex remains a vehicle for self-discovery throughout life. It begins in adolescence when eroticism is dominated by fantasy, attraction, and masturbation and continues to reveal private aspects of the self during the many decades of regular or intermittent partner sexual behaviors and into the wistful final alone years.

2.8 The Second Principle of Clinical Sexuality

Sexual experience is a dynamic ever-evolving process. It changes in the short and in the long term in response to numerous biological, psychological, interpersonal, economic, and social factors. Individuals change psychologically, physically, and sexually over time as they mature, take on new responsibilities, and experience loss, personal dilemmas, and illness.

Changes in one person invariably impact on the partner. Therapeutic interventions can be immediately effective because of the responsiveness of the balance of the couple's delicate interactions between sexual identity components and sexual function characteristics.

The second principle illustrates a limitation of medicine's traditional reliance on designing interventions for individuals. For the treatment of coupled individuals, it is useful to expand this paradigm so that the clinician recognizes that forces emanating from the partner can render a therapy that has been scientifically demonstrated to be efficacious ineffective.

2.9 The Sexual Equilibrium

The second principle explains why the sexual fate of an individual entering into a monogamous relationship is not determined by his or her precommitment sexual capacities. Once that person enters into the new sexual equilibrium, what he or she experiences will heavily depend on the interplay between the person's and the partner's component characteristics (Table 2.1).

Table 2.1 The interaction of the sexual components in any sexual equilibrium

Partner A		Partner B
Gender identity	↔	Gender identity
Orientation	↔	Orientation
Intention	↔	Intention
Sexual desire	↔	Sexual desire
Ease of arousal	↔	Ease of arousal
Orgasmic pattern	↔	Orgasmic pattern
Pain-free penetration	↔	Pain-free penetration

The interaction of these components determines the frequency of sexual behavior, what sexual acts they share, how orgasm is attained, and their sexual psychological satisfaction. The sexual equilibrium of each couple has unique features. Some individuals come to know that different levels of satisfaction occur with different partners over their lifetimes. Clinicians have to be alert to the possibility that some patients who request interventions for improving sexual capacity are not planning to use them with the apparent partner. These men and women may have a more satisfying sexual equilibrium with someone who is unknown to the partner, whether or not they have sex with their mate.

2.10 What Is Sensuality?

Satisfying functional sex requires the abandonment of ordinary daily preoccupations and the substitution of a focus on bodily sensations. Sensuality is not how a person looks. It is what a person is capable of doing and feeling during sex. Sensuality has two faces. The readily appreciated face is the capacity to experience the preoccupying sensations of a kiss, lick, a touch, a breast or genital caress, and penetration. The more subtle face of sensuality is the person's interest in transporting the partner to this realm where pleasure predominates.

2.11 An Ideal Life of Sexual Pleasure

High on the list of hoped for personal expectations from life is to have, at least for an extended period of time, a diet of emotionally satisfying sex [6]. It is as though individuals collectively know that sex can be wonderful and that it is a vehicle to feel and express love. In the last analysis, sex may be the easy way to access the much more difficult to describe subject of love [7]. Particularly in clinical medicine, where the topic of love is generally avoided, sex may be a surrogate topic for love.

A satisfying sexual life diminishes the sense that one has been cheated by life. Wonderful sex creates a comforting, stabilizing sense of happiness. People learn from it that in being a part of someone else, they not only do not lose their individuality by loving but their individuality is essential to their blissful sensual excursions. Satisfying sensual sex prevents envy of other people's sexual experiences because people sense that "It could not get better than this."

2.12 Sexual Health Is Only Potential

Recurrently satisfying sensuous interactions—sexual health—is a developmental achievement. It is not guaranteed for men or women by their biological normality, their sex-positive attitudes, or past history of sensuality. While physicians prefer to biologically intervene with sexual dysfunctions, to do so without paying attention to the psychological, interpersonal, and cultural contexts of a patient's life will often disappoint the patient and the doctor. Comprehending the potentials of sex to enhance lives ironically helps clinicians to understand these three contexts.

Sex is important because it has the capacity:

1. To please
2. To stabilize
3. To physically satisfy
4. To emotionally satisfy
5. To improve self-understanding
6. To improve understanding of the partner
7. To heighten the experience of being loved and loving
8. To enhance life through reproduction

Patients with sexual difficulties can be assumed to be currently lacking in the attainment of these potentials. Some have never, even briefly, attained them. Many have attained and lost them.

2.13 Sources of Distress

Modern criteria for sexual diagnoses require that the patient or the couple experience distress about their difficulty. While rating scales can be used to quantify distress [8] and are vital to clinical sexual research, numbers explain the intensity but not the sources of the distress. The right side of Table 2.2 clarifies the subjective contributions to the distress. These are obviously just the inverse of the positive potentials of sex. Understanding the reasons for the distress in these terms, whether or not they are explicitly stated, helps in the establishment of a trusting relationship with the patient.

2.14 Two Subtleties About the Sexual History

2.14.1 The Clinician's Audition

Our contact with the patient begins with our taking a sexual history [9]. There have been many seminal writings published on this important topic since 1970 [10–12]. The clinician should realize, however, that the initial evaluation is a mutual process. The doctor is evaluating the sexual complaint by searching for the correct diagnosis and beginning to ascertain the pathogenesis and factors that may shape the approach to therapy. The individual patient, or the couple, all the while is assessing the clinician's warmth, interest, understanding of their distress, and competence. Some initial evaluations are not followed by treatment. Some treatments are not continued for a reasonable duration. Doctors may be baffled when patients do not return or do not follow their recommendations. One of the possibilities that may be considered is that the clinicians may have flunked the patient's evaluation of them. The goal of the sexual history taking from the patient's perspective is the establishment of a hope-generating trusting alliance with the doctor. There will be no therapy, despite an accurate diagnosis and a state-of-the-art treatment plan, if the clinician fails the audition inconspicuously conducted by the patient.

Table 2.2 Positive and negative potential of sex

Positive potentials	Negative potentials
To please	To displease
To stabilize	To destabilize
To physically satisfy	To physically frustrate
To emotionally satisfy	To emotionally frustrate
To improve self-understanding	To prevent self-understanding
To improve understanding of the partner	To obscure understanding of the partner
To feel loved and loving	To feel empty—unloved and uncaring
To enhance life through reproduction and parenthood	To prevent the pleasures of reproduction and parenthood

2.14.2 There Is No Such Thing as a Complete Sexual History

The specifics of the sexual history vary, of course, with the presenting problem, the specialty of the clinician, the presumptions about the likely sources of the problem, and the patient's capacity to talk about the matter. Despite the inherent pressure clinicians feel to gather a lot of information at the first encounter, there is no such thing as a complete sexual history. For example, a gynecologist and a psychologist may each be thorough in their assessments, but the details that will emerge will be quite different. The sexual history and the doctor's ability to formulate the pathogenesis of the problem are evolving processes. This is more apparent among mental health professionals, but is nonetheless true as well among urologists, gynecologists, and pelvic floor specialists. As a general guideline to attaining a comprehensive sexual history, clinicians can recall the concept of the sexual equilibrium. Eventually, the history should reveal the individual's sexual identity components and sexual functional capacities. It should clarify the partner's capacities and how they interact. It is asking too much of any clinician to obtain a picture of all of this by the end of the first meeting.

Understanding the patient's distress and disappointment with their sexual problem, although it takes only a brief moment or two, generates moments of empathy and one-sided psychological intimacy. This seems to be how many clinicians pass their audition with very high marks. With this achieved, the doctors can turn their attention to helping the patient to improve.

References

1. Berry M. The history and evolution of sex therapy and its relationship to psychoanalysis. Int J Appl Psychoanal Stud. 2013;10(1):53–74.
2. Levine S. The first principle of clinical sexuality. J Sex Med. 2007;4:853–4.
3. Perelman M. The sexual tipping point: a mind/body model for sexual medicine. J Sex Med. 2009;6(3):629–32.
4. Levine S. Psychological intimacy: the pathway to love. In: Levine S, editor. Demystifying love: plain talk for the mental health professional. New York: Routledge; 2006.
5. Kleinplatz P. Lessons from great lovers. In: Levine SR, Levine SR, editors. Handbook of clinical sexuality for mental health professionals. 2nd ed. New York: Routledge; 2010. p. 57–72.
6. Byers E. Relationship satisfaction and sexual satisfaction: a longitudinal study of individuals in long-term relationships. J Sex Res. 2005;42(2):113–18.
7. Levine S. Barriers to loving: a clinician's perspective. New York: Routledge; 2013.
8. Derogatis L, Clayton A, Lewis-D'Agostino D, Wunderlich G, Fu Y. Validation of the female sexual distress scale-revised for assessing distress in women with hypoactive sexual desire disorder. J Sex Med. 2008;5(2):357–64.
9. Althof S, Rosen R, Perelman M, Rubio Aurioles E. Standard operating procedures for taking a sexual history. J Sex Med. 2013;10(1):26–35.
10. Masters W, Johnson V. Human sexual inadequacy. Boston: Little Brown; 1970.
11. Maurice W. Sexual medicine in primary care. St. Louis, MO: Mosby; 1999.
12. Althof S, Rosen R, Perelman M, Rubio Aurioles E. Standard operating procedure for taking a sexual history. Journal of Sexual Medicine. 2013, 10(1): 26–35.

The Impact of the Environment on Sexual Health

3

James M. Dupree and Gavin M. Langille

3.1 Introduction

There is a great deal of interest regarding environmental influences that potentially affect sexual health and fertility, as reflected by the large body of literature on the topic. Patients with sexual dysfunction or infertility are often quite motivated to assess and ameliorate these conditions, and the readily apparent nature of environmental factors in everyday life inevitably makes them a target for modification. Despite numerous studies examining environmental factors that may play a role in sexual health and fertility, widespread randomized controlled trials are limited. The issues contributing to this lack of robust data include difficulty controlling for environmental factors and a lack of consensus regarding suitable study end points. Widespread public interest in the impact of environmental factors fuels coverage from the lay press, often generating news based on inconclusive scientific discourse.

In this chapter, we review the impact of the environment on the sexual health of men and women.

J.M. Dupree, M.D., M.P.H. (✉)
Department of Urology, University of Michigan Medical Center, 3875 Taubman Center/SPC 5330, 1500 E. Medical Center Drive, Ann Arbor, MI 48109-5330, USA
e-mail: jim.dupree@gmail.com

G.M. Langille, M.D., F.R.C.S.C.
Dalhousie University, Saint John, NB, Canada

It is worth noting from the outset that sexual health is challenging to define, because what might be considered a healthy sexual lifestyle in one culture may be viewed as unhealthy in another [1]. Additionally, in women, sexual function is challenging to measure. Unlike female fecundity/fertility and hormones, measurement of "healthy" sexual functioning currently lacks the objective measures we use to assess the former metrics, in contrast to the availability of these measures in men. Nevertheless, in this chapter, we summarize the available literature on the impact of environment on sexual function in both genders; the majority of the female-specific discussion in this chapter will focus on fertility due to a paucity of research on the impact of the environment on sexual function, libido, and sexual satisfaction in women. In the studies discussed below, the terms fertility and fecundity are often used interchangeably, but in their classic definitions, fertility refers to the ability to produce a live offspring while fecundity refers to the ability to conceive [2].

3.2 Obesity

People with a body mass index (BMI) between 25 and 30 kg/m^2 are defined as overweight, while those with a BMI >30 kg/m^2 are obese [3]. As of 2010 in the United States, over one third of the population is obese [4].

L.I. Lipshultz et al. (eds.), *Management of Sexual Dysfunction in Men and Women*, DOI 10.1007/978-1-4939-3100-2_3

There is a clear relationship between obesity in women and impaired fertility. Women with increased BMI have a higher risk of menstrual disorders, miscarriages, impaired fecundity, and pregnancy outcomes [5]. A study of women with a BMI >25 or a pregnancy weight >80 kg took twice as long to achieve a pregnancy [6]. Additionally, weight loss interventions have been shown to improve menstrual cycle regularity, ovulation, and fecundity [7].

Two studies have investigated the potential relationship between obesity and female sexual dysfunction. In the first, 45 obese women were age-matched to 30 healthy controls. The study found a negative correlation between BMI and orgasm and between weight and sexual satisfaction; women with higher BMI reported lower rates of orgasms ($p=0.007$), and women with higher weights reported less satisfaction ($p=0.03$) [8]. However, on the more global female sexual function index (FSFI) scale, there were no significant differences between obese and normal weight women (mean FSFI score of 22.1 ± 4.3 versus 23.1 ± 3.7, respectively, $p=0.74$). The diagnosed rates of female sexual dysfunction (defined as an FSFI score of ≤ 26.55) were 86 % in obese women and 83 % in controls (no significant difference). A second study of 64 obese women and 27 age-matched controls similarly showed no significant differences in FSFI scores ($p=0.29$) and rates of female sexual dysfunction of 50 % and 41 % in the obese and control groups, respectively ($p=0.34$) [9].

Between 1981 and 2008, the global incidence of obesity rose from 4.8 to 9.8 % in men [10]. The rise in obesity rates in males beginning in childhood and extending into their reproductive years is especially troubling, and data regarding the effects of obesity on semen parameters are conflicting. A meta-analysis by MacDonald et al. showed no correlation between semen parameters and BMI [11]. However, a meta-analysis by Sermondade et al. demonstrated an increased chance of abnormal semen parameters in overweight and obese men [odds ratio (confidence interval) for azoospermia or oligospermia of 1.11 (1.01–1.21) for overweight, 1.28 (1.06–1.55) for obese, and 2.0 (1.59–2.62) for morbidly obese men] [12]. Data from the LIFE study by Eisenberg et al. showed an inverse correlation between waist circumference and semen volumes and concentrations [13].

Testosterone levels in obese men are lower compared to men with a lower BMI [14], attributed in part to an increase in aromatization of testosterone to estrogen in adipose tissue [15]. In addition, obesity contributes to a diagnosis of "metabolic syndrome" along with hypertension, insulin resistance, elevated triglycerides, and low levels of high-density lipoprotein, which has a negative impact on erectile function [16–18]. Dyslipidemia has also been shown to negatively impact sperm morphology [19]. The adipose tissue surrounding the testes in obese patients may impair fertility through elevated scrotal temperatures, and surgical removal of the suprapubic fat pad in such patients has resulted in increased sperm concentration and motility in a series of 22 patients [20].

3.3 Diet

Due to complex cultural and financial considerations, many countries are shifting consumption toward a "western" diet characterized by large portions of refined grains, sugars, and red meats while being low in fresh fruits and vegetables, a combination widely considered unhealthy [21]. A healthy diet contributes to both physical and mental health and is important for avoidance of obesity, diabetes, and cardiovascular disease [22]. Obese patients have a significantly increased risk of developing depression [23], a well-known risk factor for sexual dysfunction [24, 25].

While some studies have suggested that a woman's prepregnancy diet can affect fetal health [26], few studies have directly investigated potential links between female diet and fertility [22]. However, the first trimester is likely the time where the embryo's health is most directly related to the mother's diet and nutrition [22]. Numerous investigations of the impact of vitamins, particularly folic acid and other B-group vitamins on neural tube development, have led to an understanding of their impact on fetal health [27].

However, fewer studies about vitamins and their impact on fertility exist. The study of a large prospective cohort of 18,555 women did show that women taking folic acid and other B-group vitamins had a lower risk of infertility [28].

Erectile dysfunction (ED) is more commonly diagnosed in men with obesity, diabetes, and cardiovascular disease, as well as other comorbid conditions [29]. A randomized controlled trial of 145 obese men found a significant improvement in erectile function as assessed using the IIEF-5 questionnaire for those enrolled in a weight loss program employing diet and exercise [30]. In regard to male fertility, a case-control study of 30 men showed that infertile males had a lower intake of fruits and vegetables, with a higher intake of red meats [31]. Similarly, a study of 189 men showed an inverse relationship between red meat intake and total sperm count [32]. An observational study of 188 men showed that those who avoided a western diet had increased sperm motility [33].

3.4 Exercise

While exercise is generally considered a healthy endeavor, in excess, it can impair fertility in women. As far back as 1986, a population-based case-control study of 187 infertile women and 419 parous controls showed that vigorous exercise lasting more than 60 min per day could increase a women's risk for infertility associated with abnormal ovulation [34]. Female athletes show significantly more menstrual cycle irregularity as compared to sedentary women (1–44 % irregular cycles versus 2–5 % irregular cycles, respectively) [5]. Additionally, being underweight (defined as a BMI < 19) has been shown to reduce a woman's fecundity by up to fourfold [6]. In their study, Hassan and Killick found that underweight women took an average of 29 months to achieve a pregnancy, as compared to 6.8 months for women of normal weight [6]. However, for obese women with polycystic ovary syndrome, women engaging in moderate exercise were more likely to resume ovulation [35].

The Massachusetts Male Aging Study followed 593 men for 8 years; men who regularly exercised showed a 30 % decreased risk of developing ED [36]. Aerobic exercise has been shown to improve semen concentration, motility, and morphology as seen in a 14-week study of 60 men using a home treadmill routine of moderate intensity [37]. A study of 222 men aged 18–22 found that a higher ratio of exercise to television watching actually improved sperm concentration and total sperm count [37]. However, vigorous cycling was shown to increase reactive oxygen species and worsen semen parameters [38]. In obese men, regular exercise increased serum testosterone levels and improved erectile function [39].

Patients should be counseled that regular aerobic exercise of moderate intensity is likely beneficial for the maintenance of fertility and sexual function while a complete lack or excess of physical activity is likely to be detrimental.

3.5 Smoking

Although tobacco use in the western world has decreased over the past several decades, the smoking rate in the United States remains at almost 20 % [40]. Tobacco use has been associated with many health conditions including lung cancer, heart disease, and, more recently, infertility. However, public knowledge of smoking as a cause of infertility is significantly lower than knowledge about the link between smoking and lung cancer and heart disease [41]. Using a population-based sample, Hull and colleagues found that women who smoked were 54 % more likely to have a fecundity delay of greater than 12 months, as compared to nonsmokers [42]. This relationship also appears to be dose-dependent, with heavy smokers having worse fertility [6]. A review of 13 studies found that 12 of the 13 studies demonstrated a negative impact of smoking on fecundity [43]. Biologically, smoking has been associated with lowered ovarian reserve, lower estrogen levels, higher follicle-stimulating hormone levels, and earlier menopause in women, all likely contributing to the increased primary and secondary infertility seen among female smokers [44].

Similarly, male smokers demonstrate impaired semen volume [45], concentration, motility [46], and morphology [46]. However, the effects of smoking in men on pregnancy rates have been more difficult to elucidate [47]. The mechanisms underlying the effects of tobacco on semen parameters are thought to be based on elevated nitric oxide, which results in an impaired acrosome reaction and lower sperm motility, while elevated lipid peroxidation compromises the sperm plasma membrane [48].

Smokers have a 40 % higher rate of ED than nonsmokers, which varies in a dose-dependent manner [49]. The increased risk of ED in smokers is derived from the endothelial and atherosclerotic insults resulting in end organ damage [50]. Former smokers have significantly less ED than active smokers, indicating that smoking cessation can result in improved erectile dysfunction [51].

3.6 Alcohol

When consumed by women during pregnancy, alcohol is well known to be a teratogen [22]. But separate from its effect on the fetus, both moderate (<100 g per week) and heavy (>100 g per week) alcohol consumptions have also been associated with female infertility. A multicenter case-control study of 1050 infertile women and 3833 parous controls found that both moderate and high alcohol intakes were associated with a 60 % increased risk of infertility [52]. It appeared that ovulatory dysfunction was the likely etiology of infertility among the women with heavy alcohol intake.

Regarding sexual function in women, there is a dose-dependent response between blood alcohol levels and genital response, with high blood alcohol levels associated with decreased genital responsiveness. Assessment of genital responsiveness, however, is complicated by an increased subjective sense of arousal in the setting of increased alcohol consumption, even when the objective genital response is impaired [53].

Although it has long been known that alcohol in moderate amounts can increase libido in men [54], when consumed in larger quantities, it causes ED [55]. Chronic alcohol use can induce ED by multiple factors including peripheral nerve damage and hypogonadism [56]. Central disruption of the gonadal axis has also been proposed [57]. Alcohol abuse and depression have been extensively linked, with alcohol being a known precipitant for depressive episodes [58]. In turn, depression is a known risk factor for erectile dysfunction [59]. The absolute effect of alcohol on semen parameters remains controversial in the literature to date. Ethanol intake has been shown to reversibly decrease sperm morphology, although pregnancy rates remain unaffected at the population level [60]. Among heavy drinkers (ethanol intake >80 g per day), 78.8 % had abnormal semen analyses [61].

3.7 Illicit Drugs

Marijuana and cocaine use have been associated with increased rates of infertility in women. In a case-control study of 150 infertile women, marijuana use increased the risk of infertility by about 70 %, especially when used in the year preceding attempted pregnancy [62]. Cocaine use also is also associated with increased infertility rates [62].

There are few published data about the impact of illicit drugs on sexual function in women. It is generally thought that chronic use of most illicit drugs leads to decreased sexual response in women [63]. Additionally, using illicit drugs has been associated with increased risky sexual behavior, as well as an increased risk of STIs and unwanted pregnancies [63].

Narcotic use and abuse in men has deleterious effects on testosterone levels and erectile function. Chronic narcotic use decreases serum testosterone, luteinizing hormone, follicle-stimulating hormone, and libido [64]. Erectile function is also negatively affected by narcotic use [65].

The legalization of marijuana in parts of the United States and elsewhere [66] highlights the importance for awareness of its deleterious effects on sperm motility [67], as well as decreased luteinizing hormone [68] and testosterone levels [69]. Interestingly, ED was not noted among a large cohort of marijuana users [70]. Cocaine has been shown to impair sperm concentration, motility, and morphology, and heroin has also been shown to negatively affect semen parameters [71, 72].

Testosterone supplementation is a well-known male contraceptive; an international study using intramuscular testosterone enanthate produced azoospermia in 65 % of men within 4 months [73]. Despite this, a survey of 387 urologists revealed that 25 % of respondents would actually prescribe testosterone in an attempt to ameliorate infertility, apparently unaware of the actual effects of testosterone on semen quality [74].

3.8 Male Gonads and Temperature

Elevated testicular temperature has a deleterious effect on testicular function [75]. Common causes for a hyperthermic testicular environment include febrile illness [76], saunas [77], warmer weather [78], and, as previously discussed, increased insulation of the testes by adipose tissue [79]. Heat exposure associated with sitting in an automobile for periods of >3 h per day also significantly prolonged the time to achieve a pregnancy [80]. The use of tight underwear, often a topic of inquiry from patients, does not appear to be detrimental to male fertility or sexual function [81]. The studies on these areas are a continued source of debate with little in the way of consensus on the role of temperature effects on male gonadal function.

3.9 Testicular Exposure to Electromagnetic Radiation

There is evidence that the)radiofrequency electromagnetic radiation (RF-EMR) produced by cellular telephones can adversely affect sperm motility and morphology [82]. In a study of ten men, the level of sperm DNA fragmentation was increased in men using cellular telephones for more than 4 h per day, exacerbated by storage of the phone in the trouser pocket [83]. A study by Agarwal et al. demonstrated decreased motility of ejaculated sperm after exposure to RF-EMR [84]. Although robust randomized controlled trials are lacking, the available data suggest that minimization of gonadal RF-EMR exposure is advisable.

3.10 Maternal Age

The age of first maternity is increasing. According to the Centers for Disease Control and Prevention, the average age of first birth for women increased from 21.4 years in 1970 to 25.0 years in 2006 [85]. This is thought to result from a variety of factors including changes in marriage patterns, educational and career opportunities, and contraceptive use [86]. Increasing age is a clear risk factor for infertility, with women over 35 often taking significantly longer to achieve a pregnancy [87], thought to be related to higher menstrual cycle irregularity, chromosomal abnormalities, and a decrease in oocyte quality as women age [87].

3.11 The Built Environment

Although the literature is very limited, a brief discussion of the impact of the built environment on sexual health is necessary. The built environment refers to the physical structures that people live in and around, as well as the neighborhood environment [88]. "Riskscapes" describe geographic areas with low incomes and an excess of poor land use, neighborhood stressors, and limited access to healthcare resources or healthy land uses such as parks and open spaces [88]. Research into the effect of the built environment has found that adolescent residents of riskscapes have higher rates of sexually transmitted infections (STIs), unprotected sexual activities, and unintended pregnancies [88]. Additionally, women in these areas are at increased risk for sexual assault [88]. Riskscapes may also be associated with increased stress and fatigue among women for these reasons, and any environmental condition that induces stress or fatigue can lower sexual desire [1].

3.12 Conclusion

There exists a breadth of environmental influences on male and female sexual function and reproductive health. The available literature supports promotion of sexual and reproductive function through a healthy lifestyle with attention to diet and exercise while limiting tobacco, alcohol, and illicit drugs that negatively impact sexual function when possible. Future trials of higher quality are required to further elucidate the role of additional environmental factors on sexual and reproductive health.

References

1. Bancroft J. Impact of environment, stress, occupational, and other hazards on sexuality and sexual behavior. Environ Health Perspect. 1993;101 Suppl 2:101–7.
2. Buck GM, Sever LE, Batt RE, Mendola P. Life-style factors and female infertility. Epidemiology. 1997;8:435–41.
3. Bray GA. Overweight is risking fate. Definition, classification, prevalence, and risks. Ann N Y Acad Sci. 1987;499:14–28.
4. Moyer VA, U.S. Preventive Services Task Force. Screening for and management of obesity in adults: U.S. Preventive Services Task Force recommendation statement. Ann Intern Med. 2012;157:373–8.
5. Kelly-Weeder S, O'Connor A. Modifiable risk factors for impaired fertility in women: what nurse practitioners need to know. J Am Acad Nurse Pract. 2006;18: 268–76.
6. Hassan MA, Killick SR. Negative lifestyle is associated with a significant reduction in fecundity. Fertil Steril. 2004;81:384–92.
7. Norman RJ, et al. Improving reproductive performance in overweight/obese women with effective weight management. Hum Reprod Update. 2004;10: 267–80.
8. Yaylali GF, Tekekoglu S, Akin F. Sexual dysfunction in obese and overweight women. Int J Impot Res. 2010;22:220–6.
9. Kadioglu P, et al. Obesity might not be a risk factor for female sexual dysfunction. BJU Int. 2010;106: 1357–61.
10. Finucane MM, et al. National, regional, and global trends in body-mass index since 1980: systematic analysis of health examination surveys and epidemiological studies with 960 country-years and 9.1 million participants. Lancet. 2011;377:557–67.
11. MacDonald AA, Herbison GP, Showell M, Farquhar CM. The impact of body mass index on semen parameters and reproductive hormones in human males: a systematic review with meta-analysis. Hum Reprod Update. 2010;16:293–311.
12. Sermondade N, et al. BMI in relation to sperm count: an updated systematic review and collaborative meta-analysis. Hum Reprod Update. 2013;19:221–31.
13. Eisenberg ML, et al. The relationship between male BMI and waist circumference on semen quality: data from the LIFE study. Hum Reprod. 2014;29:193–200.
14. Zumoff B, et al. Plasma free and non-sex-hormone-binding-globulin-bound testosterone are decreased in obese men in proportion to their degree of obesity. J Clin Endocrinol Metab. 1990;71:929–31.
15. Cohen PG. Aromatase, adiposity, aging and disease. The hypogonadal-metabolic-atherogenic-disease and aging connection. Med Hypotheses. 2001;56:702–8.
16. Montorsi F, et al. Erectile dysfunction prevalence, time of onset and association with risk factors in 300 consecutive patients with acute chest pain and angiographically documented coronary artery disease. Eur Urol. 2003;44:360–4; Discussion 364–5.
17. Roumeguere T, Wespes E, Carpentier Y, Hoffmann P, Schulman CC. Erectile dysfunction is associated with a high prevalence of hyperlipidemia and coronary heart disease risk. Eur Urol. 2003;44:355–9.
18. Gorgel SN, Gorgel A, Sefik E. Sexual function in male patients with metabolic syndrome and effective parameters on erectile dysfunction. Int Braz J Urol. 2014;40:56–61.
19. Schisterman EF, et al. Lipid concentrations and semen quality: the LIFE study. Andrology. 2014;2:408–15.
20. Shafik A, Olfat S. Lipectomy in the treatment of scrotal lipomatosis. Br J Urol. 1981;53:55–61.
21. Bonaccio M, Iacoviello L, de Gaetano G, Moli-Sani I. The Mediterranean diet: the reasons for a success. Thromb Res. 2012;129:401–4.
22. Homan GF, Davies M, Norman R. The impact of lifestyle factors on reproductive performance in the general population and those undergoing infertility treatment: a review. Hum Reprod Update. 2007;13:209–23.
23. Hryhorczuk C, Sharma S, Fulton SE. Metabolic disturbances connecting obesity and depression. Front Neurosci. 2013;7:177.
24. Kennedy SH, Rizvi S. Sexual dysfunction, depression, and the impact of antidepressants. J Clin Psychopharmacol. 2009;29:157–64.
25. Mathew RJ, Weinman ML. Sexual dysfunctions in depression. Arch Sex Behav. 1982;11:323–8.
26. Moore VM, Davies MJ. Diet during pregnancy, neonatal outcomes and later health. Reprod Fertil Dev. 2005;17:341–8.
27. Anderson K, Nisenblat V, Norman R. Lifestyle factors in people seeking infertility treatment – a review. Aust N Z J Obstet Gynaecol. 2010;50:8–20.
28. Chavarro JE, Rich-Edwards JW, Rosner BA, Willett WC. Diet and lifestyle in the prevention of ovulatory disorder infertility. Obstet Gynecol. 2007;110:1050–8.
29. Meldrum DR, et al. Lifestyle and metabolic approaches to maximizing erectile and vascular health. Int J Impot Res. 2012;24:61–8.

30. Collins CE, et al. Improvement in erectile function following weight loss in obese men: the SHED-IT randomized controlled trial. Obes Res Clin Pract. 2013;7:e450–4.
31. Mendiola J, et al. Food intake and its relationship with semen quality: a case-control study. Fertil Steril. 2009; 91:812–18.
32. Afeiche MC, et al. Meat intake and reproductive parameters among young men. Epidemiology. 2014; 25:323–30.
33. Gaskins AJ, Colaci DS, Mendiola J, Swan SH, Chavarro JE. Dietary patterns and semen quality in young men. Hum Reprod. 2012;27:2899–907.
34. Green BB, Daling JR, Weiss NS, Liff JM, Koepsell T. Exercise as a risk factor for infertility with ovulatory dysfunction. Am J Public Health. 1986;76: 1432–6.
35. Huber-Buchholz MM, Carey DG, Norman RJ. Restoration of reproductive potential by lifestyle modification in obese polycystic ovary syndrome: role of insulin sensitivity and luteinizing hormone. J Clin Endocrinol Metab. 1999;84:1470–4.
36. Johannes CB, et al. Incidence of erectile dysfunction in men 40 to 69 years old: longitudinal results from the Massachusetts male aging study. J Urol. 2000;163: 460–3.
37. Rosety-Rodriguez M, et al. Home-based treadmill training improved seminal quality in adults with type 2 diabetes. Actas Urol Esp. 2014;38:589–93.
38. Maleki BH, Tartibian B, Vaamonde D. The effects of 16 weeks of intensive cycling training on seminal oxidants and antioxidants in male road cyclists. Clin J Sport Med. 2014;24:302–7.
39. Khoo J, et al. Comparing effects of low- and high-volume moderate-intensity exercise on sexual function and testosterone in obese men. J Sex Med. 2013;10:1823–32.
40. Bunn Jr PA. Worldwide overview of the current status of lung cancer diagnosis and treatment. Arch Pathol Lab Med. 2012;136:1478–81.
41. Practice Committee of American Society for Reproductive Medicine. Smoking and infertility. Fertil Steril. 2008;90:S254–9.
42. Hull MG, North K, Taylor H, Farrow A, Ford WC. Delayed conception and active and passive smoking. The Avon Longitudinal Study of Pregnancy and Childhood Study Team. Fertil Steril. 2000;74:725–33.
43. Hughes EG, Brennan BG. Does cigarette smoking impair natural or assisted fecundity? Fertil Steril. 1996;66:679–89.
44. U.S. Department of Health and Human Services. Women and smoking: a report of the surgeon general. Atlanta, GA: U.S. Department of Health and Human Services; 2001 http://www.cdc.gov/tobacco/data_statistics/sgr/2001/complete_report/index.htm.
45. Pasqualotto FF, Sobreiro BP, Hallak J, Pasqualotto EB, Lucon AM. Cigarette smoking is related to a decrease in semen volume in a population of fertile men. BJU Int. 2006;97:324–6.
46. Kunzle R, et al. Semen quality of male smokers and nonsmokers in infertile couples. Fertil Steril. 2003;79:287–91.
47. Stewart TM, Liu DY, Garrett C, Brown EH, Baker HW. Recruitment bias in studies of semen and other factors affecting pregnancy rates in fertile men. Hum Reprod. 2009;24:2401–8.
48. Ghaffari MA, Rostami M. Lipid peroxidation and nitric oxide levels in male smokers' spermatozoa and their relation with sperm motility. J Reprod Infertil. 2012;13:81–7.
49. He J, et al. Cigarette smoking and erectile dysfunction among Chinese men without clinical vascular disease. Am J Epidemiol. 2007;166:803–9.
50. McVary KT, Carrier S, Wessells H, Subcommittee on Smoking and Erectile Dysfunction Socioeconomic Committee, Sexual Medicine Society of North America. Smoking and erectile dysfunction: evidence based analysis. J Urol. 2001;166:1624–32.
51. Mannino DM, Klevens RM, Flanders WD. Cigarette smoking: an independent risk factor for impotence? Am J Epidemiol. 1994;140:1003–8.
52. Grodstein F, Goldman MB, Cramer DW. Infertility in women and moderate alcohol use. Am J Public Health. 1994;84:1429–32.
53. Rosen R. Alcohol and drug effects on sexual response: human experimental and clinical studies. Annu Rev Sex Res. 1991;2:119–49.
54. Abel EL. A review of alcohol's effects on sex and reproduction. Drug Alcohol Depend. 1980;5:321–32.
55. Miller NS, Gold MS. The human sexual response and alcohol and drugs. J Subst Abus Treat. 1988;5:171–7.
56. Taniguchi N, Kaneko S. [Alcoholic effect on male sexual function]. Nihon Rinsho. 1997;55:3040–4.
57. Kim JH, et al. Suppression by ethanol of male reproductive activity. Brain Res. 2003;989:91–8.
58. Vaillant GE. Is alcoholism more often the cause or the result of depression? Harv Rev Psychiatry. 1993;1: 94–9.
59. Seftel AD, Sun P, Swindle R. The prevalence of hypertension, hyperlipidemia, diabetes mellitus and depression in men with erectile dysfunction. J Urol. 2004;171:2341–5.
60. La Vignera S, Condorelli RA, Balercia G, Vicari E, Calogero AE. Does alcohol have any effect on male reproductive function? A review of literature. Asian J Androl. 2013;15:221–5.
61. Pajarinen J, Savolainen V, Perola M, Penttila A, Karhunen PJ. Polymorphism in the cytochrome P450 2E1 gene and alcohol-induced disorders of human spermatogenesis. Int J Androl. 1996;19:314–22.
62. Mueller BA, Daling JR, Weiss NS, Moore DE. Recreational drug use and the risk of primary infertility. Epidemiology. 1990;1:195–200.
63. Palha AP, Esteves M. Drugs of abuse and sexual functioning. Adv Psychosom Med. 2008;29:131–49.
64. Rajagopal A, Vassilopoulou-Sellin R, Palmer JL, Kaur G, Bruera E. Hypogonadism and sexual dysfunction in male cancer survivors receiving chronic

opioid therapy. J Pain Symptom Manag. 2003;26: 1055–61.
65. Deyo RA, et al. Prescription opioids for back pain and use of medications for erectile dysfunction. Spine. 2013;38:909–15.
66. Room R. Legalizing a market for cannabis for pleasure: Colorado, Washington, Uruguay and beyond. Addiction. 2014;109:345–51.
67. Whan LB, West MC, McClure N, Lewis SE. Effects of delta-9-tetrahydrocannabinol, the primary psychoactive cannabinoid in marijuana, on human sperm function in vitro. Fertil Steril. 2006;85:653–60.
68. Vescovi PP, et al. Chronic effects of marihuana smoking on luteinizing hormone, follicle-stimulating hormone and prolactin levels in human males. Drug Alcohol Depend. 1992;30:59–63.
69. Kolodny RC, Masters WH, Kolodner RM, Toro G. Depression of plasma testosterone levels after chronic intensive marihuana use. N Engl J Med. 1974;290:872–4.
70. Smith AM, et al. Cannabis use and sexual health. J Sex Med. 2010;7:787–93.
71. Bracken MB, et al. Association of cocaine use with sperm concentration, motility, and morphology. Fertil Steril. 1990;53:315–22.
72. Ragni G, De Lauretis L, Bestetti O, Sghedoni D, Gambaro V. Gonadal function in male heroin and methadone addicts. Int J Androl. 1988;11:93–100.
73. World Health Organization Task Force on Methods for the Regulation of Male Fertility. Contraceptive efficacy of testosterone-induced azoospermia and oligozoospermia in normal men. Fertil Steril. 1996;65:821–9.
74. Ko EY, Siddiqi K, Brannigan RE, Sabanegh Jr ES. Empirical medical therapy for idiopathic male infertility: a survey of the American Urological Association. J Urol. 2012;187:973–8.
75. Jung A, Schuppe HC. Influence of genital heat stress on semen quality in humans. Andrologia. 2007;39:203–15.
76. Sergerie M, Mieusset R, Croute F, Daudin M, Bujan L. High risk of temporary alteration of semen parameters after recent acute febrile illness. Fertil Steril. 2007;88(970):e971–7.
77. Saikhun J, Kitiyanant Y, Vanadurongwan V, Pavasuthipaisit K. Effects of sauna on sperm movement characteristics of normal men measured by computer-assisted sperm analysis. Int J Androl. 1998;21:358–63.
78. Levine RJ, et al. Differences in the quality of semen in outdoor workers during summer and winter. N Engl J Med. 1990;323:12–6.
79. Shafik A, Olfat S. Scrotal lipomatosis. Br J Urol. 1981;53:50–4.
80. Thonneau P, Ducot B, Bujan L, Mieusset R, Spira A. Effect of male occupational heat exposure on time to pregnancy. Int J Androl. 1997;20:274–8.
81. Munkelwitz R, Gilbert BR. Are boxer shorts really better? A critical analysis of the role of underwear type in male subfertility. J Urol. 1998;160:1329–33.
82. Wdowiak A, Wdowiak L, Wiktor H. Evaluation of the effect of using mobile phones on male fertility. Ann Agric Environ Med. 2007;14:169–72.
83. Rago R, et al. The semen quality of the mobile phone users. J Endocrinol Investig. 2013;36:970–4.
84. Agarwal A, et al. Effects of radiofrequency electromagnetic waves (RF-EMW) from cellular phones on human ejaculated semen: an in vitro pilot study. Fertil Steril. 2009;92:1318–25.
85. Matthews TJ, Hamilton BE. Delayed childbearing: more women are having their first child later in life. NCHS Data Brief. 2009;21:1–8.
86. Mathews TJ, Hamilton BE. Mean age of mother, 1970–2000. Nat Vital Stat Rep. 2002;51:1–13.
87. Practice Committee of the American Society for Reproductive Medicine. Aging and infertility in women: a committee opinion. Fertil Steril. 2002;78: 215–19.
88. Satcher D, Okafor M, Dill LJ. Impact of the built environment on mental and sexual health: policy implications and recommendations. ISRN Public Health. 2012;2012:7.

Multicultural Sensitivity in the Treatment of Sexual Dysfunction

4

Kathryn S.K. Hall

4.1 Sexual Dysfunction Cross-Culturally

Sexual dysfunctions as defined by Western diagnostic standards, or at least the symptoms of dysfunction, occur globally with prevalence rates that are similar to those in North America [1]. The fact that these specific sexual difficulties occur around the world should not be surprising given that the basic mechanics of sex do not change from one culture to another. Unfortunately, the epidemiologic surveys to date have not provided a measure of whether Western-defined sexual dysfunctions are more, less, or differently distressing across diverse cultures.

An examination of help-seeking behaviors may shed light on the sexual problems that are most problematic within a culture, although this will likely result in an underestimate of the prevalence of those problems. Across cultures, premature ejaculation (PE) is one of the most frequently reported sexual complaints for which men seek help [1, 2]. In Western cultures, PE may signify problems with control [3], while in many Eastern cultures, it is simply experienced as an abrupt termination of sexual pleasure [4]. Men from Westernized cultures may be interested in learning how to pace sexual arousal and delay ejaculation until their partner has experienced orgasm, whereas men from Eastern cultures might be more amenable to medication to prolong ejaculatory latency [3, 4]. Other anxieties related to ejaculation (nocturnal emissions, guilt about masturbation) account for a high number of patients reporting to sexual health clinics in India and areas in the Middle East [2, 4] and often outrank erectile dysfunction as a presenting complaint. These concerns underscore a cultural belief in the life-enhancing properties of conserving semen, a belief that is not universally shared [5].

While low sexual desire is the most frequent complaint of women in the West, in more male-centric cultures, vaginismus is the primary sexual complaint for which women seek help [6]. The prevalence of vaginismus in non-Western cultures has been attributed to the high premium placed on virginity and the fact that vaginismus interferes with intercourse (and therefore with male pleasure) and can significantly hinder reproduction [7].

K.S.K. Hall, Ph.D. (✉)
Hall Watter Institute, 20 Nassau St. Suite 411, Princeton, NJ 08542, USA
e-mail: kathrynhall@comcast.net

L.I. Lipshultz et al. (eds.), *Management of Sexual Dysfunction in Men and Women*, DOI 10.1007/978-1-4939-3100-2_4

4.2 The Impact of Culture

Culture influences sexual dysfunction in three important ways:

1. The way in which distress is experienced.
2. The way in which symptoms cluster into syndromes.
3. The diagnostic process by which syndromes are recognized as problematic [8].

In the West, for example, low sexual desire in women is often accompanied by a high rate of refusing sex, a low rate of initiating sex, and an overall reduction in the frequency of sex. Paradoxically, when sex occurs, it is usually pleasurable. Because sex is often equated with love in committed relationships, her low desire will be distressing for the woman (and her partner). Western-trained clinicians will readily recognize this cluster of symptoms as low sexual desire. In other cultures such as South Korea, a wife's consent and desire are not deemed necessary for the occurrence of sex, as sexual frequency is dictated by the husband's desire. South Korean women with low desire may engage in frequent but unwanted sex. Sexual aversion or disgust as well as anger at her spouse and disdain for men in general may result [9]. Typically, this symptom constellation would be unfamiliar to a Western-trained clinician, and the sexual issue would in all probability remain hidden behind the overt hostility.

4.3 Assessment

Western-based classification systems are based on a biopsychosocial model of human sexuality [10] and emphasize the pleasure/performance aspects of sexual functioning, our linear view of the sexual response (desire-arousal-orgasm), and the individualism inherent in the culture (e.g., the individual nature of the diagnosis and the individual basis of the distress criterion). Recently a circular model of sexual response has been proposed which described female arousal and desire interacting in a cyclical and mutually reinforcing fashion. This model emphasized the importance of sexual and emotional satisfaction and intimacy in driving women's sexual behavior [11]. However, in many parts of the world, sex is not a private act (not even necessarily an intimate act) between consenting participants but is a matter of concern for extended families and communities. While an emphasis on male sexual pleasure is universal, female sexual pleasure is more often a neglected dimension of sexuality rather than a prime motivator. Spirituality is very important in many cultures, yet it is often neglected in Western formulations of healthy sexuality and good sexual functioning [12].

Culturally sensitive assessment requires the clinician to understand the presentation of symptoms from the patient's perspective, recognizing that this perspective is strongly influenced by the culture in which the patient was raised. At present, the best practice is a diagnostic interview as there are limitations to using standard assessment tools. The majority of questionnaires designed to assess sexual function were developed for and standardized on Western populations. When cross-cultural validation has been attempted, significant differences in the factor structure of the questionnaires have been found along with translation difficulties [13–16]. When seeing clients from non-Western cultures, it is suggested that assessment measures be used with caution (e.g., following up with the patient to ensure that the meaning of the questions is clear). However, an overreliance on paper and pencil tests or questionnaires may be off-putting to certain cultural groups [17].

The diagnostic interview is the keystone of a successful and culturally sensitive assessment. It is important to listen carefully to how the problem is described ("I have ruined myself." "My vagina is locked.") as this will provide information regarding the patient's cultural perspective and will help frame treatment options. The cultural context of the problem will involve understanding the patient's causal attributions as well as the consequences of a successful or unsuccessful resolution of the problem. Ask: *What do you think is causing this problem? What have you tried to do to remedy it? What will happen if you cannot fix this problem? What do you expect will happen when the problem is fixed?* The culturally sensitive patient assessment is augmented by an awareness of the resources available to the individual or couple, as well as of the cultural impediments to treatment.

4.4 Treatment

Cultural sensitivity requires that adaptations be made to the way that sexual medicine and sex therapy are practiced. In some cases, very little modification will be required, while in others, major modifications and greater sensitivity are necessary. In extreme cases it may not be advisable to provide treatment. Given that sex therapy and sexual medicine are predicated on the belief that men and women have equal rights to enjoy and to consent (or not) to sex, it is the status of women within the culture that often provides the measure of whether or not Western interventions, even with modifications, are warranted. If the basic assumption of consent cannot be met, treatment should not be offered. If a woman is highly valued and respected within her intimate relationship (marriage) but is not recognized as an equal within the larger culture, her status in the marriage can pave the way for successful and ethical treatment of sexual dysfunction. For example, there are reports of intracavernosal injection (ICI) being given to young Iranian men unable to quickly consummate their marriage due to extreme anxiety [4]. In the traditional and patriarchal culture of rural Iran, it is assumed that an unconsummated marriage is an even greater liability for the wife as compared to her husband, as he would have the option of remarriage not typically open to her. However, even in rural Iran, if there is a great age disparity between the partners or a high probability of divorce, ICI is not offered, as the basic assumption of consent cannot be met. In the West, the standard for consent is much higher and would typically involve including the wife in the treatment process, thus actively seeking her consent and participation.

4.5 Case Example

The case of a young couple from the Middle East with unconsummated marriage illustrates cultural variations in sex therapy, as well as a multidisciplinary approach to treatment. The couple was referred to sex therapy by an infertility clinic. The husband worried that he could not "break" his wife's hymen (his statement of the problem). He was concerned that his history of masturbation had weakened him (his causal attribution) as he lost his erection just prior to intromission. The young man was concerned that his wife's family would soon intervene to end the marriage (the consequence if the problem is not corrected). The couple tried unsuccessfully to have intercourse on those mornings when the husband awoke with an erection (what they had tried to do to solve the problem). Instead of challenging "irrational" beliefs, the sex therapist worked with the patient to see if his erectile weakness could be remedied. The patient was prescribed a PDE5i by his primary care physician. The sex therapist gave him exercises to help him gain confidence in his erectile ability and learn to regain an erection should he suffer erectile failure. The patient abstained (for the most part) from ejaculating when doing the exercises due to his belief that conserving semen would strengthen him. The patient and his wife were referred to a gynecologist, who explained female genital anatomy and the physiology of arousal during an external pelvic examination. The patient and his wife were surprised to find that the hymen was not a hard membrane completely covering the vagina as they had both assumed. Sex therapy-assigned vaginal dilation exercises were carried out by the husband, using his fingers (dilators were considered to be a violation of his wife's virginity). While standard sex therapy practice is to give the wife control of the pace and timing of the dilation exercises (and she does them first), it was culturally important that the husband take the lead. As his ability to get and maintain an erection improved, the patient was reassured that he had not caused lasting damage to himself. The dilation exercises reassured the couple that penetration was possible and would not cause unbearable pain. Sex therapy exercises included relaxation techniques and instructions on foreplay. In 8 weeks the couple was able to have intercourse and therapy ended.

Too often a patient's culture is viewed as an impediment to treatment, but it may also provide valuable resources for dealing with sexual problems. Patients' religious faiths may sustain them in a marriage while sexual difficulties are being worked through. Extended family members are also resources, especially in collectivist cultures. I have previously described a case involving a Pakistani couple in which the wife's parents, highly invested in the success of the marriage, provided housekeeping and babysitting support so that their daughter and son-in-law could do sex therapy homework [12]. Others have described cases where extended family members have attended sex therapy sessions so that they could be informed of the couple's progress. This assuages their anxiety, buys time for the distressed couple, and often enlists the family's cooperation in providing time and privacy for sex therapy homework or other sexual activities [7]. The patient can often be enlisted to help problem solve culturally accepted treatment modifications. A not infrequent example would be Orthodox Jewish patients offering to contact their rabbi regarding permission to masturbate to ejaculation if the treatment required it.

At present, sexual medicine has little to offer women seeking to improve their desire and pleasure. These cases may warrant a referral to sex therapy. The referring clinician's endorsement of sex therapy (and if possible, the sex therapist) is often essential to the referral being accepted and acted upon. While Western medicine is more easily accepted by other cultures, psychotherapy and sex therapy are quite literally foreign concepts. Conversely men and women from cultures where women enjoy equal status with men (e.g., Scandinavia) are excellent candidates for sex therapy, as the value that is placed on female sexual pleasure equals that for men.

4.6 Sexual and Cultural Minority Patients

The challenge inherent in diagnosing and treating sexual problems is compounded for patients who are both sexually and culturally in the minority (e.g., gays and lesbians from Eastern cultures, as well as trans individuals from almost any cultural group). The minority stress experienced by such patients is often severe and may manifest as physical as well as psychological ailments [18]. In these cases referring a patient to a support group regarding their sexual minority status can help when their family of origin or community has rejected them.

4.7 Cultural Sensitivity Is Good Clinical Practice

Cultural and ethnic minorities are an underserved population in sexual health. Only a small proportion of minority patients experiencing sexual problems ask their physicians for help, and an even smaller percentage of physicians inquire about sexual problems [19]. Additionally, many minority patients do not return for follow-up appointments or drop out of treatment early [20]. It is important to make sexual health services accessible for all members of the population who are in need.

Following good clinical practice guidelines in a nonjudgmental and flexible manner will allow for the treatment of most, but not all, patients from diverse cultural backgrounds. The practice of sexual medicine is enhanced by a respect for a patient's culture, whether that culture is similar or different from that of the treating clinician.

References

1. Laumann EO, Paik A, Glasser DB, et al. A cross-national study of subjective sexual well-being among older women and men: findings from the global study of sexual attitudes and behaviors. Arch Sex Behav. 2006;35:143–59.
2. Verma KK, Khaitan BK, Singh OP. The frequency of sexual dysfunctions in patients attending a sex

therapy clinic in North India. Arch Sex Behav. 1998;27:309–14.
3. Kempeneers P, Andrianne R, Bauwens S, Georis I, Pairoux J-F, Blairy S. Functional and psychological characteristics of Belgian men with premature ejaculation and their partners. Arch Sex Behav. 2012; 42(1):51–66.
4. Zargooshi J, Rahmanian E, Motaee H, Kohzadi M, Nourizad S. Culturally based sexual problems in traditional sections of Kermanshah, Iran. In: Hall KSK, Graham CA, editors. The cultural context of sexual pleasure and problems: psychotherapy with diverse clients. New York: Routledge; 2013. p. 136–54.
5. Ramanathan V, Weerakoon P. Sexuality in India: ancient beliefs, present day problems, and future approaches to management. In: Hall KSK, Graham CA, editors. The cultural context of sexual pleasure and problems: psychotherapy with diverse clients. New York: Routledge; 2013. p. 173–96.
6. Yasan A, Gurgen F. Marital satisfaction, sexual problems and the possible difficulties on sex therapy in traditional Islamic culture. J Sex Marital Ther. 2009; 35:68–75.
7. Sungur M. The role of cultural factors in the course and treatment of sexual problems: failures, pitfalls, and successes in a complicated case from Turkey. In: Hall KSK, Graham CA, editors. The cultural context of sexual pleasure and problems: psychotherapy with diverse clients. New York: Routledge; 2013. p. 308–32.
8. Hughes CC. The glossary of culture-bound syndromes in the DSM-IV: a critique. Transcult Psychiatry. 1998; 35:413–21.
9. Youn G. Challenges facing sex therapy in Korea. In: Hall KSK, Graham CA, editors. The cultural context of sexual pleasure and problems: psychotherapy with diverse clients. New York: Routledge; 2013. p. 156–69.
10. Bancroft J. Human sexuality and its problems. 3rd ed. London: Elsevier; 2009.
11. Basson R. The female sexual response: a different model. J Sex Marital Ther. 2000;26(1):51–65.
12. Hall KSK, Graham CA. Culturally sensitive sex therapy: the need for shared meanings in the treatment of sexual problems. In: Binik YM, Hall KSK, editors. Principles and practice of sex therapy. 5th ed. New York: The Guilford Press; 2014. p. 334–58.
13. Graham CA, Ramos R, Bancroft J, Maglaya C, Farley TMM. The effects of steroidal contraceptives on the well-being and sexuality of women: a double-blind, placebo-controlled, two centre study of combined and progestogen-only methods. Contraception. 1995; 52:363–9.
14. Lim TO, Das A, Rampal S, Zaki M, Sahabudin RM, Rohan MJ, Isaacs S. Cross cultural adaptation and validation of the English version of the international index of erectile function (IIEF) for use in Malaysia. Int J Impot Res. 2003;15:329–36.
15. Quirk FH, Heiman JH, Rosen RC, Laan E, Smith MD, Boolell M. Development of a sexual function questionnaire for clinical trials of female sexual dysfunction. J Womens Health Gend Based Med. 2002;11: 277–89.
16. Rellini AH, Nappi RE, Vaccaro P, Ferdeghini F, Abbiati I, Meston CM. Validation of the McCoy female sexuality questionnaire in an Italian sample. Arch Sex Behav. 2005;34:641–7.
17. Kelly S, Shelton J. African American couples and sex. In: Hall KSK, Graham CA, editors. The cultural context of sexual pleasure and problems: psychotherapy with diverse clients. New York: Routledge; 2013. p. 48–83.
18. Nichols M. Same-sex sexuality from a global perspective. In: Hall KSK, Graham CA, editors. The cultural context of sexual pleasure and problems: psychotherapy with diverse clients. New York: Routledge; 2013. p. 23–46.
19. Moreira E, Brock G, Glasser D, et al. Help-seeking behaviour for sexual problems: the global study of sexual attitudes and behaviors. Int J Clin Pract. 2005;59:6–16.
20. Barrett MS, Chua W-J, Crits-Christoph P, Gibbons MB, Casiano D, Thompson D. Early withdrawal from mental health treatment: implications for psychotherapy practice. Psychotherapy. 2008;45: 247–67.

Part I

Sexual Dysfunction in the Male

Anatomy and Physiology of Erection, Ejaculation, and Orgasm

5

F. Andrew Celigoj, R. Matthew Coward, Matthew D. Timberlake, and Ryan P. Smith

5.1 Introduction

The first known descriptions of penile physiology and erectile dysfunction were described in 2000 BC on Egyptian papyrus. Hippocrates later reported on multiple cases of erectile dysfunction and attributed it to excessive horseback riding. Aristotle hypothesized that the penile erection was facilitated by the influx of air into the penis and that three nerve branches carried spirit and energy to the penis [1, 2]. Leonardo da Vinci observed during the sixteenth century that men undergoing execution by hanging often had reflexogenic erections, on examination finding that a large amount of blood was present within the penis as opposed to air [1, 2]. In a similar fashion, John Hunter made some of the first endeavors to characterize the physiology of ejaculation over 200 years ago. Since that time, ejaculatory dysfunction has become recognized as the most prevalent subclass of male sexual dysfunction [3]. In comparison, the anatomy and physiology of orgasm remain incompletely characterized. Many advances have been made since these classical theorists first proposed the mechanisms behind male sexual function, and the contemporary knowledge of the anatomy and physiology of male sexual function is reviewed in the following text.

5.1.1 Stages of Sexual Response

The human sexual response cycle was first described by Masters and Johnson in 1966 [4] and was later expanded upon by Kaplan [5] and Levin [6]. The sexual response cycle can be described using a four-stage model characterizing the physiologic responses to sexual stimulation: desire, arousal, orgasm, and resolution. Although these occur on a continuum, it is easier to describe them as separate phases. During the desire stage, vascular changes including increased heart rate, blood pressure, and penile tumescence occur. Fluid is secreted from bulbourethral (Cowper's) and periurethral (Littre's) glands, lubricating the urethra. The arousal stage continues to the threshold of orgasm. Changes seen during the desire stage are intensified. Breathing, heart rate, and blood pressure continue to increase, and muscle spasms begin in the face, hands, and feet. The orgasm phase is the third and

Dr. Coward is a consultant for American Medical Systems and Coloplast

F.A. Celigoj, M.D. • M.D. Timberlake, M.D.
R.P. Smith, M.D. (✉)
Department of Urology, University of Virginia, PO Box 800422, Charlottesville, VA 22908, USA
e-mail: rps2k@virginia.edu

R.M. Coward, M.D.
Department of Urology, University of North Carolina, Chapel Hill, NC, USA

L.I. Lipshultz et al. (eds.), *Management of Sexual Dysfunction in Men and Women*, DOI 10.1007/978-1-4939-3100-2_5

shortest stage. This is the climax of the sexual response cycle characterized by a peak in heart rate, blood pressure, and respiratory rate. This stage is characterized by the emission of seminal fluid, followed by the involuntary muscle contractions of the bulbospongiosus and ischiocavernosus muscles, resulting in ejaculation. This is accompanied by a sudden, euphoric sensation and release of sexual tension. Resolution is the final stage, during which time the physiologic changes observed previously return to their baseline. It is during this stage that penile detumescence occurs, followed by a post-orgasmic refractory period during which recovery is necessary before a male is capable of reaching orgasm again.

5.2 Anatomy and Physiology of Erection

5.2.1 Functional Anatomy of the Penis

The penis is composed of three cylindrical structures: the dorsally paired corpora cavernosa and the ventral corpus spongiosum (Fig. 5.1). The corpora cavernosa are two spongy cylinders separated by a midline, incomplete septum and housed within the tunica albuginea. The bilaminar tunica albuginea surrounds both corpora cavernosa and is a thick envelope composed of organized type I and III collagen interlaced with elastin. The elastic fibers allow

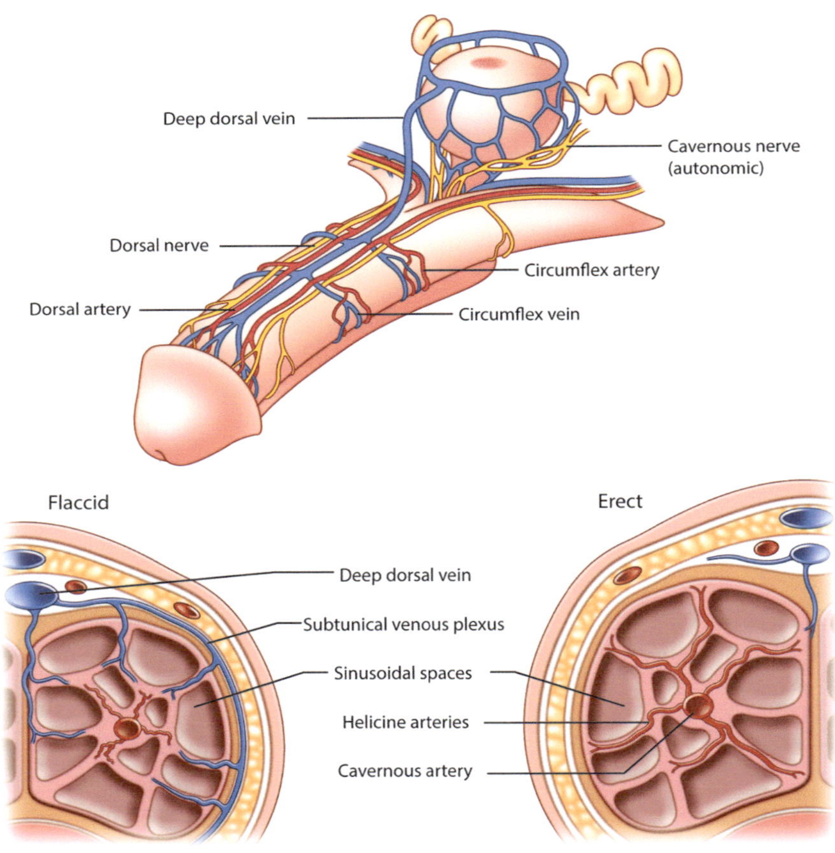

Fig. 5.1 Anatomy of the major arteries, veins, and innervation of the penis. Inset: demonstration of the veno-occlusive mechanism. In the flaccid state, there is minimal inflow via the helicine arteries and venous return is abundant. During the erection phase, relaxation of corporal smooth muscle and arterioles increases blood flow. This leads to compression of the subtunical venous plexus by the tunica albuginea (not pictured) limiting the outflow of blood

for tunical expansion during penile tumescence, while collagen contains and protects the penile spongy erectile tissue, provides rigidity, and participates in the veno-occlusive mechanism through compression of the emissary veins that traverse the tunica albuginea and connect the erectile tissue with the dorsal vein. In contrast, the corpus spongiosum lacks a complete outer layer, ensuring a low-pressure system upon erection and allowing for the expulsion of semen during ejaculation [2, 7]. Within the tunica albuginea is an array of interconnected sinusoids separated by smooth muscle trabeculae with surrounding connective and loose areolar tissue. Each corpus cavernosum is comprised of a complex network of endothelium-lined sinusoids and cavernous smooth muscle, which permit inflow of arterial blood during erection. The fundiform ligament, arising from Colles' fascia, and the suspensory ligaments, which are derived from Buck's fascia, provide external penile support. The corpora cavernosa ultimately diverge proximally into the crura of the penis and attach to the ischiopubic rami [2, 7].

5.2.2 Neurovascular Anatomy of the Penis

The primary source of penile arterial blood supply is from the internal pudendal artery, the terminal branch of the anterior trunk of the internal iliac artery. Accessory arteries to the penis may arise from the external iliac, obturator, vesical, and femoral arteries. In some men, these accessory arteries comprise the dominant or solitary vascular supply to the corpora cavernosa [8, 9]. The internal pudendal artery transitions to the common penile artery after giving off a perineal branch. The three branches of the penile artery are the dorsal, bulbourethral, and cavernous arteries, with the dorsal artery being primarily responsible for engorgement of the glans penis during erection. The bulbourethral artery supplies the bulbar urethra and corpus spongiosum and the cavernous artery gives off the many tortuous helicine arteries that supply the trabecular erectile tissue and sinusoids. These helicine arteries are constricted in the flaccid state, but dilate to allow for rapid arterial inflow during erection (Fig. 5.1) [2, 7].

Venous drainage from the corpora cavernosa and the corpus spongiosum parallels the arterial supply, with venous channels intercommunicating variably. Superficial venous drainage is accomplished by multiple subcutaneous veins, which unite to form the superficial dorsal vein and empty into the saphenous veins. Emissary veins, arising from the corpora cavernosa and corpus spongiosum, drain dorsally through the tunica albuginea to the deep dorsal vein, laterally to the circumflex veins, and ventrally to periurethral veins. More proximal emissary veins join to form the cavernous and crural veins [2, 7]. The veno-occlusive mechanism of maintaining blood in the penis during erection relies upon the compression of these tunical emissary veins as the corpora fill and become engorged with blood (Fig. 5.1).

The innervation of the penis is comprised of both autonomic and somatic nerves (Fig. 5.2). Parasympathetic innervation arises from the second, third, and fourth sacral vertebral spinal segments (S2–S4). Preganglionic parasympathetic fibers pass to the pelvic plexus and are joined by sympathetic nerves from the superior hypogastric plexus. The cavernous nerves are branches of the pelvic plexus that innervate the corpora cavernosa and corpus spongiosum and are easily injured during extirpative surgery of the prostate, bladder, and rectum. Sympathetic nervous input to the penis arises from the 11th thoracic through the second lumbar spinal segments and travels through the lumbar splanchnic nerves to the inferior mesenteric and superior hypogastric plexuses. Fibers travel within the hypogastric nerves to the pelvic plexus [2, 10–12]. Stimulation of the pelvic plexus and the cavernous nerves results in erection. In contrast, stimulation of the sympathetic trunk results in detumescence [10, 13].

Penile sensory pathways originate in the penile skin, urethra, corpora cavernosa, and glans (Fig. 5.2). These nerve endings converge to form bundles of the dorsal nerve of the penis, which later joins with additional cutaneous genital nerves to form the pudendal nerve. The pudendal

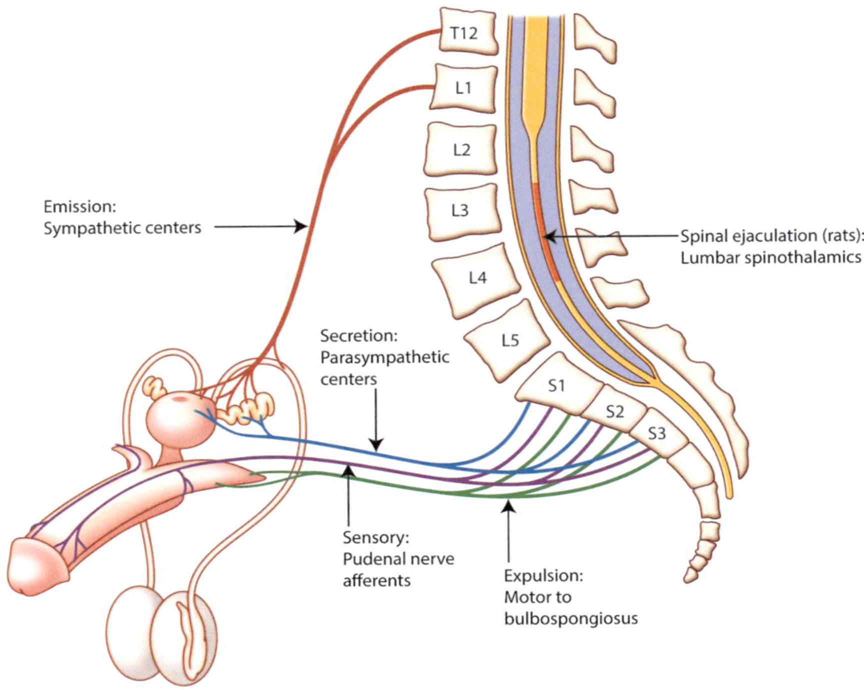

Fig. 5.2 Neural pathways involved in ejaculation. Sensory input is delivered to the spinal cord via branches of the pudendal nerve. Autonomic nerves are involved with emission of seminal fluid, while motor input to the bulbospongiosus muscles causes expulsion. Spinothalamic nerves are involved with integrating this complex signaling

nerve enters the spinal cord via the S2–S4 nerve roots and terminates in the central gray region of the lumbosacral spinal cord. The pudendal nerve stimulates contraction of the bulbocavernosus and ischiocavernosus muscles, which are essential for the rhythmic propulsion necessary for ejaculation and erectile rigidity, respectively [2, 10–12, 14, 15]. Studies of the dorsal nerve have shown that it maintains both erectile and ejaculatory function via somatic and autonomic components [16]. Supraspinal pathways also provide integration and processing of various afferent inputs (visual, olfactory, genital stimulation) involved in the initiation and maintenance of erection. The medial amygdala, medial preoptic area, paraventricular nucleus, periaqueductal gray, and ventral tegmentum are all associated with sexual function [2, 17–19].

5.2.3 Physiology of Erection

Erection of the penis is a neurovascular event involving sinusoidal relaxation, arterial dilation, and venous compression governed by hormonal and psychological influences. In the flaccid state, the intracorporeal smooth muscle is tonically contracted. This semi-contracted state permits enough arterial flow to allow for nutritional support and is resultant of myogenic activity, adrenergic input, and endothelial factors including prostaglandin $F_{2\alpha}$ and endothelins [2, 20–22]. Upon sexual stimulation, nerve impulses result in the release of neurotransmitters from the cavernous nerve terminals, leading to cavernous, arterial, and arteriolar wall smooth muscle relaxation. Nitric oxide is the principal neurotransmitter regulating penile erection and is released during nonadrenergic, noncholinergic neurotransmission and from the vascular endothelium [7, 23, 24]. Nitric oxide within the smooth muscle activates a soluble guanylyl cyclase, which then raises the intracellular concentration of the second messenger cyclic guanosine monophosphate (cGMP) [16, 23, 25, 26]. The resultant increase in cGMP, via downstream effects on certain proteins and ion channels, leads to a drop in cytosolic free calcium and relaxes the cavernous smooth muscle. Cyclic adenosine monophosphate (cAMP), like cGMP, represents another intracellular second messenger mediating smooth muscle relaxation. Through activation of specific protein kinases, protein phosphorylation leads to opening of potassium channels, closing of calcium channels, and sequestration of intracellular calcium [2, 7]. Relaxation of the trabecular smooth muscle increases sinusoidal compliance, promoting the tissue filling and expansion [7]. Lue succinctly and accurately summarized the cascade of events that follows: (1) dilation of the arteries and arterioles results in increased diastolic and systolic blood flow within the corpora; (2) sinusoidal expansion results in sequestration of the incoming blood flow; (3) compression of the subtunical venous plexuses between the tunica albuginea and peripheral sinusoids decreases venous outflow; (4) distension of the tunica albuginea to its limiting capacity further decreases venous outflow via occlusion of the emissary veins; (5) subsequent increases in P_{02} to approximately 90 mmHg and a rise in intracavernosal pressure to approximately 100 mmHg results in elevation of the dependent penis; and (6) contraction of the ischiocavernosus muscles further raises intracavernosal pressure to several hundred millimeters of mercury [2].

Norepinephrine, released from sympathetic nerve terminals, has been accepted as the principal neurotransmitter controlling detumescence. Along with prostaglandin $F_{2\alpha}$ and endothelins, these neurotransmitters activate receptors on smooth muscle cells, leading to a cascade of events translating into increased intracellular calcium concentrations and smooth muscle contraction [2, 20–22]. Detumescence is initiated at the molecular level when cGMP is hydrolyzed to GMP by phosphodiesterases, principally phosphodiesterase type 5, allowing smooth muscle to regain its tone. Coordination of muscle activity through the process of erection and detumescence is facilitated by the presence of gap junctions in the membrane of adjacent muscle cells. These intercellular channels allow the exchange of ions and other second messengers [7, 27, 28].

5.3 Endocrine Influences on Male Sexual Function

The hypothalamic-pituitary-gonadal (HPG) axis plays a critical role in the growth and development of the male reproductive tract and secondary sexual characteristics. For example, testosterone has well-established effects on libido and sexual behavior including sexual interest, frequency of sexual acts, and nocturnal erection [29]. Hypogonadism represents a frequently recognized entity in men who struggle with erectile dysfunction and diminished libido. Indeed, the prevalence of androgen deficiency has been estimated to be 38.7 % in men ≥45 years of age presenting to primary care physicians [30]. The diagnosis of hypogonadism may coincide with associated ailments known to negatively impact sexual function, including the metabolic syndrome, hypertension, type 2 diabetes mellitus, visceral adiposity, insulin resistance, and depression [31, 32].

At a molecular level, androgens promote endothelial cell survival, reduce endothelial expression of pro-inflammatory markers, and inhibit proliferation and intimal migration of vascular smooth muscle cells. Low androgen levels are associated with apoptosis of endothelial cells and smooth muscle cells [2, 33]. Testosterone and dihydrotestosterone may also assist with penile artery and cavernous smooth muscle relaxation [2, 34]. Men on androgen ablation therapy for prostate cancer frequently report poor libido and erectile function. In animal models, castration decreases arterial flow, induces venous leakage, reduces the erectile response to stimulation of the cavernous nerve, and increases the α-adrenergic response of penile smooth muscle [2, 35–38].

Hyperprolactinemia has similarly been associated with reproductive and sexual dysfunction. Elevated prolactin levels inhibit central dopaminergic activity and gonadotropin-releasing hormone secretion, resulting in lower circulating levels of testosterone. This may translate to diminished libido, erectile dysfunction, delayed or inability to achieve orgasm, galactorrhea, gynecomastia, and fertility impairment [2, 39]. Thyroid dysfunction (hyper- and hypothyroidism) may also affect sexual function, as hyperthyroidism has been associated with diminished libido, whereas hypothyroidism results in reduced circulating testosterone and elevated prolactin levels, contributing to erectile dysfunction [2].

5.4 Orgasm and Ejaculation

5.4.1 Anatomy and Physiology of Ejaculation

Antegrade ejaculation is a reflex requiring the complex interaction of somatic, sympathetic, and parasympathetic pathways (Fig. 5.2). It can be separated into two closely timed events: the emission phase and the expulsion phase [40]. Emission occurs due to sympathetic and parasympathetic outflow causing a release of seminal fluid from the prostate, seminal vesicles, and ampullae of the vas deferens into the prostatic urethra, along with closure of the bladder neck [41, 42]. Studies have shown that emission is a result of alpha-adrenergic receptor stimulation by norepinephrine from thoracolumbar sympathetic outflow [43–45]. Disruption of these pathways (i.e., surgical, pharmacological) results in impairment of emission [45].

Following emission, expulsion of seminal fluid from the urethra is due to coordinated contractions of the striated bulbospongiosus and ischiocavernosus muscles while the bladder neck remains closed [41]. The ejaculatory reflex is controlled by motor branches of the pudendal nerve [41] with the cell bodies of these somatic motor neurons being located in the ventral horn of the lumbosacral spinal cord in Onuf's nucleus [41, 42].

The ejaculatory reflex is controlled by central pattern generators at the spinal level [42]. These central pattern generators, also called lumbar spinothalamic cells, modulate the excitatory and inhibitory supraspinal inputs, which are integrated with sensory input from the dorsal nerve of the penis. These interneurons coordinate the activation of somatic and autonomic spinal centers responsible for ejaculation [46, 47]. Ejaculation is not dependent on supraspinal input, as the majority of men with spinal cord injuries above T10 are able to ejaculate with vibratory or manual stimulation [48, 49].

Supraspinal pathways modulate the ejaculatory reflex. Studies have shown that during ejaculation, the brain centers with the highest activity level include the mesodiencephalic region, the lateral central tegmental field, and the parafascicular nucleus [50]. Stimulation of the medial preoptic area elicits contractions of the bulbocavernosus muscles observed during ejaculation and orgasm [51]. Neurotransmitters play an important role in regulating ejaculation. Studies have shown that activation of serotonin 5HT1A receptors promotes ejaculation, while 5HT1B delays ejaculation [52]. Activation of dopamine receptors D2 and D3 promotes ejaculation [53–56]. Endogenous and exogenous opioids (i.e., tramadol) exhibit an inhibitory effect [57]. The complex interplay between the systems modulates the ejaculatory reflex and serves as a focal point for therapeutic intervention.

5.4.2 Anatomy and Physiology of Male Orgasm

Male orgasm represents a distinct, cortical event that is experienced cognitively and emotionally, and it is mediated through the sensory neurons in the pelvis in response to the striated muscle contractions and expulsion of semen during ejaculation [3]. It may be triggered by genital stimulation, but also by sleep, stimulation of other parts of the body, fantasy, medications, and vibratory stimulation. Orgasm is associated with increased pressure in the posterior urethra, sensory stimuli arising from the verumontanum, and contraction of the urethral bulb and accessory sexual organs [3]. Positron emission tomography studies during orgasm have shown brain activations mainly in the anterior lobe of the cerebellar vermis and deep cerebellar nuclei and deactivations in the left ventromedial and orbitofrontal cortex. While these are similar between genders, in men there is additional activation in the periaqueductal gray matter [58]. Oxytocin levels have been shown to increase in association with orgasm in both genders. Prolactin secretion similarly increases after orgasm and has been proposed as a marker for male orgasm. Oxytocin may contribute to the post-orgasmic refractory period in men whereas prolactin may serve as a neuroendocrine reproductive reflex or as a feedback mechanism modulating dopaminergic systems in the central nervous system [59, 60].

5.5 Summary

The understanding and appreciation of the anatomy and physiology of erection, ejaculation, and orgasm will serve as a cornerstone for the development of new therapies for male sexual dysfunction. Characterization of these pathways and their associated dysfunction remains a critical area of research as exemplified by our limited understanding of orgasm. Until that time, the therapeutic armamentarium available to our patients will be limited by our lack of scientific basis for treatment. A thorough understanding of the anatomy and physiology of these systems is critical to the sexual health practitioner. As captured above, the complex interplay of psychology and physiology in male sexual function necessitates treatment using an integrated approach, combining the benefits of pharmacotherapy, sex and psychotherapy, and surgery.

Acknowledgment Dr. Celigoj, Dr. Timberlake and Dr. Smith report no conflict of interest.

References

1. Brenot PH. Male impotence-a historical perspective. Paris: L'Esprit du Temps; 1994.
2. Lue TF. Physiology of penile erection and pathophysiology of erectile dysfunction. In: Wein A, Kavoussi LR, Novick AC, Partin AW, Peters CA, editors. Campbell-Walsh urology, vol. 1. 10th ed. Philadelphia: Elsevier Health Sciences; 2011. p. 688–720.
3. Rowland D, McMahon CG, Abdo C, Chen J, Jannini E, Waldinger MD, et al. Disorders of orgasm and ejaculation in men. J Sex Med. 2010;7(4 Pt 2):1668–86. PubMed PMID: 20388164.
4. Masters WH, Johnson VE. Reproductive biology research foundation (U.S.). Human sexual response. 1st ed. Boston: Little, Brown; 1966. vol. 8, 366 pp.
5. Kaplan HS. The new sex therapy; active treatment of sexual dysfunctions. New York: Brunner/Mazel; 1974. vol. 16, 544 pp.
6. Levin R. An orgasm is…who defines what an orgasm is? Sex Relat Ther. 2004;19:101–7.
7. Lue TF. Erectile dysfunction. N Engl J Med. 2000;342(24):1802–13. PubMed PMID: 10853004.
8. Breza J, Aboseif SR, Orvis BR, Lue TF, Tanagho EA. Detailed anatomy of penile neurovascular structures: surgical significance. J Urol. 1989;141(2):437–43. PubMed PMID: 2913372.
9. Droupy S, Hessel A, Benoit G, Blanchet P, Jardin A, Giuliano F. Assessment of the functional role of accessory pudendal arteries in erection by transrectal color Doppler ultrasound. J Urol. 1999;162(6):1987–91. PubMed PMID: 10569553.
10. Bella AJ, Brant WO, Lue TF. Microscopic anatomy of erectile function. In: Carson C, Kirby RS, Goldstein IG, Wyllie MG, editors. Textbook of erectile dysfunction. 2nd ed. New York, NY: Informa Healthcare USA, INC; 2009. p. 28–34.
11. Lue TF, Zeineh SJ, Schmidt RA, Tanagho EA. Neuroanatomy of penile erection: its relevance to iatrogenic impotence. J Urol. 1984;131(2):273–80. PubMed PMID: 6422055.
12. Steers WD, Mallory B, de Groat WC. Electrophysiological study of neural activity in penile nerve of the rat. Am J Physiol. 1988;254(6 Pt 2): R989–1000. PubMed PMID: 3381920.
13. Giuliano F, Rampin O. Neural control of erection. Physiol Behav. 2004;83(2):189–201. PubMed PMID: 15488539.
14. Halata Z, Munger BL. The neuroanatomical basis for the protopathic sensibility of the human glans penis. Brain Res. 1986;371(2):205–30. PubMed PMID: 3697758.
15. McKenna KE. Central control of penile erection. Int J Impot Res. 1998;10 Suppl 1:S25–34. PubMed PMID: 9669218.
16. Burnett AL, Tillman SL, Chang TS, Epstein JI, Lowenstein CJ, Bredt DS, et al. Immunohistochemical localization of nitric oxide synthase in the autonomic

innervation of the human penis. J Urol. 1993;150(1):73–6. PubMed PMID: 7685426.
17. Arnow BA, Desmond JE, Banner LL, Glover GH, Solomon A, Polan ML, et al. Brain activation and sexual arousal in healthy, heterosexual males. Brain. 2002;125(Pt 5):1014–23. PubMed PMID: 11960892.
18. Mallick HN, Manchanda SK, Kumar VM. Sensory modulation of the medial preoptic area neuronal activity by dorsal penile nerve stimulation in rats. J Urol. 1994;151(3):759–62. PubMed PMID: 8309001.
19. Marson L, Platt KB, McKenna KE. Central nervous system innervation of the penis as revealed by the transneuronal transport of pseudorabies virus. Neuroscience. 1993;55(1):263–80. PubMed PMID: 7688882.
20. Gondre M, Christ GJ. Endothelin-1-induced alterations in phenylephrine-induced contractile responses are largely additive in physiologically diverse rabbit vasculature. J Pharmacol Exp Ther. 1998;286(2): 635–42. PubMed PMID: 9694914.
21. Italiano G, Calabro A, Spini S, Ragazzi E, Pagano F. Functional response of cavernosal tissue to distension. Urol Res. 1998;26(1):39–44. PubMed PMID: 9537695.
22. Saenz de Tejada I, Kim N, Lagan I, Krane RJ, Goldstein I. Regulation of adrenergic activity in penile corpus cavernosum. J Urol. 1989;142(4):1117–21. PubMed PMID: 2795742.
23. Ignarro LJ, Bush PA, Buga GM, Wood KS, Fukuto JM, Rajfer J. Nitric oxide and cyclic GMP formation upon electrical field stimulation cause relaxation of corpus cavernosum smooth muscle. Biochem Biophys Res Commun. 1990;170(2):843–50. PubMed PMID: 2166511.
24. Saenz de Tejada I, Goldstein I, Azadzoi K, Krane RJ, Cohen RA. Impaired neurogenic and endothelium-mediated relaxation of penile smooth muscle from diabetic men with impotence. N Engl J Med. 1989;320(16):1025–30. PubMed PMID: 2927481.
25. Pickard RS, Powell PH, Zar MA. The effect of inhibitors of nitric oxide biosynthesis and cyclic GMP formation on nerve-evoked relaxation of human cavernosal smooth muscle. Br J Pharmacol. 1991 104(3):755–9. PubMed Pubmed Central PMCID: 1908248.
26. Pickard RS, Powell PH, Zar MA. Nitric oxide and cyclic GMP formation following relaxant nerve stimulation in isolated human corpus cavernosum. Br J Urol. 1995;75(4):516–22. PubMed PMID: 7788263.
27. Campos de Carvalho AC, Roy C, Moreno AP, Melman A, Hertzberg EL, Christ GJ, et al. Gap junctions formed of connexin43 are found between smooth muscle cells of human corpus cavernosum. J Urol. 1993;149(6):1568–75. PubMed PMID: 8388962.
28. Christ GJ, Brink PR, Melman A, Spray DC. The role of gap junctions and ion channels in the modulation of electrical and chemical signals in human corpus cavernosum smooth muscle. Int J Impot Res. 1993;5(2):77–96. PubMed PMID: 7688635.
29. Mulligan T, Schmitt B. Testosterone for erectile failure. J Gen Intern Med. 1993;8(9):517–21. PubMed PMID: 8410427.
30. Mulligan T, Frick MF, Zuraw QC, Stemhagen A, McWhirter C. Prevalence of hypogonadism in males aged at least 45 years: the HIM study. Int J Clin Pract. 2006;60(7):762–9. PubMed Pubmed Central PMCID: 1569444.
31. Corona G, Mannucci E, Forti G, Maggi M. Hypogonadism, ED, metabolic syndrome and obesity: a pathological link supporting cardiovascular diseases. Int J Androl. 2009;32(6):587–98. PubMed PMID: 19226407.
32. Corona G, Monami M, Rastrelli G, Aversa A, Tishova Y, Saad F, et al. Testosterone and metabolic syndrome: a meta-analysis study. J Sex Med. 2011;8(1):272–83. PubMed PMID: 20807333.
33. Mirone V, Imbimbo C, Fusco F, Verze P, Creta M, Tajana G. Androgens and morphologic remodeling at penile and cardiovascular levels: a common piece in complicated puzzles? Eur Urol. 2009;56(2):309–16. PubMed PMID: 19147269.
34. Waldkirch E, Uckert S, Schultheiss D, Geismar U, Bruns C, Scheller F, et al. Non-genomic effects of androgens on isolated human vascular and nonvascular penile erectile tissue. BJU Int. 2008;101(1):71–5. discussion 5. PubMed PMID: 17868421.
35. Mills TM, Stopper VS, Wiedmeier VT. Effects of castration and androgen replacement on the hemodynamics of penile erection in the rat. Biol Reprod. 1994;51(2):234–8. PubMed PMID: 7948478.
36. Penson DF, Ng C, Cai L, Rajfer J, Gonzalez-Cadavid NF. Androgen and pituitary control of penile nitric oxide synthase and erectile function in the rat. Biol Reprod. 1996;55(3):567–74. PubMed PMID: 8862773.
37. Traish AM, Munarriz R, O'Connell L, Choi S, Kim SW, Kim NN, et al. Effects of medical or surgical castration on erectile function in an animal model. J Androl. 2003;24(3):381–7. PubMed PMID: 12721214.
38. Traish AM, Park K, Dhir V, Kim NN, Moreland RB, Goldstein I. Effects of castration and androgen replacement on erectile function in a rabbit model. Endocrinology. 1999;140(4):1861–8. PubMed PMID: 10098525.
39. Leonard MP, Nickel CJ, Morales A. Hyperprolactinemia and impotence: why, when and how to investigate. J Urol. 1989;142(4):992–4. PubMed PMID: 2795758.
40. Johnson RD. Descending pathways modulating the spinal circuitry for ejaculation: effects of chronic spinal cord injury. Prog Brain Res. 2006;152:415–26. PubMed PMID: 16198717.
41. Giuliano F, Clement P. Neuroanatomy and physiology of ejaculation. Annu Rev Sex Res. 2005;16:190–216. PubMed PMID: 16913292.
42. Giuliano F, Clement P. Physiology of ejaculation: emphasis on serotonergic control. Eur Urol. 2005; 48(3):408–17. PubMed PMID: 15996810.

43. Anton PG, McGrath JC. Further evidence for adrenergic transmission in the human vas deferens. J Physiol. 1977;273(1):45–55. PubMed Pubmed Central PMCID: 1353725.
44. Bruschini H, Schmidt RA, Tanagho EA. Studies on the neurophysiology of the vas deferens. Investig Urol. 1977;15(2):112–6. PubMed PMID: 903209.
45. Kedia K, Markland C. The effect of pharmacological agents on ejaculation. J Urol. 1975;114(4):569–73. PubMed PMID: 1235380.
46. Borgdorff AJ, Bernabe J, Denys P, Alexandre L, Giuliano F. Ejaculation elicited by microstimulation of lumbar spinothalamic neurons. Eur Urol. 2008;54(2):449–56. PubMed PMID: 18394782.
47. Truitt WA, Coolen LM. Identification of a potential ejaculation generator in the spinal cord. Science. 2002;297(5586):1566–9. PubMed PMID: 12202834.
48. Kafetsoulis A, Brackett NL, Ibrahim E, Attia GR, Lynne CM. Current trends in the treatment of infertility in men with spinal cord injury. Fertil Steril. 2006;86(4):781–9. PubMed PMID: 16963042.
49. Sonksen J, Biering-Sorensen F, Kristensen JK. Ejaculation induced by penile vibratory stimulation in men with spinal cord injuries. the importance of the vibratory amplitude. Paraplegia. 1994;32(10):651–60. PubMed PMID: 7831070.
50. Holstege G. Central nervous system control of ejaculation. World J Urol. 2005;23(2):109–14. PubMed PMID: 15875196.
51. Marson L. Lesions of the periaqueductal gray block the medial preoptic area-induced activation of the urethrogenital reflex in male rats. Neurosci Lett. 2004;367(3):278–82. PubMed PMID: 15337249.
52. Waldinger MD, Zwinderman AH, Schweitzer DH, Olivier B. Relevance of methodological design for the interpretation of efficacy of drug treatment of premature ejaculation: a systematic review and meta-analysis. Int J Impot Res. 2004;16(4):369–81. PubMed PMID: 14961051.
53. Bitran D, Thompson JT, Hull EM, Sachs BD. Quinelorane (LY163502), a D2 dopamine receptor agonist, facilitates seminal emission, but inhibits penile erection in the rat. Pharmacol Biochem Behav. 1989;34(3):453–8. PubMed PMID: 2533690.
54. Eaton RC, Markowski VP, Lumley LA, Thompson JT, Moses J, Hull EM. D2 receptors in the paraventricular nucleus regulate genital responses and copulation in male rats. Pharmacol Biochem Behav. 1991; 39(1):177–81. PubMed PMID: 1833780.
55. Ferrari F, Giuliani D. Behavioral effects induced by the dopamine D3 agonist 7-OH-DPAT in sexually-active and -inactive male rats. Neuropharmacology. 1996;35(3):279–84. PubMed PMID: 8783202.
56. Hull EM, Eaton RC, Markowski VP, Moses J, Lumley LA, Loucks JA. Opposite influence of medial preoptic D1 and D2 receptors on genital reflexes: implications for copulation. Life Sci. 1992;51(22):1705–13. PubMed PMID: 1359367.
57. Bar-Or D, Salottolo KM, Orlando A, Winkler JV, Tramadol ODTSG. A randomized double-blind, placebo-controlled multicenter study to evaluate the efficacy and safety of two doses of the tramadol orally disintegrating tablet for the treatment of premature ejaculation within less than 2 minutes. Eur Urol. 2012;61(4):736–43. PubMed PMID: 21889833.
58. Georgiadis JR, Reinders AA, Paans AM, Renken R, Kortekaas R. Men versus women on sexual brain function: prominent differences during tactile genital stimulation, but not during orgasm. Hum Brain Mapp. 2009;30(10):3089–101. PubMed PMID: 19219848.
59. Carmichael MS, Warburton VL, Dixen J, Davidson JM. Relationships among cardiovascular, muscular, and oxytocin responses during human sexual activity. Arch Sex Behav. 1994;23(1):59–79. PubMed PMID: 8135652.
60. Kruger TH, Haake P, Chereath D, Knapp W, Janssen OE, Exton MS, et al. Specificity of the neuroendocrine response to orgasm during sexual arousal in men. J Endocrinol. 2003;177(1):57–64. PubMed PMID: 12697037.

6 Urologic and Clinical Evaluation of the Male with Erectile Dysfunction

Boback M. Berookhim, Alexander W. Pastuszak, Natan Bar-Chama, and Mohit Khera

6.1 Introduction

Among reported sexual dysfunctions in men, erectile dysfunction (ED) is the most frequently treated worldwide [1]. It is defined as the recurrent or consistent inability to obtain and/or maintain a penile erection sufficient for satisfactory sexual performance [2]. Erectile dysfunction has significant negative effects on the quality of life of both the patient and his partner, affecting the patient's emotional and psychological well-being, and is associated with poor relationship satisfaction, negative general health perceptions, and role limitations [3, 4]. Temporary ED is a fairly common phenomenon and is often related to transient life circumstances, disappearing after resolution of the underlying circumstances. However, it is generally accepted that men with ED symptoms present for at least 3 months should undergo a medical evaluation [1, 5].

6.2 Epidemiology

Estimates on the prevalence of ED on a worldwide basis are highly variable, as a result of varying study methodologies, questionnaires, and tools used for surveys, as well as differences in the definition of ED. It is estimated that at least 20 million men in the United States suffer from ED [6]. The landmark Massachusetts Male Aging Study (MMAS) was among the first studies to report on ED in a standardized fashion and has described a combined prevalence of any degree of ED in 52 % of men over the age of 40 [7]. The study further reported an increase in the rate of moderate to severe/complete ED from 22 to 49 % between the ages of 40 and 70 years. More recently, the National Social Life, Health, and Aging Project (NSHAP) performed a survey evaluation of over 1450 American men to evaluate sexual issues in older adults and reported ED in 31 % of men 57–64 years old and 45 % of men 65–74 years old, with an adjusted odds ratio of 1.83 comparing these two age groups [8]. The prevalence of ED appears to be similar among different ethnic groups, with one study reporting a 22 % rate of ED in white men

B.M. Berookhim, M.D., M.B.A.
Department of Urology, Lenox Hill Hospital, New York, NY, USA

A.W. Pastuszak, M.D., Ph.D.
Baylor College of Medicine, Division of Male Reproductive Medicine and Surgery, Center for Reproductive Medicine, Scott Department of Urology, Houston, TX, USA

M. Khera, M.D., M.B.A. (✉)
Scott Department of Urology, Baylor College of Medicine, Houston, TX, USA
e-mail: mkhera@bcm.edu

N. Bar-Chama, M.D.
Department of Urology, Mount Sinai School of Medicine, New York, NY, USA

L.I. Lipshultz et al. (eds.), *Management of Sexual Dysfunction in Men and Women*, DOI 10.1007/978-1-4939-3100-2_6

over 40 years, a 24 % rate among black men, and a 20 % rate among Hispanic men [9].

6.3 Classifications of Erectile Dysfunction

Erection is the result of a complex physiologic interaction of psychological, neuronal, hormonal, vascular, and cavernous smooth muscle systems, with derangements in any one system predisposing to ED. Although often multifactorial in nature, ED is further classified according to its origin: psychogenic, vasculogenic, endocrinologic, neurogenic, and drug induced (Table 6.1).

Table 6.1 Classification of erectile dysfunction and selected causes

Classifications	Specific causes
Psychogenic	Interpersonal factors Anxiety/anxiety disorders Disorders of sexual intimacy
Vasculogenic	Arteriogenic Cardiovascular disease Endothelial dysfunction Venogenic
Endocrinologic	Hypogonadism Hyperprolactinemia Hypothyroidism Hyperthyroidism
Neurogenic	Supraspinal Brain tumor Cerebrovascular accident Parkinson's disease Dementia Temporal epilepsy Spinal Multiple sclerosis Spinal cord injury Transverse myelitis Myelodysplasia Lumbar disc disease Iatrogenic (secondary to spinal surgery) Peripheral Lower motor neuron lesions Diabetes mellitus Trauma Radical pelvic surgery
Drug induced	Antihypertensives Psychotropics Antiandrogens 5-α reductase inhibitors Digoxin

Psychogenic (nonorganic) ED is predominantly or exclusively related to psychological or interpersonal factors [10]. It is an adrenergic-mediated phenomenon and is frequently partner related, performance related, or associated with psychological distress [11]. Psychogenic ED is a diagnosis of exclusion, once physical (organic) factors have been ruled out, and the clinical features include sudden onset ED, with intermittency of function or a situational nature to the erectile problems, as well as reports of good nocturnal erections, as well as difficulty with achieving orgasm [12].

ED and cardiovascular disease (CVD) share common risk factors, leading to the concept that vasculogenic ED is another manifestation of vascular disease [13]. One survey of over 7500 patients with hypertension and diabetes demonstrated ED in nearly 70 % of patients with either hypertension or diabetes alone and in 78 % of patients with both conditions [14]. Furthermore, a report of over 2400 patients has demonstrated each of these comorbidities to be independently associated with ED [15]. Age-adjusted odds ratios of having ED were 4.0 in diabetics, 1.58 in patients with hypertension, 1.63 in men with high cholesterol, 2.63 in men with peripheral vascular disease, and 2.5 among smokers.

ED is also a strong predictor of subsequent cardiovascular events. Data from a meta-analysis of over 45,000 participants from seven cohort studies reported a relative risk (RR) of coronary events in men with ED of 1.47 [16]. Among patients participating in the Prostate Cancer Prevention Trial (PCPT), incident ED was associated with a 25 % increased likelihood of subsequent cardiovascular events during the 5-year study follow-up. Men with either incident or prevalent ED during the study period were at a 45 % increased risk of cardiovascular events [17]. Additionally, ED may be an independent marker of cardiovascular events and all-cause mortality after adjusting for age, weight, hypertension, diabetes, hyperlipidemia, and cigarette smoking [18].

With respect to endocrinologic ED, the effect of androgens, specifically testosterone, on sexual desire, interest, and orgasmic function has been well established. Additionally, androgens play a role in overall erectile function and may maintain the fibroelastic properties of penile tissue [19, 20]. However, low serum testosterone has not been clearly linked to the presence or severity of ED [21–23]. Similarly, hyperprolactinemia has been shown to be associated with low libido, while clear association with erectile function remains the subject of debate [5, 24].

Neurogenic ED occurs secondary to neurologic impairment in either the central nervous system or peripheral nerves and is relatively uncommon in the overall population. It results from strokes, dementia, Parkinson's disease, central nervous system tumors, spinal cord injury, multiple sclerosis, as well as lower motor neuron lesions caused by trauma, major pelvic pathologies, and pelvic surgery, including radical prostatectomy and cystoprostatectomy [25].

Drug-induced ED has been reported with a number of different drug classes, including antihypertensives, psychotropics, antiandrogens, 5-α reductase inhibitors, and digoxin.

6.4 Additional Risk Factors for Erectile Dysfunction

In addition to the risk factors reported in the classification of ED above, benign prostatic hypertrophy (BPH) and lower urinary tract symptoms (LUTS) have also been linked to ED [26]. LUTS are an independent predictor of ED, with increasing prevalence of ED with increases in LUTS severity [27, 28]. The pathophysiology of these comorbid conditions is not entirely understood, but may be the same [29].

6.5 Clinical Evaluation of the Male with Erectile Dysfunction

6.5.1 History and Physical Examination

The initial evaluation of ED must include a complete medical, sexual, and psychosocial history [30]. The medical history must evaluate for the potential roles of the associated medical conditions described above with respect to ED and will help to differentiate between organic and psychogenic causes of ED, although the clinician must consider a psychogenic component in all forms of ED. A detailed sexual history is critically important, aimed at determining the severity, onset, and duration of the ED, and serves to provide additional information as to the potential etiology of ED. Erectile rigidity and sustainability should also be evaluated, and the patient should be queried as to the presence of nocturnal erections, which can further distinguish between organic and psychogenic causes. A psychosocial assessment is essential, given the association between ED and overall quality of life and relationship quality, confidence, self-esteem, and depression [31]. Identification of personal barriers to treatment and resistance to therapy in the ED patient may also facilitate effective treatment [32].

Given the often sensitive subject matter, clinicians should consider using validated questionnaires to ease into the conversation with an ED patient and to provide objective assessment of erective function. Such questionnaires include the gold standard International Index of Erectile Function (IIEF) and the abridged, five-item version of the IIEF, the Sexual Health Inventory for Men (SHIM) [33, 34]. The SHIM is one of the most common validated instruments for evaluation of ED severity and is specifically intended as an office screening tool for ED [35]. In scoring the SHIM, lower scores portend worse ED with classification into five severity grades: no ED (SHIM score 22–25), mild [17–21], mild to moderate [12–16], moderate [8–11], and severe [1–7].

In addition to the history of the patient presenting with ED, evaluation of the partner can serve to improve satisfaction for both partners, may improve compliance with ED therapy, and can potentially improve erectile function outcomes [36–39]. In the case of heterosexual relationships, male erectile function and female sexual function are interdependent, and one can assume that the same relationship could be demonstrated in same-sex couples. Sexual dysfunction in the partner may cause distress in the patient and can generate partner avoidance and antipathy, leading to overt sexual dysfunction [40].

Physical examination in men with ED is recommended, but not always necessary, as the examination infrequently reveals a specific etiology of ED, according to the International Consultation on Sexual Medicine (ICSM) committee [30]. Nevertheless, a standard general physical exam, with particular focus on the cardiovascular examination (including evaluation of blood pressure, heart rate, and peripheral pulses), should be performed. Furthermore, a focused genital examination, evaluating the penis for lesions, scars, tunical plaques, and meatal position, as well as examination of the testes for size, consistency, and presence of masses, is warranted. Digital rectal examination should be performed in the appropriately aged man.

6.5.2 Laboratory Testing

As noted from the physical examination, lab testing should be focused and is aimed at diagnosing medical conditions associated with ED. The ICSM committee recommends testing which includes fasting blood glucose, a lipid profile, and serum testosterone levels, with optional examinations such as thyroid function testing based on the clinical scenario [30, 41]. Glycosylated hemoglobin (hemoglobin A1c) is strongly associated with ED (OR 3.19) and can be considered in lieu of fasting blood glucose to screen for diabetes mellitus or in men with known diabetes mellitus [42]. The Princeton III Consensus, a multispecialty conference aimed at optimizing sexual function and promoting cardiovascular health, issued a statement that all men over the age of 30 with organic ED should be considered at increased CVD risk unless further evaluation suggests otherwise [43]. The Princeton Consensus recommends a resting electrocardiogram and serum creatinine level in addition to the previously described testing in men without known CVD. Abnormalities in these and the laboratory studies described above should prompt referral to either a primary care physician or cardiologist for further evaluation.

6.5.3 Adjunctive Testing

The various diagnostic tests used in the evaluation of the patient with erectile dysfunction are described below. A brief summary is provided in Table 6.2.

6.5.3.1 Nocturnal Penile Tumescence Monitoring

Nocturnal penile tumescence (NPT) monitoring, used to study nocturnal erectile quality and to aid in the distinction between psychogenic ED and organic ED, may be used in a sleep laboratory setting [44]. Nocturnal monitoring evaluates the rigidity, number, and duration of erectile events during sleep [45]. While potentially relevant

Table 6.2 Adjunctive testing in the evaluation of erectile dysfunction

Diagnostic modality	Role in evaluation
Nocturnal penile tumescence monitoring	Presence of nocturnal erections Primarily of historical use
Biothesiometry	Penile vibratory sensation Not specific to erectile dysfunction
Penile Doppler ultrasonography	Assessment of vasculogenic erectile dysfunction Noninvasive, office-based procedure
Dynamic infusion cavernosometry and cavernosography	Definitive study to confirm arteriogenic or venogenic erectile dysfunction Primarily of historical use
Selective internal pudendal angiography	Anatomic evaluation of arterial inflow to the penis No data on functional outcomes Invasive
Endothelial reactivity testing	Presence of endothelial dysfunction May guide overall cardiovascular assessment

from a research standpoint, nocturnal testing is generally not helpful in predicting treatment response in these patients. Therefore, its routine use for diagnostic purposes is limited.

6.5.3.2 Biothesiometry

Although it is not directly associated with erectile function and rigidity, a subset of patients presenting with ED will report decreased penile sensitivity. Biothesiometry can be used for assessment of somatic nerve sensitivity in these patients and may be of use in the evaluation of ED [46]. Vibratory stimuli are administered on the fingertips as a control site and at various locations throughout the penis, with stepwise increases in amplitude until the patient reports sensation of the stimulus. Biothesiometry may be useful in the diagnosis of neurogenic ED, particularly in patients with distal/peripheral neuropathies as seen in diabetes mellitus, although frequently patients with neurogenic ED, such as those after radical pelvic surgery, will report no sensory changes due to the absence of a sensory component to the periprostatic cavernous nerves. Patients presenting with abnormal biothesiometry results will frequently be referred for more invasive and in-depth neurological studies, including measurement of somatosensory evoked potentials.

6.5.4 Vascular Evaluation

Vascular evaluation is used in the patient with ED in order to help define whether the cause is due to arterial insufficiency or veno-occlusive dysfunction.

6.5.4.1 Historical Testing

The penile brachial pressure index (PBI) refers to the ratio of penile systolic to brachial systolic pressure value and has been used to evaluate for the presence of significant hemodynamic occlusion proximal to the penile arteries contributing to ED. There are, however, concerns about the validity of this technique secondary to significant interobserver variability and the false-positive diagnosis of arterial insufficiency. As such, the use of PBI in the evaluation of ED is primarily of historical significance [47, 48].

Intracavernosal injection (ICI) testing, performed by injection of vasodilatory drugs combined with genital or audiovisual stimulation, is the simplest way to assess organic erectile function. After injection, the erectile response is evaluated by a clinician, who can rate both erectile rigidity and response duration. Failure to obtain a rigid erection may indicate vascular disease, but may also be the result of excessive anxiety during ICI testing [49]. The primary value of ICI testing is to define a functional veno-occlusive mechanism in men who develop a rigid and sustained erection and historically was performed without ultrasonography [50].

6.5.4.2 Penile Doppler Ultrasonography

Modern approaches to evaluation of erectile function frequently utilize penile Doppler ultrasound (PDU), a reliable and noninvasive method for evaluating ED. It provides a physiologic diagnosis and can help guide therapy in patients with a poor response to oral ED therapy, can help differentiate between psychogenic ED and vascular ED, and suggests the need for cardiovascular evaluation in the man with vasculogenic ED without overt CVD risk factors [51]. An erection is induced using ICI with vasoactive medications, and rigidity and sustainability of the erection are noted. With the patient in supine position, the penis is scanned and the location of the left and right cavernosal arteries is identified (Fig. 6.1). Peak systolic velocity (PSV), end diastolic velocity (EDV), and resistive indices (RI) ($RI = PSV - EDV/PSV$) are measured. The penis is further evaluated to observe for the presence of tunical plaque (Peyronie's disease), fibrosis, and calcification.

Various cutoffs have been suggested for normal PSV values, but it is generally accepted that the patients with PSV below 25 cm/s have evidence of arteriogenic ED, with a sensitivity of 100 % and specificity of 86 % among patients with abnormalities on pudendal angiography [52, 53]. Veno-occlusive dysfunction is evaluated using EDV, in the presence of normal arterial

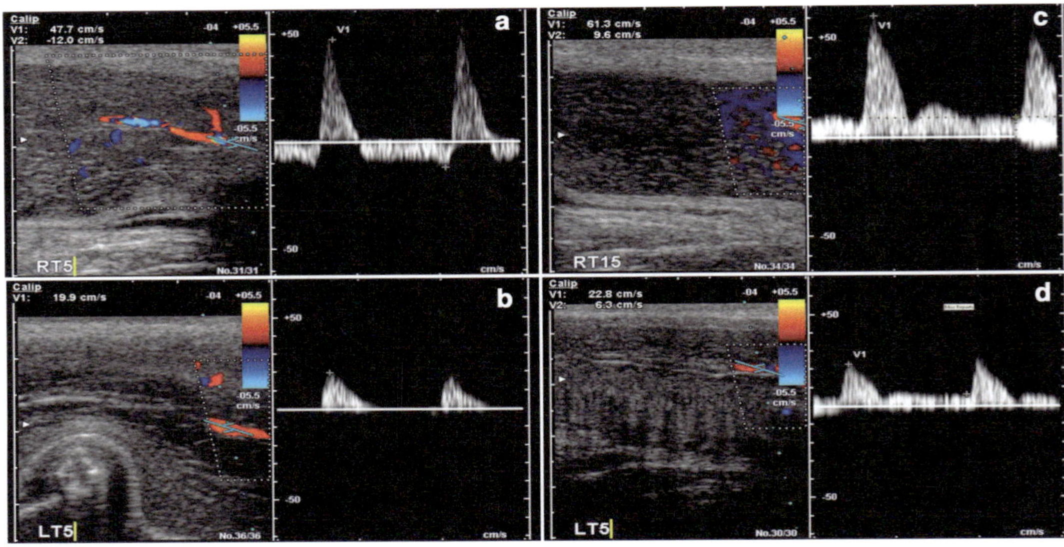

Fig. 6.1 Penile duplex ultrasound evaluation of erectile dysfunction. (**a**) Normal penile duplex US, with peak systolic velocity (PSV) of 47.7 cm/s (V2). The *left panel* represents the US image with the Doppler measure set over an artery. The *right panel* demonstrates the vascular flow trace. (**b**) Arterial insufficiency, with a PSV of 19.9 cm/s (V1). (**c**) Venous leak, with an end diastolic velocity (EDV) of 9.6 cm/s (V2). No evidence of arterial insufficiency is noted with a PSV of 61.3 cm/s. (**d**) Both arterial insufficiency (PSV 22.8 cm/s) and venous leak (EDV 6.3 cm/s)

inflow. Generally, EDV of greater than 5 cm/s is accepted as the measurement at which corporal veno-occlusive dysfunction is present [51, 54]. Given concerns for the specificity of EDV alone for the diagnosis of veno-occlusive ED in patients with arterial insufficiency, RI has been used with a threshold of less than 0.75 considered abnormal [51, 55]. Ultimately, however, the quality of the erection attained with ICI must be taken into account in analyzing the EDV values during PDU. Men with significant anxiety associated with testing may not achieve an erection during the study, but may present with a delayed, rigid erection following testing. These patients are unlikely to have true veno-occlusive dysfunction and likely have a significant psychogenic/anxiety component to their ED.

6.5.4.3 Dynamic Infusion Cavernosometry and Cavernosography

Dynamic infusion cavernosometry and cavernosography (DICC) is the most accurate assessment of erectile hemodynamics. Given the availability and relative ease of PDU, and the specialized equipment and training needed to perform DICC, its clinical use is limited primarily to young, healthy men with a history of perineal or pelvic trauma being considered for penile revascularization. Cavernosometry involves placement of a butterfly needle in each corporal body, with one connected to a pressure transducer and the other to a server-controlled pump for heparinized saline infusion [56, 57]. After induction of erection, the parameters recorded include the equilibrium pressure (mmHg) within the corpus cavernosum; the cavernosal artery inflow gradient (mmHg), which is the difference between brachial artery systolic pressure and the cavernosal artery occlusion pressure and measured on both sides; flow to maintain, defined as the flow of saline required to maintain a given intracorporal pressure; and intracorporal pressure decay. If the cavernosometry demonstrates veno-occlusive dysfunction, cavernosography may be performed, where radiopaque dye is injected intracavernosally and a radiograph is obtained in order to demonstrate the site of venous drainage (Fig. 6.2).

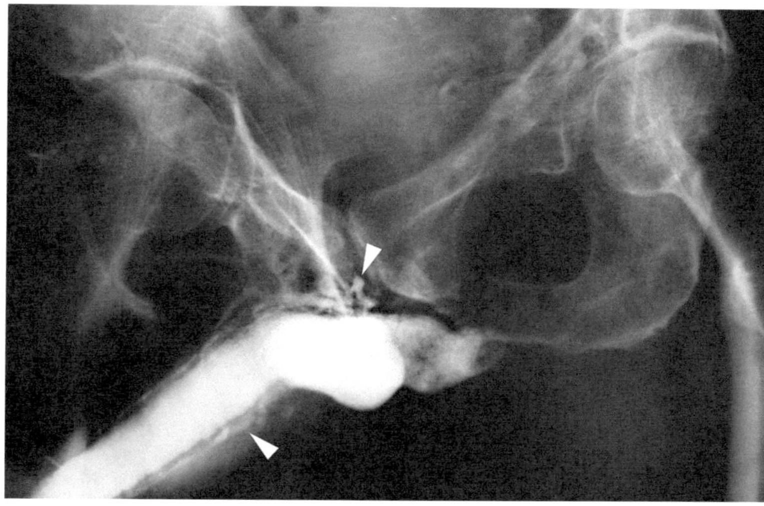

Fig. 6.2 Penile cavernosography. Penile cavernosogram demonstrating venous leak (*white arrows*). Courtesy of Irving J. Fishman, MD

Standardized data for DICC results are not available. However, generally used normal values are cavernosal artery occlusion pressure less than 30 mmHg, flow to maintain of less than 5 ml/min, and a pressure decay of less than 45 mmHg over 30 s [57].

6.5.4.4 Selective Internal Pudendal Arteriography

Penile arteriography is of limited use as a diagnostic modality for ED. It is an anatomic study that does not assess erectile function and is required in patients under consideration for penile revascularization surgery. A technically challenging and invasive procedure, pudendal/penile angiography requires an interventional radiologist with skill at cannulating both the internal pudendal arteries and the inferior epigastric arteries, which are used for revascularization [51]. Arterial inflow to the penis should be maximized using an intracavernosally delivered vasoactive agent, usually administered prior to contrast injection.

6.5.4.5 Endothelial Reactivity Testing

Recent studies have sought to analyze the presence of endothelial dysfunction as a precursor to overt CVD/atherosclerosis in patients presenting with ED. Increased flow and the resultant vasodilation in the penile arteries necessary for erection are mediated largely through nitric oxide (NO) produced by the endothelium. Endothelial dysfunction in patients with ED, but without evidence of other significant CVD, has been found within the penile vasculature but not within the small arteries of the forearm, suggesting that dysfunction occurs earlier within the penile endothelium than in other vascular beds [58]. In addition, increasing arterial stiffness, as evaluated with increasing pulse pressures, is associated with arteriogenic ED [59]. As a result, a number of diagnostic modalities have been used to assess endothelial function, including nonspecific serum markers (e.g., endothelin-1, interleukin 6, tumor necrosis factor-α, and C-reactive protein), analysis of flow-mediated dilation of the brachial artery (requiring ultrasound measurement of dilation in the brachial artery after arterial occlusion and administration of nitroglycerine—primarily a research modality), and office-based reactive hyperemia peripheral arterial tonometry (RH-PAT). The published literature provides conflicting information as to the utility of RH-PAT testing in the evaluation of men with possible vascular ED as part of their overall cardiovascular assessment [60, 61].

6.6 Conclusions

ED is a highly prevalent condition noted in the aging male and can be associated with a variety of different etiologies. Patients with vasculogenic ED are at risk for CVD and warrant further evaluation as deemed necessary on history, on physical examination, and with vascular testing. Diagnostic testing can be useful in clarifying the etiology of ED and should be used with a clear clinical indication and question which can help to clarify treatment options and long-term prognosis.

References

1. Porst H, Burnett A, Brock G, Ghanem H, Giuliano F, Glina S, et al. SOP conservative (medical and mechanical) treatment of erectile dysfunction. J Sex Med. 2013;10(1):130–71.
2. Consensus NIH. Conference. Impotence. NIH consensus development panel on impotence. JAMA. 1993;270(1):83–90.
3. Litwin MS, Nied RJ, Dhanani N. Health-related quality of life in men with erectile dysfunction. J Gen Intern Med. 1998;13(3):159–66.
4. Shabsigh R, Klein LT, Seidman S, Kaplan SA, Lehrhoff BJ, Ritter JS. Increased incidence of depressive symptoms in men with erectile dysfunction. Urology. 1998;52(5):848–52.
5. Lewis RW, Fugl-Meyer KS, Corona G, Hayes RD, Laumann EO, Moreira Jr ED, et al. Definitions/epidemiology/risk factors for sexual dysfunction. J Sex Med. 2010;7(4 Pt 2):1598–607.
6. Lue TF. Erectile dysfunction. N Engl J Med. 2000;342(24):1802–13.
7. Feldman HA, Goldstein I, Hatzichristou DG, Krane RJ, McKinlay JB. Impotence and its medical and psychosocial correlates: results of the Massachusetts male aging study. J Urol. 1994;151(1):54–61.
8. Lindau ST, Schumm LP, Laumann EO, Levinson W, O'Muircheartaigh CA, Waite LJ. A study of sexuality and health among older adults in the United States. N Engl J Med. 2007;357(8):762–74.
9. Laumann EO, West S, Glasser D, Carson C, Rosen R, Kang JH. Prevalence and correlates of erectile dysfunction by race and ethnicity among men aged 40 or older in the United States: from the male attitudes regarding sexual health survey. J Sex Med. 2007; 4(1):57–65.
10. Rosen RC. Psychogenic erectile dysfunction. Classification and management. Urol Clin North Am. 2001;28(2):269–78.
11. Lizza EF, Rosen RC. Definition and classification of erectile dysfunction: report of the nomenclature committee of the international society of impotence research. Int J Impot Res. 1999;11(3):141–3.
12. Deveci S, O'Brien K, Ahmed A, Parker M, Guhring P, Mulhall JP. Can the international index of erectile function distinguish between organic and psychogenic erectile function? BJU Int. 2008;102(3):354–6.
13. Sullivan ME, Thompson CS, Dashwood MR, Khan MA, Jeremy JY, Morgan RJ, et al. Nitric oxide and penile erection: is erectile dysfunction another manifestation of vascular disease? Cardiovasc Res. 1999;43(3):658–65.
14. Giuliano FA, Leriche A, Jaudinot EO, de Gendre AS. Prevalence of erectile dysfunction among 7689 patients with diabetes or hypertension, or both. Urology. 2004;64(6):1196–201.
15. Martin-Morales A, Saenz de Tejada I, Rodriguez-Vela L, Jimenez-Cruz JF, Burgos-Rodriguez R. Prevalence and independent risk factors for erectile dysfunction in Spain: results of the epidemiologia de la disfuncion erectil masculina study. J Urol. 2001;166(2):569–74 (Discussion 74–5).
16. Guo W, Liao C, Zou Y, Li F, Li T, Zhou Q, et al. Erectile dysfunction and risk of clinical cardiovascular events: a meta-analysis of seven cohort studies. J Sex Med. 2010;7(8):2805–16.
17. Thompson IM, Tangen CM, Goodman PJ, Probstfield JL, Moinpour CM, Coltman CA. Erectile dysfunction and subsequent cardiovascular disease. JAMA. 2005;294(23):2996–3002.
18. Gupta BP, Murad MH, Clifton MM, Prokop L, Nehra A, Kopecky SL. The effect of lifestyle modification and cardiovascular risk factor reduction on erectile dysfunction: a systematic review and meta-analysis. Arch Intern Med. 2011;171(20):1797–803.
19. Traish AM, Park K, Dhir V, Kim NN, Moreland RB, Goldstein I. Effects of castration and androgen replacement on erectile function in a rabbit model. Endocrinology. 1999;140(4):1861–8.
20. Traish AM, Toselli P, Jeong SJ, Kim NN. Adipocyte accumulation in penile corpus cavernosum of the orchiectomized rabbit: a potential mechanism for veno-occlusive dysfunction in androgen deficiency. J Androl. 2005;26(2):242–8.
21. Rhoden EL, Teloken C, Sogari PR, Souto CA. The relationship of serum testosterone to erectile function in normal aging men. J Urol. 2002;167(4):1745–8.
22. Corona G, Mannucci E, Mansani R, Petrone L, Bartolini M, Giommi R, et al. Aging and pathogenesis of erectile dysfunction. Int J Impot Res. 2004; 16(5):395–402.
23. Isidori AM, Buvat J, Corona G, Goldstein I, Jannini EA, Lenzi A, et al. A critical analysis of the role of testosterone in erectile function: from pathophysiology to treatment-a systematic review. Eur Urol. 2014;65(1):99–112.
24. Corona G, Mannucci E, Fisher AD, Lotti F, Ricca V, Balercia G, et al. Effect of hyperprolactinemia in male patients consulting for sexual dysfunction. J Sex Med. 2007;4(5):1485–93.

25. Saenz de Tejada I, Angulo J, Cellek S, Gonzalez-Cadavid N, Heaton J, Pickard R, et al. Pathophysiology of erectile dysfunction. J Sex Med. 2005;2(1):26–39.
26. Berookhim B, Steinway M, Bar-Chama N, Seftel A. Benign prostatic hyperplasia evaluation, association with sexual dysfunction, treatment, and practice patterns according to physician specialty. Curr Prostate Rep. 2009;7(1):25–31.
27. Braun MH, Sommer F, Haupt G, Mathers MJ, Reifenrath B, Engelmann UH. Lower urinary tract symptoms and erectile dysfunction: co-morbidity or typical "aging male" symptoms? Results of the "cologne male survey". Eur Urol. 2003;44(5): 588–94.
28. Blanker MH, Bohnen AM, Groeneveld FP, Bernsen RM, Prins A, Thomas S, et al. Correlates for erectile and ejaculatory dysfunction in older Dutch men: a community-based study. J Am Geriatr Soc. 2001; 49(4):436–42.
29. Glina S, Glina FP. Pathogenic mechanisms linking benign prostatic hyperplasia, lower urinary tract symptoms and erectile dysfunction. Ther Adv Urol. 2013;5(4):211–8.
30. Hatzichristou D, Rosen RC, Derogatis LR, Low WY, Meuleman EJ, Sadovsky R, et al. Recommendations for the clinical evaluation of men and women with sexual dysfunction. J Sex Med. 2010;7(1 Pt 2):337–48.
31. McCabe MP, Althof SE. A systematic review of the psychosocial outcomes associated with erectile dysfunction: does the impact of erectile dysfunction extend beyond a man's inability to have sex? J Sex Med. 2013;11:347–63.
32. Perelman MA. Psychosocial evaluation and combination treatment of men with erectile dysfunction. Urol Clin North Am. 2005;32(4):431–45, vi.
33. Rosen RC, Riley A, Wagner G, Osterloh IH, Kirkpatrick J, Mishra A. The international index of erectile function (IIEF): a multidimensional scale for assessment of erectile dysfunction. Urology. 1997;49(6):822–30.
34. Rosen RC, Cappelleri JC, Smith MD, Lipsky J, Pena BM. Development and evaluation of an abridged, 5-item version of the international index of erectile function (IIEF-5) as a diagnostic tool for erectile dysfunction. Int J Impot Res. 1999; 11(6):319–26.
35. Cappelleri JC, Rosen RC. The sexual health inventory for men (SHIM): a 5-year review of research and clinical experience. Int J Impot Res. 2005; 17(4):307–19.
36. Fisher WA, Eardley I, McCabe M, Sand M. Erectile dysfunction (ED) is a shared sexual concern of couples II: association of female partner characteristics with male partner ED treatment seeking and phosphodiesterase type 5 inhibitor utilization. J Sex Med. 2009;6(11):3111–24.
37. Jiann BP, Su CC, Tsai JY. Is female sexual function related to the male partners' erectile function? J Sex Med. 2013;10(2):420–9.
38. Moskovic DJ, Mohamed O, Sathyamoorthy K, Miles BJ, Link RE, Lipshultz LI, et al. The female factor: predicting compliance with a post-prostatectomy erectile preservation program. J Sex Med. 2010;7(11):3659–65.
39. Corona G, Petrone L, Mannucci E, Magini A, Lotti F, Ricca V, et al. Assessment of the relational factor in male patients consulting for sexual dysfunction: the concept of couple sexual dysfunction. J Androl. 2006;27(6):795–801.
40. Althof SE, Leiblum SR, Chevret-Measson M, Hartmann U, Levine SB, McCabe M, et al. Psychological and interpersonal dimensions of sexual function and dysfunction. J Sex Med. 2005;2(6):793–800.
41. Ghanem HM, Salonia A, Martin-Morales A. SOP: physical examination and laboratory testing for men with erectile dysfunction. J Sex Med. 2012;10:108–10.
42. Weinberg AE, Eisenberg M, Patel CJ, Chertow GM, Leppert JT. Diabetes severity, metabolic syndrome, and the risk of erectile dysfunction. J Sex Med. 2013;10:3102–9.
43. Nehra A, Jackson G, Miner M, Billups KL, Burnett AL, Buvat J, et al. The Princeton III consensus recommendations for the management of erectile dysfunction and cardiovascular disease. Mayo Clin Proc. 2012;87(8):766–78.
44. Wasserman MD, Pollak CP, Spielman AJ, Weitzman ED. The differential diagnosis of impotence. The measurement of nocturnal penile tumescence. JAMA. 1980;243(20):2038–42.
45. Bradley WE, Timm GW, Gallagher JM, Johnson BK. New method for continuous measurement of nocturnal penile tumescence and rigidity. Urology. 1985;26(1):4–9.
46. Bemelmans BL, Hendrikx LB, Koldewijn EL, Lemmens WA, Debruyne FM, Meuleman EJ. Comparison of biothesiometry and neuro-urophysiological investigations for the clinical evaluation of patients with erectile dysfunction. J Urol. 1995;153(5):1483–6.
47. Aitchison M, Aitchison J, Carter R. Is the penile brachial index a reproducible and useful measurement? Br J Urol. 1990;66(2):202–4.
48. Mahe G, Leftheriotis G, Picquet J, Jaquinandi V, Saumet JL, Abraham P. A normal penile pressure cannot rule out the presence of lesions on the arteries supplying the hypogastric circulation in patients with arterial claudication. Vasc Med. 2009;14(4):331–8.
49. Aversa A, Rocchietti-March M, Caprio M, Giannini D, Isidori A, Fabbri A. Anxiety-induced failure in erectile response to intracorporeal prostaglandin-E1 in non-organic male impotence: a new diagnostic approach. Int J Androl. 1996;19(5):307–13.
50. Virag R, Frydman D, Legman M, Virag H. Intracavernous injection of papaverine as a diagnostic and therapeutic method in erectile failure. Angiology. 1984;35(2):79–87.
51. Sikka SC, Hellstrom WJ, Brock G, Morales AM. Standardization of vascular assessment of erectile dysfunction: standard operating procedures for duplex ultrasound. J Sex Med. 2012;10:120–9.

52. Lue TF, Hricak H, Marich KW, Tanagho EA. Vasculogenic impotence evaluated by high-resolution ultrasonography and pulsed Doppler spectrum analysis. Radiology. 1985;155(3):777–81.
53. Quam JP, King BF, James EM, Lewis RW, Brakke DM, Ilstrup DM, et al. Duplex and color Doppler sonographic evaluation of vasculogenic impotence. AJR Am J Roentgenol. 1989;153(6):1141–7.
54. Benson CB, Aruny JE, Vickers Jr MA. Correlation of duplex sonography with arteriography in patients with erectile dysfunction. AJR Am J Roentgenol. 1993;160(1):71–3.
55. Wilkins CJ, Sriprasad S, Sidhu PS. Colour Doppler ultrasound of the penis. Clin Radiol. 2003;58(7):514–23.
56. Vardi Y, Glina S, Mulhall JP, Menchini F, Munarriz R. Cavernosometry: is it a dinosaur? J Sex Med. 2008;5(4):760–4.
57. Glina S, Ghanem H. SOP: corpus cavernosum assessment (cavernosography/cavernosometry). J Sex Med. 2013;10(1):111–4.
58. Kaiser DR, Billups K, Mason C, Wetterling R, Lundberg JL, Bank AJ. Impaired brachial artery endothelium-dependent and -independent vasodilation in men with erectile dysfunction and no other clinical cardiovascular disease. J Am Coll Cardiol. 2004; 43(2):179–84.
59. Corona G, Mannucci E, Lotti F, Fisher AD, Bandini E, Balercia G, et al. Pulse pressure, an index of arterial stiffness, is associated with androgen deficiency and impaired penile blood flow in men with ED. J Sex Med. 2009;6(1):285–93.
60. Aversa A, Francomano D, Bruzziches R, Pili M, Natali M, Spera G, et al. The application of digital pulse amplitude tonometry to the diagnostic investigation of endothelial dysfunction in men with erectile dysfunction. Andrologia. 2011;43(1):9–15.
61. Mehta A, Miner M, Sigman M. Assessment of EndoPAT scores in men with vasculogenic and nonvasculogenic erectile dysfunction. Int J Clin Pract. 2013;67(1):46–51.

7 Urologic/Clinical Treatment of Erectile Dysfunction

Nishant Patel and T. Mike Hsieh

7.1 Introduction

The treatment of erectile dysfunction (ED) has advanced over the past century. Prior to the 1960s, when ED was thought to be of psychogenic or unknown etiology, treatments consisted of testosterone supplementation or psychiatric evaluation and treatment. With advancements in the understanding of vascular, neurologic, and hormonal physiology of erectile function, a multitude of pharmacologic and surgical treatments have emerged (Fig. 7.1) [1].

Overall, the use of oral phosphodiesterase type 5 inhibitors (PDE5i's) is the most common treatment for ED. Other treatment options include lifestyle modifications to address comorbid conditions, testosterone supplementation for androgen-deficient men, intracavernosal injection (ICI) therapy, intraurethral medications, vacuum and constriction devices, penile prosthetic surgery, alternative therapies, and psychotherapy. Combining psychosocial and medical treatment will offer individualized therapy and assist patients in understanding their individual conditions.

N. Patel, M.D. • T.M. Hsieh, M.D. (✉)
Department of Urology, University of California, San Diego, San Diego, CA, USA
e-mail: tmikehsieh@ucsd.edu

7.2 Lifestyle Modification

Normal erectile function relies on the interaction of vascular, neurologic, hormonal, and psychologic mechanisms. Comorbidities such as coronary artery disease, peripheral vascular disease, hypertension, diabetes, and the metabolic syndrome are implicated as risk factors in developing ED. Additionally, a number of lifestyle risk factors have been associated with ED, including reduced physical activity, tobacco use, alcohol consumption, and obesity [2]. Thus, physician-directed counseling and modification of these risk factors can positively impact erectile function. For instance, in a group of patients where a strong association between cigarette smoking and degree of ED was observed, smoking cessation improved ED in up to a quarter of the population [3]. In a randomized study of obese patients, those men who adopted lifestyle changes including reduced caloric intake and increased physical activity reported an increase of three points on the International Index of Erectile Function (IIEF), a validated instrument for the assessment of erectile function [4].

Several mechanisms explaining the beneficial effect of physical activity and weight reduction on erectile function have been proposed, including improvement in endothelial cell function, decreased inflammation, increased serum testosterone, and improvements in mood and affect [5].

L.I. Lipshultz et al. (eds.), *Management of Sexual Dysfunction in Men and Women*, DOI 10.1007/978-1-4939-3100-2_7

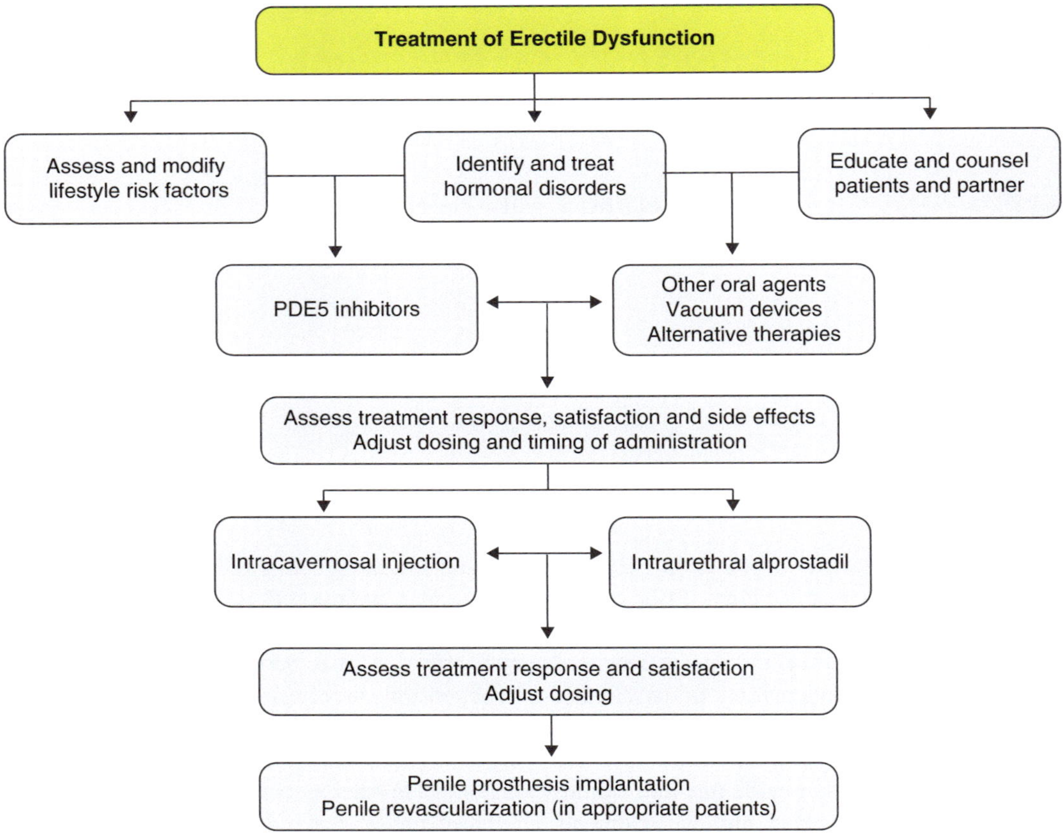

Fig. 7.1 Algorithm for the clinical treatment of erectile dysfunction (PDE5—phospho-diesterase type 5)

However, definitive clinical and basic science evidence is often lacking to confirm the favorable association between lifestyle changes and improvement in erectile function. A recent meta-analysis demonstrated improved IIEF scores after only 6 weeks of lifestyle modification and pharmacotherapy for cardiovascular risk factors [6]. However, other reports suggest lifestyle changes may take 12–24 months to achieve maximal clinical results, and proven pharmacotherapy should not be withheld pending these changes [4]. Sensible lifestyle goals for the man with ED include increasing exercise, reducing weight to achieve a BMI less than 30 kg/m^2, instituting a "heart-healthy" diet, and tobacco cessation [5, 7].

7.3 Testosterone Supplementation

Testosterone has well-defined roles in maintaining libido, supporting fertility, and sustaining adequate erectile function, through the stimulation of genes that increase nitric oxide synthase (NOS) expression [8]. Testosterone supplementation is recommended only in those men with ED who have androgen deficiency and are no longer interested in reproduction. Most clinicians agree that men who will likely benefit from testosterone therapy have serum testosterone levels of <300 ng/dL. However, calculating bioavailable or free testosterone might provide a more accurate measurement [9]. Testosterone monotherapy in men with ED and a serum total testosterone concentration <300 ng/dL has been shown to improve mean IIEF scores by six points after 1 year of therapy [10]. In men aged >65 years with androgen deficiency, combination therapy with PDE5i's and testosterone supplementation has been successful when PDE5i's alone were ineffective [11].

Testosterone is available in several preparations and can be taken orally, intramuscularly, transdermally (patch or gel), or buccally or implanted subcutaneously [12]. Prior to initiating testosterone supplementation, several baseline parameters should be assessed including serum prostate-specific antigen (PSA), complete blood count (CBC), lipid profile, and liver function tests, and a digital rectal examination performed. According to manufacturer's product inserts, testosterone supplementation has the potential to exacerbate certain conditions such as untreated prostate or breast cancer, uncontrolled congestive heart failure, polycythemia (hematocrit >52 %), severe sleep apnea, severe dyslipidemia, or severe prostatic bladder outlet obstruction and can affect patients at risk for pulmonary edema. Therefore, testosterone supplementation in these patients warrants extra attention and should be implemented after thorough evaluation and treatment of underlying conditions. Repeat serum testosterone levels after initiating therapy are necessary to assess for potential over- and undertreatment, together with assessment of the patient's hypogonadal symptoms. A patient's clinical response may not correlate with serum testosterone levels, and attempting to achieve supratherapeutic testosterone levels is not recommended. Some authors suggest discontinuing testosterone replacement if no clinical benefit is seen 3 months into therapy [13]. Potential adverse effects should be identified including acne, gynecomastia, progression of urinary symptoms, prostate cancer progression in both treated and untreated men, polycythemia, dyslipidemia, and hepatitis. Therefore, monitoring of PSA, CBC, lipid profile, and liver function tests is requisite at six-month intervals.

7.4 Oral Phosphodiesterase Type 5 Inhibitors

Per American Urologic Association (AUA) guidelines, unless contraindicated, oral PDE5i's constitute first-line therapy for the treatment of ED [14]. The US Food and Drug Administration (FDA) has approved five PDE5i's for the treatment of ED to date: sildenafil citrate tablets (Viagra®, Pfizer, Inc), vardenafil hydrochloride tablets (Levitra®, Bayer Pharma AG), vardenafil hydrochloride orally disintegrating tablets (Staxyn®, Bayer Pharma AG), tadalafil tablets (Cialis®, Lilly LLC), and, recently, avanafil tablets (Stendra®, Vivus, Inc.) (Table 7.1). The mechanism of action of PDE5i's is to inhibit phosphodiesterase 5, the enzyme responsible for metabolizing cGMP, which is produced by guanylate cyclase under the influence of nitric oxide. Increased levels of cGMP result in relaxation of erectogenic smooth muscle in the corpora cavernosa, improving cavernosal blood flow and resulting in penile erections [15]. PDE5i's do not result in spontaneous erections and require sexual stimulation for efficacy, as this generates 3′5′-cGMP, the substrate for PDE5.

Overall, PDE5i's are effective in 65 % of patients with efficacy defined as resulting in an erection sufficient for vaginal penetration, of 65 % [16]. The choice of PDE5i depends on the patient's frequency of intercourse while balancing efficacy with individual side effect profiles. An assessment of a couple's "sexual script" can help determine which drug is given based on timing and need [17]. For patients engaging in occasional sexual activity at a defined time, on-demand dosing is ideal, whereas those men engaging in frequent activity might benefit from daily PDE5i use. The various PDE5i's vary in terms of onset of action, duration of effect, absorption efficacy, and side effect profiles.

Sildenafil was the first PDE5i introduced for the treatment of ED in 1998. It is effective 30–60 min after administration and has a mean duration of action of 4–8 h, although efficacy may extend up to 12 h. Dosing is available in 25, 50, and 100 mg pills, with the usual starting dose at 50 mg

Table 7.1 Food and Drug Administration (FDA)—approved oral PDE5-inhibitor drugs

	Sildenafil	Vardenafil	Tadalafil	Avanafil
Dosage	25, 50, and 100 mg. Start with 50 mg	2.5, 5, 10, and 20 mg. Start with 10 mg 10 mg—orally disintegrating	2.5, 5, 10, and 20 mg. 2.5 and 5 mg daily dosing. Start with 10 mg	50, 100, and 200 mg. Start with 100 mg
Onset of action (min)	30–60	30	45	15
Duration (h)	4–8	4–8	Up to 36	6
Efficacy (%)	>65	>65	>65	>65
Side effects	Headache, flushing, dyspepsia, nasal congestion, abnormal vision	Flushing, nasal congestion, headache, abnormal vision	Flushing, back pain, myalgia, headache, dyspepsia, facial flushing	Flushing, nasal congestion, back pain
Contraindications	Nitrates, recent cardiovascular events. Caution with alpha-blockers	Nitrates, alpha-blockers, type 1 and 3 antiarrhythmics, prolonged QT interval	Nitrates, recent cardiovascular events. Caution with alpha-blockers	Nitrates, recent cardiovascular events. Caution with alpha-blockers
Fatty food	Reduced absorption	Reduced absorption	No effect	Reduced absorption

[1]. If taken with a high fat meal (>57 % fat), sildenafil's rate of absorption is reduced, translating to prolonged onset times or decreased efficacy. Therefore, administration while fasting is recommended. The most common side effects of sildenafil include headache (16 %), flushing (10 %), and dyspepsia (7 %). Other less common adverse reactions include nasal congestion, vision changes, and diarrhea [18].

Vardenafil, introduced in 2003, is effective within 30 min of administration and is available in 2.5, 5, 10, and 20 mg doses, with 10 mg representing the most common starting dose. In vitro, vardenafil inhibits PDE5 at concentrations tenfold lower than does sildenafil, although this may not correlate with clinical response. Vardenafil shares the same decreased absorption as sildenafil when taken with high fat meals. Flushing and nasal congestion are more common with vardenafil (9–11 %) [19]. The orally disintegrating preparation of vardenafil (Staxyn) is available in a 10 mg dose, can be taken with a high fat meal with no impact on absorption, and attains higher plasma concentrations than film-coated tablets. Neither form of vardenafil should be administered to patients taking type 1 or 3 antiarrhythmic drugs or those with congenital QT interval prolongation [20].

Tadalafil, introduced in 2003, may be administered in an on-demand fashion or daily. Available in 2.5, 5, 10, and 20 mg doses, on-demand dosing should begin at 10 mg, with a maximum of 20 mg. While tadalafil has a longer time to onset than sildenafil or vardenafil (45 min), its effects may last up to 36 h and are not impacted by the fat content of food [21]. In 2008, tadalafil was approved for daily use for ED, with a dose of 2.5–5 mg. This regimen, ideal for couples desiring frequent spontaneous sexual activity, is well tolerated, with improvements in IIEF scores [22]. Tadalafil has also recently been approved for treating men with lower urinary tract symptoms secondary to BPH at a dose of 5 mg daily [23]. More than the other PDE5i's, tadalafil exhibits the higher incidence of back pain and myalgia, thought to be secondary to cross-reactivity with PDE11, found in skeletal muscle.

Lastly, avanafil, introduced in 2013, has shown greater selectivity for PDE5 than the other agents and can be effective within 15 min of administration. The absorption of avanafil is reduced with a high fat meal, and its duration of action is short—6 h. Avanafil displays a low prevalence (<6 %) of common PDE5i adverse effects [24]. Other PDE5i's, namely, udenafil and mirodenafil, are approved for use in Korea, while lodenafil is in clinical trials.

An absolute contraindication to the use of all PDE5i's is in patients taking organic nitrates or nitric oxide donors (nitroglycerin, isosorbide dinitrate, amyl nitrates) for angina within a period of 2 weeks, as concomitant use may result in severe and life-threatening hypotension. Men taking alpha-blockers for bladder outlet obstruction are also at risk for hypotension when taking PDE5i's, and combination therapy of alpha-blockers and PDE5i's should be used with caution. Interestingly, low-dose daily tadalafil (2.5–5 mg) is also FDA approved for the treatment of lower urinary tract symptoms secondary to benign prostatic hyperplasia. Sildenafil and vardenafil have a risk of blurry vision from PDE6 cross-reactivity, and rare sudden loss of vision secondary to nonarteritic anterior optic neuropathy (NAION) may occur, although this pathology has not been directly linked to PDE5i's [25]. The pharmacokinetics of PDE5i's are not greatly affected by alcohol, although refraining from alcohol is suggested given the link between alcohol consumption and ED. However, if alcohol is taken, studies have shown that PDE5i's do not potentiate alcohol's hypotensive effects. A lower dose of PDE5i may be needed in patients taking steroid production inhibitors (ketoconazole), macrolide antibiotics, and HIV protease inhibitors (ritonavir) or those with history of liver and renal dysfunction [1].

The major reasons for nonresponse to PDE5i are poor patient understanding of medication usage and a lack of PDE5i efficacy. Patients require adequate counseling on the timing of administration related to food intake, need for sexual stimulation, timing of onset of each agent, and an understanding of potential side effects. Men should attempt a single PDE5i agent at least 4 times prior to dose escalation. No convincing data exists to support switching PDE5i after failure with one correctly administered agent, although changing agents due to drug intolerance is likely to be beneficial [26].

7.5 Other Oral Treatments

Dopamine within the periventricular nucleus of the brain plays a role in the central control of erections. Apomorphine is a centrally acting dopaminergic agent that is taken sublingually on demand in doses of 2, 4, and 6 mg and is of particular interest in treating psychogenic ED. Side effects include nausea, headache, dizziness, and, rarely, syncopal events. Apomorphine has shown the best efficacy in patients with mild to moderate ED [27]. Bremelanotide is a synthetic analogue of alpha-melanocyte stimulating hormone, which activates melanocortin receptors 3 and 4. This activation is thought to regulate sexual behavior and erectile function. Studies of bremelanotide administered subcutaneously appear to increase libido and initiate erections, but the drug is not currently approved for commercial use [28].

Oral phentolamine mesylate is an alpha-adrenergic receptor antagonist. In erectile physiology, the alpha-1 adrenoreceptor's downstream effects result in contraction of smooth muscle and detumescence via phospholipase C. One study demonstrated 40 mg of phentolamine to be efficacious in men with mild to moderate ED, with side effects including headache, facial flushing, and nasal congestion [29]. Yohimbine hydrochloride, a derivative from the bark of the yohimbe tree, acts as an alpha-2 adrenoreceptor antagonist and is administered at 5.4 mg three times daily. Adverse reactions include hypertension, tachycardia, and anxiety, and yohimbe has no proven efficacy in men with organic ED compared to placebo [30]. Acting via serotonin receptors, trazodone, with a known side effect of priapism, has been studied in the setting of ED, but clinical evidence demonstrating efficacy is lacking.

7.6 Intraurethral Alprostadil

After failure of oral therapies, second-line agents such as ICIs and intraurethral suppositories are indicated. Alprostadil is a synthetic vasodilator that mimics naturally occurring prostaglandin E1. Alprostadil binds to adenylate cyclase and increases cyclic AMP, which results in relaxation of erectogenic smooth muscle. MUSE® (Medicated Urethral System for Erections, Meda Pharmaceuticals, Inc.) is an intraurethral alprostadil suppository placed into the distal urethra (Fig. 7.2). The drug is absorbed through the

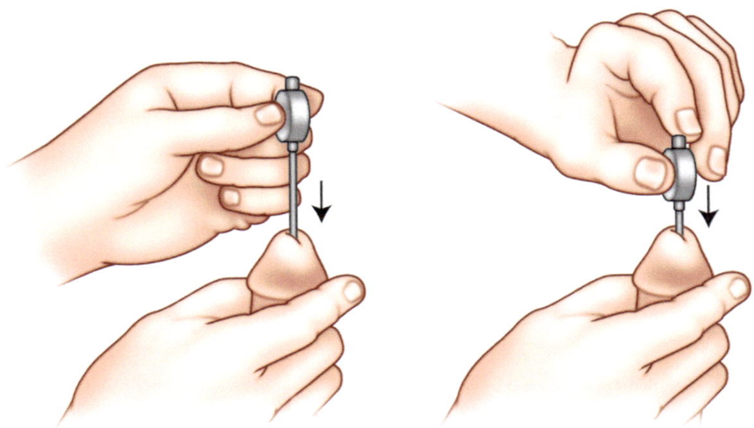

Fig. 7.2 Insertion method for MUSE® intraurethral alprostadil pellet

urethral mucosa and into the corpora cavernosa and acts within 20 min of administration. The suppositories are available in 125, 250, 500, and 1000 mcg, and recent literature supports a starting dose of 500 mcg, as this has shown higher efficacy than lower doses without a significant increase in adverse events [31]. Men with neurogenic ED should be started on the lowest possible dose. Approximately 50 % of men respond to MUSE, and among those, 70 % have erections sufficient for penetration [32]. Adverse effects include priapism, penile/urethral pain, headache, dizziness, and syncope. Since a 3 % risk of hypotension and syncope has been reported, especially in men with a venous leak component to their ED, it is recommended that the first dose of MUSE be administered under supervision of a healthcare provider [32]. If the female partner is pregnant, a condom is recommended when using MUSE. Studies have demonstrated that intraurethral alprostadil, in combination with a PDE5i or penile constriction device, is more effective than alprostadil alone [33].

7.7 Intracavernosal Injections

As another second-line therapy, ICI of vasoactive agents allows for on-demand erections within 5–15 min (Fig. 7.3). Efficacy rates range from 70 to 90 %, with satisfaction rates ranging from 87 to 93.5 % [1]. Several agents are used alone or in combination to achieve an optimal response. Injectable alprostadil is available as Edex (Auxilium Pharmaceuticals, LLC) and Caverject (Pfizer, Inc.) as monotherapy. Side effects include penile pain (11 %), local hematoma, priapism (2 %), and penile fibrosis (1 %) [34]. Papaverine is a nonspecific phosphodiesterase inhibitor, resulting in increased intracellular levels of cAMP and cGMP. Papaverine has a lower risk of penile pain than alprostadil, but higher risk of priapism and fibrosis (10–12 %). Phentolamine inhibits alpha-adrenergic receptors and inhibits detumescence. Its side effects include hypotension, nasal congestion, reflex tachycardia, and dyspepsia. Bi-Mix, a mixture of papaverine and phentolamine; Tri-Mix, a mixture of papaverine, phentolamine, papaverine, and prostaglandin E1; and Quad-mix, consisting of Tri-Mix with the addition of atropine or forskolin, all result in efficacy rates of 80–90 % [35]. The distinct advantage of the above mixtures includes decreased volume for injection and potential superiority versus prostaglandin E1, alone in treating ED due to venous leak. Vasoactive intestinal polypeptide (VIP) has been studied for ICI, but has poor results as monotherapy. A mixture of VIP with phentolamine (Invicorp) exhibits greater efficacy (80 %) than VIP alone and is currently approved in other countries [36].

Dose titration should begin at the lowest possible dose, especially in men with neurogenic ED. Initial dosing under a healthcare provider's

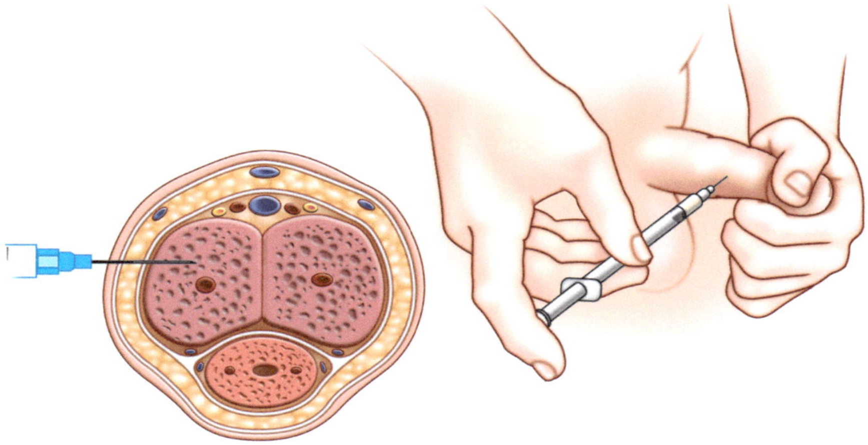

Fig. 7.3 Injection method for intracavernosal injection. The patient performs self-injection of a vasoactive agent directly into the penile corpora cavernosa

supervision is recommended to ensure proper technique (including partner education) and determine appropriate dose. Contraindications for ICI include men at risk for priapism (prior events, sickle cell anemia), poor manual dexterity, significant coagulopathy, and the use of monoamine oxidase inhibitors (to prevent severe hypertension if an alpha agonist is necessary during a priapism event) [37]. Men with recurring priapism secondary to ICI are managed with dose reduction and a phenylephrine kit for self-treatment.

7.8 Vacuum Erection Device

In men who fail, cannot tolerate, or have contraindications to PDE5i or ICI, a vacuum erection device (VED) offers a good noninvasive option and represents another second-line ED treatment option. A VED works by creating a vacuum around the penis, resulting in expansion of the corpora cavernosa and increased inflow of blood. Placement of a penile constriction ring diminishes outflow of blood and prevents penile detumescence. The VED consists of a plastic cylinder and a pump source to generate negative pressure (Fig. 7.4). After an erection is achieved, the constriction band is placed at the penile base, and the device removed. Recent reviews suggest efficacy rates range from 75 to 91 % in achieving erection sufficient for penetration and satisfaction rates ranging from 65 to 80 % [38].

VEDs display a low rate of complications, including bruising, interference with ejaculation secondary to the constrictive ring, numbness, and penile pain. Men on anticoagulants may experience increased ecchymosis and should use caution. The device is of particular interest in post-prostatectomy penile rehabilitation, as early VED use may improve cavernosal tissue oxygenation and erections and facilitate earlier sexual intercourse postoperatively [39]. Additionally, combination of a VED with PDE5i, ICI, or MUSE has been shown to increase efficacy and patient-partner satisfaction [40, 41].

7.9 Surgical Treatments

For patients with ED who fail first- and second-line treatments, a third-line treatment is penile prosthetic surgery. After replacing the normal erectile tissue with the prosthesis, the corporal tissue is altered and the potential for smooth muscle relaxation is eliminated, making "natural"

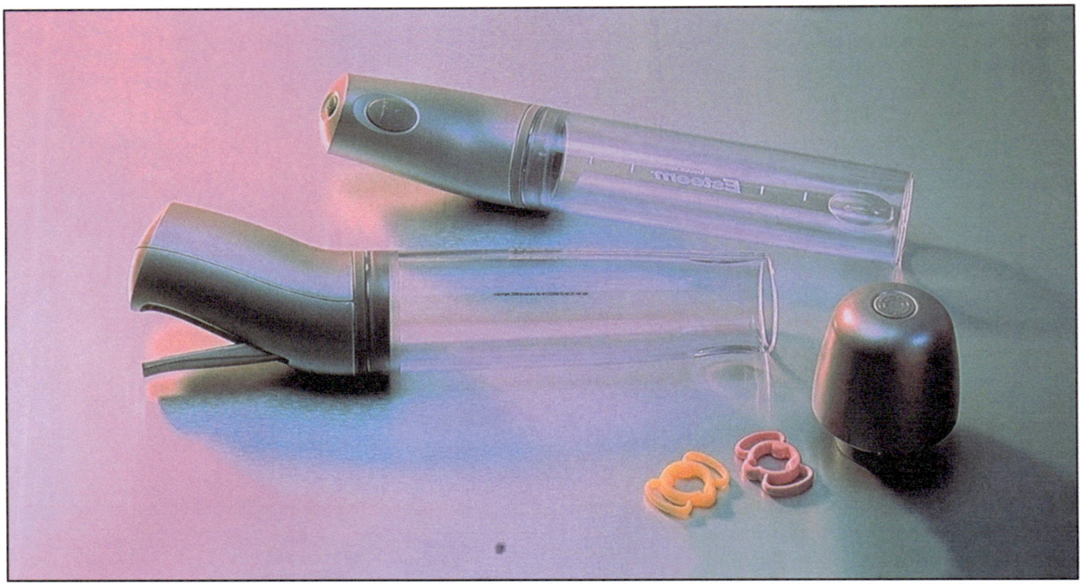

Fig. 7.4 Commercially available vacuum erection device with either manual or electric pump and constriction bands. With permission from Timm Medical Technologies, Inc.

erections impossible after prosthesis placement. Adequate counseling is necessary regarding penile prosthesis options, risk of erosion or infection, need for subsequent operations, penile shortening, and proper use of the device. Satisfaction rates as high as 85 % for the patient and 76 % for his partner have been reported [42]. The two main types of prostheses are non-inflatable (malleable) and inflatable. Non-inflatable devices are semirigid and manipulate to an erect position for sexual activity. The advantages of a non-inflatable device include a low rate of mechanical failure and less need for manual dexterity. However, malleable prostheses carry an increased risk of erosion and chronic pain [43]. Inflatable prostheses are available in two- or three-piece configurations. The three-piece inflatable prosthesis is most commonly used and consists of paired corporal cylinders, an abdominal fluid reservoir, and a scrotal pump. It provides a flaccid state at baseline, and activating the scrotal pump allows fluid to transfer from the abdominal reservoir to the cylinders, resulting in an increase in penile girth and rigidity. A release valve on the pump then transmits fluid back to the reservoir (Fig. 7.5). Compared to malleable devices, inflatable prostheses have a higher rate of mechanical failure (6–15 % at 5 years) [44] yet more lifelike function.

Complications of penile prosthesis placement include bleeding, infection (2–4 % of cases), mechanical failure, injury to vascular or bowel structures, erosion, and penile shortening. Erosion and infection usually require explantation of some or all of the prosthesis. Reimplantation of another device after infection may be performed after the infection resolves or during the explantation procedure to preserve penile length [45].

Surgeries to either limit venous outflow or increase arterial inflow are appealing in theory, but currently have limited clinical utility. The AUA recommends against surgeries to restrict venous outflow and recommends penile arterial reconstructive surgery for men <55 years old, nonsmokers, nondiabetics, without venous leak, and with a focal stenosis of the internal pudendal artery [46]. Complications of revascularization include glans hyperemia, thrombosis of the anastomoses, scarring, and hernia [47].

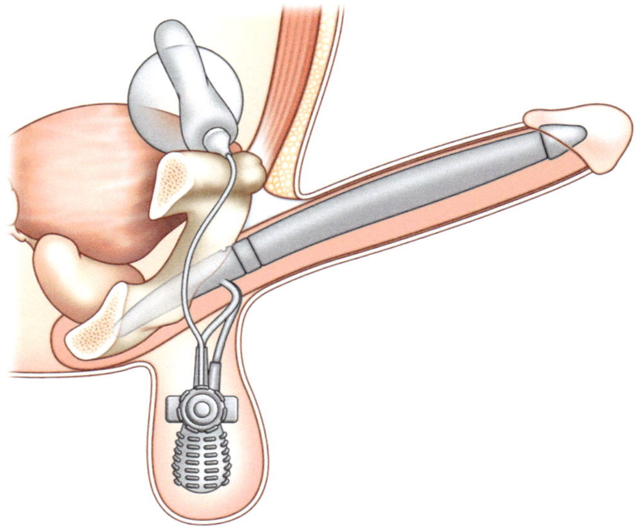

Fig. 7.5 The three-piece inflatable penile prosthesis consisting of paired corporal cylinders, an abdominal fluid reservoir, and a scrotal pump

7.10 Alternative Therapies

Throughout history, a myriad of alternative therapies have been employed to treat ED, including herbal formulations (gingko, ginseng), L-arginine, hypnotherapy, pelvic floor physiotherapy, biofeedback, and acupuncture [48]. Unfortunately, randomized controlled trials are lacking in comparing herbal therapies to well-established pharmacotherapy. A small study randomizing men with ED to acupuncture and hypnosis versus placebo demonstrated improvements in sexual function in the treatment group, but these were not significantly different from the control group [49]. Since most of these therapies are patient driven, they are best employed in conjunction with evidence-based pharmacotherapy.

7.11 Psychotherapy

While medical therapies are aimed at treating the underlying pathophysiologic mechanisms of ED, a psychogenic component exists for all types of ED. Effectively addressing these psychogenic issues is essential in maximizing sexual outcomes for the couple. A Japanese study demonstrated that ED was significantly associated with depression and anxiety status [50]. The pharmacologic treatment of depression and anxiety often carries undesired sexual side effects. Psychotherapy can aid in overcoming psychosocial barriers, making clinical treatments for ED more effective. The goals of psychotherapy include identifying and addressing resistances to medical intervention, reducing or eliminating performance anxiety, understanding the context for a couple's sexual activity, and implementing education and modification of sexual scripts [51]. A meta-analysis evaluating the effectiveness of psychological interventions for the treatment of ED compared to the clinical treatments described above demonstrated that group therapy improves ED and that psychotherapy in addition to PDE5i's was more effective than pharmacotherapy alone [52]. As the clinical treatment of ED advances, physicians can maximize effectiveness by addressing the patient as a whole with appropriate psychosocial interventions.

FUTURE THERAPIES—addressed in Chap. 12 (A. Burnett).

7.12 Summary Statement

The physician treating erectile dysfunction has a large armamentarium of clinical treatments to utilize in a step-wise fashion if initial therapies fail. A thorough assessment of psychosocial factors will aid in maximizing the benefit of these therapies.

References

1. Hatzimouratidis K, Amar E, Eardley I, et al. Guidelines on male sexual dysfunction: erectile dysfunction and premature ejaculation. Eur Urol. 2010;57:804–14.
2. Lewis RW, Fugl-Meyer KS, Corona G, et al. Definitions/epidemiology/risk factors for sexual dysfunction. J Sex Med. 2010;7:1598–607.
3. Pourmand G, Alidaee MR, Rasuli S, et al. Do cigarette smokers with erectile dysfunction benefit from stopping?: a prospective study. BJU Int. 2004;94:1310–3.
4. Esposito K, Giugliano F, Di Palo C, et al. Effect of lifestyle changes on erectile dysfunction in obese men: a randomized controlled trial. JAMA. 2004;291:2978–84.
5. Glina S, Sharlip ID, Hellstrom WJ. Modifying risk factors to prevent and treat erectile dysfunction. J Sex Med. 2013;10:115–9.
6. Gupta BP, Murad MH, Clifton MM, et al. The effect of lifestyle modification and cardiovascular risk factor reduction on erectile dysfunction: a systematic review and meta-analysis. Arch Intern Med. 2011;171:1797–803.
7. Mozaffarian D, Wilson PW, Kannel WB. Beyond established and novel risk factors: lifestyle risk factors for cardiovascular disease. Circulation. 2008;117:3031–8.
8. Jacob BC. Testosterone replacement therapy in males with erectile dysfunction. J Pharm Pract. 2011;24:298–306.
9. Bhasin S, Cunningham GR, Hayes FJ, et al. Testosterone therapy in men with androgen deficiency syndromes: an endocrine society clinical practice guideline. J Clin Endocrinol Metab. 2010;95:2536–59.
10. Karazindiyanoglu S, Cayan S. The effect of testosterone therapy on lower urinary tract symptoms/bladder and sexual functions in men with symptomatic late-onset hypogonadism. Aging Male. 2008;11:146–9.
11. Shamloul R, Ghanem H, Fahmy I, et al. Testosterone therapy can enhance erectile function response to sildenafil in patients with PADAM: a pilot study. J Sex Med. 2005;2:559–64.
12. Fabbri A, Giannetta E, Lenzi A, et al. Testosterone treatment to mimic hormone physiology in androgen replacement therapy. A view on testosterone gel and other preparations available. Expert Opin Biol Ther. 2007;7:1093–106.
13. Wang C, Nieschlag E, Swerdloff R, et al. Investigation, treatment, and monitoring of late-onset hypogonadism in males: ISA, ISSAM, EAU, EAA, and ASA recommendations. Eur Urol. 2009;55:121–30.
14. Montague DK, Jarow JP, Broderick GA, et al. Chapter 1: The management of erectile dysfunction: an AUA update. J Urol. 2005;174:230–9.
15. Goldstein I, Lue TF, Padma-Nathan H, et al. Oral sildenafil in the treatment of erectile dysfunction. Sildenafil study group. N Engl J Med. 1998;338:1397–404.
16. Carson CC. Phosphodiesterase type 5 inhibitors: state of the therapeutic class. Urol Clin North Am. 2007;34:507–15.
17. Dunn ME, Althof SE, Perelman MA. Phosphodiesterase type 5 inhibitors' extended duration of response as a variable in the treatment of erectile dysfunction. Int J Impot Res. 2007;19:119–23.
18. Viagra (sildenafil) package insert. 2013.
19. Vardenafil (Levitra) package insert. 2013.
20. Staxyn (vardenafil ODT) package insert. 2013.
21. Tadalafil (Cialis) package insert. 2013.
22. Rajfer J, Aliotta PJ, Steidle CP, et al. Tadalafil dosed once a day in men with erectile dysfunction: a randomized, double-blind, placebo-controlled study in the US. Int J Impot Res. 2007;19:95–103.
23. Porst H, Kim ED, Casabe AR, et al. Efficacy and safety of tadalafil once daily in the treatment of men with lower urinary tract symptoms suggestive of benign prostatic hyperplasia: results of an international randomized, double-blind, placebo-controlled trial. Eur Urol. 2011;60:1105–13.
24. Burke RM, Evans JD. Avanafil for treatment of erectile dysfunction: review of its potential. Vasc Health Risk Manag. 2012;8:517–23.
25. Bella AJ, Brant WO, Lue TF, et al. Non-arteritic anterior ischemic optic neuropathy (NAION) and phosphodiesterase type-5 inhibitors. Can J Urol. 2006;13:3233–8.
26. Kendirci M, Tanriverdi O, Trost L, et al. Management of sildenafil treatment failures. Curr Opin Urol. 2006;16:449–59.
27. Mohee A, Bretsztajn L, Eardley I. The evaluation of apomorphine for the treatment of erectile dysfunction. Expert Opin Drug Metab Toxicol. 2012;8:1447–53.
28. Eardley I, Donatucci C, Corbin J, et al. Pharmacotherapy for erectile dysfunction. J Sex Med. 2010;7:524–40.
29. Padma-Nathan H, Goldstein I, Klimberg I, et al. Long-term safety and efficacy of oral phentolamine mesylate (Vasomax) in men with mild to moderate erectile dysfunction. Int J Impot Res. 2002;14:266–70.
30. Teloken C, Rhoden EL, Sogari P, et al. Therapeutic effects of high dose yohimbine hydrochloride on organic erectile dysfunction. J Urol. 1998;159:122–4.

31. Costa P, Potempa AJ. Intraurethral alprostadil for erectile dysfunction: a review of the literature. Drugs. 2012;72:2243–54.
32. Padma-Nathan H, Hellstrom WJ, Kaiser FE, et al. Treatment of men with erectile dysfunction with transurethral alprostadil. Medicated urethral system for erection (MUSE) study group. N Engl J Med. 1997;336:1–7.
33. Mydlo JH, Volpe MA, Macchia RJ. Initial results utilizing combination therapy for patients with a suboptimal response to either alprostadil or sildenafil monotherapy. Eur Urol. 2000;38:30–4.
34. Linet OI, Ogrinc FG. Efficacy and safety of intracavernosal alprostadil in men with erectile dysfunction. The Alprostadil Study Group. N Engl J Med. 1996;334:873–7.
35. Perimenis P, Konstantinopoulos A, Perimeni PP, et al. Long-term treatment with intracavernosal injections in diabetic men with erectile dysfunction. Asian J Androl. 2006;8:219–24.
36. Dinsmore WW, Wyllie MG. Vasoactive intestinal polypeptide/phentolamine for intracavernosal injection in erectile dysfunction. BJU Int. 2008;102:933–7.
37. Porst H. Current perspectives on intracavernosal pharmacotherapy for erectile dysfunction. Int J Impot Res. 2000;12 Suppl 4:S91–100.
38. Brison D, Seftel A, Sadeghi-Nejad H. The resurgence of the vacuum erection device (VED) for treatment of erectile dysfunction. J Sex Med. 2013;10:1124–35.
39. Raina R, Agarwal A, Ausmundson S, et al. Early use of vacuum constriction device following radical prostatectomy facilitates early sexual activity and potentially earlier return of erectile function. Int J Impot Res. 2006;18:77–81.
40. Canguven O, Bailen J, Fredriksson W, et al. Combination of vacuum erection device and PDE5 inhibitors as salvage therapy in PDE5 inhibitor nonresponders with erectile dysfunction. J Sex Med. 2009;6:2561–7.
41. John H, Lehmann K, Hauri D. Intraurethral prostaglandin improves quality of vacuum erection therapy. Eur Urol. 1996;29:224–6.
42. Holloway FB, Farah RN. Intermediate term assessment of the reliability, function and patient satisfaction with the AMS700 Ultrex penile prosthesis. J Urol. 1997;157:1687–91.
43. Zermann DH, Kutzenberger J, Sauerwein D, et al. Penile prosthetic surgery in neurologically impaired patients: long-term followup. J Urol. 2006;175:1041–4 (discussion 1044).
44. Montague DK. Penile prosthesis implantation in the era of medical treatment for erectile dysfunction. Urol Clin North Am. 2011;38:217–25.
45. Mulcahy JJ. Penile prosthesis infection: progress in prevention and treatment. Curr Urol Rep. 2010;11:400–4.
46. Hellstrom WJ, Montague DK, Moncada I, et al. Implants, mechanical devices, and vascular surgery for erectile dysfunction. J Sex Med. 2010; 7:501–23.
47. Kawanishi Y, Kimura K, Nakanishi R, et al. Penile revascularization surgery for arteriogenic erectile dysfunction: the long-term efficacy rate calculated by survival analysis. BJU Int. 2004;94:361–8.
48. Aung HH, Dey L, Rand V, et al. Alternative therapies for male and female sexual dysfunction. Am J Chin Med. 2004;32:161–73.
49. Aydin S, Ercan M, Caskurlu T, et al. Acupuncture and hypnotic suggestions in the treatment of non-organic male sexual dysfunction. Scand J Urol Nephrol. 1997;31:271–4.
50. Sugimori H, Yoshida K, Tanaka T, et al. Relationships between erectile dysfunction, depression, and anxiety in Japanese subjects. J Sex Med. 2005;2:390–6.
51. Althof SE, Wieder M. Psychotherapy for erectile dysfunction: now more relevant than ever. Endocrine. 2004;23:131–4.
52. Melnik T, Soares BG, Nasello AG. The effectiveness of psychological interventions for the treatment of erectile dysfunction: systematic review and meta-analysis, including comparisons to sildenafil treatment, intracavernosal injection, and vacuum devices. J Sex Med. 2008;5:2562–74.

8 The Impact of Lifestyle Modification on Erectile Dysfunction

Phil Bach and Robert E. Brannigan

8.1 Introduction

Major insights into the physiology of erections and the pathophysiology of erectile dysfunction (ED) were gleaned from work during the 1980s and 1990s. Most notably, the discovery of nitric oxide (NO) as a signaling molecule responsible for erection was crucial in not only helping understand the role of endothelial dysfunction in ED but also in driving the development of phosphodiesterase-5 (PDE-5) inhibitors as a first-line treatment for ED. Since then, numerous studies have linked ED with disease states that also affect endothelial function, such as cardiovascular disease (CVD), hypertension, diabetes mellitus, metabolic syndrome, and obesity [1, 2]. Furthermore, an increased prevalence of ED has been associated with lifestyle issues such as smoking, lack of physical activity, and psychosocial factors including depression [1, 2]. This chapter will examine the links between lifestyle and ED and explore the impact of lifestyle modifications in improving ED.

P. Bach, M.D.
Division of Urology, Faculty of Medicine and Dentistry, University of Alberta, Edmonton, AB, Canada

R.E. Brannigan, M.D. (✉)
Department of Urology, Feinberg School of Medicine, Northwestern University, Galter Pavilion, Suite 20-150, 675 N Saint Clair, Chicago, IL 60611, USA
e-mail: r-brannigan@northwestern.edu

8.2 Risk Factors for ED

While it is difficult to definitively establish causality between various comorbidities and ED, there are clear and strong associations between ED and other health factors (Fig. 8.1). The Massachusetts Male Aging Study (MMAS) was an observational, community-based survey of men aged 40–70 conducted between 1987 and 1989 in and around Boston, Massachusetts. Investigators found that after adjusting for age, there was a higher probability of ED in men with a history of heart disease, hypertension, diabetes, and cigarette smoking [1]. Subsequent studies have reaffirmed these findings. A recent cross-sectional, population-based survey study of 108,477 men aged 45 years and older in New South Wales also found a higher risk of moderate-to-severe ED in men with high body mass index (BMI), smoking history, heart disease, and hypertension [2].

8.2.1 Links Between ED and CVD

Numerous studies have documented strong links between ED and CVD, with many now considering ED and CVD to be different manifestations of the same pathophysiology. Montorsi et al. [3] studied 300 men with angiographically documented coronary artery disease (CAD) and found that 49 % had ED using the International Index of Erectile Function (IIEF), a validated survey

L.I. Lipshultz et al. (eds.), *Management of Sexual Dysfunction in Men and Women*, DOI 10.1007/978-1-4939-3100-2_8

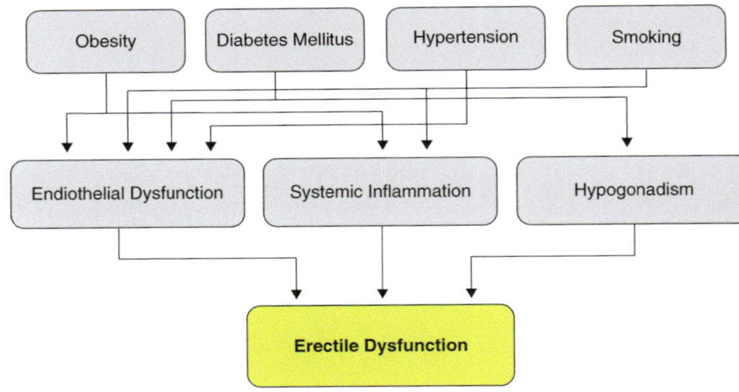

Fig. 8.1 Pathogenic factors contributing to penile endothelial dysfunction/erectile dysfunction

measure of erectile function [3]. Of the 147 men with coexisting ED and CAD, 67 % reported having ED symptoms an average of 39 months prior to the onset of CAD symptoms, suggesting a relatively short interval between the onset of the two conditions [3]. Montorsi's findings were corroborated by a prospective study in which 19 % (9/47) of men with vasculogenic ED were found to have angiographically, documented, but clinically asymptomatic, CAD [4].

Two meta-analyses have evaluated whether ED could be used as a predictor of CVD in men. Vlachopoulos et al. [5] conducted a meta-analysis of 14 studies comprising 92,757 patients with a mean follow-up of 6.1 years and demonstrated that men with ED had a 44 % increased risk for total cardiovascular events, 62 % increased risk for myocardial infarction, 39 % increased risk for cerebrovascular events, and a 25 % increased risk for all-cause mortality [5]. Similarly, a smaller meta-analysis of 12 prospective cohort studies comprising of 36,744 men found that those with ED had a significantly increased risk of 48 % for CVD, 46 % for coronary heart disease (CHD), 35 % for stroke, and 19 % for all-cause mortality [6]. The results from both studies support the hypothesis that ED is an important marker of silent CVD.

Theories aiming to explain the strong association between ED and CVD are based on similarities in the pathophysiologies of the two conditions. The physiology of penile erections is heavily dependent on the integrity of the endothelium, whose ability to release nitric oxide (NO) and other factors promotes relaxation of corporal smooth muscle, an increase in penile arterial inflow, and a decrease in penile venous outflow. This cascade contributes to corporal cavernosal engorgement, with resultant increases in the intracavernosal pressures and, ultimately, penile erection. Disruptions in normal endothelial function result in decreased secretion of NO, impaired vasodilatation, and, ultimately, decreased penile blood flow during erection. Similarly, the pathophysiology of CVD is thought to be related to endothelial dysfunction, leading to decreased NO release and, ultimately, atherosclerosis and decreased blood flow (see Fig. 8.1). While the pathophysiology of both ED and CVD is systemic, penile arteries (1–2 mm) are much smaller than coronary arteries (3–4 mm) and may therefore manifest endothelial dysfunction and atherosclerosis prior to the coronary circulation, resulting in much more significant reductions in blood flow in the penis than in the heart [7].

8.3 Impact of Lifestyle Modification on ED

It is well established that modifying CVD risk factors can improve CVD symptoms and risk profile, raising the possibility of a benefit from therapeutic lifestyle interventions in the setting of ED as well (Table 8.1).

8.3.1 ED and Obesity/Physical Activity

A number of studies have described a strong association between ED and obesity. The MMAS found that men with baseline obesity and a

Table 8.1 Summary of studies examining lifestyle modifications and effect on ED

Author	Study design	Intervention	Effect on ED
Esposito et al. [10]	Single-blind prospective randomized controlled trial	Increased physical activity and reduced caloric intake	Improvement in ED (IIEF scores 13.9–17)
Lamina et al. [11]	Prospective cohort study in hypertensive patients	Eight-week exercise program	Improvement in ED (IIEF scores 11.5–15.1)
Cheng et al. [12]	Meta-analysis	Physical activity	Dose-dependent improvement in erectile function with increased physical activity
Wessells et al. [20]	Prospective randomized controlled trial in type 1 DM men	Intensive glycemic control	Decreased rates of ED with better glycemic control
Cordero et al. [24]	Cross-sectional observational study	Treatment of HTN with beta-blocking agent for ≥6 months	Blood pressure control associated with lower prevalence of ED
Pourmand et al. [30]	Prospective cohort study	Smoking cessation	Improvement in ED in 25 % of men who stopped smoking

sedentary lifestyle have a significantly higher incidence of ED [8]. However, obese men who had initiated regular moderate to vigorous exercise were able to decrease their risk of developing ED [8]. In a multivariate analysis conducted in the Health Professionals Follow-Up Study, a cohort study of 22,086 American men aged 40–75, obesity was found to increase the risk of developing ED as a function of BMI [9]. Compared to men with BMI under 25 kg/m^2, those with a BMI 25–26.9 kg/m^2 had a 19 % increased risk of developing ED, while those with a BMI 27–29.9 kg/m^2 had a 33 % increased risk of developing ED [9]. In contrast, physical activity was inversely associated with ED [9].

Esposito et al. [10] conducted a randomized, single-blind trial of 110 men with a mean BMI of 36 kg/m^2 and with ED (mean IIEF score 13.7). Men with other comorbidities such as hypertension, diabetes, and hyperlipidemia were excluded from the study. The intervention group was given specific advice on how to lose at least 10 % of their body weight through increased physical activity and by reducing caloric intake, whereas the control group was simply given general information about healthy food choices and exercise. After 2 years, the intervention group had a statistically significant decrease in BMI (36.9–31.2 kg/m^2) compared with the controls (36.4–35.7 kg/m^2) and statistically significant increases in physical activity (48–195 min/week vs. 51–84 min/week) and IIEF scores (13.9–17 vs. 13.5–13.6) when compared to the control group [10]. Approximately one third of men in the intervention group had IIEF scores above 22, suggesting that they had regained their erectile function [10]. Multivariate analysis revealed that changes in body mass and physical activity were independently associated with changes in IIEF scores [10]. More recently, Lamina et al. [11] conducted a prospective cohort study examining the effects of exercise on ED in hypertensive patients. Twenty-two hypertensive patients with ED aged 50–70 were assigned an 8-week exercise program and compared to age-matched controls. Similar to the prior study, the authors found a significant improvement in IIEF scores in the exercise group compared to the control group (IIEF 11.50±5.30–15.14±4.92 vs. 8.10±4.02–8.95±3.90) [11]. A meta-analysis examining seven cross-sectional studies found not only a negative correlation between physical activity and ED (OR 0.53, 99 % CI 0.31-0.91) but also identified a dose–response relationship between physical activity and ED, with higher levels of activity resulting in a lower incidence of ED (OR 1 for low activity, OR 0.63, 99 % CI 0.43-0.93 for moderate activity, and OR 0.42, 99 % CI 0.22-0.82 for high activity) [12].

The explanation for the relationship between ED and obesity revolves around the effect of inflammation on endothelial function. Chronic inflammation contributes significantly to the pathogenesis of obesity and the metabolic syndrome; excessive calorie intake and physical inactivity lead to overproduction of pro-inflammatory cytokines including C-reactive protein (CRP), tumor necrosis factor-alpha (TNF-α), and interleukin-6 (IL-6) [13]. In turn, these cytokines lead to a persistent state of low-grade inflammation that impairs endothelial function, most notably by decreasing the bioavailability of endothelial NO and initiating a cascade of events ultimately leading to atherosclerosis [14]. Support for this hypothesis can be found in the significantly higher CRP levels detected in men with ED compared to those without when controlled for age and comorbidities [15], as well as the association between CRP levels and penile arterial disease severity as measured via penile Doppler ultrasound in men with ED [16]. Furthermore, in Lamina et al.'s [11] study, men in the exercise group with significantly higher IIEF scores after exercise also had significantly lower CRP levels when compared to the control group [11].

8.3.2 ED and Diabetes Mellitus

The prevalence of ED among diabetic men ranges from 35 to 90 % [17]. In a multivariable regression analysis from the Health Professionals Follow-Up Study, men with type 1 and 2 diabetes were both at significantly higher risk of developing ED compared to nondiabetic men (RR 3.0, 95 % CI 1.5–5.9 for type 1, and RR 1.3, 95 % CI 1.1–1.5 for type 2) [18]. Additionally, risk of ED in type 2 diabetics increased with duration of diabetes (RR 1.7, 95 % CI 1.1–2.7 in men with >20 years of disease) [18]. In their cross-sectional study of diabetic men in Israel, Kalter-Leibovici et al. [19] observed severe ED in 30.5 % of diabetic men and found association between worsening ED severity and both advancing patient age and diabetes duration [19].

While no published trials directly comparing the impact of glycemic control on ED are available, numerous studies offer indirect evidence that good glycemic control may improve ED symptoms. In the Diabetes Control and Complications Trial, 761 type 1 diabetic men were randomized to either intensive glycemic control or conventional glycemic control between 1983 and 1989 and treated until 1993. The men were divided into two cohorts: the primary prevention cohort, which consisted of 366 men who had a disease duration of 1–5 years without evidence of microvascular complications, and the secondary intervention cohort, which consisted of 395 men who had a disease duration of 1–15 years and evidence of nonproliferative retinopathy and/or microalbuminuria. In 2003, an ancillary study using a validated ED questionnaire was conducted on 571 men (295 men from the primary prevention cohort and 280 men from the secondary intervention cohort) and found a significantly decreased rate of ED in the intensive glycemic control group compared to the conventional glycemic control group for the secondary intervention cohort (12.8 vs. 30.8 %, $p=0.001$) [20]. Of note, on multivariate analysis, the risk of developing ED was significantly associated with mean hemoglobin A1c (HbA1c); with a 55 % increased adjusted odds of ED symptoms in the secondary intervention cohort and a 21.5 % increased adjusted odds of ED symptoms in the primary prevention cohort for every 10 % increase in mean HbA1c [20]. Used as a measure for glycemic control, another small study of 78 men with type 2 diabetes found a significant inverse relationship between HbA1c levels and erectile function and identified HbA1c as an independent predictor of erectile function [21].

The pathophysiology of ED in diabetes is thought to be multifactorial. Beyond the endothelial dysfunction that presages macrovascular atherosclerotic disease, microvascular complications lead to nerve ischemia and subsequent damage, causing both autonomic and peripheral neuropathy. Penile innervation via the dorsal and perineal nerves includes not only sympathetic and parasympathetic nerves, but also motor and sensory somatic nerves. Impaired parasympathetic stimulation from autonomic neuropathy impedes smooth muscle relaxation within the corpora cavernosa and can lead to ED [17]. Diabetic peripheral neuropathy can impair the transmission of both sensory impulses from the penile shaft and glans to the reflexogenic erectile center and motor impulses to the bulbocavernosus and ischiocavernosus muscles responsible for preventing venous outflow from the cavernous bodies during erection [17]. Finally, diabetes is frequently associated with hypogonadism, with 20 % of diabetic men having a low total testosterone level below 8 nmol/L and 31 % of diabetic men having a borderline low testosterone level between 8 and 12 nmol/L [22].

8.3.3 ED and Hypertension

As an important risk factor for CVD and a contributor to systemic endothelial dysfunction, hypertension is also a risk factor for ED. The MMAS found hypertension to be directly associated with an increased risk of ED [1] while a cross-sectional analysis of the 2126 American men in the National Health and Nutrition Examination Survey (NHANES) found the age-adjusted prevalence of ED to be 27.7 % in men with treated hypertension and 15.1 % in men with untreated hypertension [23].

In contrast, in a cross-sectional, observational study of 1242 hypertensive men, Cardero et al. [24] assessed the impact on ED of treating hypertension for over 6 months with beta-blockade and found that blood pressure control resulted in a lower prevalence of ED independent of age, medical treatments, and CVD [24]. The favorable impact of beta-blockade on ED was most pronounced with nebivolol, especially in younger patients [24]. A separate study of 1007 patients also found that treatment of hypertension with nebivolol specifically resulted in a lower prevalence of ED [25]. The improvement in ED seen in the two studies may be related to nebivolol's unique ability to function as a vasodilator by potentiating NO release.

The higher prevalence of ED found in men with treated hypertension compared to those with untreated hypertension in the NHANES study shows how antihypertensive medications can contribute to ED. Many antihypertensive medications, such as diuretics, nonselective beta-blockers, and alpha-2 blockers, are known to contribute to ED, whereas angiotensin-converting enzyme inhibitors and calcium channel blockers typically do not have adverse effects on erectile function [26].

8.3.4 ED and Smoking

Various clinical and epidemiological studies have identified a relationship between smoking and ED. Prospective results from the MMAS found that after adjusting for age and other covariates, baseline cigarette smokers had a significantly higher risk of developing moderate or complete ED (24 vs. 14 %, $p=0.01$) when compared to non-smokers [27]. In this study, cigar smoking and passive exposure to cigarette smoke were also significant predictors of ED [27]. A secondary analysis of a cross-sectional survey of 4462 Vietnam War veterans also found a significant association between smoking and ED that held even after accounting for confounders (adjusted OR 1.5, 95 % CI 1.0–2.2) [28]. A recent meta-analysis of eight studies including 28,856 patients found an overall odds ratio of ED of 1.51 (95 % CI 1.34–1.71) in current smokers and 1.29 (95 % CI 1.07–1.47) in former smokers when compared to non-smokers [29].

Pourmand et al. [30] conducted the first prospective trial examining the beneficial impact of smoking cessation on ED. Smokers with ED who requested nicotine replacement therapy (NRT) and who had no concurrent risk factors (such as hypertension, dyslipidemia, diabetes, psychiatric disorders, or illicit drug history) were assessed with IIEF questionnaires before initiating NRT and after 1 year of follow-up. While a significant correlation between ED severity and level of exposure to smoking was observed, an improvement in ED in 25 % of men who stopped smoking compared to none in those who continued smoking was also seen [30].

A more recent study compared penile tumescence using penile plethysmography in men who were able to successfully stop smoking during an 8-week smoking cessation program with those who relapsed and found a significant improvement in both penile tumescence response and time to reach maximum sexual arousal in those men with successful cessation who did not relapse [31].

The etiology of smoking's deleterious effects on erectile function is not entirely understood, but is thought to be secondary to endothelial dysfunction. Smoking causes an increase in reactive oxygen species that are directly detrimental to endothelial cells, leading to an exacerbation in oxidative stress and a decreased bioavailability of NO required for smooth muscle relaxation in the corpora cavernosa [32].

8.3.5 ED and Psychosocial Factors

Psychosocial factors such as anxiety and depression have been closely associated with ED and are thought to contribute to up to 40 % of cases, though it is unclear whether ED is the cause or result of these psychosocial factors [33, 34]. In the MMAS, a strong association was found between men with depressive symptoms and ED (OR 2.03, 95 % CI 1.39–2.96) [1]. Even after multifactorial regression analysis controlling for confounding factors such as age, CVD, medical conditions, and physical activity, men with depressive symptoms were 1.82 times more likely to have moderate-to-severe ED compared to those without depressive symptoms [1]. A prospective Finnish study of 1683 men aged 50–70 years attempted to assess the relationship between ED and depressive symptoms and found the relationship to be bidirectional [35]. The study found a higher incidence of ED in men with depressive symptoms (59/1000 person-years, 95 % CI 39–90) than in those without depressive symptoms (37/1000 person-years, 95 % CI 32–43) as well as a higher incidence of depression in men with ED (20/1000 person-years, 95 % CI 13–30) than in those without ED (11/1000 person-years, 95 % CI 8–14) [35].

While there appears to be a strong relationship between depression and ED, there is a paucity of robust data on the effects of lifestyle modifications in depression and ED. In fact, a major repercussion of the medical therapies used in managing depression is ED. A prospective study examining the effects of various selective serotonin reuptake inhibitors (SSRIs) on sexual function in 344 men with normal baseline sexual function found de novo ED incidence rates of 16.8 %, 34.1 %, 9.5 %, and 15.8 % for men taking fluoxetine, paroxetine, fluvoxamine, and sertraline, respectively [36].

Although the evidence consists of a few small studies with significant heterogeneity, sex therapy and psychotherapy do appear to have a positive impact on ED. Sex psychotherapy focuses on treating anxiety and psychosocial factors by utilizing a number of techniques such as desensitization, sex education, interpersonal therapy, rational-emotive therapy, and communications training. A prospective trial of 23 couples presenting with a primary complaint of ED found a significant improvement in ED following implementation of sex psychotherapy that was sustained after 6 months [37], while a recent systematic review and meta-analysis of 100 patients showed that group psychotherapy and sex group therapy were effective in reducing ED when compared to no treatment (RR 0.40, 95 % CI 0.17–0.98, $p=0.05$) [38]. Furthermore, evidence from the meta-analysis suggests that psychotherapy may have synergistic effects in reducing ED when combined with commonly used medical therapies such as sildenafil citrate (RR 0.46, 95 % CI 0.24–0.88, $p=0.02$ compared to sildenafil citrate-only group) [38].

8.4 Summary and Conclusion

While difficult to definitively establish causality, numerous studies have shown strong correlations between ED and lifestyle diseases such as CVD, obesity, diabetes, hypertension, and smoking. The common link between these clinical entities appears to be endothelial dysfunction that, due to the smaller size of the penile arteries, manifests as ED prior to the onset of symptomatic CVD. Obesity, diabetes, hypertension, and smoking, which are all risk factors for CVD, double as risk factors for ED and contribute to endothelial dysfunction through chronic low-grade inflammation.

Modifications of risk factors related to obesity, diabetes, hypertension, smoking, and psychosocial factors have been shown to improve or have been associated with improved erectile function. The links between ED and lifestyle diseases open an important avenue for healthcare professionals to explore in managing ED. Lifestyle modifications and a multidimensional approach that incorporates psychosocial factors represent important interventions that can improve ED and should be among first-line recommendations for the treatment of ED.

References

1. Feldman HA, Goldstein I, Hatzichristou DG, Krane RJ, McKinlay JB. Impotence and its medical and psychosocial correlates: results of the Massachusetts male aging study. J Urol. 1994;151(1):54–61.
2. Weber MF, Smith DP, O'Connell DL, Patel MI, de Souza PL, Sitas F, et al. Risk factors for erectile dysfunction in a cohort of 108 477 Australian men. Med J Aust. 2013;199(2):107–11.
3. Montorsi F, Briganti A, Salonia A, Rigatti P, Margonato A, Macchi A, et al. Erectile dysfunction prevalence, time of onset and association with risk factors in 300 consecutive patients with acute chest pain and angiographically documented coronary artery disease. Eur Urol. 2003;44(3):360–4.
4. Vlachopoulos C, Rokkas K, Ioakeimidis N, Aggeli C, Michaelides A, Roussakis G, et al. Prevalence of asymptomatic coronary artery disease in men with vasculogenic erectile dysfunction: a prospective angiographic study. Eur Urol. 2005;48(6):996–1002.
5. Vlachopoulos CV, Terentes-Printzios DG, Ioakeimidis NK, Aznaouridis KA, Stefanadis CI. Prediction of cardiovascular events and all-cause mortality with erectile dysfunction: a systematic review and meta-analysis of cohort studies. Circ Cardiovasc Qual Outcomes. 2013;6(1):99–109.
6. Dong JY, Zhang YH, Qin LQ. Erectile dysfunction and risk of cardiovascular disease: meta-analysis of prospective cohort studies. J Am Coll Cardiol. 2011; 58(13):1378–85.
7. Gandaglia G, Briganti A, Jackson G, Kloner RA, Montorsi F, Montorsi P, et al. A systematic review of the association between erectile dysfunction and cardiovascular disease. Eur Urol. 2013 (in press).
8. Derby CA, Mohr BA, Goldstein I, Feldman HA, Johannes CB, McKinlay JB. Modifiable risk factors and erectile dysfunction: can lifestyle changes modify risk? J Urol. 2000;56(2):302–6.
9. Bacon CG, Mittleman MA, Kawachi I, Giovannucci E, Glasser DB, Rimm EB. A prospective study of risk factors for erectile dysfunction. J Urol. 2006;176(1): 217–21.
10. Esposito K, Giugliano F, Di Palo C, Giugliano G, Marfella R, D'Andrea F, et al. Effect of lifestyle changes on erectile dysfunction in obese men: a randomized controlled trial. JAMA. 2004;291(24): 2978–84.
11. Lamina S, Okoye CG, Dagogo TT. Therapeutic effect of an interval exercise training program in the management of erectile dysfunction in hypertensive patients. J Clin Hypertens (Greenwich). 2009;11(3): 125–9.
12. Cheng JY, Ng EM, Ko JS, Chen RY. Physical activity and erectile dysfunction: meta-analysis of population-based studies. Int J Impot Res. 2007; 19(3):245–52.
13. Vlachopoulos C, Rokkas K, Ioakeimidis N, Stefanadis C. Inflammation, metabolic syndrome, erectile dysfunction, and coronary artery disease: common links. Eur Urol. 2007;52(6):1590–600.
14. Trepels T, Zeiher AM, Fichtlscherer S. The endothelium and inflammation. Endothelium. 2006;13(6): 423–9.
15. Yao F, Huang Y, Zhang Y, Dong Y, Ma H, Deng C, et al. Subclinical endothelial dysfunction and low-grade inflammation play roles in the development of erectile dysfunction in young men with low risk of coronary heart disease. Int J Androl. 2012;35(5):653–9.
16. Billups KL, Kaiser DR, Kelly AS, Wetterling RA, Tsai MY, Hanson N, et al. Relation of C-reactive protein and other cardiovascular risk factors to penile vascular disease in men with erectile dysfunction. Int J Impot Res. 2003;15(4):231–6.
17. Malavige LS, Levy JC. Erectile dysfunction in diabetes mellitus. J Sex Med. 2009;6(5):1232–47.
18. Bacon CG, Hu FB, Giovannucci E, Glasser DB, Mittleman MA, Rimm EB. Association of type and duration of diabetes with erectile dysfunction in a large cohort of men. Diabetes Care. 2002;25(8): 1458–63.
19. Kalter-Leibovici O, Wainstein J, Ziv A, Harman-Bohem I, Murad H, Raz I, Israel Diabetes Research Group (IDRG) Investigators. Clinical, socioeconomic, and lifestyle parameters associated with erectile dysfunction among diabetic men. Diabetes Care. 2005;28(7):1739–44.
20. Wessells H, Penson DF, Cleary P, Rutledge BN, Lachin JM, McVary KT, Schade DS, Sarma AV, Diabetes Control and Complications Trial/Epidemiology of Diabetes Interventions and Complications Research Group. Effect of intensive glycemic therapy on erectile function in men with type 1 diabetes. J Urol. 2011;185(5):1828–34.
21. Romeo JH, Seftel AD, Madhun ZT, Aron DC. Sexual function in men with diabetes type 2: association with glycemic control. J Urol. 2000;163(3):788–91.
22. Kapoor D, Aldred H, Clark S, Channer KS, Jones TH. Clinical and biochemical assessment of hypogonadism in men with type 2 diabetes: correlations with bioavailable testosterone and visceral adiposity. Diabetes Care. 2007;30(4):911–7.
23. Selvin E, Burnett AL, Platz EA. Prevalence and risk factors for erectile dysfunction in the US. Am J Med. 2007;120(2):151–7.

24. Cordero A, Bertomeu-Martinez V, Mazon P, Facila L, Gonzalez-Juanatey JR. Erectile dysfunction may improve by blood pressure control in patients with high-risk hypertension. Postgrad Med. 2010; 122(6):51–6.
25. Cordero A, Bertomeu-Martinez V, Mazon P, Facila L, Bertomeu-Gonzalez V, Conthe P, et al. Erectile dysfunction in high-risk hypertensive patients treated with beta-blockade agents. Cardiovasc Ther. 2010;28(1):15–22.
26. Lue T. Physiology of penile erection and pathophysiology of erectile dysfunction. In: Wein A, editor. Campbell-Walsh urology. 10th ed. Philadelphia: Elsevier-Saunders; 2012. p. 688–720.
27. Feldman HA, Johannes CB, Derby CA, Kleinman KP, Mohr BA, Araujo AB, et al. Erectile dysfunction and coronary risk factors: prospective results from the Massachusetts male aging study. Prev Med. 2000; 30(4):328–38.
28. Mannino DM, Klevens RM, Flanders WD. Cigarette smoking: an independent risk factor for impotence? Am J Epidemiol. 1994;140(11):1003–8.
29. Cao S, Yin X, Wang Y, Zhou H, Song F, Lu Z. Smoking and risk of erectile dysfunction: systematic review of observational studies with meta-analysis. PLoS One. 2013;8(4), e60443.
30. Pourmand G, Alidaee MR, Rasuli S, Maleki A, Mehrsai A. Do cigarette smokers with erectile dysfunction benefit from stopping?: a prospective study. BJU Int. 2004;94(9):1310–3.
31. Harte CB, Meston CM. Association between smoking cessation and sexual health in men. BJU Int. 2012;109(6):888–96.
32. Tostes RC, Carneiro FS, Lee AJ, Giachini FR, Leite R, Osawa Y, et al. Cigarette smoking and erectile dysfunction: focus on NO bioavailability and ROS generation. J Sex Med. 2008;5(6):1284–95.
33. Melman A, Tiefer L, Pedersen R. Evaluation of first 406 patients in urology department based center for male sexual dysfunction. Urology. 1988;32(1):6–10.
34. McCabe M, Althof SE, Assalian P, Chevret-Measson M, Leiblum SR, Simonelli C, Wylie K. Psychological and interpersonal dimensions of sexual function and dysfunctions. J Sex Med. 2010;7(1):327–36.
35. Shiri R, Koskimaki J, Tammela T, Hakkinen J, Auvinen A, Hakama M. Bidirectional relationship between depression and erectile dysfunction. J Urol. 2007;177:669–73.
36. Montejo-gonzàlez AL, Llorca G, Izquierdo JA, Ledesma A, Bousono M, Calcedo A, Carrasco JL, Ciudad J, Daniel E, De LA Gandara J, Derecho J, Franco M, Gomez MJ, Macias JA, Martin T, Perez V, Sanchez JM, Sanchez S, Vicens E. Fluoxetine, paroxetine, sertraline, and fluvoxamine in a prospective, multicenter, and descriptive clinical study of 344 patients. J Sex Marital Ther. 1997; 23(3):176–94.
37. Wylie K. Treatment outcome of brief couple therapy in psychogenic male erectile disorder. Arch Sex Behav. 1997;26(5):527–45.
38. Melnik T, Soares BG, Nasello AG. The effectiveness of psychological interventions of the treatment of erectile dysfunction: systematic review and meta-analysis, including comparisons to sildenafil treatment, intracavernosal injection, and vacuum devices. J Sex Med. 2008;5(11):2562–74.

Erectile Dysfunction in the Setting of Prostate Cancer

9

Mary K. Samplaski and Kirk C. Lo

9.1 Introduction

Prostate cancer (PCa) has a wide range of pathologies and treatment modalities, many of which can negatively affect erectile function. The incidence of erectile dysfunction (ED) after treatment for PCa ranges from 14 to 89 % after surgery [1] and 2–56 % after radiation therapy [2]. The National Institutes of Health (NIH) defines erectile dysfunction (ED) as "the consistent inability to obtain or maintain an erection satisfactory for sexual performance" [3]. However, the phrase "sexual performance" is vague and does not mention the use of erectogenic aids. It is clear that there are individual patient-related, disease-related, treatment-related, and psychological factors that compromise erectile function in the setting of PCa. In addition, PCa continues to be diagnosed in younger men, in whom potency preservation is an important consideration [4, 5].

M.K. Samplaski, M.D.
Department of Surgery, Institute of Urology, University of Southern California, Los Angeles, CA, USA

K.C. Lo, M.D., F.R.C.S.C. (✉)
Division of Urology, Department of Surgery, Mount Sinai Hospital, Faculty of Medicine, Institute of Medical Science, University of Toronto, 60 Murray Street, 6th floor, Box# 19, Toronto, ON, Canada, M5T 3L9
e-mail: klo@mtsinai.on.ca

9.2 Baseline Erectile Function

Pretreatment erectile function is a predictor of posttreatment erectile function in men treated for PCa [6, 7]. However, there are many factors that play into pretreatment erectile function, including age and comorbidities. Age is a significant risk factor for both PCa and ED [8], and men with PCa may already be experiencing an age-related decline in erection quality [9]. In the 2008 Prostate Cancer Outcomes Study, a significant relationship was found between age and sexual function following nerve sparing radical prostatectomy (RP), ranging from 61 % of men <55 years of age to 18 % of men >65 years having functional erections [10]. Related to age are comorbidities and body mass index (BMI), type 2 diabetes, and depression—all confounders of baseline ED [7].

Further, the psychological distress associated with a cancer diagnosis and proximity to treatment may skew evaluation of a patient's true baseline erectile function [11]. In this way, validated questionnaires may not accurately represent male sexual function. Indeed, there are men whose scores on validated questionnaires decline after PCa treatment who still consider themselves fully sexually functional [12–14]. Finally, there is wide variability on baseline erectogenic aid use in the literature, and clearly an unbiased assessment of a man's pretreatment

L.I. Lipshultz et al. (eds.), *Management of Sexual Dysfunction in Men and Women*, DOI 10.1007/978-1-4939-3100-2_9

erectile function will allow for more realistic expectations for erectile outcomes after PCa treatment.

9.3 Setting Realistic Expectations

Clinicians are responsible for preemptively addressing sexual function prior to any PCa treatment and setting realistic posttreatment expectations. Ideally this topic should be addressed with both the patient and his partner [15] and should encompass evaluation of pretreatment sexual function, individualized treatment, and clinician factors such as medical and surgical experience [16]. There is also substantial variation in the definition of posttreatment ED [12]. A 2009 meta-analysis found that most of the published literature "does not meet strict criteria for reporting posttreatment erectile function," although even in this article, "strict criteria" were not defined [17]. In addition, outcomes for erectile function are often reported only for a small proportion of men undergoing treatment [17]. In light of these factors, it may be challenging to provide patients with realistic expectations; however, every effort should be made to set expectations based on individual patient circumstances.

9.4 Surgical Issues

Predisposing factors for post-radical prostatectomy (RP) ED include age, preoperative erectile function, comorbidities [18], prostate-specific antigen (PSA), race, BMI, and intended treatment details [19]. Briganti et al. [18] developed a risk-stratification tool, grouping men into low, intermediate, and high risk for postoperative ED. The 3-year erectile function recovery rates were 85 %, 59 %, and 37 %, respectively. This scheme has been applied to men undergoing robot-assisted RP with similar predictive outcomes [6].

The etiology of ED after RP is likely due to mechanical injury to the corporal cavernosal nerve plexus [20]. Nerve sparing is recommended when men have normal preoperative erectile function and organ-confined disease [21]. However, functional outcomes are not always optimal, and a meta-analysis comparing potency rates after treatment for PCa demonstrated that the probability of maintaining erectile function after nerve sparing RP was 34 % at 1 year and 25 % at 2 years and for standard RP was 25 % at 1 year and 2 years [2].

The discrepancy between desired and actual outcomes appears to be related to other surgical factors, as even during nerve-sparing procedures, the cavernous nerves are affected by direct trauma, stretching, heating, ischemia, and local inflammation [22, 23]. This results in neuropraxia, a temporary blockage of nerve transmission, despite anatomically intact nerves. In addition, damage to the accessory pudendal arteries [24] and development of venous leak after RP appears to further impair recovery of erectile function [16, 25, 26]. Men with venous leak are more likely to experience ED, with 9 % of men with venous leak having erections sufficient for intercourse, as opposed to 47 % of those without [27]. In addition, men with venous leak have been shown to be less likely to respond to phosphodiesterase type 5 inhibitors (PDE5-Is) [28].

The loss of daily and nocturnal erections typical of the post-RP recovery period may result in chronically decreased cavernosal oxygenation and erectile tissue damage from the production of proapoptotic factors within the corpora [16, 25, 29]. The presence of TGF-β1 [30, 31] and hypoxia inducible factor-1α [30] and the overexpression of endothelin-1 type B receptor [32] strongly suggest that hypoxia plays a role in the physiology of ED. Histologically supporting this, an increase in corporal fibrosis and collagen deposition after RP has been demonstrated in humans, with a corresponding decrease in elastic and smooth muscle fibers [29].

9.5 Radiation Issues

While many men believe that radiation will have reduced effects on sexual function, ED rates seem to be similar between radiation and RP patients [33]. Across radiation treatment modalities, brachytherapy may result in a slightly higher preservation of erectile function versus external beam radiotherapy (EBRT) [34]. While possibly multifactorial, the predominant etiology of radiation-induced impotence is from vascular damage to the cavernosal nerves [35–37]. This effect is progressive, and there is oftentimes a lag between the administration of therapy and development of adverse effects, evidenced histologically by the development of cavernosal fibrosis for 3 years after radiotherapy [33].

After radiotherapy for PCa, decreased frequency and intensity of erections have been reported in 2–56 % of men [38–40]. Specifically, a meta-analysis [2] looking at maintaining erectile function found that for brachytherapy the probability was 76 % at 1 year, for brachytherapy plus EBRT 60 %, and for EBRT alone 55 %. Two recent prospective trials have observed a 30–40 % incidence of ED in EBRT-treated men [36, 41]. After brachytherapy, ED rates have ranged from 5 to 51 %, with the highest rates seen after combination EBRT and brachytherapy [42–44].

Factors that play a role in the development of post-radiotherapy ED include age, comorbidities, previous pelvic surgery, medications, pretreatment sexual function, hormonal treatment [44], and the presence of lower urinary tract symptoms [45]. Interestingly, while there is some conflicting evidence, most studies suggest that the radiation dose received by the corpora cavernosa and/or penile bulb is not related to the development of post-radiotherapy ED [36]. However, it is rational that reducing the volume of tissue irradiated may reduce the likelihood of developing ED, as with intensity-modulated radiation therapy or proton beam radiotherapy [46–48].

In addition, emerging evidence suggests that some men may be genetically predisposed to developing post-radiation ED. Certain TGF-β1 single-nucleotide polymorphism genotypes have been associated with the development of ED and rectal bleeding in patients treated with radiotherapy for PCa, possibly due to a propensity for developing fibrosis [49]. Gene therapy to target neurotropic factors to promote neuronal regeneration is promising, but still in development [50]. Similarly, studies using erythropoietin as a neuromodulatory agent have found increased recovery of erections [51].

9.6 Posttreatment Recovery of Erectile Function

Erectile function improves for up to 48 months after RP [12, 52–54]. The timeline is not uniform, and factors associated with quicker recovery include younger age, pre-RP sexual function, nerve sparing, and surgeon experience [15]. The ability to obtain an erection, either spontaneously or with PDE5-I support, within 3 months of a RP is an excellent prognostic indicator for long-term erectile function [52]. ED after radiotherapy seems to develop during the first 2 years, and plateaus from then on [36, 41].

The hypoxia theory has raised hope that erectile function can be improved by oxygenating the cavernosal tissue during neuropraxia, resulting in penile rehabilitation efforts. However, there is little consensus regarding the best approach [55, 56]. Strategies investigated, either alone or in combination, include PDE5-Is, intracavernosal injections (ICI), intraurethral prostaglandin, or vacuum erection devices (VED) [57]. PDE5-Is have gained popularity as they improve oxygenation to the corporal bodies by maintaining nitric oxide-mediated vasodilation, thereby inhibiting collagen synthesis, maintaining penile elasticity, and preserving endothelial and cavernosal functions [30, 58, 59]. Animal models have shown that the PDE5-I sildenafil promotes smooth muscle preservation and ameliorates fibrosis through the modulation of extracellular matrix and tissue growth factor gene expression after bilateral cavernosal nerve resection [60].

While the use of penile rehabilitation programs is common, much of the available data are extrapolated from either in vitro or animal studies [16, 25]. In spite of these limitations, the International Consensus of Sexual Medicine (ICSM) recommends that clinicians counsel men on the possibility of postoperative ED and options for rehabilitation, including PDE5-Is, ICI, intraurethral prostaglandin, VED, or neuromodulatory devices [16], although the optimal treatment protocol remains undefined [25, 61–63]. Men who are most likely to recover erectile function using a penile rehabilitation protocol after RP are those <55 years of age with a preoperative International Index of

Erectile Function (IIEF) score of >22 [64]. In addition, even men undergoing nonnerve-sparing procedures should be considered candidates for penile rehabilitation, as these men may also benefit [65, 66].

In a series of post-RP men using postoperative PDE5-Is at a high-volume center, the 3-year erectile function recovery rates were higher in men using PDE5-Is compared with those who did not (73 vs. 37 %) [18]. Corroborating this, a randomized, double-blind, placebo-controlled study demonstrated that in men with normal preoperative erectile function undergoing RP, nightly sildenafil for 36 weeks resulted in the return of spontaneous erections in 27 % of men versus 4 % of controls, as well as improvement in IIEF scores [62]. While both of these studies support the use of PDE5-Is, the optimal dosing schedule remains unknown. While this study supports nightly PDE5-I use, other data suggest that on-demand use of a PDE5-Is as efficacious as daily use [25].

Management strategies for recovery of erectile function after radiation therapy (RT) are derived predominantly from the RP literature and are primarily based on PDE5-Is. Two randomized, double-blind trials of men developing ED after RT have demonstrated an increase in IIEF scores and also more men reporting successful intercourse (55 vs. 18 %) after treatment with sildenafil [67, 68]. Similar results have been found using tadalafil, with more men reporting successful intercourse with treatment (48 vs. 9 %) [39, 40]. Early treatment with PDE5-Is in the setting of RT seems to be optimal [69].

In men in whom PDE5-Is are ineffective, ICI may be attempted [16, 25, 70]. From a physiologic perspective, if we hypothesize that therapies that increase corporal oxygen will be the most efficacious, then erections induced by the VED or urethral prostaglandin may be less functional [71]. However, VED use in early penile rehabilitation has resulted in higher IIEF and SHIM scores and no loss in stretched penile length [72].

Finally, dietary supplements with endothelial nitric oxide synthase (eNOS) have shown promise in the treatment of ED not related to RP. L-arginine has been shown to increase eNOS [71], and pycnogenol stimulates the conversion of L-arginine to nitric oxide by eNOS [73]. Four trials consistently demonstrated increased patient-reported erectile function with these supplements [74–77]. In light of this, one protocol for post-RP penile rehabilitation includes dietary supplementation with L-arginine and pycnogenol [71].

9.7 Penile Prosthesis

Men failing medical therapy for ED after treatment for PCa may be candidates for penile prosthesis [78, 79]. These are rarely used, as a recent review found that for a group of 68,558 men treated with either surgery or radiation for PCa, the penile implant utilization rate was 0.78 % [79]. This is not due to a lack of technical feasibility, and implants can safely be placed in men who have had a RP [69] with minimal morbidity [71] and high patient satisfaction rates [79–81]. Conversely, patients who have already had a three-piece inflatable penile implant placed can safely undergo either open- or robot-assisted RP [82, 83]. Finally, the concurrent performance of a nonnerve-sparing RP and placement of a penile prosthesis has been reported [84], although this is not standard of care.

9.8 Testosterone Supplementation

There is evidence that testosterone (T) may regulate NO formation [85] and cavernosal PDE5 expression [85–87], helping to maintain penile innervation [85]. In addition, preoperative serum T levels have been shown to correlate with post-RP erectile function [88]. Because of this, there has been some interest in T replacement in men with ED and PCa. The role of T replacement in this population is hotly debated though, given concerns that dormant PCa cells will be stimulated by T. There are several retrospective studies supporting the relative safety of T replacement in men after RP and its benefits to sexual function without leading to a clinically significant increase in PSA [89–92]. Regardless, T replacement in these men should be accompanied by a thorough and frank discussion about the risks and benefits, and close monitoring during treatment.

It is clear that androgen deprivation therapy, either as primary therapy or adjunctive to surgical or radiation, negatively impacts erections. There is also emerging evidence that androgen deprivation therapy may be associated with a reduced response to PDE5-Is [93, 94]. In light of this, it has been speculated that a combination of PDE5-I and T therapy may be beneficial in penile rehabilitation, a concept that is being tested in a randomized trial (NCT00848497). The data from this and other trials will help to guide the role of T in the treatment of ED in men with PCa.

9.9 Psychosexual Counseling

The shock of receiving a PCa diagnosis and the ensuing uncertainties of cancer prognosis, treatment, and treatment-related physical changes has been associated with increased patient anxiety [95], cardiovascular events, and suicide [96, 97]. This anxiety may correlate with erectile function, as men with cancer after prostate biopsy have been shown to have a decrease in scores on all IIEF domains [98]. The impact on sexual function of carrying a diagnosis of PCa without undergoing treatment will likely become increasingly prominent with the increasing use of active surveillance protocols [99]. Because of this, sexual counseling is an important aspect of both therapy and prevention of ED. Patients should be informed of the possible sequelae of treatment on their sexual functioning.

Increasing evidence shows that any penile rehabilitation program should include sexual counseling. Without counseling, up to half of men will not even fill the PDE5-I prescription given to them, and a large percentage of those that do will stop taking the medication after not seeing a result [100]. Further studies have shown that in men using ICI for post-RP penile rehabilitation, those receiving sexual counseling reported higher scores on multiple IIEF domains, the lowest discontinuation rate, and the highest degree of couple satisfaction when compared with men not receiving sexual counseling [101]. Finally, men in couples undergoing sexual counseling after radiation therapy or surgery for PCa had increased use of erectogenic aids and showed improvements in overall distress, male global sexual function, and female global sexual function as assessed using the IIEF and Female Sexual Function Index (FSFI) [102].

The literature suggests that most oncologic professionals are reluctant to address sexuality and the majority of sexologic professionals do not feel that they have adequate expertise to discuss cancer and its treatment effects [103, 104]. It is likely that a more formalized collaborative effort would improve patient care fostering a more educated experience of what to expect after treatment, avoid misconceptions, obtain education about the available therapies, and an understanding about their options for sexual dysfunction after PCa treatment (Fig. 9.1) [66].

9.10 Conclusions

ED in the setting of PCa is a common problem. The etiology of ED in the setting of PCa appears to be multifactorial, with some sexual dysfunction being present at the time of diagnosis as a function of age and comorbid conditions, some arising from the diagnosis itself and some being treatment related. A more sophisticated understanding of the etiology of PCa-related ED would allow for more individualized therapy. The literature is inconsistent on its definition of "normal" erectile function both before and after PCa treatment, and validated sexual function questionnaires should be utilized consistently to track progress. Clinicians should frankly discuss the known risk factors for and predictors of recovery of erectile function in men being treated for PCa, and patients should be given individualized outcomes based on their baseline erectile function, factors related to each treatment modality, surgeon-specific factors, and timing. In this way, patients can have the most realistic expectations for their recovery.

After treatment, there are no optimal penile rehabilitation strategies, although the literature supports a proactive approach. The optimal

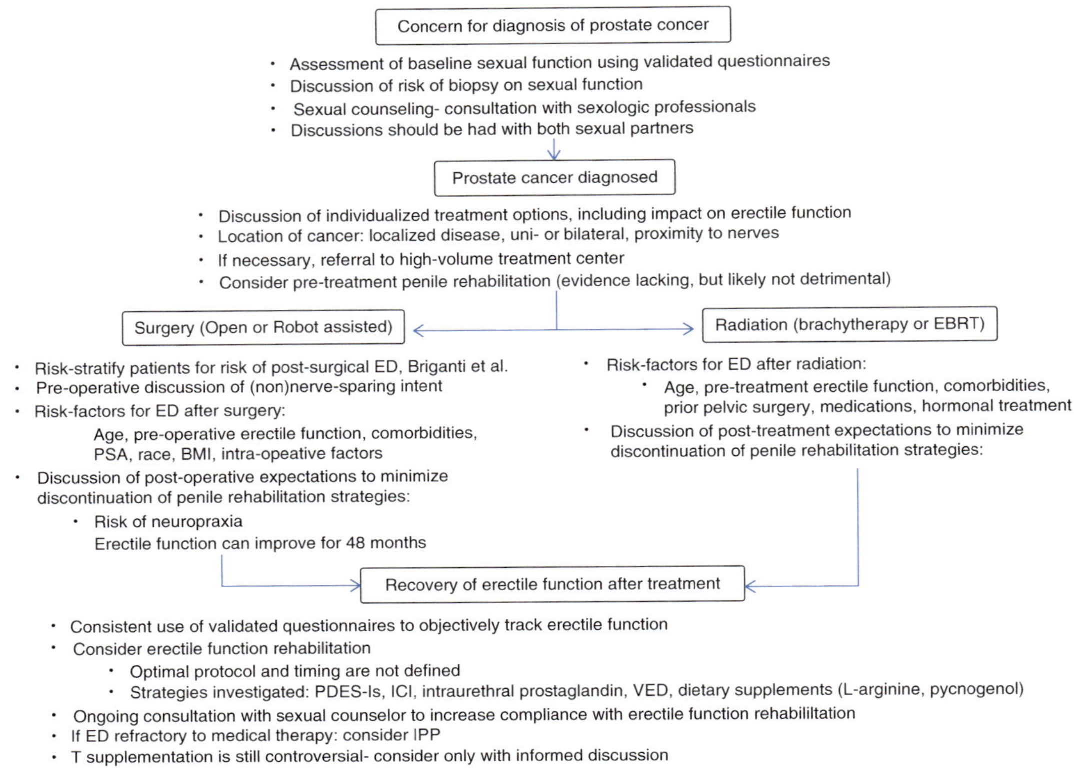

Fig. 9.1 Algorithm for preservation of erectile function in men with prostate cancer. Pre-diagnosis, treatment-related, and posttreatment erectile function rehabilitation factors should be considered to preserve erectile function in these patients and provide them with accurate expectations

regimen for post-PCa treatment-related ED is still evolving. Emerging evidence for the use of oral agents and genetic predispositions is compelling. Testosterone replacement in these men may eventually play a role but presently should be considered experimental. Finally, evidence supports a multidisciplinary approach including sexual and psychiatric counseling to optimally manage these men.

References

1. Raina R, Pahlajani G, Agarwal A, Jones S, Zippe C. Long-term potency after early use of a vacuum erection device following radical prostatectomy. BJU Int. 2010;106:1719–22.
2. Robinson JW, Moritz S, Fung T. Meta-analysis of rates of erectile function after treatment of localized prostate carcinoma. Int J Radiat Oncol Biol Phys. 2002;54:1063–8.
3. NIH Consensus Conference. Impotence. NIH consensus development panel on impotence. JAMA. 1993;270:83–90.
4. Merrill RM, Sloan A. Risk-adjusted incidence rates for prostate cancer in the United States. Prostate. 2012;72:181–5.
5. Sidana A, Hernandez DJ, Feng Z, Partin AW, Trock BJ, Saha S, et al. Treatment decision-making for localized prostate cancer: what younger men choose and why. Prostate. 2012;72:58–64.
6. Novara G, Ficarra V, D'Elia C, Secco S, De Gobbi A, Cavalleri S, et al. Preoperative criteria to select patients for bilateral nerve-sparing robotic-assisted radical prostatectomy. J Sex Med. 2010;7:839–45.
7. Salomon G, Isbarn H, Budaeus L, Schlomm T, Briganti A, Steuber T, et al. Importance of baseline potency rate assessment of men diagnosed with clinically localized prostate cancer prior to radical prostatectomy. J Sex Med. 2009;6:498–504.
8. Salonia A, Burnett AL, Graefen M, Hatzimouratidis K, Montorsi F, Mulhall JP, et al. Prevention and management of postprostatectomy sexual dysfunctions. Part 1: choosing the right patient at the right time for the right surgery. Eur Urol. 2012;62:261–72.

9. Walz J, Perrotte P, Suardi N, Hutterer G, Jeldres C, Benard F, et al. Baseline prevalence of erectile dysfunction in a prostate cancer screening population. J Sex Med. 2008;5:428–35.
10. Penson DF, McLerran D, Feng Z, Li L, Albertsen PC, Gilliland FD, et al. 5-year urinary and sexual outcomes after radical prostatectomy: results from the prostate cancer outcomes study. J Urol. 2008;179:S40–4.
11. Kim DS, Chung YG, Kim DJ, Park KK, Chung MS, Lee DH, et al. Optimal timing to evaluate prediagnostic baseline erectile function in patients undergoing robot-assisted radical prostatectomy. J Sex Med. 2012;9:602–7.
12. Burnett AL, Aus G, Canby-Hagino ED, Cookson MS, D'Amico AV, Dmochowski RR, et al. Erectile function outcome reporting after clinically localized prostate cancer treatment. J Urol. 2007;178:597–601.
13. Teloken P, Valenzuela R, Parker M, Mulhall J. The correlation between erectile function and patient satisfaction. J Sex Med. 2007;4:472–6.
14. Briganti A, Gallina A, Suardi N, Capitanio U, Tutolo M, Bianchi M, et al. What is the definition of a satisfactory erectile function after bilateral nerve sparing radical prostatectomy? J Sex Med. 2011;8:1210–7.
15. Salonia A, Zanni G, Gallina A, Briganti A, Sacca A, Suardi N, et al. Unsuccessful investigation of preoperative sexual health issues in the prostate cancer "couple": results of a real-life psychometric survey at a major tertiary academic center. J Sex Med. 2009;6:3347–55.
16. Mulhall JP, Bella AJ, Briganti A, McCullough A, Brock G. Erectile function rehabilitation in the radical prostatectomy patient. J Sex Med. 2010;7:1687–98.
17. Tal R, Alphs HH, Krebs P, Nelson CJ, Mulhall JP. Erectile function recovery rate after radical prostatectomy: a meta-analysis. J Sex Med. 2009; 6:2538–46.
18. Briganti A, Gallina A, Suardi N, Capitanio U, Tutolo M, Bianchi M, et al. Predicting erectile function recovery after bilateral nerve sparing radical prostatectomy: a proposal of a novel preoperative risk stratification. J Sex Med. 2010;7:2521–31.
19. Alemozaffar M, Regan MM, Cooperberg MR, Wei JT, Michalski JM, Sandler HM, et al. Prediction of erectile function following treatment for prostate cancer. JAMA. 2011;306:1205–14.
20. Walsh PC, Donker PJ. Impotence following radical prostatectomy: insight into etiology and prevention. 1982. J Urol. 2002;167:1005–10.
21. Heidenreich A, Bellmunt J, Bolla M, Joniau S, Mason M, Matveev V, et al. EAU guidelines on prostate cancer. Part 1: screening, diagnosis, and treatment of clinically localised disease. Eur Urol. 2011;59:61–71.
22. Masterson TA, Serio AM, Mulhall JP, Vickers AJ, Eastham JA. Modified technique for neurovascular bundle preservation during radical prostatectomy: association between technique and recovery of erectile function. BJU Int. 2008;101:1217–22.
23. Burnett AL. Rationale for cavernous nerve restorative therapy to preserve erectile function after radical prostatectomy. Urology. 2003;61:491–7.
24. Secin FP, Touijer K, Mulhall J, Guillonneau B. Anatomy and preservation of accessory pudendal arteries in laparoscopic radical prostatectomy. Eur Urol. 2007;51:1229–35.
25. Hatzimouratidis K, Burnett AL, Hatzichristou D, McCullough AR, Montorsi F, Mulhall JP. Phosphodiesterase type 5 inhibitors in postprostatectomy erectile dysfunction: a critical analysis of the basic science rationale and clinical application. Eur Urol. 2009;55:334–47.
26. Tal R, Valenzuela R, Aviv N, Parker M, Waters WB, Flanigan RC, et al. Persistent erectile dysfunction following radical prostatectomy: the association between nerve-sparing status and the prevalence and chronology of venous leak. J Sex Med. 2009;6:2813–9.
27. Mulhall JP, Slovick R, Hotaling J, Aviv N, Valenzuela R, Waters WB, et al. Erectile dysfunction after radical prostatectomy: hemodynamic profiles and their correlation with the recovery of erectile function. J Urol. 2002;167:1371–5.
28. Mulhall J, Barnas J, Aviv N, Anderson M, Parker M. Sildenafil citrate response correlates with the nature and the severity of penile vascular insufficiency. J Sex Med. 2005;2:104–8.
29. Iacono F, Giannella R, Somma P, Manno G, Fusco F, Mirone V. Histological alterations in cavernous tissue after radical prostatectomy. J Urol. 2005;173:1673–6.
30. Leungwattanakij S, Bivalacqua TJ, Usta MF, Yang DY, Hyun JS, Champion HC, et al. Cavernous neurotomy causes hypoxia and fibrosis in rat corpus cavernosum. J Androl. 2003;24:239–45.
31. Hu WL, Hu LQ, Song J, Li SW, Zheng XM, Cheng B, et al. Fibrosis of corpus cavernosum in animals following cavernous nerve ablation. Asian J Androl. 2004;6:111–6.
32. Vignozzi L, Filippi S, Morelli A, Ambrosini S, Luconi M, Vannelli GB, et al. Effect of chronic tadalafil administration on penile hypoxia induced by cavernous neurotomy in the rat. J Sex Med. 2006;3:419–31.
33. Potosky AL, Davis WW, Hoffman RM, Stanford JL, Stephenson RA, Penson DF, et al. Five-year outcomes after prostatectomy or radiotherapy for prostate cancer: the prostate cancer outcomes study. J Natl Cancer Inst. 2004;96:1358–67.
34. Snyder KM, Stock RG, Buckstein M, Stone NN. Long-term potency preservation following brachytherapy for prostate cancer. BJU Int. 2012;110:221–5.
35. Zelefsky MJ, Eid JF. Elucidating the etiology of erectile dysfunction after definitive therapy for prostatic cancer. Int J Radiat Oncol Biol Phys. 1998;40:129–33.

36. van der Wielen GJ, Mulhall JP, Incrocci L. Erectile dysfunction after radiotherapy for prostate cancer and radiation dose to the penile structures: a critical review. Radiother Oncol. 2007;84:107–13.
37. Akbal C, Tinay I, Simsek F, Turkeri LN. Erectile dysfunction following radiotherapy and brachytherapy for prostate cancer: pathophysiology, prevention and treatment. Int Urol Nephrol. 2008;40:355–63.
38. Bottomley D, Ash D, Al-Qaisieh B, Carey B, Joseph J, St Clair S, et al. Side effects of permanent I125 prostate seed implants in 667 patients treated in Leeds. Radiother Oncol. 2007;82:46–9.
39. Incrocci L, Slagter C, Slob AK, Hop WC. A randomized, double-blind, placebo-controlled, crossover study to assess the efficacy of tadalafil (Cialis) in the treatment of erectile dysfunction following three-dimensional conformal external-beam radiotherapy for prostatic carcinoma. Int J Radiat Oncol Biol Phys. 2006;66:439–44.
40. Incrocci L, Slob AK, Hop WC. Tadalafil (Cialis) and erectile dysfunction after radiotherapy for prostate cancer: an open-label extension of a blinded trial. Urology. 2007;70:1190–3.
41. Pinkawa M, Gagel B, Piroth MD, Fischedick K, Asadpour B, Kehl M, et al. Erectile dysfunction after external beam radiotherapy for prostate cancer. Eur Urol. 2009;55:227–34.
42. Sanda MG, Dunn RL, Michalski J, Sandler HM, Northouse L, Hembroff L, et al. Quality of life and satisfaction with outcome among prostate-cancer survivors. N Engl J Med. 2008;358:1250–61.
43. Potters L, Torre T, Fearn PA, Leibel SA, Kattan MW. Potency after permanent prostate brachytherapy for localized prostate cancer. Int J Radiat Oncol Biol Phys. 2001;50:1235–42.
44. Incrocci L, Jensen PT. Pelvic radiotherapy and sexual function in men and women. J Sex Med. 2013;10 Suppl 1:53–64.
45. Lehrer S, Cesaretti J, Stone NN, Stock RG. Urinary symptom flare after brachytherapy for prostate cancer is associated with erectile dysfunction and more urinary symptoms before implantation. BJU Int. 2006;98:979–81.
46. Slater JD, Rossi Jr CJ, Yonemoto LT, Bush DA, Jabola BR, Levy RP, et al. Proton therapy for prostate cancer: the initial Loma Linda University experience. Int J Radiat Oncol Biol Phys. 2004;59: 348–52.
47. Kao J, Turian J, Meyers A, Hamilton RJ, Smith B, Vijayakumar S, et al. Sparing of the penile bulb and proximal penile structures with intensity-modulated radiation therapy for prostate cancer. Br J Radiol. 2004;77:129–36.
48. Buyyounouski MK, Horwitz EM, Price RA, Hanlon AL, Uzzo RG, Pollack A. Intensity-modulated radiotherapy with MRI simulation to reduce doses received by erectile tissue during prostate cancer treatment. Int J Radiat Oncol Biol Phys. 2004;58:743–9.
49. Peters CA, Stock RG, Cesaretti JA, Atencio DP, Peters S, Burri RJ, et al. TGFB1 single nucleotide polymorphisms are associated with adverse quality of life in prostate cancer patients treated with radiotherapy. Int J Radiat Oncol Biol Phys. 2008;70: 752–9.
50. Chung E, Brock GB. Emerging and novel therapeutic approaches in the treatment of male erectile dysfunction. Curr Urol Rep. 2011;12:432–43.
51. Burnett AL, Allaf ME, Bivalacqua TJ. Erythropoietin promotes erection recovery after nerve-sparing radical retropubic prostatectomy: a retrospective analysis. J Sex Med. 2008;5:2392–8.
52. Mulhall JP. Defining and reporting erectile function outcomes after radical prostatectomy: challenges and misconceptions. J Urol. 2009;181:462–71.
53. Rabbani F, Schiff J, Piecuch M, Yunis LH, Eastham JA, Scardino PT, et al. Time course of recovery of erectile function after radical retropubic prostatectomy: does anyone recover after 2 years? J Sex Med. 2010;7:3984–90.
54. Bannowsky A, Schulze H, van der Horst C, Seif C, Braun PM, Junemann KP. Nocturnal tumescence: a parameter for postoperative erectile integrity after nerve sparing radical prostatectomy. J Urol. 2006;175:2214–7.
55. Mulhall JP, Bivalacqua TJ, Becher EF. Standard operating procedure for the preservation of erectile function outcomes after radical prostatectomy. J Sex Med. 2013;10:195–203.
56. Tal R, Teloken P, Mulhall JP. Erectile function rehabilitation after radical prostatectomy: practice patterns among AUA members. J Sex Med. 2011;8: 2370–6.
57. Teloken P, Mesquita G, Montorsi F, Mulhall J. Post-radical prostatectomy pharmacological penile rehabilitation: practice patterns among the international society for sexual medicine practitioners. J Sex Med. 2009;6:2032–8.
58. Musicki B, Burnett AL. eNOS function and dysfunction in the penis. Exp Biol Med. 2006;231: 154–65.
59. Nehra A, Goldstein I, Pabby A, Nugent M, Huang YH, de las Morenas A, et al. Mechanisms of venous leakage: a prospective clinicopathological correlation of corporeal function and structure. J Urol. 1996;156:1320–9.
60. Sirad F, Hlaing S, Kovanecz I, Artaza JN, Garcia LA, Rajfer J, et al. Sildenafil promotes smooth muscle preservation and ameliorates fibrosis through modulation of extracellular matrix and tissue growth factor gene expression after bilateral cavernosal nerve resection in the rat. J Sex Med. 2011;8:1048–60.
61. Montorsi F, Brock G, Lee J, Shapiro J, Van Poppel H, Graefen M, et al. Effect of nightly versus on-demand vardenafil on recovery of erectile function in men following bilateral nerve-sparing radical prostatectomy. Eur Urol. 2008;54:924–31.
62. Padma-Nathan H, McCullough AR, Levine LA, Lipshultz LI, Siegel R, Montorsi F, et al. Randomized, double-blind, placebo-controlled study of postoperative

nightly sildenafil citrate for the prevention of erectile dysfunction after bilateral nerve-sparing radical prostatectomy. Int J Impot Res. 2008;20:479–86.
63. Bannowsky A, Schulze H, van der Horst C, Hautmann S, Junemann KP. Recovery of erectile function after nerve-sparing radical prostatectomy: improvement with nightly low-dose sildenafil. BJU Int. 2008;101:1279–83.
64. Gallina A, Ferrari M, Suardi N, Capitanio U, Abdollah F, Tutolo M, et al. Erectile function outcome after bilateral nerve sparing radical prostatectomy: which patients may be left untreated? J Sex Med. 2012;9:903–8.
65. Garcia-Cardoso J, Vela R, Mahillo E, Mateos-Caceres PJ, Modrego J, Macaya C, et al. Increased cyclic guanosine monophosphate production and endothelial nitric oxide synthase level in mononuclear cells from sildenafil citrate-treated patients with erectile dysfunction. Int J Impot Res. 2010;22:68–76.
66. Salonia A, Burnett AL, Graefen M, Hatzimouratidis K, Montorsi F, Mulhall JP, et al. Prevention and management of postprostatectomy sexual dysfunctions part 2: recovery and preservation of erectile function, sexual desire, and orgasmic function. Eur Urol. 2012;62:273–86.
67. Incrocci L, Koper PC, Hop WC, Slob AK. Sildenafil citrate (Viagra) and erectile dysfunction following external beam radiotherapy for prostate cancer: a randomized, double-blind, placebo-controlled, cross-over study. Int J Radiat Oncol Biol Phys. 2001;51:1190–5.
68. Incrocci L, Hop WC, Slob AK. Efficacy of sildenafil in an open-label study as a continuation of a double-blind study in the treatment of erectile dysfunction after radiotherapy for prostate cancer. Urology. 2003;62:116–20.
69. Schiff JD, Bar-Chama N, Cesaretti J, Stock R. Early use of a phosphodiesterase inhibitor after brachytherapy restores and preserves erectile function. BJU Int. 2006;98:1255–8.
70. Mulhall J, Land S, Parker M, Waters WB, Flanigan RC. The use of an erectogenic pharmacotherapy regimen following radical prostatectomy improves recovery of spontaneous erectile function. J Sex Med. 2005;2:532–40. discussion 40–2.
71. Park DL, Aron M, Rewcastle JC, Boyd SD, Gill IS. A model for managing erectile dysfunction following prostate cancer treatment. Curr Opin Urol. 2013;23:129–34.
72. Kohler TS, Pedro R, Hendlin K, Utz W, Ugarte R, Reddy P, et al. A pilot study on the early use of the vacuum erection device after radical retropubic prostatectomy. BJU Int. 2007;100:858–62.
73. Vardi Y, Appel B, Jacob G, Massarwi O, Gruenwald I. Can low-intensity extracorporeal shockwave therapy improve erectile function? A 6-month follow-up pilot study in patients with organic erectile dysfunction. Eur Urol. 2010;58:243–8.
74. Aoki H, Nagao J, Ueda T, Strong JM, Schonlau F, Yu-Jing S, et al. Clinical assessment of a supplement of Pycnogenol® and L-arginine in Japanese patients with mild to moderate erectile dysfunction. Phytother Res. 2012;26:204–7.
75. Ledda A, Belcaro G, Cesarone MR, Dugall M, Schonlau F. Investigation of a complex plant extract for mild to moderate erectile dysfunction in a randomized, double-blind, placebo-controlled, parallel-arm study. BJU Int. 2010;106:1030–3.
76. Stanislavov R, Nikolova V, Rohdewald P. Improvement of seminal parameters with Prelox: a randomized, double-blind, placebo-controlled, cross-over trial. Phytother Res. 2009;23:297–302.
77. Stanislavov R, Nikolova V. Treatment of erectile dysfunction with pycnogenol and L-arginine. J Sex Marital Ther. 2003;29:207–13.
78. Montague DK. Penile prosthesis implantation for end-stage erectile dysfunction after radical prostatectomy. Rev Urol. 2005;7 Suppl 2:S51–7.
79. Tal R, Jacks LM, Elkin E, Mulhall JP. Penile implant utilization following treatment for prostate cancer: analysis of the SEER-Medicare database. J Sex Med. 2011;8:1797–804.
80. Menard J, Tremeaux JC, Faix A, Pierrevelcin J, Staerman F. Erectile function and sexual satisfaction before and after penile prosthesis implantation in radical prostatectomy patients: a comparison with patients with vasculogenic erectile dysfunction. J Sex Med. 2011;8:3479–86.
81. Tefilli MV, Dubocq F, Rajpurkar A, Gheiler EL, Tiguert R, Barton C, et al. Assessment of psychosexual adjustment after insertion of inflatable penile prosthesis. Urology. 1998;52:1106–12.
82. Deho F, Salonia A, Briganti A, Zanni G, Gallina A, Rokkas K, et al. Anatomical radical retropubic prostatectomy in patients with a preexisting three-piece inflatable prosthesis: a series of case reports. J Sex Med. 2009;6:578–83.
83. Choi KH, Lee SH, Jung WS, Chung BH. Robot-assisted radical prostatectomy in a patient with a preexisting three-piece inflatable penile prosthesis. Korean J Urol. 2010;51:70–2.
84. Ramsawh HJ, Morgentaler A, Covino N, Barlow DH, DeWolf WC. Quality of life following simultaneous placement of penile prosthesis with radical prostatectomy. J Urol. 2005;174:1395–8.
85. Khera M. Androgens and erectile function: a case for early androgen use in postprostatectomy hypogonadal men. J Sex Med. 2009;6 Suppl 3:234–8.
86. Morelli A, Filippi S, Mancina R, Luconi M, Vignozzi L, Marini M, et al. Androgens regulate phosphodiesterase type 5 expression and functional activity in corpora cavernosa. Endocrinology. 2004;145:2253–63.
87. Morelli A, Corona G, Filippi S, Ambrosini S, Forti G, Vignozzi L, et al. Which patients with sexual dysfunction are suitable for testosterone replacement therapy? J Endocrinol Investig. 2007;30:880–8.

88. Kim SC, Song C, Kim W, Kang T, Park J, Jeong IG, et al. Factors determining functional outcomes after radical prostatectomy: robot-assisted versus retropubic. Eur Urol. 2011;60:413–9.
89. Agarwal PK, Oefelein MG. Testosterone replacement therapy after primary treatment for prostate cancer. J Urol. 2005;173:533–6.
90. Khera M, Grober ED, Najari B, Colen JS, Mohamed O, Lamb DJ, et al. Testosterone replacement therapy following radical prostatectomy. J Sex Med. 2009;6:1165–70.
91. Leibowitz RL, Dorff TB, Tucker S, Symanowski J, Vogelzang NJ. Testosterone replacement in prostate cancer survivors with hypogonadal symptoms. BJU Int. 2010;105:1397–401.
92. Pastuszak AW, Pearlman AM, Lai WS, Godoy G, Sathyamoorthy K, Liu JS, et al. Testosterone replacement therapy in patients with prostate cancer after radical prostatectomy. J Urol. 2013;190:639–44.
93. Wilke DR, Parker C, Andonowski A, Tsuji D, Catton C, Gospodarowicz M, et al. Testosterone and erectile function recovery after radiotherapy and long-term androgen deprivation with luteinizing hormone-releasing hormone agonists. BJU Int. 2006;97:963–8.
94. Teloken PE, Ohebshalom M, Mohideen N, Mulhall JP. Analysis of the impact of androgen deprivation therapy on sildenafil citrate response following radiation therapy for prostate cancer. J Urol. 2007; 178:2521–5.
95. Dale W, Bilir P, Han M, Meltzer D. The role of anxiety in prostate carcinoma: a structured review of the literature. Cancer. 2005;104:467–78.
96. Bill-Axelson A, Garmo H, Lambe M, Bratt O, Adolfsson J, Nyberg U, et al. Suicide risk in men with prostate-specific antigen-detected early prostate cancer: a nationwide population-based cohort study from PCBaSe Sweden. Eur Urol. 2010;57:390–5.
97. Fang F, Keating NL, Mucci LA, Adami HO, Stampfer MJ, Valdimarsdottir U, et al. Immediate risk of suicide and cardiovascular death after a prostate cancer diagnosis: cohort study in the United States. J Natl Cancer Inst. 2010;102:307–14.
98. Helfand BT, Glaser AP, Rimar K, Zargaroff S, Hedges J, McGuire BB, et al. Prostate cancer diagnosis is associated with an increased risk of erectile dysfunction after prostate biopsy. BJU Int. 2013;111:38–43.
99. Klotz L. Active surveillance for favorable-risk prostate cancer: background, patient selection, triggers for intervention, and outcomes. Curr Urol Rep. 2012;13:153–9.
100. Salonia A, Gallina A, Zanni G, Briganti A, Deho F, Sacca A, et al. Acceptance of and discontinuation rate from erectile dysfunction oral treatment in patients following bilateral nerve-sparing radical prostatectomy. Eur Urol. 2008;53:564–70.
101. Titta M, Tavolini IM, Dal Moro F, Cisternino A, Bassi P. Sexual counseling improved erectile rehabilitation after non-nerve-sparing radical retropubic prostatectomy or cystectomy—results of a randomized prospective study. J Sex Med. 2006;3:267–73.
102. Canada AL, Neese LE, Sui D, Schover LR. Pilot intervention to enhance sexual rehabilitation for couples after treatment for localized prostate carcinoma. Cancer. 2005;104:2689–700.
103. Incrocci L. Talking about sex to oncologists and cancer to sexologists. J Sex Med. 2011;8:3251–3.
104. Stead ML, Fallowfield L, Brown JM, Selby P. Communication about sexual problems and sexual concerns in ovarian cancer: qualitative study. BMJ. 2001;323:836–7.

Commentary: Erectile Dysfunction in the Setting of Prostate Cancer

Christian J. Nelson

As Samplaski and Lo highlight in the preceding chapter, a diagnosis of erectile dysfunction (ED) in the prostate cancer patient can be challenging to manage. Not only does the etiology of prostate cancer-related ED differ from that in most cases of ED, relating more directly to treatment for the cancer, it is often accompanied by psychological ramifications that can be further debilitating and are magnified as a result of the cancer diagnosis and treatment. However, the psychological impact of prostate cancer, its treatment, and the subsequent physical effects are often overlooked. As such, the treatment challenges of prostate cancer-related ED are further multiplied by the presence of a significant psychological burden in these men. Often, a treatment approach focused exclusively on medical or surgical therapies will have suboptimal results. Therefore, it is imperative that clinicians consider the psychological impact of ED in men with prostate cancer and appropriately treat or refer men they are unable to manage themselves.

In the following commentary, Nelson looks under the proverbial hood of the man with ED related to prostate cancer, pointing out the key psychological factors—depression and anxiety—that are often present concomitantly with ED in these patients and the resultant avoidance of sexual behaviors and negative impact on relationships. The stark reality of a contribution from psychological factors to sexual dysfunction broadly, and even more significantly in men with prostate cancer, should be considered and addressed in all patients towards the goal of optimized treatment using a multidisciplinary approach.

The Editors

Christian J. Nelson, Ph.D.
Memorial Sloan Kettering Cancer Center,
New York, NY, USA

Commentary

It is important to understand that men with erectile dysfunction (ED) often experience comorbid depression and anxiety [1–5]. In one study of 120 men presenting to a sexual medicine clinic, 33 % reported high levels of depression and anxiety with major depression being the most common [6]. Of note, only about one third of these men were identified by their urologist as having a psychological concern, highlighting the need for medical care givers to ask about psychological sequelae of ED [6]. In another study of 103 men with ED, 63 % had a detectable psychiatric diagnosis including depressive symptoms in 25.2 %, anxiety disorders in 11.7 %, depression anxiety in 6.8 %, and personality disorders in 5.8 % [7].

Depressive Symptoms Related to ED

The association between ED and depression has been demonstrated in a number of well-designed population-based studies of aging men in the USA, Finland, Brazil, Japan, and Malaysia [2, 3, 8]. Data from the Massachusetts Male Aging Study (MMAS) confirm that men 40–70 years old with clinically significant depressive symptoms are nearly two times more likely to report ED compared to their nondepressed peers, controlling for important sociodemographic and medical factors [9]. ED is associated with a higher incidence of depressive symptoms independent of age, marital status, and comorbid medical conditions [1]. The association between ED and depression is considered a bidirectional relationship in which the two conditions reinforce each other in a “downward spiral” [9]. When focusing on prostate cancer, some authors have argued that depression or distress related to ED is mitigated as patients focus on the lifesaving nature of treatment [10]. Nevertheless, data confirms the presence of depressive symptoms, ED bother, and loss of masculine identity in men with ED following prostate cancer treatments [11, 12].

Anxiety and Sexual Performance

Anxiety is also an important concern in men with ED and can play a role in the maintenance of ED. For many men, erectile problems will heighten sexual anxieties due to increased concerns about erectile response leading up to and during sexual encounters [5]. This heightened focus on performance and feeling self-conscious are cognitive distractions that exacerbate problems with arousal and performance [13, 14]. These pressures increase the likelihood of failure and reinforce the pressure to perform during successive encounters, resulting in a vicious cycle of failure and escalating performance anxiety [5]. Ultimately, the anticipation of failure may cause avoidance of sex altogether, which may also detrimentally impact other aspects of intimacy in his relationship.

Relationship Impact

Not surprisingly, both patients and partners are impacted by the changes that ED may have on their relationships and must adjust to those changes individually and as a couple. Regret and feelings of loss are reported by both men and their partners in the face of sexual dysfunction [15]. Partner and relationship factors are important considerations in assessing men’s reactions to ED, the impact of a cancer diagnosis, and the impact ED may have on their psychological well-being and quality of life.

Avoidance

Given the psychological consequences of ED, it is not surprising that many men have difficulty accepting they have ED and delay pursuing treatment [16]. Although the embarrassment related to ED may be mitigated in men whose ED is caused by a medical condition such as prostate cancer, many men delay seeking treatment, hoping their ED will improve spontaneously. Only 50 % of men who report an interest in ED treatment actually pursue it [17]. Additionally, a growing body of literature is showing that compliance with ED treatments is poor. Disappointment, shame, and relationship strain may impact men's ability to commit to and sustain the use of ED medications, and current data indicate that 50–80 % of men discontinue use of medical interventions (i.e., pills, injections, vacuum devices) for ED within a year [18, 19]. Phosphodiesterase 5 inhibitors (PDE5-Is) are used as first-line therapy in about 90 % of men who seek ED treatment; however, despite being safe and effective, discontinuation rates are 30–50 % [20–23]. Although men may stop ED treatment for a number of reasons, those who develop a pattern of avoidance may be particularly prone to poor adherence. This type of avoidance can be especially damaging in the context of prostate cancer and penile rehabilitation. Avoidance may cause men to miss the post-prostatectomy treatment window that maximizes the impact of penile rehabilitation, which may then lead to chronic ED, further prolonging or exacerbating the negative effects of a man's ED on emotional and relational well-being.

Case Example

James is a 64-year-old man who was diagnosed with early stage, intermediate risk prostate cancer. He had a difficult time deciding on a treatment option and wanted to avoid treatment altogether. He was concerned about how prostate cancer treatment would impact his sexual function, and his first priority was to maintain his erections. James' doctors all agreed that treatment was needed and encouraged him repeatedly to be treated. Despite these persistent recommendations, James continued to decline treatment. Finally, through the urging of his wife and family, he decided to have a radical prostatectomy. With regard to cancer treatment, the surgery was a success. However, James experienced ED following prostatectomy and reported significant distress and depressive symptoms related to his ED. While initially motivated to participate in a penile rehabilitation program, he quickly began avoiding penile injections and withdrew physically and emotionally from his wife. This created marital conflict, leading to an increase in his personal distress as well as increased anxiety related to intimate situations.

The reaction that James had to his ED and the resulting impact on his relationship is relatively typical for men with ED following prostate cancer treatment. Even though they are thankful the cancer was successfully treated, men often experience ED, which leads to shame, embarrassment, and emotional distress. These psychosocial ramifications highlight the importance of working with mental health professionals to mitigate these issues in the context of sexual dysfunction following cancer treatment. James worked with a psychologist to help address his depression and avoidance using techniques from Acceptance and Commitment Therapy with the primary goal of reducing James' avoidance of penile injections and engaging in sexual situations. Using this approach, James began to use the penile injections at the rate suggested for penile rehabilitation, and he was able to reconnect with his wife on an intimate level. These two successes then led to reduced distress and relationship tension. Eventually, James recovered erectile function several months after his prostatectomy and no longer needed treatment for ED.

References

1. Shabsigh R, et al. Increased incidence of depressive symptoms in men with erectile dysfunction. Urology. 1998;52(5):848–52.
2. Araujo AB, et al. The relationship between depressive symptoms and male erectile dysfunction: cross-sectional results from the Massachusetts Male Aging Study. Psychosom Med. 1998;60(4):458–65.
3. Shiri RR, et al. Bidirectional relationship between depression and erectile dysfunction. J Urol. 2007; 177(2):669–73.
4. Perelman MA. Erectile dysfunction and depression: screening and treatment. Urol Clin North Am. 2011;38(2):125–39.
5. Hedon F. Anxiety and erectile dysfunction: a global approach to ED enhances results and quality of life. Int J Impot Res. 2003;15(Suppl 2):S16-9.
6. Lee IC, et al. The prevalence and influence of significant psychiatric abnormalities in men undergoing comprehensive management of organic erectile dysfunction. Int J Impot Res. 2000;12(1):47–51.
7. Mallis D, et al. Psychiatric morbidity is frequently undetected in patients with erectile dysfunction. J Urol. 2005;174(5):1913–6.

8. Nicolosi A, et al. A population study of the association between sexual function, sexual satisfaction and depressive symptoms in men. J Affect Disord. 2004;82(2):235–43.
9. Araujo AB, et al. The relationship between depressive symptoms and male erectile dysfunction: cross-sectional results from the Massachusetts Male Aging Study. Psychosom Med. 1998;60(4): 458–65.
10. Penson DF, et al. Is quality of life different for men with erectile dysfunction and prostate cancer compared to men with erectile dysfunction due to other causes? Results from the ExCEED data base. J Urol. 2003;169(4):1458–61.
11. Nelson CJ, Mulhall JP, Roth AJ. The association between erectile dysfunction and depressive symptoms in men treated for prostate cancer. J Sex Med. 2011;8(2):560–6.
12. Nelson CJ, et al. Sexual bother following radical prostatectomyjsm. J Sex Med. 2010;7(1 Pt 1):129–35.
13. Hale VE, Strassberg DS. The role of anxiety on sexual arousal. Arch Sex Behav. 1990;19(6): 569–81.
14. Beck JG, Barlow DH. The effects of anxiety and attentional focus on sexual responding—II: Cognitive and affective patterns in erectile dysfunction. Behav Res Ther. 1986;24(1):19–26.
15. Resendes LA, McCorkle R. Spousal responses to prostate cancer: an integrative review. Cancer Invest. 2006;24(2):192–8.
16. de Boer BJ, et al. The prevalence of bother, acceptance, and need for help in men with erectile dysfunction. J Sex Med. 2005;2(3):445–50.
17. Salonia A, et al. Does educational status affect a patient's behavior toward erectile dysfunction? J Sex Med. 2008;5(8):1941–8.
18. Schover LR, et al. Defining sexual outcomes after treatment for localized prostate carcinoma (see comment). Cancer. 2002;95(8):1773–85.
19. Sundaram CP, et al. Long-term follow-up of patients receiving injection therapy for erectile dysfunction. Urology. 1997;49(6):932–5.
20. Huang SA, Lie JD. Phosphodiesterase-5 (PDE5) inhibitors in the management of erectile dysfunction. P t. 2013;38(7):407–19.
21. Jiann BP, et al. Compliance of sildenafil treatment for erectile dysfunction and factors affecting it. Int J Impot Res. 2006;18(2):146–9.
22. Klotz T, et al. Why do patients with erectile dysfunction abandon effective therapy with sildenafil (Viagra)? Int J Impot Res. 2005;17(1):2–4.
23. Perelman MA. Psychosocial evaluation and combination treatment of men with erectile dysfunction. Urol Clin North Am. 2005;32(4):431–45.

Peyronie's Disease and Other Anatomical Disorders

10

Shahin T. Chandrasoma and Martin K. Gelbard

10.1 Introduction

Disorders of penile anatomy can result in a variety of problems with sexual function, ranging from purely physical issues with regard to size, shape, or rigidity to psychologic impairment—embarrassment, loss of confidence, alteration in body image, and depression. There are three clinical conditions that comprise this group: Peyronie's disease, congenital penile curvature or chordee, and hypospadias. The prime focus of this chapter will be on Peyronie's disease (PD), as it is the most common of the three. Congenital curvature and hypospadias are present throughout life and unless particularly severe are not often regarded as abnormal unless commented on by a partner. Peyronie's disease, however, is an acquired condition that alters baseline sexual function and can result in severe psychological effects.

Peyronie's disease is named after Francois Gigot de la Peyronie, physician and battlefield surgeon to the court of Louis XV. He was credited with the first medical article describing a "ram's horn" curvature of the penis associated with palpable subcutaneous nodules, though written descriptions of a similar observation date to the sixteenth century and earlier.

Peyronie's disease can cause painful erection, difficulty maintaining an erection, curvature, indentation, or twisting of the penis, and loss of penile length and girth. Congenital curvature, comparatively, is associated with an otherwise normal penis that curves laterally, ventrally, or dorsally. Dorsal or upward curvature is the most common presentation of PD and the least common congenital deformity. Hypospadias, a congenital condition wherein the urethra variably exits the penis proximally and ventrally to the tip of the glans, can be associated with ventral or downward bending as well. All three conditions can cause sexual dysfunction via physical or psychological effects on the patient and/or his partner.

10.2 Prevalence and Genetic Patterns

Though it has been identified in all races, PD is most common in men of Northern European ancestry. The prevalence of PD varies considerably, depending on the cohort studied: from 0.39 % based on diagnoses within Rochester County, Minnesota [1], to 20.3 % based on cases identified in diabetic men with erectile dysfunction [2]. Another study showed 7.9 % prevalence

S.T. Chandrasoma, M.D.
Skyline Urology, 2601 W Alameda Ave,
Los Angeles, CA, USA

M.K. Gelbard, M.D. (✉)
Clinical Faculty, Skyline Urology, University of California, Los Angeles, 2601 West Alameda Avenue, Burbank, CA 91505, USA
e-mail: mgelbard@uamg.net

L.I. Lipshultz et al. (eds.), *Management of Sexual Dysfunction in Men and Women*, DOI 10.1007/978-1-4939-3100-2_10

among patients with erectile dysfunction [3]. A large general Internet-based survey of 11,420 subjects found a 0.5 % prevalence [4], while a different general survey of 4432 men measured prevalence at 3.2 % [5]. A survey of 647 men between 50 and 70 showed a 7.1 % prevalence [6], and another study of 534 men over 40 being screened for prostate cancer identified 8.9 % with the diagnosis [7].

10.3 Natural History and Pathology

Of the disorders covered in this chapter, only PD is acquired; as such, its development tends to follow a predictable pattern or so-called natural history. In some cases it follows an obvious coital injury, which can range from pain and/or a cracking, popping sensation during intercourse up to frank penile fracture with detumescence and appearance of a hematoma. In those cases of penile fracture, whether treated surgically or by observation, alteration of penile shape and palpable penile induration are usually apparent soon after the event. By comparison, presentation may be delayed for a year or more after less violent injuries.

Although trauma is a known inciting event, the clinical fact is that most patients present without any history of penile injury. Roughly only half of affected patients complain of penile pain or a history of painful erections, though in some cases a period of painful erections precedes the appearance of bending or palpable nodules. In other cases penile curvature is reported as coming "out of the blue," with patients describing the surprise they experience when they notice that their morning erection has suddenly taken a turn in a new direction.

Most cases of PD evolve over a period of 12–18 months before stabilizing. Since most cases follow this progression, there is a clinical distinction between early and late PD. Pain, if present, is usually associated only with this early formative phase and in most cases tends to resolve spontaneously with the passage of time. Following the cessation of pain and/or stabilization of evolving deformity, most patients will experience relatively little change in their condition. As will be described in more detail below, this late phase is characterized by the presence of stable, mature scarring of the penile tunica albuginea, the dense collagenous wall of the corpus cavernosum. Significant variation in this pattern has been recognized, however. In 217 men followed for a mean of 14.5 months, Mulhall et al. found that curvature worsened in 48 %, improved in 12 %, and stabilized in 40 % [8]. Similarly, some patients will continue to experience erectile pain for several years into the course of the disorder, though this is rare.

Congenital curvature is generally first noted at puberty. Most cases will exhibit little change over subsequent years, though occasionally the bend will increase slightly over time, perhaps due to the mild trauma experienced on the concave side from straightening the penis during intercourse. Many patients with hypospadias severe enough to cause downward curvature will have had corrective surgery by the time they reach puberty. This experience carries its own unique psychological effects, though some authors feel that surgical correction prior to puberty in general decreases emotional strain relative to the condition.

PD has been characterized as a wound healing disorder of the tunica albuginea [9]. The earliest histologic changes observed are fibrin deposition within the tunica and a round cell inflammatory infiltrate in the areolar layer just deep to it. These findings are thought to represent the initial subclinical trauma and the consequent inflammatory response and are consistent with the usual early, transient painful phase, mediated by inflammatory cytokines. For unknown reasons, the wound healing response engendered by these events is not properly regulated, persisting and causing an inappropriate amount of scarring. The net result is that most patients with PD will develop permanently scarred regions of the tunica. By producing firm areas, or plaques, the normal pliancy of the tunica albuginea is limited. Peyronie's plaque can range from areas of reversible inflammation (early PD) to permanently scarred tissue (late PD). Regardless of their composition, plaques alter the shape of the erect corpora cavernosa. Like cellophane tape on the wall of a balloon, they prevent symmetrical inflation and result in a bent, shortened, indented, or otherwise misshapen erection.

All sexually active men experience some degree of wear and tear on vulnerable areas of the erectile mechanism. Both the structural arrangement of the corpora and the inherent elasticity of its connective tissues counteract the mechanical stress imposed by intercourse. But by the time men reach the sixth decade of life, tunical elasticity is waning. The median age for the appearance of PD is 55. Fibrin deposition in the tunica, the earliest microscopic change associated with PD, is a common finding on autopsy studies in asymptomatic men. While many men develop areas of fibrin deposition, only a small percentage will experience progression to plaque formation. There is no generally accepted explanation as to what factors or situations stimulate this progression, though it is thought that some men are genetically susceptible, as PD can occur in families and is closely associated with Dupuytren's contractures, a hereditary condition causing similar fascial scarring in the palm of the hand. PD has also been associated with the presence of the human leukocyte antigen DQ5 locus, Paget's disease of bone, diabetes, hyperlipidemia, hypertension, heart disease, the use of beta blockers, smoking, low testosterone, penile instrumentation, radical prostatectomy, and penile injection therapy.

10.4 Presentation and Clinical Findings

Though identifiable by puberty, congenital curvature without hypospadias often will not become apparent until the patient becomes sexually active, if the bend is severe enough to interfere with intercourse. Hypospadias with or without curvature is usually identified at birth. Peyronie's disease, however, most often presents in the fifth or sixth decade of life, though it occasionally occurs as early as the third decade. There appear to be two common modes of presentation: painful erections followed by the onset of penile bend and/or indent and the rather abrupt appearance of change in penile shape without antecedent pain. Only about 50 % of new PD patients complain of pain. Although many patients become aware of a hardened platelike or nodular region below the skin ("Peyronie's plaque"), recognition of a plaque—which can be tender to touch—is not commonly the initial presentation. Some PD patients can recall a specific traumatic coital event that precipitated the problem, though in most cases there is no clear-cut history of such an event.

There are a variety of subjective responses seen in PD patients in addition to pain: erectile dysfunction, which can be psychogenic and/or organic via interference with passive venocclusion, embarrassment, anger, shame, loss of confidence, change in self-image, withdrawal, loss of intimacy, and depression. Recently, a statistically validated questionnaire was developed to identify and quantitate the subjective bother associated with PD. The disabling psychological effects of this condition are now recognized as particularly prevalent; one study showed clinically significant depression in 48 % of unselected men with this diagnosis [10].

Objective findings in Peyronie's patients include bending, indentation, and or twisting of the erect penis, loss of length or girth, and the presence of lumps or plaques palpable when flaccid. Changes in girth can be unilateral (indentation), bilateral ("hourglass deformity"), or segmental (distal taper or diameter loss beyond a plaque). Areas of diameter loss compromise column rigidity of the shaft and can produce buckling or so-called "hinge" effects. Often, passive elasticity or the unrestricted ability to stretch the flaccid penis is impaired in PD.

10.5 Diagnosis

Hypospadias is readily diagnosed by finding that the urethral opening or meatus is located more proximally on the penis than the tip of the glans. *Congenital penile curvature* can be identified when curvature has been present since puberty and is not associated with penile plaque, pain, and loss of elasticity or girth. The diagnosis of *Peyronie's disease* can be made clinically without the need for imaging or laboratory studies in most patients based on the history and physical findings noted above. Very rarely the diagnosis is in question, as penile phlebothromboses (Mondor's syndrome) or malignant tumor infiltration of the corpora can also produce painful nodules in the penis. Mondor's syndrome does not tend to cause curvature, while tumor infiltration will change the shape of the erection in addition to causing an atypical pattern of continual pain rather than erectile pain. In these cases MRI is helpful in differentiating the diagnosis. Despite the ability to diagnose most cases without such studies, imaging and measurement of objective findings in PD are essential for careful clinical management.

The first step in clinical management of PD is obtaining a detailed history, covering the patient's perceptions of the various symptoms and findings noted above. To this should be added the disease duration, whether there was a history of preceding coital trauma, and whether there is a personal of family history of Dupuytren's contractures of the hand or plantar fibromatoses (Ledderhose disease). Other conditions felt to contribute to PD include diabetes, beta-blocker use, and a history of urethral or prostate surgery. The Peyronie's Disease Questionnaire (PDQ) is a statistically validated instrument for the documentation of psychologic bother and is a helpful adjunct to the screening history [11].

Detailed and directed physical examination should be performed and should include the stretched length of the flaccid penis, usually measured from the pubic symphysis to the penile corona. Plaque location and configuration likewise should be identified, though detailed measurement of plaque size is not clinically reliable or helpful in the management of these patients. We find it helpful to comment on the preservation or absence of passive stretch or extensibility. Complaints about sensory change are rare but if present can be evaluated with biothesiometry of vibratory thresholds.

There are a variety of ways to document penile deformity. This step is mandatory, as patients' subjective estimation of their curvature is inaccurate. Photos submitted by patients can be helpful, and there is even a smartphone app for quantifying the degree of bending. Bending and other shape issues can be most reliably measured and documented following intracavernosal injection of vasoactive compounds such as prostaglandin E1 or Trimix. Goniometer measurement in this setting is sufficient in some cases, though most clinicians will do this as part of a penile duplex Doppler ultrasound examination. The value of this examination is that in addition to identifying the location of the primary plaque or the area most contributing to the deformity, it can determine whether the calcified plaque is present and whether there is any associated vasculogenic erectile dysfunction. A recent survey of 220 men with mean age 55 years showed 69.5 % had vasculogenic erectile dysfunction: 10 % with arterial insufficiency, 43.2 % with venocclusive dysfunction, and 16.3 % with both [12].

Plaque calcification can also be assessed with xeroradiography or low kilovoltage radiography (50 KV at 50MAs) utilizing film in a light tight paper jacket without an image intensification cassette. In those rare cases where other causes of penile induration are present, MRI imaging can be helpful. Laboratory testing is generally not necessary, though based on reports on the association of PD with low testosterone, some clinicians will obtain screening testosterone levels.

10.6 Treatment

There is no nonsurgical treatment for hypospadias or congenital curvature. While the management of hypospadias is beyond the scope of this article, surgery for congenital curvature involves surgical plication of the corpora, which is discussed below.

A variety of medications, surgery, and stretching devices have been used in the treatment of Peyronie's disease. Even extracorporeal shock waves, as administered for kidney stones, have been tested. Until large multi-institutional international studies were recently completed, there was little consensus among urologists as to what constituted an optimal approach. Even with the robust data generated from those studies, there are still widely varying opinions on best practices. This is due in part to deficiencies of earlier studies and in part to the wide variation in presentation from one individual to another, ranging from the pain of early inflammation in some patients to later stage shrinkage or curvature in others.

To evaluate the efficacy of PD treatments, the evolution of the disease in the absence of therapy should be known. Erections can be painful during the first 6 months or early phase of the disorder, though about half of patients have minimal or no pain initially. Eventually, pain tends to resolve on its own as PD enters the second or chronic stable phase. Unfortunately, bending does not usually follow the same resolving course as pain—in the majority of men, angulation present in the latter stages of PD usually persists. Bending may worsen or progress after this point, and spontaneous resolution is rare. Factors associated with a tendency for bending to persist are the presence of Dupuytren's contractures in the hand, the presence of plaque calcification, and severe penile angulation (>45°). Understanding this "natural history" provides a basis for comparison of outcomes from various treatment modalities. Despite the well-documented course of untreated PD, there exist a number of deficiencies in much of Peyronie's clinical literature; the quality of evidence supporting nonsurgical treatment varies considerably.

10.7 Medications

Until recently, nonsurgical or "medical therapy" was thought to give best results during the early phase of PD, while correction of curvature associated with chronic second stage scarring required surgery. Traditionally, medications were employed early in the initial inflammatory stage with surgery indicated later where loss of sexual function accompanied persistent penile deformity.

This view was based on the mechanism of action of early medical therapy. Though never well characterized by exhaustive basic science, medical therapy was intended to reduce the inflammatory response or inhibit the deposition of new scar tissue. On the other hand, effective pharmacologic manipulation of established or chronic scar has been an elusive goal until recently. Data from clinical trials of collagenase clostridium histolyticum (CCH) have shown statistically meaningful improvement both in curvature and subjective function in men with stable chronic disease of >1 year duration. While starting treatment early is always a good principle, the use of CCH is changing the traditional timing of nonsurgical treatment. For the first time, men with long-standing deformity may expect improvement in many cases with nonsurgical therapy.

There are a number of medications and remedies that have been used off-label in the treatment of PD [13]. Some of the most commonly used agents are:

- Vitamin E: this antioxidant has been widely used in the treatment of PD since 1948, though evidence of its efficacy is lacking.
- Potassium para-aminobenzoate (POTABA): related to B complex vitamins and can theoretically increase the supply of oxygen to inflamed tissues. There are no good randomized controlled trial data demonstrating efficacy in PD treatment, and the high doses frequently recommended may cause digestive upset.
- Colchicine: a medication used for many years in the treatment of gout, colchicine has anti-inflammatory properties and interferes with collagen (scar) synthesis. There is weak evidence for efficacy in PD in clinical trials, and it can cause diarrhea and should not be used in patients who are on statins (cholesterol-lowering drugs) due to the risk of muscle inflammation.
- Tamoxifen: a nonsteroidal antiestrogen that may inhibit scar-producing cells. Clinical evidence for the use in PD is weak—it was unable to outperform placebo.
- Acetyl carnitine: appears to reduce cellular damage due to inflammation. Clinical trials in PD patients have shown minimal effects.
- L-Arginine: an amino acid supplement that is a precursor to a nitric oxide, a neurotransmitter critical for erection, and thought to inhibit fibrosis or scarring.

- Pentoxifylline: a nonselective phosphodiesterase inhibitor that improves red blood cell circulation in vascular disorders and may help to locally reduce scarring following inflammation.
- Verapamil: blocks the delivery of scar tissue precursors into an area of wound healing. Penetration into penile plaque has not been proven when used as a topical ointment. Injection directly into the plaques has shown varying degrees of success—some clinical trials have shown benefit, while others found it did not outperform placebo.
- Interferon-α (IFN-α): a signaling protein that plays a role in human immune responses by inhibiting cellular proliferation. IFN-α was the first anti-PD drug to be tested in a multi-institutional clinical trial, where comparison to placebo showed a small effect on curvature reduction. It has a tendency to produce systemic flu-like symptoms.

10.8 Biological Agents in Peyronie's Disease

The only treatment specifically approved by the US Food and Drug Administration in the management of Peyronie's disease is CCH, a proprietary combination of two enzymes found in cell-free filtrates from cultures of the bacterium *Clostridium histolyticum*. This mix of powerful enzymes is highly specific for collagen, the molecular constituent of scar tissue. It is capable of dissolving this scar tissue at normal body temperature and pH, reducing the curving or distorting effect scar creates in the penile corpora cavernosa. That it is highly specific for collagen and binds it tightly at the injection site without a tendency to spread through tissues contributes to its safety profile. It has been FDA approved for the treatment of Dupuytren's contractures of the hand since 2011, and in December 2013 it was approved for the use in PD. This biologic agent (it is not technically a drug) is in a completely new class compared to the existing therapeutic agents discussed above. Because it is the first nonsurgical treatment to be tested extensively for safety and efficacy in international multi-institutional clinical trials, it is supported by evidence gathered under more stringent and exacting conditions than in any other study of PD treatment to date [14].

The quality of clinical trial data supporting the use of nonsurgical therapy for the treatment of curvature and subjective bother due to PD has been graded in a recent comprehensive survey [15]. The authors found that the highest level of evidence supporting this approach came from the use of either CCH or IFN-α.

10.9 Other Minimally Invasive Treatment Modalities

Traction therapy, conducted using mechanical stretching devices, is proposed to work by the induction of plaque remodeling via tensile stress. Studies have shown it can have a modest impact on penile curvature and length when used regularly, but can be uncomfortable and inconvenient. The mechanism of action whereby shock wave therapy can influence PD has not been defined, and meta-analyses of pooled clinical outcomes have failed to confirm efficacy.

10.10 Surgical Management of Peyronie's Disease

In cases refractory to minimally invasive treatment, surgical intervention may be considered. The approach is dictated by the location, direction, and severity of curvature, the presence of plaque calcification, and the presence or absence of concurrent or underlying erectile dysfunction. Typically, surgical management is reserved for patients who are in the chronic stable phase of the disease, with curvature significant enough to preclude penetration during intercourse [16]. Based on results of CCH in chronic stable Peyronie's disease, the indications for surgery can be modified to include chronic stable PD patients with heavy plaque calcification or those who have failed a course of CCH.

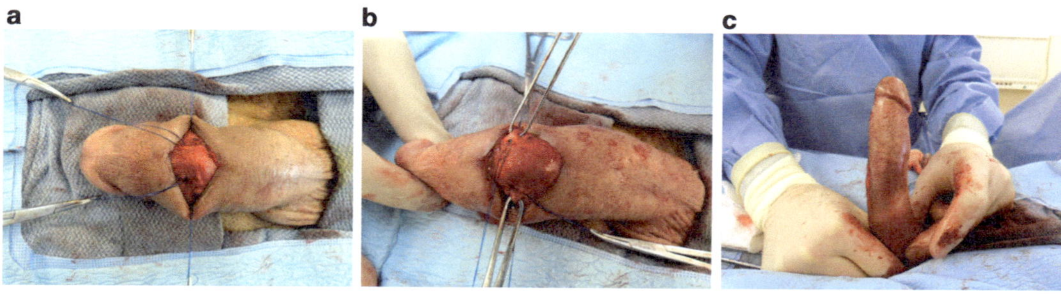

Fig. 10.1 Nesbit plication. (**a**) Exposure of the ventral penis after artificial erection, followed by (**b**) clamping of penile tissue in the area of curvature to define the degree of plication needed. Suture is then placed to cinch the tissue and straighten the penis, contributing to (**c**) the final result

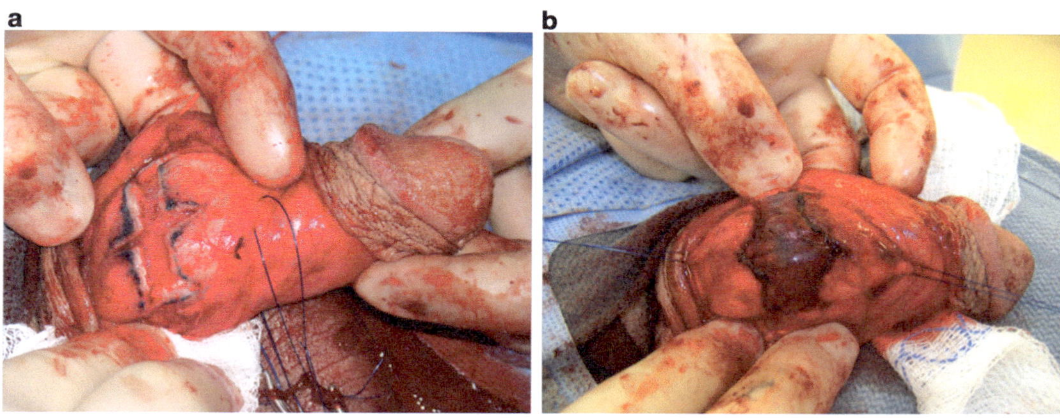

Fig. 10.2 Peyronie's plaque incision and grafting. (**a**) Relaxing incision of a PD plaque with (**b**) placement of autologous temporalis fascia graft with watertight closure

Lesser degrees of bending due to PD can be corrected surgically with simple plication opposite the point of bending (Fig. 10.1). This is also the preferred method for correcting congenital curvature regardless of severity. It is also indicated for the surgical correction of ventral PD, as grafting procedures for this condition often compromises erectile rigidity. These procedures can be done with either suture plication or removal of a small ellipse of tunica followed by closure. Plication procedures will shorten the penis and may cause indentation, sensory change, or reduced erectile rigidity.

For more pronounced curvature or complex deformities involving indentation or diameter loss, incision of the contracture and grafting is more effective (Fig. 10.2). We have had good results using autologous temporalis fascia, though many other graft materials have been employed successfully as well. The plaque is incised and the contracture expanded, removing spicules of sub-tunical calcifications if they are present using relaxing incisions. Usually several grafts are required, which are sutured in place for a watertight closure. This procedure can also cause penile shortening, sensory change, and loss of erectile rigidity.

Patients with underlying erectile dysfunction at baseline may elect graftless straightening at the time of inflatable penile prosthesis placement.

In this procedure the PD plaque is incised with short staggered incisions that expand the contracture; much like is accomplished by meshing a split-thickness skin graft.

10.11 Conclusion

Peyronie's disease is one of the most common disorders of penile anatomy in the adult population. Unlike hypospadias or congenital curvature, PD is acquired in adult life so it tends to have a powerful secondary psychological effect. Historically, medical management of PD left much to be desired; surgical management of Peyronie's disease was considered the gold standard. With regulatory approval of CCH, we now have a reliable intermediate option, as CCH is highly effective at correction of mild to moderate bends without the shortening and other complications seen with surgery. Future directions of study will include a better understanding of wound healing and its disorders, while contemporary practice will continue to recognize the powerful psychologic and relational issues created by this challenging disorder.

References

1. Lindsay MB, Schain DM, Grambsch P, Benson RC, Beard CM, Kurland LT. The incidence of Peyronie's disease in Rochester, Minnesota, 1950 through 1984. J Urol. 1991;146(4):1007–9.
2. Arafa M, Eid H, El-Badry A, Ezz-Eldine K, Shamloul R. The prevalence of Peyronie's disease in diabetic patients with erectile dysfunction. Int J Impot Res. 2007;19(2):213–7 [Epub 2006 Aug 17].
3. El-Sakka AI. Prevalence of Peyronie's disease among patients with erectile dysfunction. Eur Urol. 2006;49(3):564–9 [Epub 2005 Dec 19].
4. Dibenedetti DB, Nguyen D, Zografos L, Ziemiecki R, Zhou X. A population-based study of Peyronie's disease: prevalence and treatment patterns in the United States. Adv Urol. 2011;2011:282503 [Epub 2011 Oct 23].
5. Schwarzer U, Sommer F, Klotz T, Braun M, Reifenrath B, Engelmann U. The prevalence of Peyronie's disease: results of a large survey. BJU Int. 2001;88(7):727–30.
6. La Pera G, Pescatori ES, Calabrese M, Boffini A, Colombo F, Andriani E, Natali A, Vaggi L, Catuogno C, Giustini M, Taggi F, SIMONA Study Group. Peyronie's disease: prevalence and association with cigarette smoking. A multicenter population-based study in men aged 50–69 years. Eur Urol. 2001; 40(5):525–30.
7. Mulhall JP, Creech SD, Boorjian SA, Ghaly S, Kim ED, Moty A, Davis R, Hellstrom W. Subjective and objective analysis of the prevalence of Peyronie's disease in a population of men presenting for prostate cancer screening. J Urol. 2004;171(6 Pt 1):2350–3.
8. Mulhall JP, Schiff J, Guhring P. An analysis of the natural history of Peyronie's disease. J Urol. 2006;175(6):2115–8; discussion 2118.
9. Mulhall JP. Implications of basic science research in Peyronie's disease. In: Levine L, editor. Peyronie's disease: a guide to clinical management. Totowa, NJ: Humana Press Inc.; 2007. p. 39–57.
10. Nelson CJ, Diblasio C, Kendirci M, Hellstrom W, Guhring P, Mulhall JP. The chronology of depression and distress in men with Peyronie's disease. J Sex Med. 2008;5(8):1985–90 [Epub 2008 June 28].
11. Hellstrom WJ, Feldman R, Rosen RC, Smith T, Kaufman G, Tursi J. Bother and distress associated with Peyronie's disease: validation of the Peyronie's disease questionnaire. J Urol. 2013;190(2):627–34 [Epub 2013 Jan 31].
12. Serefoglu EC, Trost L, Sikka SC, Hellstrom WJ. The direction and severity of penile curvature does not have an impact on concomitant vasculogenic erectile dysfunction in patients with Peyronie's disease. Int J Impot Res. 2015;27(1):6–8.
13. Levine L. Understanding Peyronie's disease. Omaha, NE: Addicus Books; 2007.
14. Gelbard M, Goldstein I, Hellstrom WJ, McMahon CG, Smith T, Tursi J, Jones N, Kaufman GJ, Carson 3rd CC. Clinical efficacy, safety and tolerability of collagenase clostridium histolyticum for the treatment of peyronie disease in 2 large double-blind, randomized, placebo controlled phase 3 studies. J Urol. 2013;190(1):199–207 [Epub 2013 Jan 31].
15. Jordan GH, Carson CC, Lipshultz LI. Minimally invasive treatment of Peyronie's disease: evidence-based progress. BJU Int. 2014;114(1):16–24.
16. Gelbard M. Correction of penile curvature using tunica albuginea plication, flaps, and expansion with fascial grafts. In: Ehrlich R, Alter G, editors. Reconstructive and plastic surgery of the external genitalia: adult and pediatric. Philadelphia: W.B. Saunders Company; 1999. p. 479–88.

Commentary: Peyronie's Disease and Other Anatomical Disorders

Christian J. Nelson

When considered superficially, Peyronie's disease and other conditions that result in penile curvature or deformity may be considered "minor" issues in a man's sexual health. After all, penile curvature is often imminently treatable, whether using medication or via a surgical approach, and minor penile curvature may not be so severe as to impact sexual function. Often, little consideration is given to the psychological ramifications of conditions that alter penile anatomy. This may be in part due to the private nature of these conditions and the reluctance of men to talk about them. One should also not overlook the fact that the physicians treating these conditions—urologists—often approach them from a physical perspective, seeking to address the condition directly with the assumption that this will result in cure.

In the preceding chapter, the organic etiologies and treatment approaches to penile deformities, in particular Peyronie's disease, are laid out in detail. What most clinicians do not consider, however, is the significant psychological impact that Peyronie's disease can have on affected men, with many of these men having depressive symptoms and relationship issues attributable to their penile deformity. The following commentary, however, outlines the current knowledge on the psychological impact of Peyronie's disease, showing just how potently affected these men can be. Knowing that penile deformity can significantly alter a man's psychological perspectives and deeply affect his relationships is worthwhile for the clinician and should prompt a discussion with the patient about these often overlooked aspects of these conditions. Only by understanding the global impact of penile deformity on the patient's condition can appropriate, truly curative, treatment be implemented.

The Editors

Christian J. Nelson, Ph.D.
Memorial Sloan Kettering Cancer Center, New York, NY, USA

Commentary

It should not be surprising that many men experience distress related to Peyronie's disease (PD). Gelbard and colleagues were the first to characterize the psychological impact of PD in 1990 [1]. They conducted a survey of 97 men with PD that included an assessment of "psychological effects" and reported that 77 % indicated a psychological impact from their PD. Of these men, 36 % indicated that the psychological impact remained the same and did not improve with time, while 36 % said that is worsened [1]. Even of the men who had improvement in their PD symptoms, up to half indicated that they worried about the PD "frequently" or "all the time."

A study by Smith and colleagues supports the results of the Gelbard study. Smith et al. discovered that over 80 % of men reported "emotional difficulties" related to their PD [2]. Importantly, 50 % of men endorsed relationship problems due to PD. Smith and colleagues also identified possible predictors of this distress. The presence of relationship problems and loss of penile length were significant and independent predictors of emotional problems due to PD. Likewise, emotional difficulties and the inability to have intercourse were independent predictors of relationship problems. To address these psychological problems, the authors suggested that physicians integrate a psychosocial evaluation early in the assessment phase of PD to facilitate referrals for appropriate mental health therapy [2].

Nelson and colleagues sought to specifically assess the level of depression that men with PD experience. In 92 patients with PD, 48 % of men reported clinically meaningful depression (26 % moderate; 21 % severe) [3]. Men who were single and self-reported greater loss of penile length were more likely to also report depressive symptoms. In support of the Gelbard study discussed above, the analyses showed that depression remained consistently high over time, regardless of length of time since diagnosis of PD. The authors argue that physicians should go beyond the role of treating the PD and facilitate proper evaluation and treatment of the emotional and relationship ramifications of the disease [3].

Rosen and colleagues conducted a qualitative study to better understand men's experience with PD, highlighting important concerns among men with PD [4]. Men reported significant distress related to the physical appearance of their penis. Regardless of the severity of their PD, the psychological distress was consistently high for all affected men. Some men expressed that "even looking at or touching their penis was unpleasant." Men with PD described feelings of shame and inadequacy and discussed how PD impacted their masculinity, stating that they felt like "less of a man" as a consequence of their penile deformity. Men reported a decreased sense of sexual attractiveness, sexual interest, and sexual confidence. As a result, patients were hesitant to initiate sexual relations with a partner, while single men avoided dating. The feelings of bother in men with PD were extreme and highly distressing [4].

All men reported a significant decrease in their sexual satisfaction since the onset of PD. Many reported that PD impacted other aspects of their sexuality as well and endorsed an increase in performance anxiety in addition to difficulties with erection, ejaculation, or other aspects of sexual function [4]. Practically all men with PD were afraid that they were not satisfying their partners sexually, although none had sought counseling together with their partners. Importantly, men reported a sense of social stigmatization and isolation. Many men with PD found it hard to discuss this condition with their health care professionals, their partners, or their friends, leaving them feeling chronically stigmatized and socially isolated over time.

Case Study

Bob was a 45-year-old man who developed PD. During a sexual encounter with his wife, he stated that he "injured his penis" followed by a significant amount of pain and bleeding. Following this penile injury, he reported about 30 degrees of curvature. He presented to a sexual medicine clinic for treatment of his PD, and at the time his wife strongly suggested he see a mental health professional. He and his wife reported that he was depressed as a result of the PD and that he was spending less time with his family, which included his wife and his two young children. Bob indicated that he did not enjoy playing with his children, that he felt "different" than other men, and that he could not talk about his PD with anyone because he was fearful of what they would say and who they might tell. He was started on intralesional verapamil injections to treat the PD, and during this time, he continued to report significant frustration related to his PD. He continued to feel isolated and felt like he had a "disease" that no one had heard about and the treatment for which was like some "medieval torture."

He eventually agreed to see a psychologist to address his PD-related distress. Bob's therapy focused on helping the patient reengage in sexual relations with his wife. He was afraid to attempt intercourse because he feared reinjuring his penis and was anxious that he would not be able to please his wife sexually or that his attempts would end in failure. His therapy also focused on helping him feel less isolated. He eventually identified one friend who he could confide in about his PD, providing an important sounding board in the recovery process. Eventually, Bob's depression lifted during treatment, and he was able to see that there were many important and meaningful aspects of his life and that he could continue to have a meaningful sex life with his wife.

References

1. Gelbard MK, Dorey F, James K. The natural history of Peyronie's disease. J Urol. 1990;144(6):1376–9.
2. Smith JF, et al. Risk factors for emotional and relationship problems in Peyronie's disease. J Sex Med. 2008;5(9):2179–84.
3. Nelson CJ, et al. The chronology of depression and distress in men with Peyronie's disease. J Sex Med. 2008;5(8):1985–90.
4. Rosen R, et al. Impact of Peyronie's disease on sexual and psychosocial functioning: qualitative findings in patients and controls. J Sex Med. 2008;5(8):1977–84.

The Future of Erectile Dysfunction Therapy I: Implementation of Translational Research

11

Michael Pan and Jason R. Kovac

11.1 Introduction

Erectile dysfunction (ED), defined as the inability to develop and maintain a penile erection satisfactory for sexual intercourse, is a widespread clinical problem. The prevalence of ED increases with age, and up to 77.5 % of men aged 75 and older are affected [1]. Current pharmacological options such as phosphodiesterase 5 inhibitors (PDE5i's), while effective, do not produce satisfactory results for many men [2]. Indeed, the success rates for sildenafil, the first and prototypical PDE5i, are up to 82 % [2]. For the many men with ED that do not respond to PDE5i's, including those who have undergone non-nerve-sparing radical prostatectomy, there remain few nonsurgical or minimally invasive treatment options for their ED.

Current practice involves the use of intracavernosal injections (ICI) and intraurethral suppositories using vasodilator medications as second-line therapies and surgical implantation of inflatable penile prostheses (IPP) to treat ED refractory to pharmacotherapy as third-line treatment. Understanding the various biochemical pathways involved in erectile function is critically important for the development of novel therapies, as deficient and/or malfunctioning pathways represent targets for therapeutic intervention. Currently, available treatment modalities often address only the symptoms of ED but fail to definitively and durably correct the underlying pathophysiology.

Several novel therapies target the reversal and/or prevention of the underlying endothelial and vascular dysfunction and nerve injury that are major components of ED pathophysiology. While many physicians understand the need for more options for the effective management of ED, these have yet to be put into practice. This chapter focuses on several promising potential and novel treatment modalities including nanoparticles, shockwave therapy, stem cells, tissue engineering, and gene therapy.

11.2 Nanoparticles

Nanoparticles represent a novel and exciting field in the treatment of ED. Friedman et al. [3] in 2008 described a novel nanoparticle delivery platform using a hydrogel- and nitrite-containing glass composites for delivery of small peptides and small molecules, including nitric oxide (NO), to tissues [3, 4]. Physiologically, the NO and

M. Pan, M.D.
Baylor College of Medicine, Scott Department of Urology, Houston, TX, USA

J.R. Kovac, M.D., Ph.D. (✉)
Urology of Indiana, 12188-A North Meridian Street, Suite 200, Carmel, IN 46032, USA
e-mail: jason.r.kovac@gmail.com

L.I. Lipshultz et al. (eds.), *Management of Sexual Dysfunction in Men and Women*, DOI 10.1007/978-1-4939-3100-2_11

cyclic GMP (cGMP) pathway is one of the primary pathways regulating corporal smooth muscle relaxation and subsequent erection.

On a molecular scale, such a nitrite-containing platform consists of a stable amorphous solid with strong hydrogen bonds creating lattices to entrap dry NO and subsequently release it on exposure to moisture. This platform is extremely effective at generating, storing, and releasing NO [3]. Initial work has found nanoparticles constructed from sugar-derived glassy matrices to have smaller pores than those constructed from silica "sol-gel"-based matrices [5] and that by mixing glassy and "sol-gel" components together, matrix pore size can be modified to dramatically alter and fine-tune the rate of release of the particles' contents [3].

Nitric oxide is an important mediator of vasodilation throughout the body and is essential for penile erection, inducing the production of cGMP and subsequent activation of protein kinase G followed by smooth muscle relaxation in the penile vasculature. Previous studies suggest that decreases in NO production are associated with ED secondary to aging, diabetes mellitus, and cavernous nerve injury [6]. By increasing cGMP levels within the corporal cavernosal endothelial cells, administration of NO has the potential to work synergistically with PDE5i to further inhibit cGMP breakdown. Such an approach, via administration of NO-releasing nanoparticles, has the potential to improve erectile function and responsiveness to PDE5i in patients with ED.

The ability of NO-releasing nanoparticles to improve ED in animal studies has been promising. Han et al. [4] were able to construct nanoparticles capable of carrying drugs including tadalafil and sialorphin, a neutral endopeptidase inhibitor that can cause erections by potentially prolonging the activity of signaling molecules at their receptors [4, 7, 8]. Recent work used nanoparticles containing NO, sialorphin, tadalafil, and placebo that were applied as a gel to the glans penis and penile shaft of diabetic rats [4]. Rats treated with NO and sialorphin nanoparticle microspheres had spontaneous erections, and those treated with tadalafil-containing nanoparticles exhibited increased mean intracavernosal pressures (ICP) with visibly improved erectile response following cavernous nerve stimulation (CNS) [4]. Taken together, the study by Han et al. [4] proved the feasibility of creating a nanoparticle-based delivery system to transport NO and other drugs directly to the corpora cavernosa.

Another recent study of fluorescently tagged NO-releasing nanoparticle microspheres showed persistent release of NO for 4 weeks in vitro [9]. Measurement of various parameters of erectile function after CNS also found significantly increased peak penile ICP to mean arterial pressure (MAP) ratios in the microsphere and combined microsphere and sildenafil treatment groups when compared with control and sildenafil only groups [9]. The microspheres were also seen to enhance the effect of sildenafil for 3 weeks. Lastly, after injection into the corpus cavernosum of adult diabetic rats, NO microspheres did not migrate into adjacent tissues, providing further evidence for the safety of the technique [9].

In summary, nanoparticles provide a promising platform for the treatment of ED. Several characteristics of these particles lend themselves particularly well for treatment, including their stability at room temperature and minimal toxicity [3]. The ability to fine-tune the rate of release of nanoparticle contents anywhere from an initial burst to a protracted, slow release makes this platform particularly effective for drug delivery [3]. The particles also have the ability to carry various pharmacologic agents, including NO or PDE5i's, directly into desired tissue [3, 4]. Application of a gel or injection containing these nanoparticles to a specific site may also help to prevent systemic side effects, such as the headache, flushing, and congestion associated with PDE5i's [4, 10]. In addition, absorption of PDE5i's can be heavily affected by diet, and the drug is subject to first-pass metabolism by the liver, creating individual differences in serum levels among patients [4, 11]. Local application of nanoparticles can help to mitigate many of these concerns. Indeed, the glans penis may be an excellent site for such local transdermal applications given its rich venous supply and the absence of tunica albuginea that may act as a physical barrier to the corpus cavernosum [4]. Further studies are necessary, but the premise bears promise.

11.3 Stem Cells

The use of stem cell therapy)has attracted significant attention, particularly regarding its potential applications in men with post-prostatectomy ED. Currently, few options exist for patients with post-radical prostatectomy ED as a result of cavernosal nerve damage. Stem cells have the ability to divide and renew themselves over a protracted time frame while retaining the ability to differentiate into specialized cells (including endothelial, smooth muscle, and neuronal cells) and replace damaged tissues [12–23]. Stem cells can also be combined with other treatment approaches, such as tissue engineering and gene therapy, to provide increased efficacy.

The best-studied stem cells in the treatment of ED are adipose tissue-derived stem cells (ADSCs). However, stems cells obtained from muscle and bone marrow have also been evaluated [21, 24–26]. ADSCs are isolated from the stromal vascular fraction of adipose tissue. Advantages of using ADSCs in stem cell therapy include easy accessibility and plentiful supply [21]. Previous studies have documented success in rats when ADSCs were injected directly into the corpus cavernosum with improvements in ICP/MAP and increased NOS expression [27–29]. Other studies demonstrated the ability of ADSCs to partially regenerate damaged cavernous nerves [28, 30].

Recent studies have found that injection of ADSCs along with brain-derived neurotrophic factor (BDNF) and FGF2-hydrogel into the corpus cavernosum of rats with bilateral cavernosal nerve crush injury induced incrementally greater responses in ICP/MAP and increased smooth muscle/collagen ratios, neuronal NOS content, α-SMA expression, and cGMP compared to rats who received treatments with ADSCs alone [31]. Interestingly, no significant differences were observed between rats treated with FGF2-hydrogel and ADSC/BDNF compared to control rats without cavernous nerve crush injury [31]. Addition of the PDE5i udenafil to ADSCs/BDNF resulted in marked improvements in erectile function and preservation of corpus cavernosum architecture [32]. Udenafil also increased expression of VEGF, but not neuronal NOS (nNOS), indicating that inclusion of udenafil with ADSC treatment may have a synergistic effect [32].

Treatment of ED using stem cells derived from other tissues has also shown promising results. Urine-derived stem cells express mesenchymal stem cell markers, and transfection of these cells with FGF2 induces expression of the endothelial markers CD31 and von Willebrand factor (vWF) [26]. Intracavernous injection of these stem cells with and without FGF2 has shown increased expression of endothelial and smooth muscle cell markers [26]. When injected into the corpus cavernosum of rats, muscle-derived stem cells exhibited smooth muscle morphology and increased expression of α-SMA while bone marrow-derived stem cells increased smooth muscle content as well as penile nNOS, neurofilament, and cavernous endothelial content [24, 25].

In summary, stem cells appear potentially effective at improving ED, primarily in the experimental animal. More studies are required, especially in man, prior to wide-scale acceptance of the technique.

11.4 Tissue Engineering

Tissue engineering aims) to generate new tissues by using an artificial "support system" that serves as a scaffold for and stimulates tissue growth [6]. The newly formed tissue should resemble the function and structure of native tissues as closely as possible. The scaffold can be created using various materials such as decellularized xenografts, allografts, autografts, or synthetic materials that can then be seeded using stem cells and differentiated cell lines or used to stimulate growth of native tissue [6].

Current investigations using tissue engineering principles have produced exciting results with the regeneration of nerve, cavernosal, and tunica albuginea tissues [6]. Regeneration of cavernosal and tunica albuginea tissue may play a larger role in reconstruction of penile tissues after trauma, burns, or other injuries; however, tissue engineering of nerves represents a significant innovation in the treatment of ED due to cavernosal nerve injury during radical prostatectomy.

Application of tissue engineering techniques via neural tissue grafting may promote nerve regeneration and recovery of erectile function. End-to-end suturing of nerves and primary repair of the nerve are limited to bridging gaps of 5 mm [33]. Distances greater than 5 mm typically require interposed bridging materials that serve as a guide for growing axons. These engineered materials can extend the repairable gap distance to ~3 cm [33]. The current gold standard of nerve repair is autologous nerve grafting, but this approach is fraught with disadvantages including requirement of a second surgical site for nerve harvesting, damage to the harvested nerve, infection of the harvest site, and size and internal structure mismatches between the graft and target nerves [33].

With regard to the role of tissue engineering in ED, early animal studies in rats whose cavernous nerves were excised found that reconstruction of the cavernous nerve by interposition of silicone tubes seeded with Schwann cells resulted in greater erectile responses to neurostimulation compared to rats treated with Schwann cell grafts or silicone tubes alone [34]. Schwann cells are important in that they are able to stimulate regeneration of damaged nerves through the production of extracellular matrix as well as through remyelination and regeneration of axons while secreting neurotrophic factors such as the Sonic hedgehog (SHH) protein [34, 35].

SHH is essential in the maintenance of cavernous nerve architecture and likely acts through regulation of BDNF [36, 37], which enhances nerve growth through activation of the JAK/STAT pathway [38, 39]. Treatment of rats with bilateral cavernosal nerve crush injuries using linear peptide amphiphile nanofibers, a platform for extended release of SHH, promoted cavernosal nerve regeneration, suppressed penile apoptosis, and resulted in a 58 % improvement in erectile function compared to controls [36]. Peptide amphiphile nanofibers are biodegradable and are advantageous for their ability to provide directional guidance for growing axons as well as the ability to continually release proteins for an extended period [36].

Implanted tubes constructed of polycaprolactone fumarate (PCLF) have demonstrated significantly greater myelin thickness in recovering nerves compared to other materials such as poly-l-lactide acid, poly-lactic-co-glycolic acid, and oligo(polyethylene glycol) [33]. However, nerve autografts generally showed greater electrophysiological recovery and number of regenerated axons than the biomaterials studied [33].

When applied to decellularized corporal collagen scaffolds in animal studies, autologous and muscle-derived stem cell (MDSC)-derived smooth muscle and endothelial cells, as well as umbilical artery smooth muscle cells, have shown progressive regeneration of smooth muscle similar to that of native tissues [40–42]. Indeed, rabbits with their entire pendular penile corpora replaced with tissue generated using autologous smooth muscle and endothelial cell-seeded scaffolds had the ability to achieve erections rigid enough to copulate and impregnate females compared to negative controls [41].

Other studies have found that tissue engineering can regenerate the tunica albuginea as well [43]. For example, rats with Peyronie's disease underwent plaque excision and grafting using tunica albuginea grafts of human umbilical cells seeded onto sheets of human fibroblasts [43], with resulting endothelial cells forming capillary-like structures in addition to extracellular matrix produced entirely by fibroblasts [43]. Furthermore, in a model of tunica albuginea excision, grafts of porcine small intestinal mucosa seeded with ADSCs showed significant restoration of erectile function and increased endothelial and neural NOS expression compared to rats that received graft alone [44].

11.5 Gene Therapy

Gene therapy has) many exciting potential applications, from the correction of genetic defects to the repair of genetic material due to oxidative damage or other DNA injuries. Gene therapy focuses on the introduction of foreign genetic material into cells with the aim of restoring defective cellular function or suppressing aberrant cellular processes [45]. Genetic material can be delivered to the patient through a variety of methods: introduction of cells containing the desired genetic information to host tissues; insertion of genetic material into the nuclei of host cells via viruses, naked DNA transfer, cDNA liposomes, and polyethylenimine; or transfection of mesenchymal stem cells that are then implanted and allowed to divide and differentiate [6]. The penis is an excellent target for gene therapy for several reasons: its external location provides easy access to penile tissue and it can be readily isolated from the systemic circulation using a constriction band at its base, preventing systemic spread of foreign genetic material [46]. Moreover, gap junctions between cavernosal smooth muscle cells enable signal transduction even if only a small number of cells are modified [46]. Lastly, the slow turnover rate of smooth muscle cells enables the effects of any genetic modulation to persist for an extended period [46].

Major targets for gene therapy include the pathways involved in the normal erectile response including the NO-cGMP-PKG pathway (described above) as well as the modulation of endothelial and neural growth factors. Potential targets of the NO-cGMP-PKG pathway that can be upregulated include the actions of NOS, the activity of cGMP-dependent protein kinase, and suppression of the protein inhibitor of NOS [47–51]. Previous studies have shown that stem cells and myoblasts can be transfected using adenoviruses containing genetic information and implanted into the corpora cavernosa [52–54], resulting in significant increases in ICP/MAP and inducible NOS and highlighting the potential for this type of approach [52–54].

Modulation of growth factors such as BDNF and VEGF can also improve erectile function. In rats fed a high-cholesterol diet, transfection of BDNF into host cells via adenovirus resulted in increased nNOS-stained nerve fibers and higher ICP than in controls [55, 56]. Kato et al. [57, 58] have also studied a neurotrophic factor called neurturin, a member of the glial cell line-derived neurotrophic factors (GDNFs), and found that rats with cavernous nerve injury treated with neurturin had significant recovery of ICP and improved survival of major pelvic ganglion neurons [57, 58]. Transfection of VEGF-encoding genes into penile corpus cavernosal cells resulted in regeneration of smooth muscle and nerves in addition to endothelial cell hypertrophy and overall improvement in maximal ICP [59, 60].

Smad7, a protein that inhibits Smad2 and Smad3 and the TGF-β pathway, is also a potential gene therapy target for ED treatment. After intracavernosal injection of adenovirus encoding Smad7, cavernosal tissues exhibited decreased endothelial cell apoptosis and increased endothelial NOS phosphorylation, as well as increased production of extracellular matrix proteins like plasminogen activator inhibitor-1, fibronectin, collagen type I, and collagen type IV [61]. Lastly, the modulation of other targets such as superoxide dismutase and RhoA/Rho kinase and the expression of various potassium channels are promising as potential ED treatments as well [62–66]. Given this information, gene therapy appears to be poised to develop worthwhile treatments in the future, with the primary difficulty resting with selection of the most appropriate gene targets.

11.6 Alternative Therapies

A variety of other novel pharmacologic treatments are being studied as potential treatments for ED. Melatonin, an endogenous hormone produced by the pineal gland, affects sleep, direction orientation, sexual maturation, and sperm motility [67] but is also a potent antioxidant and scavenger of reactive oxygen species [68]. Melatonin is also)produced by the testes, and chronic administration of the hormone inhibits reproductive behavior in male rats [69, 70]. In addition, recent studies indicate that melatonin supplementation may prevent the development of ED in certain cases. Indeed, rats injected with 100 μg/kg of melatonin demonstrated significantly increased mating behavior frequency and decreased time to mounting and intromission compared to control rats [67]. Studies of melatonin administration in rats at a dose of 10 mg/kg injected intraperitoneally showed increased ICP and reversal of oxidative changes caused by diabetes mellitus and spinal cord injury [68, 71]. The results from these preliminary studies suggest that melatonin may play a role in preventing oxidative damage to the cavernous nerves and may have a role in ED prevention.

Other novel pharmacologic therapies include rho kinase inhibitors and valproic acid. RhoA and ROCK, the major downstream target of RhoA,) enhance calcium sensitivity and lead to smooth muscle contraction [72]. Bilateral cavernous nerve injury results in upregulation of ROCK signaling in the penis, suggesting that increased smooth muscle contraction resulting from this increased signaling may contribute to the development of ED [72]. A ROCK inhibitor administered to a bilateral cavernous nerve injury rat model showed improvement in peak ICP and ICP/MAP with restoration of NO pathway signaling and significantly fewer apoptotic cells compared to injured controls. Valproic acid, widely used in the treatment of seizure disorders and bipolar mania, can also prevent penile fibrosis and development of ED in rats with bilateral cavernous nerve injuries, suggesting another potential role for this drug [73].

11.7 Summary

This chapter has examined the role of nanoparticles, stem cells, tissue engineering, and gene therapy for the treatment of ED. While several modalities have made the advance to human studies, much work still needs to be conducted for these novel ED treatments to become part of the treatment paradigm for ED.

Acknowledgments JRK is an NIH K12 Scholar supported by a Male Reproductive Health Research Career (MRHR) Development Physician-Scientist Award (HD073917-01) from the Eunice Kennedy Shriver National Institute of Child Health and Human Development (NICHD) Program.

References

1. Saigal CS, Wessells H, Pace J, Schonlau M, Wilt TJ, Urologic Diseases in America Project. Predictors and prevalence of erectile dysfunction in a racially diverse population. Arch Intern Med. 2006;166(2):207–12. PubMed PMID: 16432090.
2. Guay AT, Perez JB, Jacobson J, Newton RA. Efficacy and safety of sildenafil citrate for treatment of erectile dysfunction in a population with associated organic risk factors. J Androl. 2001;22(5):793–7. PubMed PMID: 11545291.
3. Friedman AJ, Han G, Navati MS, Chacko M, Gunther L, Alfieri A, et al. Sustained release nitric oxide releasing nanoparticles: characterization of a novel delivery platform based on nitrite containing hydrogel/glass composites. Nitric Oxide Biol Chem. 2008;19(1):12–20. PubMed PMID: 18457680.
4. Han G, Tar M, Kuppam DS, Friedman A, Melman A, Friedman J, et al. Nanoparticles as a novel delivery vehicle for therapeutics targeting erectile dysfunction. J Sex Med. 2010;7(1 Pt 1):224–33. PubMed PMID: 19765204. Pubmed Central PMCID: 2864537.
5. Kawashita M, Tsuneyama S, Miyaji F, Kokubo T, Kozuka H, Yamamoto K. Antibacterial silver-containing silica glass prepared by sol-gel method. Biomaterials. 2000;21(4):393–8. PubMed PMID: 10656321.
6. Hakim L, Van der Aa F, Bivalacqua TJ, Hedlund P, Albersen M. Emerging tools for erectile dysfunction: a role for regenerative medicine. Nat Rev Urol. 2012;9(9):520–36. PubMed PMID: 22824778.
7. Tong Y, Tar M, Davelman F, Christ G, Melman A, Davies KP. Variable coding sequence protein A1 as a marker for erectile dysfunction. BJU Int. 2006;98(2):396–401. PubMed PMID: 16879685. Pubmed Central PMCID: 2034203.
8. Tong Y, Tar M, Melman A, Davies K. The opiorphin gene (ProL1) and its homologues function in erectile physiology. BJU Int. 2008;102(6):736–40. PubMed PMID: 18410445. Pubmed Central PMCID: 2872073.
9. Soni SD, Song W, West JL, Khera M. Nitric oxide-releasing polymeric microspheres improve diabetes-related erectile dysfunction. J Sex Med. 2013;10(8):1915–25. PubMed PMID: 23751157.
10. Alpert JS. Nanette K. Wenger: a woman's life in cardiology. Clin Cardiol. 2004;27(2):114–5. PubMed PMID: 14979635.
11. Jetter A, Kinzig-Schippers M, Walchner-Bonjean M, Hering U, Bulitta J, Schreiner P, et al. Effects of grapefruit juice on the pharmacokinetics of sildenafil. Clin Pharmacol Ther. 2002;71(1):21–9. PubMed PMID: 11823754.

12. Skolarikos A, Alargof E, Rigas A, Deliveliotis C, Konstantinidis E. Shockwave therapy as first-line treatment for Peyronie's disease: a prospective study. J Endourol. 2005;19(1):11–4. PubMed PMID: 15735375.
13. Liu J, Zhou F, Li GY, Wang L, Li HX, Bai GY, et al. Evaluation of the effect of different doses of low energy shock wave therapy on the erectile function of streptozotocin (STZ)-induced diabetic rats. Int J Mol Sci. 2013;14(5):10661–73. PubMed PMID: 23698784. Pubmed Central PMCID: 3676859.
14. Gruenwald I, Appel B, Kitrey ND, Vardi Y. Shockwave treatment of erectile dysfunction. Ther Adv Urol. 2013;5(2):95–9. PubMed PMID: 23554844. Pubmed Central PMCID: 3607492.
15. Holfeld J, Tepekoylu C, Kozaryn R, Urbschat A, Zacharowski K, Grimm M, et al. Shockwave therapy differentially stimulates endothelial cells: implications on the control of inflammation via toll-like receptor 3. Inflammation. 2014;37(1):65–70. PubMed PMID: 23948864.
16. Wang CJ, Yang YJ, Huang CC. The effects of shockwave on systemic concentrations of nitric oxide level, angiogenesis and osteogenesis factors in hip necrosis. Rheumatol Int. 2011;31(7):871–7. PubMed PMID: 20232068.
17. Zuoziene G, Laucevicius A, Leibowitz D. Extracorporeal shockwave myocardial revascularization improves clinical symptoms and left ventricular function in patients with refractory angina. Coron Artery Dis. 2012;23(1):62–7. PubMed PMID: 22107803.
18. Ciccone MM, Notarnicola A, Scicchitano P, Sassara M, Carbonara S, Maiorano M, et al. Shockwave therapy in patients with peripheral artery disease. Adv Ther. 2012;29(8):698–707. PubMed PMID: 22869515.
19. Qiu X, Lin G, Xin Z, Ferretti L, Zhang H, Lue TF, et al. Effects of low-energy shockwave therapy on the erectile function and tissue of a diabetic rat model. J Sex Med. 2013;10(3):738–46. PubMed PMID: 23253086. Pubmed Central PMCID: 3593747.
20. Vardi Y, Appel B, Kilchevsky A, Gruenwald I. Does low intensity extracorporeal shock wave therapy have a physiological effect on erectile function? Short-term results of a randomized, double-blind, sham controlled study. J Urol. 2012;187(5):1769–75. PubMed PMID: 22425129.
21. Condorelli RA, Calogero AE, Vicari E, Favilla V, Morgia G, Cimino S, et al. Vascular regenerative therapies for the treatment of erectile dysfunction: current approaches. Andrology. 2013;1(4):533–40. PubMed PMID: 23658196.
22. Zhang H, Yang R, Wang Z, Lin G, Lue TF, Lin CS. Adipose tissue-derived stem cells secrete CXCL5 cytokine with neurotrophic effects on cavernous nerve regeneration. J Sex Med. 2011;8(2):437–46. PubMed PMID: 21114767. Pubmed Central PMCID: 3176296.
23. Lin G, Banie L, Ning H, Bella AJ, Lin CS, Lue TF. Potential of adipose-derived stem cells for treatment of erectile dysfunction. J Sex Med. 2009;6 Suppl 3:320–7. PubMed PMID: 19267855. Pubmed Central PMCID: 2895916.
24. Xu LJ, Xue BX, Chen D, Gao J, Yang DR, Sun CY, et al. Isolation and passage of muscle-derived stem cells from the rat penile corpora cavernosa and induction of differentiation into smooth muscle cells. Cytotechnology. 2013;66:987–94. PubMed PMID: 24242826.
25. Ryu JK, Kim DH, Song KM, Yi T, Suh JK, Song SU. Intracavernous delivery of clonal mesenchymal stem cells restores erectile function in a mouse model of cavernous nerve injury. J Sex Med. 2014;11(2):411–23. PubMed PMID: 24251583.
26. Ouyang B, Sun X, Han D, Chen S, Yao B, Gao Y, et al. Human urine-derived stem cells alone or genetically-modified with FGF2 Improve type 2 diabetic erectile dysfunction in a rat model. PLoS One. 2014;9(3):e92825. PubMed PMID: 24663037. Pubmed Central PMCID: 3963968.
27. Huang YC, Ning H, Shindel AW, Fandel TM, Lin G, Harraz AM, et al. The effect of intracavernous injection of adipose tissue-derived stem cells on hyperlipidemia-associated erectile dysfunction in a rat model. J Sex Med. 2010;7(4 Pt 1):1391–400. PubMed PMID: 20141586. Pubmed Central PMCID: 3163604.
28. Qiu X, Villalta J, Ferretti L, Fandel TM, Albersen M, Lin G, et al. Effects of intravenous injection of adipose-derived stem cells in a rat model of radiation therapy-induced erectile dysfunction. J Sex Med. 2012;9(7):1834–41. PubMed PMID: 22548750. Pubmed Central PMCID: 3389585.
29. Piao S, Kim IG, Lee JY, Hong SH, Kim SW, Hwang TK, et al. Therapeutic effect of adipose-derived stem cells and BDNF-immobilized PLGA membrane in a rat model of cavernous nerve injury. J Sex Med. 2012;9(8):1968–79. PubMed PMID: 22642440.
30. Ying C, Hu W, Cheng B, Yang M, Zheng X, Wang X. Erectile function restoration after repair of resected cavernous nerves by adipose-derived stem cells combined with autologous vein graft in rats. Cell Mol Neurobiol. 2014;34(3):393–402. PubMed PMID: 24398902.
31. Lee SH, Kim IG, Jung AR, Shrestha KR, Lee JH, Park KD, et al. Combined effects of brain-derived neurotrophic factor immobilized poly-lactic-co-glycolic acid membrane with human adipose-derived stem cells and basic fibroblast growth factor hydrogel on recovery of erectile dysfunction. Tissue Eng A. 2014;20:2446–54. PubMed PMID: 24673637.
32. Jeong HH, Piao S, Ha JN, Kim IG, Oh SH, Lee JH, et al. Combined therapeutic effect of udenafil and adipose-derived stem cell (ADSC)/brain-derived neurotrophic factor (BDNF)-membrane system in a rat model of cavernous nerve injury. Urology. 2013;81(5):1108 e7–14. PubMed PMID: 23522997.
33. Daly WT, Knight AM, Wang H, de Boer R, Giusti G, Dadsetan M, et al. Comparison and characterization of multiple biomaterial conduits for peripheral nerve

repair. Biomaterials. 2013;34(34):8630–9. PubMed PMID: 23937914.
34. May F, Weidner N, Matiasek K, Caspers C, Mrva T, Vroemen M, et al. Schwann cell seeded guidance tubes restore erectile function after ablation of cavernous nerves in rats. J Urol. 2004;172(1):374–7. PubMed PMID: 15201814.
35. Bhatheja K, Field J. Schwann cells: origins and role in axonal maintenance and regeneration. Int J Biochem Cell Biol. 2006;38(12):1995–9. PubMed PMID: 16807057.
36. Angeloni NL, Bond CW, Tang Y, Harrington DA, Zhang S, Stupp SI, et al. Regeneration of the cavernous nerve by Sonic hedgehog using aligned peptide amphiphile nanofibers. Biomaterials. 2011;32(4): 1091–101. PubMed PMID: 20971506. Pubmed Central PMCID: 2993249.
37. Bond CW, Angeloni N, Harrington D, Stupp S, Podlasek CA. Sonic Hedgehog regulates brain-derived neurotrophic factor in normal and regenerating cavernous nerves. J Sex Med. 2013;10(3):730–7. PubMed PMID: 23237228. Pubmed Central PMCID: 3593960.
38. Bella AJ, Lin G, Tantiwongse K, Garcia M, Lin CS, Brant W, et al. Brain-derived neurotrophic factor (BDNF) acts primarily via the JAK/STAT pathway to promote neurite growth in the major pelvic ganglion of the rat: part I. J Sex Med. 2006;3(5):815–20. PubMed PMID: 16942526.
39. Lin G, Bella AJ, Lue TF, Lin CS. Brain-derived neurotrophic factor (BDNF) acts primarily via the JAK/STAT pathway to promote neurite growth in the major pelvic ganglion of the rat: part 2. J Sex Med. 2006;3(5):821–7, discussion 8–9. PubMed PMID: 16942527.
40. Song LJ, Xu YM, Li C, Fu Q, Cui L, Hu XY. Construction of cavernosum smooth muscle using umbilical artery smooth muscle cells seeded on acellular corporal collagen matrices. Int J Androl. 2009;32(5):514–23. PubMed PMID: 18399980.
41. Chen KL, Eberli D, Yoo JJ, Atala A. Bioengineered corporal tissue for structural and functional restoration of the penis. Proc Natl Acad Sci U S A. 2010;107(8):3346–50. PubMed PMID: 19915140. Pubmed Central PMCID: 2840474.
42. Ji C, Min F, Liang W, Chen Y, Pan S, Bin L, et al. Construction of tissue-engineered corpus cavernosum with muscle-derived stem cells and transplantation in vivo. BJU Int. 2011;107(10):1638–46. PubMed PMID: 20868390.
43. Imbeault A, Bernard G, Ouellet G, Bouhout S, Carrier S, Bolduc S. Surgical option for the correction of Peyronie's disease: an autologous tissue-engineered endothelialized graft. J Sex Med. 2011;8(11):3227–35. PubMed PMID: 21718447.
44. Ma L, Yang Y, Sikka SC, Kadowitz PJ, Ignarro LJ, Abdel-Mageed AB, et al. Adipose tissue-derived stem cell-seeded small intestinal submucosa for tunica albuginea grafting and reconstruction. Proc Natl Acad Sci U S A. 2012;109(6):2090–5. PubMed PMID: 22308363. Pubmed Central PMCID: 3277542.
45. Burnett AL. Erectile dysfunction management for the future. J Androl. 2009;30(4):391–6. PubMed PMID: 18802198.
46. Hatzimouratidis K. Editorial comment on: smooth-muscle-specific gene transfer with the human maxi-K channel improves erectile function and enhances sexual behavior in atherosclerotic cynomolgus monkeys. Eur Urol. 2009;56(6):1066. PubMed PMID: 19167151.
47. Bivalacqua TJ, Champion HC, Mehta YS, Abdel-Mageed AB, Sikka SC, Ignarro LJ, et al. Adenoviral gene transfer of endothelial nitric oxide synthase (eNOS) to the penis improves age-related erectile dysfunction in the rat. Int J Impot Res. 2000;12 Suppl 3:S8–17. PubMed PMID: 11002394.
48. Magee TR, Ferrini MG, Davila HH, Zeller CB, Vernet D, Sun J, et al. Protein inhibitor of nitric oxide synthase (NOS) and the N-methyl-D-aspartate receptor are expressed in the rat and mouse penile nerves and colocalize with penile neuronal NOS. Biol Reprod. 2003;68(2):478–88. PubMed PMID: 12533411.
49. Magee TR, Kovanecz I, Davila HH, Ferrini MG, Cantini L, Vernet D, et al. Antisense and short hairpin RNA (shRNA) constructs targeting PIN (protein inhibitor of NOS) ameliorate aging-related erectile dysfunction in the rat. J Sex Med. 2007;4(3):633–43. PubMed PMID: 17433082.
50. Bivalacqua TJ, Kendirci M, Champion HC, Hellstrom WJ, Andersson KE, Hedlund P. Dysregulation of cGMP-dependent protein kinase 1 (PKG-1) impairs erectile function in diabetic rats: influence of in vivo gene therapy of PKG1alpha. BJU Int. 2007;99(6):1488–94. PubMed PMID: 17355372.
51. Chang S, Hypolite JA, Velez M, Changolkar A, Wein AJ, Chacko S, et al. Downregulation of cGMP-dependent protein kinase-1 activity in the corpus cavernosum smooth muscle of diabetic rabbits. Am J Physiol Regul Integr Comp Physiol. 2004;287(4):R950–60. PubMed PMID: 15205187.
52. Bivalacqua TJ, Deng W, Kendirci M, Usta MF, Robinson C, Taylor BK, et al. Mesenchymal stem cells alone or ex vivo gene modified with endothelial nitric oxide synthase reverse age-associated erectile dysfunction. Am J Physiol Heart Circ Physiol. 2007;292(3):H1278–90. PubMed PMID: 17071732.
53. Chancellor MB, Tirney S, Mattes CE, Tzeng E, Birder LA, Kanai AJ, et al. Nitric oxide synthase gene transfer for erectile dysfunction in a rat model. BJU Int. 2003;91(7):691–6. PubMed PMID: 12699487.
54. Tirney S, Mattes CE, Yoshimura N, Yokayama T, Ozawa H, Tzeng E, et al. Nitric oxide synthase gene therapy for erectile dysfunction: comparison of plasmid, adenovirus, and adenovirus-transduced myoblast vectors. Mol Urol. 2001;5(1):37–43. PubMed PMID: 11689150.
55. Bakircioglu ME, Lin CS, Fan P, Sievert KD, Kan YW, Lue TF. The effect of adeno-associated virus mediated brain derived neurotrophic factor in an animal model of neurogenic impotence. J Urol. 2001;165(6 Pt 1):2103–9. PubMed PMID: 11371936.

56. Gholami SS, Rogers R, Chang J, Ho HC, Grazziottin T, Lin CS, et al. The effect of vascular endothelial growth factor and adeno-associated virus mediated brain derived neurotrophic factor on neurogenic and vasculogenic erectile dysfunction induced by hyperlipidemia. J Urol. 2003;169(4):1577–81. PubMed PMID: 12629419.
57. Kato R, Wolfe D, Coyle CH, Huang S, Wechuck JB, Goins WF, et al. Herpes simplex virus vector-mediated delivery of glial cell line-derived neurotrophic factor rescues erectile dysfunction following cavernous nerve injury. Gene Ther. 2007;14(18):1344–52. PubMed PMID: 17611585.
58. Kato R, Wolfe D, Coyle CH, Wechuck JB, Tyagi P, Tsukamoto T, et al. Herpes simplex virus vector-mediated delivery of neurturin rescues erectile dysfunction of cavernous nerve injury. Gene Ther. 2009;16(1):26–33. PubMed PMID: 18668142. Pubmed Central PMCID: 2615792.
59. Dall'Era JE, Meacham RB, Mills JN, Koul S, Carlsen SN, Myers JB, et al. Vascular endothelial growth factor (VEGF) gene therapy using a nonviral gene delivery system improves erectile function in a diabetic rat model. Int J Impot Res. 2008;20(3):307–14. PubMed PMID: 18273028.
60. Rogers RS, Graziottin TM, Lin CS, Kan YW, Lue TF. Intracavernosal vascular endothelial growth factor (VEGF) injection and adeno-associated virus-mediated VEGF gene therapy prevent and reverse venogenic erectile dysfunction in rats. Int J Impot Res. 2003;15(1):26–37. PubMed PMID: 12605238.
61. Song KM, Chung JS, Choi MJ, Jin HR, Yin GN, Kwon MH, et al. Effectiveness of intracavernous delivery of adenovirus encoding Smad7 gene on erectile function in a mouse model of cavernous nerve injury. J Sex Med. 2014;11(1):51–63. PubMed PMID: 24433558.
62. Bivalacqua TJ, Usta MF, Kendirci M, Pradhan L, Alvarez X, Champion HC, et al. Superoxide anion production in the rat penis impairs erectile function in diabetes: influence of in vivo extracellular superoxide dismutase gene therapy. J Sex Med. 2005;2(2):187–97, discussion 97–8. PubMed PMID: 16422885.
63. Chitaley K, Bivalacqua TJ, Champion HC, Usta MF, Hellstrom WJ, Mills TM, et al. Adeno-associated viral gene transfer of dominant negative RhoA enhances erectile function in rats. Biochem Biophys Res Commun. 2002;298(3):427–32. PubMed PMID: 12413959.
64. Christ GJ, Day N, Santizo C, Sato Y, Zhao W, Sclafani T, et al. Intracorporal injection of hSlo cDNA restores erectile capacity in STZ-diabetic F-344 rats in vivo. Am J Physiol Heart Circ Physiol. 2004;287(4):H1544–53. PubMed PMID: 15371262.
65. Christ GJ, Rehman J, Day N, Salkoff L, Valcic M, Melman A, et al. Intracorporal injection of hSlo cDNA in rats produces physiologically relevant alterations in penile function. Am J Physiol. 1998;275(2 Pt 2):H600–8. PubMed PMID: 9683449.
66. Melman A, Biggs G, Davies K, Zhao W, Tar MT, Christ GJ. Gene transfer with a vector expressing Maxi-K from a smooth muscle-specific promoter restores erectile function in the aging rat. Gene Ther. 2008;15(5):364–70. PubMed PMID: 18200069.
67. Drago F, Busa L. Acute low doses of melatonin restore full sexual activity in impotent male rats. Brain Res. 2000;878(1–2):98–104. PubMed PMID: 10996140.
68. Qiu XF, Li XX, Chen Y, Lin HC, Yu W, Wang R, et al. Mobilisation of endothelial progenitor cells: one of the possible mechanisms involved in the chronic administration of melatonin preventing erectile dysfunction in diabetic rats. Asian J Androl. 2012;14(3):481–6. PubMed MID: 22367180. Pubmed Central PMCID: 3720169.
69. Tijmes M, Pedraza R, Valladares L. Melatonin in the rat testis: evidence for local synthesis. Steroids. 1996;61(2):65–8. PubMed PMID: 8750434.
70. Yamada K, Maruyama K, Mogami S, Miyagawa N, Tsuboi M. Influence of melatonin on reproductive behavior in male rats. Chem Pharm Bull. 1992;40(8):2222–3. PubMed PMID: 1423787.
71. Tavukcu HH, Sener TE, Tinay I, Akbal C, Ersahin M, Cevik O, et al. Melatonin and tadalafil treatment improves erectile dysfunction after spinal cord injury in rats. Clin Exp Pharmacol Physiol. 2014;41(4):309–16. PubMed PMID: 24552354.
72. Hannan JL, Albersen M, Kutlu O, Gratzke C, Stief CG, Burnett AL, et al. Inhibition of Rho-kinase improves erectile function, increases nitric oxide signaling and decreases penile apoptosis in a rat model of cavernous nerve injury. J Urol. 2013;189(3):1155–61. PubMed PMID: 23021998. Pubmed Central PMCID: 4007006.
73. Hannan JL, Kutlu O, Stopak BL, Liu X, Castiglione F, Hedlund P, et al. Valproic acid prevents penile fibrosis and erectile dysfunction in cavernous nerve-injured rats. J Sex Med. 2014;11:1442–51. PubMed PMID: 24636283.

12 The Future of Erectile Dysfunction Therapy II: Novel Pharmacotherapy and Innovative Technology

Brian V. Le and Arthur L. Burnett

12.1 Introduction

Erectile dysfunction (ED) is defined by the inability to obtain and maintain a penile erection sufficient for satisfactory sexual performance [1]. It is a condition that affects the quality of life of over 150 million men worldwide [2], and in the United States, it is estimated that almost 52 % of men above age 40 experience ED [3]. A major breakthrough in ED treatment occurred in 1998 with the introduction of sildenafil, a selective phosphodiesterase-5 inhibitor (PDE5i) that potentiates the smooth muscle relaxing effects of cyclic guanosine monophosphate (cGMP), allowing for improved erectile response [4]. Since then, PDE5is have been the first line in ED therapy. However, up to 35 % of ED patients may fail to respond to these drugs and move to second- or third-line therapies which have increasing levels of invasiveness [5]; thus, the quest for improved treatments of ED is ongoing [6]. While current treatment modalities have become easier to administer, more scientifically based, and clinically accepted, they still have shortcomings including inconvenience and limited efficacy and spontaneity. Moreover, these therapies do not correct the underlying physiological problem or prevent ED, whereas an ideal therapy would. These shortcomings are well recognized, with many investigators exploring improved methods to meet this objective. Broadly speaking, such directions include novel pharmacotherapy, gene therapies, tissue engineering, and mechanical technologies. Among these directions, some notable progress has been made in the fields of stem cell therapy, gene therapy, internal pudendal artery stenting, vibratory stimulation, growth factors, and low intensity shockwave therapy. These treatment strategies together are advancing the understanding of erection physiology by identifying key molecular targets as well as prime biological constituents. Continued evaluation of these novel therapeutic modalities will bring new options for the man dealing with erectile dysfunction.

12.2 New Treatments for Erectile Dysfunction

12.2.1 Novel Pharmacotherapy

Small molecule and biologically based pharmacotherapy have been the mainstays of erectile dysfunction treatment, from oral medications to intraurethral suppositories and intracavernosal

B.V. Le, MD (✉)
Department of Urology, University of Wisconsin School of Medicine and Public Health, Madison, WI, USA
e-mail: ble6@jhmi.edu

A.L. Burnett, MD
Brady Urological Institute, Johns Hopkins School of Medicine, Baltimore, MD, USA

L.I. Lipshultz et al. (eds.), *Management of Sexual Dysfunction in Men and Women*, DOI 10.1007/978-1-4939-3100-2_12

(IC) injections. Improved understanding of the mechanisms of erection has identified new targets and avenues for modulating the erectile response. The cell signaling pathways being actively targeted pharmacologically are related to vasodilation (nitric oxide (NO)-cGMP pathways, cAMP pathways) and vasoconstriction (adrenergic pathways, endothelin receptors, angiotensin receptors, and RhoA/Rho kinase).

Given the well-established role of NO in the physiology of erections, there are numerous novel pharmacological therapies targeted at increasing endogenous NO concentrations. A diverse array of strategies is being studied including targeting catalytic enzymes, biochemical cofactors and products, and degradative enzymes. One approach targets the substrate for NO synthases through the administration of L-arginine or inhibiting arginases. Studies in rabbits and diabetic rats provide evidence for improved erectile function and decreased inflammation with administration of L-arginine and analogs [7, 8], as well as studies looking at arginase inhibition [9, 10]. However, it is unclear whether oral administration raises serum levels of L-arginine significantly in humans, although two trials demonstrated some benefit in patients with mild–moderate ED [11, 12]. Another novel strategy targets extracellular signal-related kinase (ERK), whereby inhibition improves cavernosal relaxation in diabetic mice [13]. Of particular interest is the development of guanylate cyclase activators that drive increased cGMP production independent of NO stimulation [14]. In vitro and in vivo studies have demonstrated the benefit of guanylate cyclase activators in various animal models of ED, which increase cGMP production [15, 16]. The pro-erectile effects of these agents are further enhanced with co-administration of PDE5is [17]. These agents are of particular interest in patients who may have impaired endogenous NO release, such as in neurologically impaired patients or those who have undergone prostatectomy. Besides activation of the cGMP pathway, activation of the adenylate cyclase-cAMP pathway has been targeted in the treatment of ED via alprostadil, a cAMP agonist. Adenosine itself is a potent vasodilator and promotes penile erection, although it carries a potential risk for penile fibrosis [18]. As a pharmacotherapy, adenosine is very short-lived and studies looking at intracavernosal injection in men demonstrated increased blood flow but failure to obtain full erections [19].

Strategies targeting vasoconstriction inhibition have made significant progress as well. Recent work has confirmed a major role of the RhoA/Rho-kinase signaling pathway as a dominant regulator of vascular smooth muscle contraction throughout the body as well as in the penis [20]. RhoA/Rho kinase is involved in maintaining the flaccid state through increased noradrenergic tone and has been studied in several animal models [21, 22]. A particular focus of attention for pharmacotherapeutic development is whether the actions of conceivably selective stimulatory or inhibitory binding proteins for this pathway operate in the penis and may be exploited to derive an erectile response specifically and without adverse consequences elsewhere in the body [23]. Several Rho kinase inhibitors improve erectile function in rat models of ED and may do so in the presence of inhibition of nitric oxide synthase (NOS) [24, 25]. Thus, RhoA/Rho kinase represents exciting therapeutic targets in ED. However, findings in animal models have yet to be validated with human trials. Other approaches to suppress vasoconstrictive and anti-erectile mechanisms include α-adrenoreceptor antagonists, endothelin receptor antagonists, and angiotensin receptor antagonists [26]. Several studies demonstrated that selective endothelin receptor A antagonists improve erectile function in animal models of ED [27, 28]. While angiotensin receptors are routinely targeted in the treatment of hypertension with angiotensin-converting enzyme inhibitors and angiotensin receptor blockers, there is an increasing body of evidence that purports beneficial effects on erections by improving cavernosal endothelial function [29, 30].

There is great clinical interest in the area of regenerative medicine through the use of growth factors that may offer neuroprotective and vasculoprotective interventions, improving the erectile response that is damaged by neuropathic disease or injury. An extensive body of work has been accumulated, primarily using experimental rodent models, demonstrating that various neurotrophins and angiogenic factors [i.e., nerve growth factor (NGF), acidic fibroblast growth factor (FIBP), and brain-derived neurotrophic factor (BDNF)] as well as atypical neurotrophic factors such as growth hormone, the morphogenic factor Sonic hedgehog protein (SHH), the cytokine-hormone erythropoietin, vascular endothelial growth factor (VEGF), insulin-like growth factor (IGF-1), and fibroblast growth factor (FGF) play major roles in penile neuronal functions [31–35]. The use of these growth factors is of particular interest in regenerative medicine in scenarios including post-prostatectomy ED. Sonic Hedgehog protein, for instance, promotes cavernous nerve regeneration and improves erectile function after crush injury in animal models and is believed to function in part through the actions of BDNF [36–41]. Angiogenic factors such as VEGF and erythropoietin can promote nerve regeneration, inhibit apoptosis, stimulate cell proliferation, and maintain endothelial function. Local delivery in rabbit and rodent models showed improved recovery of erectile function in castration, diabetes, hyperlipidemia, and peripheral vascular disease models of ED [19]. The idea or restoring or regenerating endogenous mechanisms for erections is certainly an appealing approach; however, human clinical trials have yet to confirm the efficacy of any particular approach.

Overall, novel pharmacotherapy continues to be a fertile ground for future ED treatments with two main approaches underway: pharmacological stimulation/inhibition of pathways involved in the erectile response and regenerative approaches aimed at reversing dysfunction associated with worsening erectile response. RhoA/Rho kinase inhibition is a particularly interesting approach that could be used synergistically with current treatments. However, like other small-molecule therapies, it continues to have the same pharmacokinetic limitations of maintaining adequate blood levels and not treating the underlying disorder. Growth factors offer the promise of reversing the underlying disorder. However, ED tends to be multifactorial and may not be adequately corrected with any one particular approach, and the magnitude of the clinical effect in humans has not been studied. Thus, more work must be done on growth factors to understand their clinical utility and role, be it a limited protective effect when a direct insult is anticipated, such as post-prostatectomy or after radiotherapy, or more widespread use in cases of mild ED.

12.2.2 Mechanical Technologies

12.2.2.1 Internal Pudendal Artery Stenting

Arterial insufficiency is one of the most common etiologies of ED as the penis can be viewed as an extension of the vascular system. Furthermore, ED progression correlates with and often precedes clinical manifestations of vascular diseases, such as coronary artery disease, atherosclerosis, and peripheral vascular disease. However, historical attempts at treating penile arterial insufficiency as a cause of ED through bypass grafts and revascularization procedures were plagued by complications and poor patient selection [26]. Given the lack of clear benefit in ED patients who most commonly suffer from venous leak, as opposed to arterial insufficiency, and the relative high risk of microsurgical vascular reconstructive procedures, the American Urological Association discourages the use of such procedures, except in select situations including otherwise healthy young men with perineal trauma or pelvic fracture [42]. More recently, there have been significant technological advances in the use of interventional procedures to both diagnose and treat stenotic vessels with low risk of complications, such as has been used in coronary artery and peripheral vascular disease. The rationale for the use of stenting in the treatment of ED is that older patients with obstructive atherosclerotic disease who fail to respond to PDE5is may have arterial insufficiency as a significant contributory factor. Furthermore, this subgroup may be identified by angiography in the iliac, internal pudendal, and cavernosal arteries. These stenotic regions are then targeted for dilation and stenting. The Zen

Trial evaluated the use of stents coated with the antiproliferative agent zotarolimus, a derivative of rapamycin (zotarolimus-eluting stent system—Medtronic, Santa Rosa, CA) in patients with internal pudendal artery stenosis [43]. In the trial, 30 patients were treated with drug-eluting stents to the internal pudendal artery after stenosis was identified. All demonstrated significant improvements in peak systolic velocity on duplex studies after the procedure with 14.4 cm/s improvement at 30 days and 22.5 cm/s at 6 months. The primary endpoint was an improvement of ≥4 points on the IIEF-6 ED domain in ≥50 % of subjects, and 59.3 % of patients met this endpoint with no significant complications. Another study looked at balloon dilation of the internal pudendal artery without stenting in a case series of three patients, and patients reported subjective improvement in erectile function [44]. Both studies sought to address the problem of pudendal artery stenosis refractory to PDE5i-mediated smooth muscle relaxation. Another group in Germany sought to treat veno-occlusive dysfunction through selective embolization of veins draining the penis. In a series of 27 patients, the authors reported embolization of the dorsal penile vein with *N*-butyl-2-cyanoacrylate and observed improvements in erectile function in 24 of 27 men with 29.6 % reporting "normal" tumescence and rigidity after the procedure [45].

12.2.2.2 Vibratory Stimulation

While previously mentioned ED therapies focus on potentiating the efferent effects of neural stimulation and downstream vascular responses, vibratory stimulation aims to stimulate afferent nerve pathways, primarily via pudendal-cavernosal reflexes [46]. Vibratory stimulation may provide penile rehabilitative effects that allow for improved erectile responses. Advances in vibratory stimulation led to the introduction and FDA clearance of a handheld vibratory stimulator in 2011. The Viberect (Reflexonic, Chambersburg, PA) provokes penile erections and ejaculation in men through stimulation of the pudendal nerve reflex [46]. Its main role is believed to be through the rehabilitation of nerve tissue through the regular afferent stimulation of nerve fibers. Animal data from male rats and dogs suggests that afferent and efferent pathways via the pudendal nerve branches contribute to the erectogenic response [47, 48]. Preliminary data from clinical trials in spinal cord injury patients [49] as well as non-spinal cord injury patients demonstrate that it is safe and may improve subjective erectile function and urinary incontinence [50], though these studies primarily assessed safety rather than efficacy. Randomized trials and carefully conducted clinical trials are still needed to fully assess the role of vibratory stimulation in the treatment of ED.

12.2.2.3 Shockwave Therapy

Low-intensity extracorporeal shockwave therapy (LI-ESWT) is a novel treatment modality that aims to restore the natural erectile mechanism to allow spontaneous erections. Low-intensity shock wave treatments allow energy transmission through tissue towards a focal point. The basis for this treatment stems from studies done on grafts that demonstrated that sustained treatments of low-intensity ultrasound energy causes micro-trauma, which stimulates enhanced angiogenesis and expression of the angiogenic factor VEGF [51]. This in turn results in improved vasculogenic responses to neural stimulation during the erectile response.

Most studies looking at LI-SWT use approximately 300 shocks per treatment point with an energy density of <0.1 mJ/mm^2 at a frequency of 120 per min, though it is not clear if this is the optimal treatment parameters [52]. Wang et al. demonstrated that LI-SWT stimulated angiogenesis-related growth factors including dNOS, VEGF, and endothelial cell proliferation factors and that the resultant neovascularization persisted for greater than 6 months [53]. This was then tested in animal models of erectile dysfunction and indeed showed enhanced VEGF expression with improved intracorporeal pressures with electrical stimulation [51].

In the first study to evaluate the feasibility and safety of LI-ESWT in humans, investigators enrolled men with ED who had a prior positive response to PDE5i therapy. The authors demonstrated safety and a stable improvement in their

IIEF-ED domain scores from 13.5 to 20.9 over the 6-month study period [54]. This same biweekly, 9-week LI-ESWT protocol was used in two additional studies: one evaluating LI-ESWT in severe ED patients who were poor PDE5i responders and a randomized, double-blind sham controlled study looking at efficacy. Both studies demonstrated feasibility and tolerability of the treatment with modest efficacy, at least in the short term [52, 55]. Such a technique is quite promising if the effects are durable. As opposed to existing pharmacotherapy, this approach attempts to counter the underlying causes of ED allowing increased spontaneity and reduced dependence on pharmacotherapy.

12.2.2.4 Mechanical Implants

It is unknown when regenerative ED therapies such as stem cell, gene, and growth factors will be clinically implemented in humans. In addition, there are still limited clinical trial data for low-intensity shockwave therapy and internal pudendal artery stenting. In the meantime, investigators have sought new ways to improve upon existing ED treatments, such as new penile implants and improvements on existing penile implant technology. Penile implants have very high user satisfaction rates and immediately restore the ability to have erections sufficient for intercourse. Researchers are exploring improvements of existing technologies using new materials, improving user experiences through easier pump manipulation, and simplifying the surgery. Other researchers are investigating shape memory materials with properties that offer improved operating characteristics for the patient and the potential of eliminating the pump and reservoir component of the inflatable penile prosthesis [56].

One approach being pursued is the use of nickel–titanium (Ni–Ti) alloys in penile prostheses. These alloys have the desired characteristics of being biocompatible and superelastic and having shape memory properties. By programming the shape memory material to have an expanded cylindrical shape in its activated state, the prosthesis can mimic the erect state of the cavernosal bodies. When deactivated, the material becomes more flexible and mimics the flaccid state. The process of activation can be through direct heat, external magnetic induction using a handheld device, or a small electrical current. In one study, the Ni–Ti alloy was directly compared to existing prosthetic devices and was found to have similar and sometimes superior mechanical properties to existing penile prosthetic devices [57]. Furthermore, since the transition changes occur with realignment at the molecular level, no hydraulic mechanism is necessary, eliminating the pump and reservoir and allowing a profile similar to current malleable devices, but with the operating characteristics of inflatable prostheses.

Mechanical technologies are quite variable in their approach to the treatment of ED. Some are rehabilitative, as in the case of shock wave therapy and vibratory stimulation, while others address the vasculogenic response or offer significant improvements over existing mechanical treatments. The main advantages of the rehabilitative approaches are that they allow spontaneity, have a low risk profile, and may avoid the use of medications. The disadvantages are the need for repeated treatment sessions using specialized equipment, and the durability of the effect and the need for re-treatment are unknown. Internal pudendal artery stenting targets a subset of ED patients that have internal pudendal artery stenosis as well as ED. The advantages are that it allows a one-time treatment to improve erections and may work with other therapeutic options. The disadvantages are that it may only work for a limited subset of ED patients and the duration of the effect is not known. Despite these limitations, mechanical approaches offer a significant alternative to biochemically based approaches that may be used in combination therapies.

12.3 Conclusions

Significant progress has been made in our understanding of the complex physiology of erections, which has allowed more scientifically based treatments to emerge. Though novel pharmacotherapies are being actively pursued, alternative approaches that aim to improve blood flow, regenerate tissue, and restore cell populations provide exciting therapeutic options for the future.

References

1. Impotence. NIH Consens Statement. 1992;10(4): 1–33.
2. Rajfer J, Magee T, Gonzalez-Cadavid N. Future strategies for treating erectile dysfunction. Rev Urol. 2002;4 Suppl 3:S48–53.
3. Feldman HA, et al. Impotence and its medical and psychosocial correlates: results of the Massachusetts male aging study. J Urol. 1994;151(1):54–61.
4. Goldstein I, et al. Oral sildenafil in the treatment of erectile dysfunction. Sildenafil Study Group. N Engl J Med. 1998;338(20):1397–404.
5. Shamloul R, Ghanem H. Erectile dysfunction. Lancet. 2013;381(9861):153–65.
6. Stein MJ, Lin H, Wang R. New advances in erectile technology. Ther Adv Urol. 2014;6(1):15–24.
7. Hupertan V, et al. Effects of nucleotides adenosine monophosphate and adenosine triphosphate in combination with L-arginine on male rabbit corpus cavernosum tissue. Int J Androl. 2012;35(6):860–6.
8. Cheng YS, et al. Argirein alleviates corpus cavernosum dysfunction by suppressing pro-inflammatory factors p66Shc and ER stress chaperone Bip in diabetic rats. J Pharm Pharmacol. 2013;65(1):94–101.
9. Bivalacqua TJ, et al. Overexpression of arginase in the aged mouse penis impairs erectile function and decreases eNOS activity: influence of in vivo gene therapy of anti-arginase. Am J Physiol Heart Circ Physiol. 2007;292(3):H1340–51.
10. Segal R, et al. Chronic oral administration of the arginase inhibitor 2(S)-amino-6-boronohexanoic acid (ABH) improves erectile function in aged rats. J Androl. 2012;33(6):1169–75.
11. Neuzillet Y, et al. A randomized, double-blind, crossover, placebo-controlled comparative clinical trial of arginine aspartate plus adenosine monophosphate for the intermittent treatment of male erectile dysfunction. Andrology. 2013;1(2):223–8.
12. Cormio L, et al. Oral L-citrulline supplementation improves erection hardness in men with mild erectile dysfunction. Urology. 2011;77(1):119–22.
13. Carneiro FS, et al. DOCA-salt treatment enhances responses to endothelin-1 in murine corpus cavernosum. Can J Physiol Pharmacol. 2008;86(6):320–8.
14. Brioni JD, et al. Activators of soluble guanylate cyclase for the treatment of male erectile dysfunction. Int J Impot Res. 2002;14(1):8–14.
15. Lasker GF, et al. The sGC activator BAY 60-2770 has potent erectile activity in the rat. Am J Physiol Heart Circ Physiol. 2013;304(12):H1670–9.
16. Gur S, Kadowitz PJ, Hellstrom WJ. Exploring the potential of NO-independent stimulators and activators of soluble guanylate cyclase for the medical treatment of erectile dysfunction. Curr Pharm Des. 2010;16(14):1619–33.
17. Albersen M, et al. Synergistic effects of BAY 60-4552 and vardenafil on relaxation of corpus cavernosum tissue of patients with erectile dysfunction and clinical phosphodiesterase type 5 inhibitor failure. J Sex Med. 2013;10(5):1268–77.
18. Wen J, et al. Increased adenosine contributes to penile fibrosis, a dangerous feature of priapism, via A2B adenosine receptor signaling. FASEB J. 2010; 24(3):740–9.
19. Decaluwe K, et al. Treatment of erectile dysfunction: new targets and strategies from recent research. Pharmacol Biochem Behav. 2013;121:146–57.
20. Mills TM, et al. Effect of rho-kinase inhibition on vasoconstriction in the penile circulation. J Appl Physiol (1985). 2001;91(3):1269–73.
21. Bivalacqua TJ, et al. RhoA/Rho-kinase suppresses endothelial nitric oxide synthase in the penis: a mechanism for diabetes-associated erectile dysfunction. Proc Natl Acad Sci U S A. 2004;101(24):9121–6.
22. Burnett AL, et al. Nitric oxide/redox-based signalling as a therapeutic target for penile disorders. Expert Opin Ther Targets. 2006;10(3):445–57.
23. Jin L, Burnett AL. RhoA/Rho-kinase in erectile tissue: mechanisms of disease and therapeutic insights. Clin Sci (Lond). 2006;110(2):153–65.
24. Decaluwe K, et al. New therapeutic targets for the treatment of erectile dysfunction. J Sex Med. 2011;8(12):3271–90.
25. Guagnini F, et al. Erectile properties of the rho-kinase inhibitor SAR407899 in diabetic animals and human isolated corpora cavernosa. J Transl Med. 2012;10:59.
26. Burnett AL. Erectile dysfunction management for the future. J Androl. 2009;30(4):391–6.
27. Xu M, et al. Comparison of sildenafil with strontium fructose diphosphate in improving erectile dysfunction against upregulated cavernosal NADPH oxidase, protein kinase Cepsilon, and endothelin system in diabetic rats. J Pharm Pharmacol. 2012;64(2):244–51.
28. Carneiro FS, et al. Activation of the ET-1/ETA pathway contributes to erectile dysfunction associated with mineralocorticoid hypertension. J Sex Med. 2008;5(12):2793–807.
29. Schlimmer N, et al. Telmisartan, ramipril and their combination improve endothelial function in different tissues in a murine model of cholesterol-induced atherosclerosis. Br J Pharmacol. 2011;163(4):804–14.
30. Kilarkaje N, et al. Role of angiotensin II and angiotensin-(1-7) in diabetes-induced oxidative DNA damage in the corpus cavernosum. Fertil Steril. 2013;100(1): 226–33.
31. Albersen M, et al. Injections of adipose tissue-derived stem cells and stem cell lysate improve recovery of erectile function in a rat model of cavernous nerve injury. J Sex Med. 2010;7(10):3331–40.
32. Podlasek CA, et al. Sonic hedgehog, the penis and erectile dysfunction: a review of sonic hedgehog signaling in the penis. Curr Pharm Des. 2005;11(31): 4011–27.
33. Castela A, et al. Differentially expressed angiogenic genes in diabetic erectile tissue—results from a microarray screening. Mol Genet Metab. 2012; 105(2):255–62.

34. Ichim TE, et al. Intracavernous administration of bone marrow mononuclear cells: a new method of treating erectile dysfunction? J Transl Med. 2013;11:139.
35. Nishimatsu H, et al. Adrenomedullin mediates adipose tissue-derived stem cell-induced restoration of erectile function in diabetic rats. J Sex Med. 2012;9(2):482–93.
36. Bond CW, et al. Sonic Hedgehog regulates brain-derived neurotrophic factor in normal and regenerating cavernous nerves. J Sex Med. 2013;10(3):730–7.
37. Castiglione F, et al. Intratunical injection of human adipose tissue-derived stem cells prevents fibrosis and is associated with improved erectile function in a rat model of Peyronie's disease. Eur Urol. 2013; 63(3):551–60.
38. He Y, et al. Transplantation KCNMA1 modified bone marrow-mesenchymal stem cell therapy for diabetes mellitus-induced erectile dysfunction. Andrologia. 2013;46:479–86.
39. Lin CS, et al. Stem-cell therapy for erectile dysfunction. Expert Opin Biol Ther. 2013;13(11):1585–97.
40. Condorelli RA, et al. Vascular regenerative therapies for the treatment of erectile dysfunction: current approaches. Andrology. 2013;1(4):533–40.
41. Bahk JY, et al. Treatment of diabetic impotence with umbilical cord blood stem cell intracavernosal transplant: preliminary report of 7 cases. Exp Clin Transplant. 2010;8(2):150–60.
42. Montague DK, et al. Chapter 1: The management of erectile dysfunction: an AUA update. J Urol. 2005;174(1):230–9.
43. Rogers JH, et al. Zotarolimus-eluting peripheral stents for the treatment of erectile dysfunction in subjects with suboptimal response to phosphodiesterase-5 inhibitors. J Am Coll Cardiol. 2012;60(25):2618–27.
44. Babaev A, Jhaveri RR. Angiography and endovascular revascularization of pudendal artery atherosclerotic disease in patients with medically refractory erectile dysfunction. J Invasive Cardiol. 2012;24(5): 236–40.
45. Aschenbach R, et al. Endovascular embolisation therapy in men with erectile impotence due to veno-occlusive dysfunction. Eur J Radiol. 2013;82(3): 504–7.
46. Tajkarimi K, Burnett AL. The role of genital nerve afferents in the physiology of the sexual response and pelvic floor function. J Sex Med. 2011;8(5): 1299–312.
47. Sachs BD, Liu YC. Maintenance of erection of penile glans, but not penile body, after transection of rat cavernous nerves. J Urol. 1991;146(3):900–5.
48. Pullen AH, Humphreys P. Protracted elevation of neuronal nitric oxide synthase immunoreactivity in axotomised adult pudendal motor neurons. J Anat. 1999;194(Pt 4):547–65.
49. Everaert K, et al. Neuroanatomy and neurophysiology related to sexual dysfunction in male neurogenic patients with lesions to the spinal cord or peripheral nerves. Spinal Cord. 2010;48(3):182–91.
50. Segal RL, Tajkarimi K, Burnett AL. Viberect penile vibratory stimulation system: evaluation of its erectogenic efficacy. Can J Urol. 2013;20(4):6844–7.
51. Gruenwald I, et al. Shockwave treatment of erectile dysfunction. Ther Adv Urol. 2013;5(2):95–9.
52. Gruenwald I, Appel B, Vardi Y. Low-intensity extracorporeal shock wave therapy—a novel effective treatment for erectile dysfunction in severe ED patients who respond poorly to PDE5 inhibitor therapy. J Sex Med. 2012;9(1):259–64.
53. Wang CJ, et al. Shock wave therapy induces neovascularization at the tendon-bone junction. A study in rabbits. J Orthop Res. 2003;21(6):984–9.
54. Vardi Y, et al. Can low-intensity extracorporeal shockwave therapy improve erectile function? A 6-month follow-up pilot study in patients with organic erectile dysfunction. Eur Urol. 2010;58(2):243–8.
55. Vardi Y, et al. Does low intensity extracorporeal shock wave therapy have a physiological effect on erectile function? Short-term results of a randomized, double-blind, sham controlled study. J Urol. 2012;187(5):1769–75.
56. Le B, Colombo A, Mustoe T, McVary K. Evaluation of novel nickel-titanium alloy for use in penile prostheses. In: AUA conference, San Diego, CA; 2012.
57. Le B, Colombo A, McVary K. Finite element simulation modeling to study the behavior of a novel shape-memory based penile prosthesis. In: SMSNA conference, New Orleans, LA; 2013.

Commentary: The Future of Erectile Dysfunction Therapy II—Novel Pharmacotherapy and Innovative Technology

Michael A. Perelman and Alexander W. Pastuszak

Men with erectile dysfunction (ED) commonly visit their physician first when seeking treatment and are often prescribed medical first-line therapy for their ED. However, these therapies are incompletely effective, and there is a growing understanding that ED, even when organic in origin, has a psychosocial component. This psychosocial contribution is often overlooked or not known by treating physicians. As a result, treatment escalation in most men with ED often remains focused on medical, and finally surgical, therapies, at which point psychotherapy is moot. It is imperative that clinicians understand that ED has psychological ramifications and do not lose sight of the positive effects of incorporating psychotherapy into the treatment of these men. Such a combined therapeutic approach may improve the response to both medical and psychotherapies and decrease the need or dosage of medical therapies.

While Burnett and Kovac focus on the future of ED therapy from a medical perspective in their chapters, a truly comprehensive understanding of the future of ED therapy incorporates an understanding of psychotherapeutic approaches as well. As such, the following commentary highlights psychosocial cultural factors and corresponding mental health approaches to ED that, when applied in combination or in lieu of medical therapies, will optimize ED therapy. A combined, collaborative approach to ED therapy, irrespective of the medical therapy, truly represents the future of ED therapy.

The Editors

Michael A. Perelman, Ph.D. (✉)
Psychiatry, Reproductive Medicine and Urology, Weill Medical College Cornell University, New York, NY, USA

Co-Director, Human Sexuality Program, The New York Presbyterian Hospital, New York, NY, USA

Founder, MAP Education and Research Fund, New York, NY, USA
e-mail: perelman@earthlink.net

Alexander W. Pastuszak, M.D., Ph.D.
Baylor College of Medicine, Division of Male Reproductive, Medicine and Surgery, Center for Reproductive Medicine, Scott Department of Urology, Houston, TX, USA

Commentary

Brian V. Le and Arthur L. Burnett's chapter provides an excellent overview of future opportunities for erectile dysfunction (ED) treatment from a biological point of view with its emphasis on the probable emergence of novel pharmacotherapies, growth factor and stem cell therapies, and mechanical technologies. Le and Burnett also touch on the potential for some of those therapies to be combined with both each other and existing medical treatments to enhance efficacy beyond what is currently available today. However, an appreciation for the additional improvements that a psychosocial-behavioral and cultural (PSBC) paradigm would provide has eluded mention in their chapter and others in this text. Such an integration is not only key to optimizing efficacy; it can also improve treatment safety as drug dosage can be reduced with the inclusion of non-pharmaceutical factors that enhance response to ED treatment. The benefits and rationale for using an integrated treatment approach were partially elucidated in chapter one and have been described extensively elsewhere [1, 2]. An integrated approach can be easily understood using a number of dual control paradigms. However, the Sexual Tipping Point (STP®) model is especially useful when it comes to illustrating integration of future medical modalities within a biopsychosocial-behavioral and cultural model (see Fig. 1.2, 1.3, 1.4). In short, the STP® model provides a conceptual framework for an optimized, integrated treatment approach for every novel future therapy summarized by Le and Burnett.

All cases of ED can be considered of "mixed" etiology, with contributions from both organic and PSBC components [3, 4]. Sachs suggests that there are "neural, neurochemical, and endocrine mechanisms whose participation in erectile function depends on the behavioral context in which erection occurs" [5]. Thus, optimal therapy for ED, and for any sexual dysfunction for that matter, should be approached with an understanding that both the physical and mental aspects of the sexual dysfunction are essential contributors to the pathology and that addressing both facets of the condition will offer the most significant improvements [6]. To provide an example using existing treatments, discontinuation rates of phosphodiesterase 5 inhibitor (PDE5i) therapies in men with ED approach 50 % [7], but 18 % of men who discontinue PDE5is have psychological factors that can readily be addressed using combination therapy [8–12]. Other psychosocial factors, including a couple's dynamics, a man's approach to sex with his partner, and the couple's expectations of the effects of the medical intervention in their love life, are often less obvious to the physician, but are nevertheless essential in restoring full sexual function and are often not considered [13]. By extrapolating from studies of men undergoing psychotherapy where erectile function improvements were observed in the absence of medication [14, 15], as well as examining response rates of ED to placebo in randomized clinical trials (RCTs), it is reasonable to predict that all of the novel treatments Le and Burnett describe could be "dose" titrated down to improve safety profiles when attention to PSBC variables is integrated into the treatment approach. Support for such integration may be found by examining early reports of adjunctive sex therapy for men suffering from organic ED who underwent penile prosthesis placement. Counseling helped set expectations and facilitated the integration of the prosthesis into the sex life of the couple and often resulted in increased patient and partner satisfaction [16–21]. Much recent work argues for an integrative treatment approach in men with ED, and steady progress towards this goal is being made [9, 11, 22–25].

A transdisciplinary approach, whether offered by a solo practitioner or a multidisciplinary team, should always be considered, even as other improvements in systems medicine stand to revolutionize treatment of ED and other sexual dysfunctions [2]. A primary care practitioner (PCP) or urologist may integrate sex counseling with the use of pharmacotherapy in their treatment of ED within the limits of their skill set and available time. The most important PSBC factors can frequently be identified during the course of a proper diagnostic interview using standard techniques for obtaining a focused sexual history and current sex status [26]. However, a collaborative approach, whether using a virtual or in-house team involving sex therapists and the patient's medical care team, will further facilitate and improve care of these patients, particularly in cases with moderate or severe psychosocial complexity where the principle etiologic factors of the patient's ED lie outside the primary provider's expertise [18, 27]. There is even evidence, which only future research will confirm, that such behavioral and cognitive interventions change brain chemistry and neuropathways in a manner that makes success more continuous and minimizes risk of relapse.

Like all medical interventions, future therapy for ED must consider and should rely on a patient-centered approach, guiding treatment based on a patient's goals [12, 18, 28]. Involvement of the patient's partner in the assessment and treatment process is almost always preferable [29]. Yet, urologists who frequently see the man for treatment alone may find it comforting that sex therapy research supports partner cooperation, rather than attendance at each office visit, as the key to treatment success [21]. Nonetheless, regardless of the development and deployment of novel effective and safe approaches to ED, all clinicians are well reminded to emphasize patient and partner pleasure and satisfaction over objective performance, as exemplified by the "Good Enough Sex" model by Metz and McCarthy [30]. Again, the use of a "sex status" examination, which focuses on identifying all the key factors relating to the patient's ED, is critical in comprehensively understanding the landscape of the patient's problem and can help to identify appropriate medical and psychosocial interventions, highlighting the utility of an integrative approach [24]. Of course, the need for patient education and regular follow-up cannot be emphasized enough regardless of treatment novelty, as these facilitate adherence to treatment [11, 31, 32].

In much the same way that Le and Burnett describe exciting targets for both selective inhibition and stimulation of binding proteins that would facilitate erectile activity without adverse consequences elsewhere in the body, psychosocial-behavioral interventions derived from traditional sex therapy, cognitive behavior therapy, and systems approaches all help optimize the efficacy of these future pharmaceutical interventions [1]. Several key signaling pathways and molecules, including nitric oxide (NO) synthases and endogenous NO levels, the angiotensin receptor, extracellular signal-related kinase (ERK), guanylate cyclase modulators, and Rho/RhoA kinase, are highlighted by Le and Burnett as novel pharmacotherapeutic targets. While these pathways and molecules are critically important in the physiologic ability to initiate and maintain an erectile response via positive and negative influences on their respective pathways, and thus the STP®, one must also consider the psychological processes acting through a cascade of central effects, which further influence the STP®. Like PDE5is, sexual stimulation (both mental and physical) will likely potentiate the action of pharmacotherapies targeting the above pathways [15], further highlighting the mind-body connection in sex.

As one contemplates an integrative model, enhancement of arousing factors and minimizing of inhibiting factors must be considered. When discussing growth factors, Le and Burnett focus on neurotrophic and angiogenic factors that are now known to play major roles in penile function and may be of particular interest in situations where damage to the cavernosal nerves occurs, such as post-prostatectomy. Similar to the considerations with pharmacotherapies, each growth factor functions by stimulating a specific physiologic pathway, resulting in improved penile function and exerting a positive influence, tipping the STP® balance scale towards greater sexual responsiveness. While penile physiology may improve using medical treatment, the psychological grief and adjustment that is often an integral part of post-prostatectomy ED [33] is clearly an inhibitor, which is often best addressed using counseling alone or in combination with pharmacotherapy [34].

Although stem cell therapies are oriented towards replacing nonfunctional tissue to restore the natural processes that facilitate erection rather than modulating existing pathways, their impact on physiology likewise integrates excitatory and inhibitory functions and fits into the STP® model, much like the effects of the other medical therapies described by Le and Burnett. Similarly, pudendal artery stenting, low-intensity extracorporeal shock wave therapy (LI-ESWT), and penile vibratory stimulation also improve penile physiology and help to maximize physical potential, but in the absence of optimized psychosocial-behavioral and cultural factors, the patient's STP® may remain closer to "Not" than "Hot," and his true potential remains unmet.

Finally, experimental design is an additional relevant factor that should be considered when evaluating all the exciting potential new treatments for ED described by Le and Burnett. Specifically, advances in understanding the placebo effect and its application to sexual disorders are important considerations [35, 36]. One of the most important elements that psychology brings to medical and pharmaceutical evaluation is the notion of placebo, placebo response, and placebo effect. We should remain mindful that these variables impact our studies and that careful scientific evaluation requires an understanding of these concepts. It is well known that responses to placebo often well exceed 20 % in RCTs evaluating ED treatments. Evidence has also surfaced in some psychiatric drug trials that the therapeutic setting and frequency of visits can account for over 50 % of observed positive responses. To what extent is this true for clinical trials in sexual medicine? It makes intuitive sense that more frequent contact and follow-up with patients may contribute to better responses, and this is supported by the relapse prevention literature [37]. In fact, this effect is even more pronounced in older adults, the very demographic more likely to be suffering from ED [36]. It would be extraordinary if we could better understand how to minimize the placebo effect, particularly in clinical trials, and maximize it during treatment! That indeed would be the type of elegant advance resulting from integration of knowledge from two seemingly disparate areas of science. Yet the benefit to researchers, clinicians, and patients alike would be both remarkable and profound.

In conclusion, it is our belief that almost every sexual experience, whether or not facilitated by a pharmaceutical (or alternative technology), could be enhanced by an increase in erotic thought, a reduction in distracting negative intrusive cognitions, and better quality and pleasing "friction." Improving these elements or more simply put increasing "friction and fantasy" has been advocated by sex therapists for decades [11]. Reciprocally, identifying and successfully targeting key signaling pathways and molecules in the manner outlined by Le and Burnett will improve the erectile capacity of men well beyond the early successes of the last 20 years. The STP® model provides a framework for understanding the subtleties of the combined and variable effects of physiology and psychobiology in sexual function. Such an understanding that addresses all factors involved in the dysfunction will truly optimize, and in the future revolutionize, treatment of ED and other sexual dysfunctions. Integrating medical therapy and counseling potentiates the individual approaches, and the sum of the parts is significantly greater than each part alone (see Fig. 1.4).

References

1. Perelman MA. Integrated sex therapy: a psychosocial-cultural perspective integrating behavioral, cognitive, and medical approaches. In: Carson CC, Kirby RS, Goldstein I, Wyllie MG, editors. Textbook of erectile dysfunction. 2nd ed. London: Informa Healthcare; 2009.
2. Perelman MA. Advocating for a transdisciplinary perspective in sexual medicine. Curr Sex Health Rep. 2015;7(1):1–2.
3. Pastuszak A. Current diagnosis and management of erectile dysfunction. Curr Sex Health Rep. 2014;6: 164–76.
4. Berry MD, Berry PD. Contemporary treatment of sexual dysfunction: reexamining the biopsychosocial model. J Sex Med. 2013;10(11):2627–43.
5. Sachs BD. Contextual approaches to the physiology and classification of erectile function, erectile dysfunction, and sexual arousal. Neurosci Biobehav Rev. 2000;24(5):541–60.
6. Perelman MA. Erectile dysfunction and depression: screening and treatment. Urol Clin N Am. 2011;38(2):125–39.

7. Althof S. Therapeutic weaving: the integration of treatment techniques. In: Levine S, editor. Handbook of clinical sexuality for mental health professionals. New York: Brunner-Routledge; 2003. p. 359–76.
8. Carvalheira AA, Pereira NM, Maroco J, Forjaz V. Dropout in the treatment of erectile dysfunction with PDE5: a study on predictors and a qualitative analysis of reasons for discontinuation. J Sex Med. 2012;9(9):2361–9.
9. Althof SE, Needle RB. Psychological factors associated with male sexual dysfunction: screening and treatment for the urologist. Urol Clin N Am. 2011;38(2):141–6.
10. Banner LL, Anderson RU. Integrated sildenafil and cognitive-behavior sex therapy for psychogenic erectile dysfunction: a pilot study. J Sex Med. 2007;4(4 Pt 2):1117–25.
11. Perelman MA. Sex coaching for physicians: combination treatment for patient and partner. Int J Impot Res. 2003;15 Suppl 5:S67–74.
12. Perelman MA. Psychosocial evaluation and combination treatment of men with erectile dysfunction. Urol Clin N Am. 2005;32(4):431–45, vi.
13. Althof SE. When an erection alone is not enough: biopsychosocial obstacles to lovemaking. Int J Impot Res. 2002;14 Suppl 1:S99–104.
14. Melnik T, Soares BG, Nasselo AG. Psychosocial interventions for erectile dysfunction. Cochrane Database Syst Rev. 2007;(3):CD004825.
15. Dunn ME, Althof SE, Perelman MA. Phosphodiesterase type 5 inhibitors' extended duration of response as a variable in the treatment of erectile dysfunction. Int J Impot Res. 2007;19(2):119–23.
16. Kramer AC, Schweber A. Patient expectations prior to coloplast titan penile prosthesis implant predicts postoperative satisfaction. J Sex Med. 2010;7(6): 2261–6.
17. Mulhall JP, Ahmed A, Branch J, Parker M. Serial assessment of efficacy and satisfaction profiles following penile prosthesis surgery. J Urol. 2003;169(4): 1429–33.
18. Berry M, Berry P. Integrative approaches to the treatment of erectile dysfunction. Curr Sex Health Rep. 2014;6:114–23.
19. McCarthy B, Fucito L. Integrating medication, realistic expectation, and therapeutic interventions in the treatment of male sexual dysfunction. J Sex Marital Ther. 2005;31:319–28.
20. Perelman MA. Rehabilitative sex therapy for organic impotence. In: Segraves T, Haeberle E, editors. Emerging dimensions of sexology. New York: Praeger Publications; 1984. p. 181–8.
21. Perelman MA. The impact of relationship variables on the etiology, diagnosis and treatment of erectile dysfunction. Adv Prim care Med Clin Update. 2007;3:3–6.
22. Wylie KR, Jones RH, Walters S. The potential benefit of vacuum devices augmenting psychosexual therapy for erectile dysfunction: a randomized controlled trial. J Sex Marital Ther. 2003;29(3):227–36.
23. Hawton K. Integration of treatments for male erectile dysfunction. Lancet. 1998;351(9095):7–8.
24. Rosen R. Medical and psychological interventions for erectile dysfunction: toward a combined treatment approach. In: Leiblum S, Rosen R, editors. Principles and practice of sex therapy. New York: Guilford Press; 2000.
25. Simopoulos EF, Trinidad AC. Male erectile dysfunction: integrating psychopharmacology and psychotherapy. Gen Hosp Psychiatry. 2013;35(1):33–8.
26. Althof SE, Rosen RC, Perelman MA, Rubio-Aurioles E. Standard operating procedures for taking a sexual history. J Sex Med. 2013;10(1):26–35.
27. Perelman M. Combination therapy for sexual dysfunction: integrating sex therapy and pharmacotherapy. In: Balon R, Segraves R, editors. Handbook of sexual dysfunction. London: Taylor and Francis; 2005. p. 13–41.
28. Montorsi F, Adaikan G, Becher E, Giuliano F, Khoury S, Lue TF, et al. Summary of the recommendations on sexual dysfunctions in men. J Sex Med. 2010; 7(11):3572–88.
29. Dean J, Rubio-Aurioles E, McCabe M, Eardley I, Speakman M, Buvat J, et al. Integrating partners into erectile dysfunction treatment: improving the sexual experience for the couple. Int J Clin Pract. 2008;62(1): 127–33.
30. Metz M, MCCarthy B. The 'good-enough sex' model for couple sexual satisfaction. Sex Relat Ther. 2007;22(3):351–62.
31. Laumann EO, Paik A, Rosen RC. The epidemiology of erectile dysfunction: results from the National Health and Social Life Survey. Int J Impot Res. 1999;11 Suppl 1:S60–4.
32. Rosen RC. Reproductive health problems in ageing men. Lancet. 2005;366(9481):183–5.
33. Wittmann D, Foley S, Balon R. A biopsychosocial approach to sexual recovery after prostate cancer surgery: the role of grief and mourning. J Sex Marital Ther. 2011;37(2):130–44.
34. Titta M, Tavolini IM, Dal Moro F, Cisternino A, Bassi P. Sexual counseling improved erectile rehabilitation after non-nerve-sparing radical retropubic prostatectomy or cystectomy—results of a randomized prospective study. J Sex Med. 2006;3(2):267–73.
35. Bradford A, Meston CM. Behavior and symptom change among women treated with placebo for sexual dysfunction. J Sex Med. 2011;8(1):191–201.
36. Rutherford BR. Deconstructing placebo response in antidepressant clinical trials placebo. New York: Columbia University/New York State Psychiatric Institute; 2013 [cited 2015 April 18].
37. McCarthy B, McDonald D. Assessment, treatment, and relapse prevention: male hypoactive sexual desire disorder. J Sex Marital Ther. 2009;35(1): 58–67.

13 Underlying Principles in Ejaculatory and Orgasmic Function and Dysfunction in the Male

Jason M. Scovell and Michael L. Eisenberg

13.1 Prevalence of Male Sexual Dysfunction

Ejaculatory and orgasmic disorders are common in men. Data from the National Health and Social Life Survey collected in 1992 estimates that 13–17 % of men experience low libido, 7–9 % are unable to achieve orgasm, and 28–32 % experience premature ejaculation [1]. The lifetime prevalence of orgasmic disorder is much greater in HIV-positive homosexual men (20–38 %) when compared to their heterosexual counterparts (0–9 %), highlighting the psychological contributions to sexual dysfunction [2, 3]. Ejaculation and orgasm are complex processes that integrate numerous neural, psychological, and physiological processes and are challenging to study. In this chapter, we discuss the current understanding of these processes and the use of state-of-the-art approaches, including animal models, neuroimaging, and genomic analysis, to better define the mechanisms of human ejaculation and orgasm.

13.2 Animal Models

Studying sexual function can pose many challenges, as sexual activity is often private and may involve multiple individuals. Animal models provide an avenue to study some of the underlying mechanisms of sexual function and dysfunction without the potential taboo of using human subjects. However, it is important to understand that findings from animal models may not always translate to the complex physiological and psychological aspects of human sexual behavior. Much of our understanding of the neurobiology of sexual behavior and function has been derived from rat models [4]. Because rats can achieve up to five ejaculations in a 30-min period, they have been proven as an effective model to test various pharmacological treatments for ejaculatory and erectile disorders. These studies have also contributed to our understanding of the neuroanatomical and neurochemical pathways important for ejaculatory response [5–8]. Our understanding of the roles of neurotransmitters and neuropeptides, including serotonin, dopamine, oxytocin, and prolactin, has largely arisen from studies in rat models [5, 6, 8, 9].

J.M. Scovell
Center for Reproductive Medicine, Scott Department of Urology, Baylor College of Medicine, Houston, TX, USA

M.L. Eisenberg, M.D. (✉)
Department of Urology, Stanford University School of Medicine, Palo Alto, CA, USA
e-mail: eisenberg@stanford.edu

L.I. Lipshultz et al. (eds.), *Management of Sexual Dysfunction in Men and Women*, DOI 10.1007/978-1-4939-3100-2_13

13.3 Neuroanatomical Modeling

Studying the neuroanatomical pathways involved in human sexual function has been limited by available techniques. Approaches have included the use of animal models [10], patients with epileptic seizures with sexual features, and the study of patients with localized brain lesions resulting in sexual symptoms [11]. Another approach has been to evaluate the effects of neurological surgery on various functional regions of the brain [12–15]. The advent of functional magnetic resonance imaging (fMRI) and positron emission tomography (PET) has played an integral role in our understanding of the neurological pathways involved in sexual arousal and orgasm. These techniques have enabled the noninvasive study of normal, healthy individuals as well as patients with sexual dysfunction. fMRI and PET imaging permit site-specific and whole-brain investigation of both the neuroanatomical pathways and the cognitive aspects of sexual function via evaluation of brain regions with increased blood flow or metabolic activity, measured as regional cerebral blood flow (rCBF) [16]. Furthermore, both approaches have a spatial resolution down to ~1–3 mm, and both provide almost real-time temporal feedback (fMRI, 2–3 s; PET, 1 min). These studies have permitted the identification of the association between male ejaculation and orgasm and brain structures including the prefrontal cortex, the ventral tegmental area, and the cerebellum [17, 18]. A deeper understanding of the neuroanatomical pathways and their response to various stimuli will be useful in identifying the underlying pathophysiology of various sexual disorders and may provide a more targeted approach for either pharmacological or psychological therapy.

13.4 Genomic Techniques

As technologies to investigate genetic variation become increasingly cost- and time effective, these techniques can provide insights into the pathways important in ejaculation and orgasm. Over the past decade, these high-throughput technologies have been instrumental in identifying single nucleotide polymorphisms (SNPs) and gene copy number variations (CNVs), permitting ever more rapid and accurate investigation into the genetic changes that underlie numerous conditions, particularly when applied using next-generation sequencing techniques that permit evaluation on a genome-wide level. SNP analysis allows for rapid and affordable screening of many patients for known nucleotide polymorphisms and can identify genetic alterations that may lead to changes in protein concentration or function, facilitating the association of these small genetic alterations with various clinical phenotypes. These approaches can be used to identify novel pathways and to add to our understanding of already described processes. Several studies have utilized SNP arrays in various populations to identify candidate genes important for sexual function, including the serotonin and dopamine receptors, as well as genes in the glutamatergic pathway [19–21]. These are discussed in more detail below.

13.5 Pathways in Ejaculation and Orgasm

Ejaculation is classically divided into three phases: emission, ejection (expulsion), and orgasm. The ejaculatory reflex occurs via communication between sensory receptors, cerebral sensory areas, spinal motor pathways, and efferent neural pathways. Proper function requires a complex interplay between many different types of neurotransmitters including serotonin, dopamine, acetylcholine, oxytocin, nitric oxide (NO), norepinephrine, and gamma-aminobutyric acid (GABA) [22]. Seminal emission is mediated via sympathetic nerves originating from T10 to L2. Coordinated contractions of the seminal vesicles and the prostate gland transfer sperm and seminal fluid into the posterior urethra. Ejection is then stimulated via somatic nerves originating from S2 to S4 and occurs through coordinated contractions of the bulbocavernosus and pelvic floor muscles, together with relaxation of the external urinary sphincter (Fig. 13.1). Simultaneously, intermittent contraction of the urethral sphincter prevents retrograde flow into the bladder [22, 25, 26].

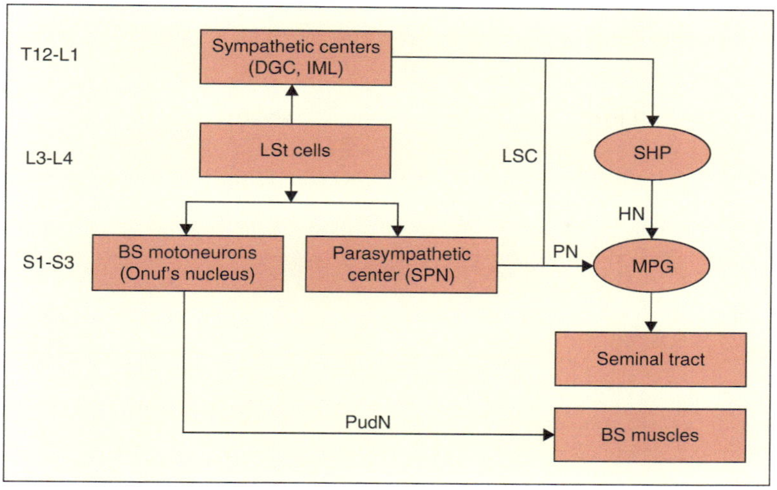

Fig. 13.1 Neural signal integration in the control of ejaculation in rats. Parasympathetic fibers project from the spinal ejaculation generator (LSt) to the sacral parasympathetic nucleus (SPN). Sympathetic fibers are projecting from the LSt to the dorsal gray commissure (DGC) and the intermediolateral cell column (IML). Sympathetics travel to the seminal tract by projections through the lumbar sympathetic chain (LSC) to the superior hypogastric plexus (SH) and then onto MPG. The bulbospongiosus (BS) motor neurons responsible for expulsion will travel to the BS muscle through the motor branch of the pudendal nerve (PudN). HN, hypogastric nerve [23]. With permission from Giuliano F, Clement P. Serotonin and premature ejaculation: from physiology to patient management. Eur Urol. 2006; 50:454–466 [24]

Control centers in the central nervous system (CNS) serve to regulate ejaculation. Structures including the posteromedial bed nucleus of the stria terminalis, the posterodorsal medial amygdaloid nucleus, the posterodorsal preoptic nucleus, and the parvicellular portion of the subparafascicular thalamus serve to inhibit ejaculation (Fig. 13.2) [27]. Molecular imaging techniques have been used to evaluate the brain for regions involved in ejaculation. One study recorded rCBF during ejaculation aided by the participant's female partner so as to minimize background noise that would have otherwise been generated by manual stimulation [18]. The authors utilized PET with a scanning interval of ~10 min, and participants performed various tasks including rest, erection, sexual stimulation, and ejaculation while their head was restrained using an adhesive band. During ejaculation, the scanning interval was shortened to 10 s. During ejaculation, the primary activation was found to be in the mesodiencephalic transition zone that includes the ventral tegmental area, which is involved in the reward pathway. A variety of other mesodiencephalic structures were also found to be activated. Interestingly, neocortical activity was increased exclusively on the right side during ejaculation. In this study, the cerebellum, involved in emotional processing, demonstrated high levels of activation [17]. However, subsequent studies have suggested that the most important events involve deactivation throughout the entire prefrontal cortex, a region critical for higher-order functions that include, but are not limited to, both self-control and working memory [17]. This finding is supported by reports documenting disinhibition and hypersexuality in individuals with damage to the prefrontal cortex [28, 29], as well as other studies demonstrating that reduced cortical activity in the prefrontal cortex associates with male sexual arousal [30]. Studies using PET imaging are limited by their suboptimal temporal resolution (~1 min) given the short duration of ejaculation, and fMRI data to assess male orgasm and ejaculation remain limited. One study utilizing fMRI to study ejaculatory function

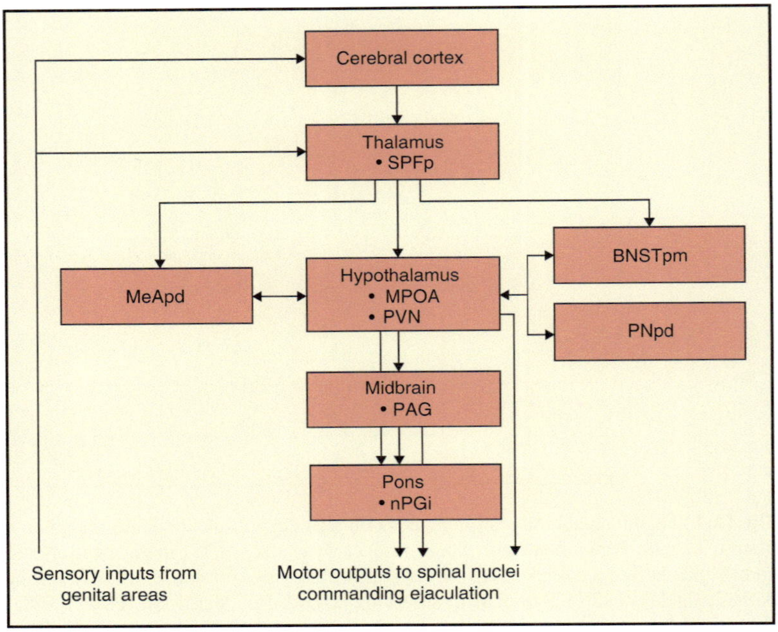

Fig. 13.2 Locations and pathways of the inhibitory central pathways of ejaculation. Gray structures are mediated by serotonin auto-/heteroreceptors. SPFp, parvicellular part of the subparafascicular thalamus; MeAPD, posterodorsal medial amygdala [23]. With permission from Giuliano F, Clement P. Serotonin and premature ejaculation: from physiology to patient management. Eur Urol. 2006; 50:454–466 [24]

primarily focused on sexual satiety and suggested that the refractory period following ejaculation may be due in part to neuronal activation of the temporal lobes, septal areas, and amygdalae [31].

Orgasm is the result of CNS processing of pudendal nerve sensory signals. Stimuli for orgasm include increased pressure in the posterior urethra, signals originating at the verumontanum, and contractions of the urethral bulb and accessory sexual organs [25]. Molecular imaging has been used to study the male orgasm and has found increased rCBF only in the right prefrontal cortex with global decreases in all other cortical regions [32]. Although current data support the roles of different neuronal regions in orgasm, there remains a need for a more complete understanding of the neuroanatomical pathways involved in the process before a cohesive understanding is reached.

Several studies have applied genomic techniques to identify candidate genes involved in male sexual dysfunction. In a small study, men with a history of depression being treated with selective serotonin reuptake inhibitors (SSRIs) were evaluated using SNP analysis to identify potential genetic risk factors for SSRI-induced sexual dysfunction [33]. Men between the ages of 18 and 40 without sexual dysfunction prior to initiation of therapy were included in the study cohort. Sexual dysfunction was evaluated using the validated self-administered Changes in Sexual Functioning Questionnaire (CSFQ) which measures changes in sexual functioning or desire [34]. The authors investigated the pharmacogenetic candidate *5-HT2A*–1438G/A and a polymorphism in the gene encoding the beta subunit of its G-protein second messenger *GNB3* C825T using polymerase chain reaction (PCR) amplification and subsequent pyrosequencing [35]. Bishop and colleagues found that a SNP in the gene coding for 5-HT_{2A} was associated with decreased desire/frequency and arousal in females, although this did not reach statistical significance in the male cohort. Despite the limitations of this study, including its retrospective nature, use of a self-administered questionnaire to assess changes in sexual function, and small sample of males included in the study, this work demonstrates the utility of identifying genetic risk factors and their potential impact on various aspects of sexual dysfunction.

A relationship between a SNP in the gene encoding the dopamine D2 receptor and sexual dysfunction in the male schizophrenic population on antipsychotic monotherapy (clozapine, risperidone, chlorpromazine, haloperidol, olanzapine) has also been observed [20]. Zhang and colleagues analyzed four candidate polymorphisms in two genes coding for the dopamine D2 receptor and endothelial nitric oxide synthase (*DRD2*, *eNOS*). Sexual symptoms were evaluated using the Arizona Sexual Experience Scale (ASEX) [36] and the five-item version of the International Index of Erectile Function (IIEF-5) [37]. Only the polymorphism *DRD2*–141C Ins/Del was associated with a lower overall ASEX score as well as lower scores in the arousal, penile erection, and orgasm (ability) questions. There was also an association between this polymorphism and a man's ability to obtain and maintain an erection.

Genes involved in the glutamatergic pathway (*GRIA3*, *GRIK2*, *GRIA1*, *GRIN3A*) have also been associated with sexual dysfunction using SNP analysis in patients with major depressive disorder (MDD) treated with citalopram [21]. These data come from a subset analysis of the NIMH Sequenced Treatment Alternatives to Relieve Depression (STAR*D) study, which was a large multicenter prospective trial including 4041 outpatients aged 18–75 at 41 clinical sites throughout the United States being treated for MDD. The primary goal of this study was to identify the effectiveness of various MDD treatment modalities [38]. The analysis performed by Perlis and colleagues focused on 68 genes chosen by expert consensus in several known pathways (serotonergic, glutamatergic, dopaminergic, adrenergic, neurotrophic, and others). The authors evaluated mutations in the entire gene as opposed to individual SNPs so as to account for linkage disequilibrium and to identify genes that may be altered by SNPs. *GRIN3A*, a gene encoding for a glutamate receptor, had the strongest association with difficulty in achieving erection. Similar to the previous study by Bishop and colleagues, mutations in the serotonergic receptor 5-HT_{2A} were also associated with erectile dysfunction. Mutations in two other genes encoding receptors in the glutamatergic pathway (*GRIA3* and *GRIK2*) carried an increased risk of 20–30 % and 30–40 % for decreased libido. An association with orgasmic difficulty was also found with *GRIA1*, another glutamate receptor. This study highlights the potential importance of the glutamatergic pathway on antidepressant-associated sexual dysfunction, which has not been studied in humans.

Kurose and colleagues performed a prospective genome-wide association study (GWAS) to evaluate the relationship between various SNPs and SSRI-induced sexual dysfunction [39]. Patients with MDD who were naïve to SSRI therapy or patients on SSRI therapy who underwent a 10-day washout period were included in the study and given paroxetine, fluvoxamine, or milnacipran. Sexual dysfunction was defined as decreased libido, delayed ejaculation, delayed orgasm, or erectile dysfunction. Genomic analysis was performed using a SNP array that identified 262,264 known SNPs, and 201 unrelated patients (106 male) were included for analysis. The authors identified 16 SNPs associated with sexual dysfunction, and of these 11 (69 %) were located in the gene encoding for the *MAM domain-containing glycosylphosphatidylinositol anchor 2* (*MDGA2*) protein. This gene and its product are not well described, but this study shows the potential value of identifying novel pathways involved in sexual dysfunction. Other studies have been less successful in linking SNPs to various sexual dysfunctions [40, 41].

13.6 Diminished Ejaculation Disorders

Diminished ejaculation disorders are a subset of male orgasmic disorders encompassing altered ejaculation and/or orgasm and include reduced semen volume, retrograde ejaculation, decreased force and sensation of ejaculation, and altered ejaculatory latency [42]. Ejaculatory latency is defined as the time it takes for a man to achieve ejaculation. For research purposes, this is often defined as the intravaginal ejaculation latency time (IELT), which utilizes vaginal penetration as the starting point from which latency time is measured. Some men struggle with the duration of their ejaculatory latency time which spans from premature to delayed to anejaculation. According to the Waldinger neurobiological hypothesis of ejaculatory control, these disorders are at the extremes of the same continuum [43]. The causes of ejaculatory latency dysfunction are numerous and include iatrogenic, psychological, and genetic. While the iatrogenic causes of ejaculatory latency dysfunction are well described, by definition, the idiopathic causes are often not well understood.

A panel of experts convened by the International Society for Sexual Medicine (ISSM) defines premature ejaculation (PE) as "...ejaculation which always or nearly always occurs prior to or within about one minute of vaginal penetration, the inability to delay ejaculation on all or nearly all vaginal penetrations, and the presence of negative personal consequences, such as distress, bother, frustration and/or the avoidance of sexual intimacy [44]." Evidence from several trials suggests that >80 % of men with lifelong PE have intravaginal ejaculatory latency times under 1 min, with the balance ejaculating in under 2 min. It is important to note that most studies are limited to heterosexual men engaging in vaginal intercourse [44]. In general, PE can be classified into two main forms: (1) lifelong (primary) and (2) acquired (secondary). The latter occurs later in life and may accompany erectile dysfunction (ED), and data suggest that up to half of men with ED also have PE [45–47].

The prevalence of PE can vary based on cultural norms and practice as well as whether or not the data come from subject self-report versus clinician diagnosis. Two commonly quoted sexual surveys estimate the prevalence of PE between 20 and 30 %. The international Global Study of Sexual Attitudes and Behaviors (GSSAB) reported a prevalence of 30 % across all age strata [45, 48], and the Premature Ejaculation Prevalence and Attitude Survey identified a rate of 23 % among men 18–70 years old [47].

Delayed ejaculation and anejaculation is poorly understood, with few studies focused on these disorders [49]. Unlike PE, delayed ejaculation is relatively rare with a prevalence of ≤3 % [42]. The etiology of delayed ejaculation is often idiopathic, although various iatrogenic causes including nervous system disorders (i.e., multiple sclerosis, diabetes mellitus, spinal cord injury) as well as drugs that affect the α-adrenergic pathway may result in delayed ejaculation [50–52]. The causes of delayed ejaculation can sometimes be identified as pathological as opposed to pathophysiological, suggesting a known etiology and a potentially treatable disease [53]. Unfortunately, the majority of cases are idiopathic, and discerning whether or not the cause is due to genetic and developmental factors as opposed to pathological disease processes is not possible. Although many hypothesize that genetics may play a role in determining a man's ejaculatory latency, a Finnish twin study suggests otherwise, finding only an influence of genetics on premature ejaculation and no genetic influence on delayed ejaculation [54].

Many of the known physiological factors influencing ejaculatory latency involve age-related changes. A decrease in penile sensitivity that develops during the male aging process is a likely contributor to delayed ejaculatory latency [55, 56]. Similarly, changes in the sensitivity of the ejaculatory reflex pathway may increase the time it takes for a man to achieve ejaculation. As discussed above, the interplay between the physical response pathways and the psychological control processes driving orgasmic and ejaculatory function is complex, and impairment of the central cognitive arousal pathway is another likely driving factor in increased ejaculatory latency [57].

Reduction or absence of ejaculate volume is another component of ejaculatory dysfunction. The majority of decreased or absent semen volume with ejaculation is due to anatomical defects, which include both congenital and acquired conditions. The most common etiology for low semen volume is retrograde ejaculation secondary to a transurethral resection of the prostate for benign prostatic hyperplasia. Other anatomical causes of decreased semen volume include defects of the nervous system, obstruction, and hypogonadism [58]. Very few studies exploring the relationship between genetics and semen volume are available. The positive relationship between GGN repeats in the androgen receptor gene and semen volume was demonstrated in a study from Sweden evaluating 220 adolescent Swedish men. Men with <23 GGN repeats had a decreased semen volume when compared to men with 23 GGN repeats (−0.6 ml, $p=0.02$) and when compared to men with >23 GGN repeats (−0.9 ml, $p=0.002$) [59]. This finding was replicated in the Latvian population with similar results. An effect of paternal origin (Latvian versus non-Latvian) on semen parameters was also shown to exist. Men with Latvian fathers had a greater sperm concentration and total sperm counts when compared to men born to non-Latvian father [60]. These data suggest a role of genetic variation in the androgen receptor gene on semen volume. Variation in other genes important in seminal fluid production has yet to be investigated, but it is tempting to speculate that semen production and volume are a function of numerous genetic variations present throughout the population.

The precise etiology of ejaculatory latency dysfunction is uncertain but likely involves the complex interplay between neurochemical, anatomic, psychological, and environmental factors. One proposed mechanism states that abnormal serotonin neurotransmitter signaling underlies altered ejaculatory latency. This hypothesis is based on the observation that stimulation of 5-HT_{1A} receptors results in shortened ejaculatory latency in rats [61]. These findings are supported by the fact that treatment with SSRIs can result in a delayed ejaculatory response in humans, suggesting that serotonin is an important factor in the male ejaculatory response [62].

Animal models have allowed researchers to study the complex role of serotonin in sexual behavior. Through a combination of SSRIs, 5-HT receptor agonists and antagonists, receptor subtypes 5-HT_{1A} and 5-HT_{1B}, have been identified as critical in ejaculatory function. Differential action at these receptors modulates ejaculation in opposing directions [63–66]. Antagonism at the 5-HT_{1A} receptor delays ejaculation, whereas agonism at the 5-HT_{1B} receptor increases ejaculatory latency. However, our understanding of the role of serotonin on ejaculatory function remains limited. One hypothesis is that some SSRIs delay the ejaculatory response through activation of serotonergic receptors in specific brain or spinal cord regions, while those SSRIs that do not seem to affect time to ejaculation (i.e., citalopram, fluvoxamine) may not act on these receptors [4].

Alternatively, cellular and neuroendocrine pathway alterations may drive the delayed ejaculatory response seen in chronic SSRI administration. In rats, a time-dependent administration of fluoxetine and paroxetine reduces oxytocin, adrenocorticotropic hormone (ACTH), and corticosterone levels in response to a 5-HT_{1A} agonist. In these studies, there was no change in 5-HT_{1A} receptor density in any region of the brain. However, levels of the G_{i1} and G_{i3} proteins, G-protein subunits important in stimulating downstream signaling pathway inhibition and activation, in the hypothalamus were reduced. Thus, it appears that 5-HT_{1A} receptors are desensitized by some SSRIs, and this desensitization may be through decreased levels of hypothalamic G-proteins [67, 68]. More specific targeting and modulation of 5-HT receptor subtypes will improve the ability to identify therapeutic targets for premature ejaculation and to avoid the potential unwanted side effect of delayed ejaculation in men with depression and normal ejaculatory latency.

SNP analysis has linked polymorphisms in the 5-HT_{2C} receptor that have been linked to men with lifelong premature ejaculation [19]. This technique has also identified an association between premature ejaculation and a mutation in the oxytocin receptor (*OXTR*), supporting the role of oxytocin in ejaculatory latency [69]. In this study Jern and colleagues studied 1517 male twin and non-twin brothers between the ages of 18 and 45 years old as a subset analysis of a larger study entitled the Genetics of Sex and Aggression, a population-based study of Finnish twins and their siblings [54]. This study looked at SNPs in the oxytocin and arginine vasopressin 1A and 1B receptor genes and their association with PE. Premature ejaculation was quantified using four questions asking about ejaculatory latency time, number of thrusts before ejaculation, frequency of anteportal ejaculation, and ejaculatory control. One SNP in *OXTR* (rs75775) was associated with differences in self-reported ejaculatory latency and perceived ejaculatory control. These findings strengthen our understanding of the role of hormonal signaling in PE.

13.7 Summary

The mechanisms underlying male ejaculatory and orgasmic disorders are not well characterized, but appear to be undergoing a renaissance due to the use of novel, contemporary techniques in their study. Animal models and patients with localized brain lesions have provided much of our understanding about the neuroanatomical and biochemical pathways important for ejaculation and orgasm. With the emergence of noninvasive techniques including molecular-level brain imaging and genetic analysis, there are opportunities to strengthen our current understanding and identify novel pathways that can lead to improved therapies. There is ample opportunity and significant need for these studies to better characterize the anatomical and physiological components required for normal ejaculatory and orgasmic function.

References

1. Laumann EO, Paik A, Rosen RC. Sexual dysfunction in the United States: prevalence and predictors. JAMA. 1999;281:537–44.
2. Catalan J, Klimes I, Day A, et al. The psychosocial impact of HIV infection in gay men. A controlled investigation and factors associated with psychiatric morbidity. Br J Psychiatry. 1992;161:774–8.
3. Catalan J, Klimes I, Bond A, et al. The psychosocial impact of HIV infection in men with haemophilia: controlled investigation and factors associated with psychiatric morbidity. J Psychosom Res. 1992;36: 409–16.
4. Chan JS, Olivier B, de Jong TR, et al. Translational research into sexual disorders: pharmacology and genomics. Eur J Pharmacol. 2008;585:426–35.
5. Kruger TH, Hartmann U, Schedlowski M. Prolactinergic and dopaminergic mechanisms underlying sexual arousal and orgasm in humans. World J Urol. 2005;23:130–8.
6. de Jong TR, Veening JG, Olivier B, et al. Oxytocin involvement in SSRI-induced delayed ejaculation: a review of animal studies. J Sex Med. 2007;4:14–28.
7. de Jong TR, Veening JG, Waldinger MD, et al. Serotonin and the neurobiology of the ejaculatory threshold. Neurosci Biobehav Rev. 2006;30:893–907.
8. Bitran D, Hull EM. Pharmacological analysis of male rat sexual behavior. Neurosci Biobehav Rev. 1987;11:365–89.
9. Hull EM, Muschamp JW, Sato S. Dopamine and serotonin: influences on male sexual behavior. Physiol Behav. 2004;83:291–307.
10. Agmo A. Male rat sexual behavior. Brain Res Brain Res Protoc. 1997;1:203–9.
11. Rees PM, Fowler CJ, Maas CP. Sexual function in men and women with neurological disorders. Lancet. 2007;369:512–25.
12. Burns JM, Swerdlow RH. Right orbitofrontal tumor with pedophilia symptom and constructional apraxia sign. Arch Neurol. 2003;60:437–40.
13. Devinsky J, Sacks O, Devinsky O. Kluver-Bucy syndrome, hypersexuality, and the law. Neurocase. 2010;16:140–5.
14. Dieckmann G, Schneider-Jonietz B, Schneider H. Psychiatric and neuropsychological findings after stereotactic hypothalamotomy, in cases of extreme sexual aggressivity. Acta Neurochir Suppl. 1988;44:163–6.
15. Freeman W. Sexual behavior and fertility after frontal lobotomy. Biol Psychiatry. 1973;6:97–104.
16. Stoleru S, Fonteille V, Cornelis C, et al. Functional neuroimaging studies of sexual arousal and orgasm in healthy men and women: a review and meta-analysis. Neurosci Biobehav Rev. 2012;36:1481–509.
17. Georgiadis JR, Reinders AA, Van der Graaf FH, et al. Brain activation during human male ejaculation revisited. Neuroreport. 2007;18:553–7.
18. Holstege G, Georgiadis JR, Paans AM, et al. Brain activation during human male ejaculation. J Neurosci Off J Soc Neurosci. 2003;23:9185–93.
19. Luo S, Lu Y, Wang F, et al. Association between polymorphisms in the serotonin 2C receptor gene and premature ejaculation in Han Chinese subjects. Urol Int. 2010;85:204–8.
20. Zhang XR, Zhang ZJ, Zhu RX, et al. Sexual dysfunction in male schizophrenia: influence of antipsychotic drugs, prolactin and polymorphisms of the dopamine D2 receptor genes. Pharmacogenomics. 2011;12:1127–36.
21. Perlis RH, Laje G, Smoller JW, et al. Genetic and clinical predictors of sexual dysfunction in citalopram-treated depressed patients. Neuropsychopharmacology. 2009;34:1819–28.
22. Courtois F, Carrier S, Charvier K, et al. The control of male sexual responses. Curr Pharm Des. 2013;19: 4341–56.
23. Wolters JP, Hellstrom WJ. Current concepts in ejaculatory dysfunction. Rev Urol. 2006;8 Suppl 4:S18–25.
24. Giuliano F, Clement P. Serotonin and premature ejaculation: from physiology to patient management. Euro Urol. 2006;50:454–66.
25. McMahon CG, Jannini E, Waldinger M, et al. Standard operating procedures in the disorders of orgasm and ejaculation. J Sex Med. 2013;10:204–29.
26. Perelman M, McMahon C, Barada J. Evaluation and treatment of the ejaculatory disorders. In: Lue T, editor. Atlas of male sexual dysfunction. Philadelphia: Current Medicine, Inc; 2004. p. 127–57.
27. Meisel RL, Sachs BD. The physiology of male sexual behavior. In: Knobil E, Neill JD, editors. The physiology of reproduction. New York: Raven; 2005. p. 3–105.
28. Damasio H, Grabowski T, Frank R, et al. The return of Phineas Gage: clues about the brain from the skull of a famous patient. Science. 1994;264:1102–5.

29. Aloni R, Katz S. A review of the effect of traumatic brain injury on the human sexual response. Brain Inj. 1999;13:269–80.
30. Montorsi F, Perani D, Anchisi D, et al. Brain activation patterns during video sexual stimulation following the administration of apomorphine: results of a placebo-controlled study. Eur Urol. 2003;43:405–11.
31. Mallick HN, Tandon S, Jagannathan NR, et al. Brain areas activated after ejaculation in healthy young human subjects. Indian J Physiol Pharmacol. 2007;51:81–5.
32. Tiihonen J, Kuikka J, Kupila J, et al. Increase in cerebral blood flow of right prefrontal cortex in man during orgasm. Neurosci Lett. 1994;170:241–3.
33. Bishop JR, Moline J, Ellingrod VL, et al. Serotonin 2A–1438 G/A and G-protein Beta3 subunit C825T polymorphisms in patients with depression and SSRI-associated sexual side-effects. Neuropsychopharmacology. 2006;31:2281–8.
34. Clayton AH, McGarvey EL, Clavet GJ. The changes in sexual functioning questionnaire (CSFQ): development, reliability, and validity. Psychopharmacol Bull. 1997;33:731–45.
35. Arranz MJ, Munro J, Owen MJ, et al. Evidence for association between polymorphisms in the promoter and coding regions of the 5-HT2A receptor gene and response to clozapine. Mol Psychiatry. 1998;3:61–6.
36. McGahuey CA, Gelenberg AJ, Laukes CA, et al. The Arizona sexual experience scale (ASEX): reliability and validity. J Sex Marital Ther. 2000;26:25–40.
37. Rosen RC, Cappelleri JC, Smith MD, et al. Development and evaluation of an abridged, 5-item version of the international index of erectile function (IIEF-5) as a diagnostic tool for erectile dysfunction. Int J Impot Res. 1999;11:319–26.
38. Rush AJ, Trivedi M, Fava M. Depression, IV: STAR*D treatment trial for depression. Am J Psychiatry. 2003;160:237.
39. Kurose K, Hiratsuka K, Ishiwata K, et al. Genome-wide association study of SSRI/SNRI-induced sexual dysfunction in a Japanese cohort with major depression. Psychiatry Res. 2012;198:424–9.
40. Jern P, Westberg L, Ankarberg-Lindgren C, et al. Associations between salivary testosterone levels, androgen-related genetic polymorphisms, and self-estimated ejaculation latency time. Sex Med. 2014;2:107–14.
41. Zuccarello D, Ghezzi M, Pengo M, et al. No difference in 5-HTTLPR and Stin2 polymorphisms frequency between premature ejaculation patients and controls. J Sex Med. 2012;9:1659–68.
42. Perelman M, McMahon C, Barada J. Evaluation and treatment of ejaculatory disorders. In: Lue TF, editor. Atlas of male sexual dysfunction. Philadelphia: Current Medicine LLC; 2004. p. 127–57.
43. Waldinger MD. The neurobiological approach to premature ejaculation. J Urol. 2002;168:2359–67.
44. McMahon CG, Althof SE, Waldinger MD, et al. An evidence-based definition of lifelong premature ejaculation: report of the international society for sexual medicine (ISSM) ad hoc committee for the definition of premature ejaculation. J Sex Med. 2008;5:1590–606.
45. Laumann EO, Nicolosi A, Glasser DB, et al. Sexual problems among women and men aged 40–80 y: prevalence and correlates identified in the global study of sexual attitudes and behaviors. Int J Impot Res. 2005;17:39–57.
46. Basile Fasolo C, Mirone V, Gentile V, et al. Premature ejaculation: prevalence and associated conditions in a sample of 12,558 men attending the andrology prevention week 2001 – a study of the Italian society of andrology (SIA). J Sex Med. 2005;2:376–82.
47. Porst H, Montorsi F, Rosen RC, et al. The premature ejaculation prevalence and attitudes (PEPA) survey: prevalence, comorbidities, and professional help-seeking. Eur Urol. 2007;51:816–23. discussion 824.
48. Nicolosi A, Laumann EO, Glasser DB, et al. Sexual behavior and sexual dysfunctions after age 40: the global study of sexual attitudes and behaviors. Urology. 2004;64:991–7.
49. Corona G, Rastrelli G, Maseroli E, et al. Sexual function of the ageing male. Best Pract Res Clin Endocrinol Metab. 2013;27:581–601.
50. Witt MA, Grantmyre JE. Ejaculatory failure. World J Urol. 1993;11:89–95.
51. Master VA, Turek PJ. Ejaculatory physiology and dysfunction. Urol Clin N Am. 2001;28:363–75. x.
52. Vale J. Ejaculatory dysfunction. BJU Int. 1999;83: 557–63.
53. Perelman MA, Rowland DL. Retarded ejaculation. World J Urol. 2006;24:645–52.
54. Johansson A, Jern P, Santtila P, et al. The genetics of sexuality and aggression (GSA) twin samples in Finland. Twin Res Hum Genet. 2013;16:150–6.
55. Rowland DL. Penile sensitivity in men: a composite of recent findings. Urology. 1998;52:1101–5.
56. Paick JS, Jeong H, Park MS. Penile sensitivity in men with premature ejaculation. Int J Impot Res. 1998;10:247–50.
57. Motofei IG, Rowland DL. Neurophysiology of the ejaculatory process: developing perspectives. BJU Int. 2005;96:1333–8.
58. Roberts M, Jarvi K. Steps in the investigation and management of low semen volume in the infertile man. Can Urol Assoc J. 2009;3:479–85.
59. Lundin KB, Giwercman YL, Rylander L, et al. Androgen receptor gene GGN repeat length and reproductive characteristics in young Swedish men. Eur J Endocrinol. 2006;155:347–54.
60. Erenpreiss J, Tsarev I, Giwercman A, et al. The impact of androgen receptor polymorphism and parental ethnicity on semen quality in young men from Latvia. Int J Androl. 2008;31:477–82.
61. Ahlenius S, Larsson K, Svensson L, et al. Effects of a new type of 5-HT receptor agonist on male rat sexual behavior. Pharmacol Biochem Behav. 1981;15:785–92.
62. Schachter M, Parkes JD. Fluvoxamine and clomipramine in the treatment of cataplexy. J Neurol Neurosurg Psychiatry. 1980;43:171–4.
63. Ahlenius S, Larsson K. Synergistic actions of the 5-HT1A receptor antagonist WAY-100635 and citalopram on male rat ejaculatory behavior. Eur J Pharmacol. 1999;379:1–6.

64. Ahlenius S, Larsson K. Evidence for an involvement of 5-HT1B receptors in the inhibition of male rat ejaculatory behavior produced by 5-HTP. Psychopharmacology. 1998;137:374–82.
65. de Jong TR, Pattij T, Veening JG, et al. Citalopram combined with WAY 100635 inhibits ejaculation and ejaculation-related Fos immunoreactivity. Eur J Pharmacol. 2005;509:49–59.
66. Hillegaart V, Ahlenius S. Facilitation and inhibition of male rat ejaculatory behaviour by the respective 5-HT1A and 5-HT1B receptor agonists 8-OH-DPAT and anpirtoline, as evidenced by use of the corresponding new and selective receptor antagonists NAD-299 and NAS-181. Br J Pharmacol. 1998;125: 1733–43.
67. Li Q, Muma NA, van de Kar LD. Chronic fluoxetine induces a gradual desensitization of 5-HT1A receptors: reductions in hypothalamic and midbrain Gi and G(o) proteins and in neuroendocrine responses to a 5-HT1A agonist. J Pharmacol Exp Ther. 1996;279:1035–42.
68. Li Q, Muma NA, Battaglia G, et al. A desensitization of hypothalamic 5-HT1A receptors by repeated injections of paroxetine: reduction in the levels of G(i) and G(o) proteins and neuroendocrine responses, but not in the density of 5-HT1A receptors. J Pharmacol Exp Ther. 1997;282:1581–90.
69. Jern P, Westberg L, Johansson A, et al. Are single nucleotide polymorphisms in the oxytocin and vasopressin 1A/1B receptor genes likely candidates for variation in ejaculatory function? BJU Int. 2012;110:E1173–80.

Commentary: Underlying Principles in Ejaculatory and Orgasmic Function and Dysfunction in the Male

Marcel Waldinger

Human ejaculatory and orgasmic control pathways are complex and our understanding of these mechanisms is still in its nascency—this is made clear in the preceding chapter by Scovell and Eisenberg. However, the growing use of sophisticated technologies to map brain regions involved in conscious and subconscious processes, including ejaculation and orgasm, and the application of cutting-edge genomic technologies to better understand how our genetic milieu regulates how we respond to sexual stimuli, are improving our grasp of these conditions faster than ever before. Nevertheless, as Waldinger astutely highlights in the following commentary, detailed observation of men with ejaculatory problems can identify details that can lead to novel classifications of these disorders. It is this intersection between sophisticated technologies that can identify molecular factors that affect ejaculation and orgasm, combined with the human touch and close observation that can parse the vagaries of these conditions that will truly permit us to understand ejaculatory and orgasmic dysfunction. With this detailed understanding will then come the ability to effectively intervene, whether it's using pharmacotherapy, surgery, or other therapies in the quiver of the mental health specialist.

The Editors

Marcel Waldinger, M.D., Ph.D.
Division Pharmacology, Department of Pharmaceutical Sciences, Faculty of BetaSciences, Utrecht University, Utrecht, The Netherlands

Practice for Psychiatry and Neurosexology, Amstelveen, The Netherlands

Commentary

In the last two decades, substantial progress has been made in understanding ejaculatory and orgasmic disorders. In vivo animal research, human clinical research, and brain imaging studies have contributed to a better neurobiological understanding of particularly premature ejaculation (PE) [1–4]. Despite this progress, for many sexologists, research and treatment of PE seem to have started (and ended) in the 1960s with Masters and Johnson, who advocated behavioral therapy in the form of the squeeze technique to the penis applied by the female partner [5]. It is still generally believed that oral drug treatment is a relatively new concept in the treatment of PE, starting with the introduction of monoamine oxidase inhibitors (MAOIs), mellaril, and clomipramine during the 1970s and becoming particularly popular since the introduction of SSRIs and dapoxetine during the 1990s [6].

In this commentary, two new concepts in the understanding of PE, particularly lifelong PE, will be reported and explained. Intriguingly, the roots of one of these concepts were partly formulated in the 1940s, but subsequently largely ignored and forgotten.

The First PE Research and the First Oral Drug for PE

Research exploring PE started long before Masters and Johnson suggested that PE was the result of self-learned behavior [7]. In 1917, the well-known psychoanalyst Karl Abraham called it "ejaculatio praecox" and postulated that it was the manifestation of unresolved unconscious conflicts [8]. However, he never systematically investigated this hypothesis. It was Bernhard Schapiro who investigated a very large number of men with complaints of PE in the 1920s and 1930s at the Institut fur Sexualwissenschaft in Berlin [9]. In the 1920s, he developed Präjaculin, which was the first oral drug for the treatment of lifelong PE [10]. Präjaculin was produced by the German company Promonta in Hamburg from 1932 until the mid-1960s [10]. In other words, oral drug treatment for PE was available more than a decade before even the first review article on PE was published by Schapiro and more than 40 years before Masters and Johnson published their squeeze technique. Bernhard Schapiro is not only the true pioneer in the research of PE; his findings, as published in 1943, are still valid today and have, 70 years after publication, also become the basis for a new concept in the understanding of PE.

Erectio Praecox

Essential to the ideas of Schapiro on PE is that he listened very carefully to the details his patients reported on PE. In this way, he was able to distinguish two PE subtypes: lifelong and acquired. At the time he called them the hypertonic (lifelong PE) and hypotonic (acquired PE) types [9]. Schapiro also noticed that, in contrast to men with acquired PE, men with lifelong PE reported little difficulty in obtaining erections [9]. He called this "erectio praecox" [9]. Notably, after his 1943 publication, the term "erectio praecox" was never quoted in the sexological literature until 2002, when Waldinger reintroduced the term, highlighting that many men with lifelong PE report this phenomenon and that it may be related to central oxytocin release [11]. However, the primary complaint of men with lifelong PE is the persistent early ejaculations. Often, these men are not even aware of how easily they achieve erections, and this is reported to the physician by their female partners.

Detumescentia Praecox

Waldinger recently reported that men with lifelong PE often have an acute and complete penile detumescence after ejaculation [12]. He called this phenomenon "detumescentia praecox" [12]. Similar to erectio praecox, this rapid penile detumescence is hardly expressed as a complaint, as men with lifelong PE are accustomed to it. Still, both phenomena should be regarded as subtle rather ego-syntonic manifestations of lifelong PE.

Hypertonic State

The presence of rapid erection and/or penile detumescence shows that lifelong PE is not only a matter of persistent early ejaculations, as believed for so many decades. As soon as these men become involved in an erotic or sexual situation, they become unwantedly overwhelmed by a "hypertonic state," an acute physical/genital state of sexual/genital hyperarousability with premature ejaculation and/or facilitated erection and/or facilitated penile detumescence [12]. This new concept, as recently formulated by Waldinger, has important consequences for the approach and treatment of men with lifelong PE.

Classification of Four PE Subtypes

Based on stopwatch measurements of the intravaginal ejaculation latency time (IELT), stopwatch-mediated epidemiological studies of the IELT, and the occurrence of PE throughout life and the frequency of complaints, Waldinger and Schweitzer proposed a new classification of four PE subtypes: lifelong PE, acquired PE, subjective PE, and variable PE [13–15]. In contrast to the very short IELTs of lifelong and acquired PE, men with subjective PE have normal or even long IELTs [16]. In variable PE, the complaints of PE occur only sometimes [16]. The hypertonic state is characteristic for lifelong PE, whereas a hypotonic state characterizes acquired PE. Subjective PE and variable PE are characterized by a normotonic state [16]. Erectio praecox and detumescentia praecox only occur in lifelong PE [12, 17].

Advantages of the New PE Classification

A major advantage of the new classification system is that males with all IELT values can be classified into one of the four PE subtypes. Yet, the new classification system also demands the existence of factors other than the IELT. By using this system, classification no longer depends on the (subjective) mental/emotional state of a man complaining of PE, but on concrete physical symptoms.

Treatment Differences Among the Four PE Subtypes

The different clinical symptoms and genital/physical tonus of the four PE subtypes obviously affect the emotions and mental coping mechanisms of these men. However, the emotional and psychological burdens in these men also depend on factors unrelated to the specific PE subtype. In other words, psychological and emotional factors are inadequate to identify and group males into the four subtypes, as affected men may suffer to the same emotional extent. Indeed, the duration of the IELT, the course in life, the frequency of occurrence, and the presence of erectio praecox and detumescentia praecox are the most important factors allowing distinction between the four PE subtypes. This is clinically relevant, as the current ISSM [18] and DSM-5 definitions [19] of PE in terms of (1) IELT duration, (2) extent of ejaculatory control, and (3) negative personal consequences appear to be inadequate to encapsulate all four PE subtypes.

Counseling and Psychoeducation

The ability to distinguish the four PE subtypes is relevant for both treatment and research. Drug therapy is frequently essential for lifelong PE and acquired PE. Preferably, this drug treatment by daily or on-demand use of oral drugs is accompanied by psychoeducation on PE and the positive and adverse effects of the drugs. Treatment of "subjective PE" should consist of counseling and psychoeducation with specific attention toward psychological and cultural factors that contribute to the conviction of a man with a normal/long IELT duration that he suffers from PE. Counseling and psychoeducation are also important for "variable PE," which is a normal variant of human ejaculatory performance. Notably, local anesthetic creams or sprays may also be indicated for men with both subjective and variable PE. It might well be that behavioral treatment in the form of the stop/start or squeeze technique will have better outcomes in subjective PE than so far has been found in lifelong or acquired PE. Future research is therefore warranted.

Psychoanalytic Research

Another issue of PE that has been often overlooked in our times is the psychodynamic consequences of PE. The new classification may constitute a solid basis for renewed psychodynamic research. The fact that lifelong PE is currently thought to be substantially influenced by neurobiological and genetic factors should not be an impairment for psychoanalytic research of these men. Psychoanalytic treatment in brain-damaged patients is one of the core elements of neuropsychoanalysis [20–22]. In this respect, (neuro)psychoanalytic analysis of men with PE, particularly those with lifelong PE, would be extremely interesting and even more so when compared with work evaluating men with subjective PE. In addition, other psychological schools of thought would each shed an improved understanding of psychosocial-behavioral and cultural components of PE etiology and impact on both men and their partner. In particular for this author, the need for additional psychoanalytic evaluation of PE is clear, not only to better understand men for in whom PE has become part of a neurotic behavioral pattern but also to elucidate epigenetic and genetic factors that contribute to the expression or maintenance of PE.

13.1 Genetic Research of the IELT

In the last decade, genetic research examining IELT in men with lifelong PE, combined with stopwatch measurements of their IELTs, has shown that persistent short IELTs are associated with at least three genetic polymorphisms of the 5-HTT gene, the 5-HT1A receptor gene, and the 5-HT2C receptor gene [23–27]. This genetic research focused on the central serotonergic system that mediates ejaculation in both male rats and humans [28]. However, the new concept of the hypertonic state in lifelong PE implies that lifelong PE is not just associated with the central serotonin system [12]. Accepting erectio praecox and detumescentia praecox as part of the phenomenology of lifelong PE implicates that other neurotransmitter systems (e.g., dopamine, oxytocin) and hormonal factors (e.g., testosterone, prolactin) also play an important role in lifelong PE [12].

Conclusion

In conclusion, according to a newly formulated concept, lifelong PE is no longer solely characterized by persistent, very short IELTs, but also by rapid erections, rapid penile detumescence, and an acute hypertonic state. Another new concept is the identification and classification of four PE subtypes. This classification system is organized such that men with all IELT values and also complaints of PE can be described. Most essential for new theoretical discoveries on PE remains the listening ear of the clinician who preferably must also have a critical mind and the gift to note subtle symptoms as very relevant for diagnosis, treatment, and research.

References

1. Olivier B, van Oorschot R, Waldinger MD. Serotonin, serotonergic receptors, selective serotonin reuptake inhibitors and sexual behaviour. Int Clin Psychopharmacol. 1998;13(suppl 6):S9–S14.
2. Olivier B, Chan JS, Pattij T, de Jong TR, Oosting RS, Veening JG, Waldinger MD. Psychopharmacology of male rat sexual behavior: modelling human sexual dysfunctions? Int J Impot Res. 2006;18(Suppl 1): S14–23.
3. Pattij T, de Jong T, Uitterdijk A, Waldinger MD, Veening JG, van der Graaf PH, Olivier B. Individual differences in male rat ejaculatory behavior: searching for models to study ejaculation disorders. Eur J Neurosci. 2005;22:724–34.
4. Georgiadis JR. Doing it … wild? On the role of the cerebral cortex in human sexual activity. Socioaffect Neurosci Psychol. 2012;2:17337.
5. Masters WH, Johnson VE. Premature ejaculation. In: Masters WH, Johnson VE, editors. Human sexual inadequacy. Boston: Little, Brown and Co.; 1970.

6. Waldinger MD, Zwinderman AH, Schweitzer DH, Olivier B. Relevance of methodological design for the interpretation of efficacy of drug treatment of premature ejaculation: a systematic review and meta-analysis. Int J Impot Res. 2004;16:369–81.
7. Perelman MA. Treatment of premature ejaculation. In: Leiblum S, Pervin L, editors. Principles and practices of sex therapy. New York: Guilford Press; 1980. p. 199–233.
8. Abraham K. Uber Ejaculatio Praecox. Z Aertzlicher Psychoanalyse. 1917;4:171–86.
9. Schapiro B. Premature ejaculation: a review of 1130 cases. J Urol. 1943;50:374–9.
10. Schapiro B. Präjaculin. Kombiniertes Epiphysen-Präparat gegen Reizzustände am Genitale und Hypererotismus. Hamburg: Chemische Farbrik Promonta G.m.b.H.; 1932.
11. Waldinger MD. The neurobiological approach to premature ejaculation. J Urol. 2002;168:2359–67.
12. Waldinger MD. Ejaculatio praecox, erectio praecox, and detumescentia praecox as symptoms of a hypertonic state in lifelong premature ejaculation: a new hypothesis. Pharmacol Biochem Behav. 2014;121: 189–94.
13. Waldinger MD, Schweitzer DH. Changing paradigms from an historical DSM-III and DSM-IV view towards an evidence based definition of premature ejaculation. Part II: Proposals for DSM-V and ICD-11. J Sex Med. 2006;3:693–705.
14. Waldinger MD. Premature ejaculation: different pathophysiologies and etiologies determine its treatment. J Sex Marital Ther. 2008;34:1–13.
15. Waldinger MD, Schweitzer DH. The use of old and recent DSM definitions of premature ejaculation in observational studies: a contribution to the present debate for a new classification of PE in the DSM-V. J Sex Med. 2008;5:1079–87.
16. Waldinger MD. History of premature ejaculation. In: Jannini EA, McMahon CG, Waldinger MD, editors. Premature ejaculation. From etiology to diagnosis and treatment. New York: Springer; 2013. p. 5–24.
17. Waldinger MD. Sexuelle Functionsstorung beim Mann: Lebenslange vorzeitige Ejaculation. In: Stirn A, Stark R, Tabbert K, Wehrum-Osinsky S, Oddo S, Hrsg. Sexualität, Krper und Neurobiologie: Grundlagen und Strungsbilder im interdisziplinären Fokus. Verlag W. Kohlhammer; 2014. p. 216–41.
18. McMahon CG, Althof S, Waldinger MD, Porst H, Dean J, Sharlip I, Adaikan PG, Becher E, Broderick GA, Buvat J, Dabees K, Giraldi A, Giuliano F, Hellstrom WJ, Incrocci L, Laan E, Meuleman E, Perelman MA, Rosen R, Rowland D, Segraves R. An evidence-based definition of lifelong premature ejaculation: report of the international society for sexual medicine (ISSM) ad hoc committee for the definition of premature ejaculation. J Sex Med. 2008;5:1590–606.
19. American Psychiatric Association. Diagnostic and Statistical Manual of Mental Disorders (DSM-5). 5th ed. Washington, DC: American Psychiatric Association; 2013.
20. Panksepp J, Solms M. What is neuropsychoanalysis? Clinically relevant studies of the minded brain. Trends Cogn Sci. 2012;16(1):6–8.
21. Axmacher N, Kessler H, Waldhauser GT. Editorial on psychoanalytical neuroscience: exploring psychoanalytic concepts with neuroscientific methods. Front Hum Neurosci. 2014;8:674.
22. Solms A. A neuropsychoanalytical approach to the hard problem of consciousness. J Integr Neurosci. 2014;13(2):173–85.
23. Waldinger MD. The need for a revival of psychoanalytic investigations into premature ejaculation. J Mens Health Gender. 2006;3:390–6.
24. Janssen PK, Bakker SC, Réthelyi J, Zwinderman AH, Touw DJ, Olivier B, Waldinger MD. Serotonin transporter promoter region (5-HTTLPR) polymorphism is associated with the intravaginal ejaculation latency time in Dutch men with lifelong premature ejaculation. J Sex Med. 2009;6(1):276–84.
25. Janssen PKC, van Schaik R, Zwinderman AH, Olivier B, Waldinger MD. The 5-HT_{1A} receptor C(1019)G polymorphism influences the intravaginal ejaculation latency time in Dutch Caucasian men with lifelong premature ejaculation. Pharmacol. Biochem Behav 2014;121:184–8.
26. Janssen PK, van Schaik R, Olivier B, Waldinger MD. The 5-HT_{2C} receptor gene Cys23Ser polymorphism influences the intravaginal ejaculation latency time in Dutch Caucasian men with lifelong premature ejaculation. Asian J Androl. 2014;16: 607–10.
27. Janssen PK, Olivier B, Zwinderman AH, Waldinger MD. Measurement errors in polymerase chain reaction are a confounding factor for a correct interpretation of 5-HTTLPR polymorphism effects on lifelong premature ejaculation: A critical analysis of a previously published meta-analysis of six studies. PLoS One. 2014;9(3):e88031.
28. Waldinger MD, Berendsen HHG, Blok BFM, Olivier B, Holstege G. Premature ejaculation and serotonergic antidepressants-induced delayed ejaculation: the involvement of the serotonergic system. Behav Brain Res. 1998;92:111–8.

14 Clinical Evaluation and Treatment of Disorders of Ejaculation

Daniel H. Williams IV and Brett A. Johnson

14.1 Introduction

Disorders of ejaculation are among the most common male sexual pathologies and affect up to 40 % of the male population. Ejaculation is separate from the psychological climax, or orgasm, although the two events often accompany one another and occur simultaneously. Orgasm is a somatosensory experience, while ejaculation is a coordinated neuromuscular reflex [1].

Sexual dysfunction is a broad and diverse entity that encompasses psychosocial, neurological, vascular, anatomical, and pharmacological problems. Ejaculatory dysfunction is a common complaint thought to affect 30–40 % of men across all age groups. It is often associated with a significant negative impact on quality of life and is often a source of relationship distress and intimacy anxiety.

D.H. Williams IV, M.D. (✉)
Department of Urology, University of Wisconsin School of Medicine and Public Health, Madison, WI, USA
e-mail: Williams@urology.wisc.edu

B.A. Johnson M.D.
Department of Urology, University of Wisconsin-Madison, 1685 Highland Ave, Madison, WI 53705, USA

14.2 Normal Ejaculation

The majority of the ejaculate is derived from the seminal vesicles, but the prostate, epididymis, vas deferens, and bulbourethral glands also contribute to the ejaculate volume. Ejaculation involves sensory stimuli, the central nervous system, and autonomic nervous pathways. It occurs in two phases—emission and expulsion.

During emission, seminal fluid is deposited in the posterior urethra. The sympathetic nervous system facilitates contraction of smooth muscles in the prostate, vas deferens, and seminal vesicles to deposit seminal fluid. The superior and inferior hypogastric sympathetic plexus is also responsible for closure of the bladder neck required for antegrade ejaculation.

The expulsion phase propels semen out of the urethra. Antegrade expulsion requires contraction of periurethral skeletal muscles, closure of the bladder neck, and relaxation of the external urethral sphincter. Except for the closure of the bladder neck, the somatic nervous system is responsible for this phase of ejaculation. The pudendal nerve activates the bulbospongiosus, ischiocavernosus, and pelvic floor muscles to mediate seminal expulsion [2]. At the level of the central nervous system, dopamine and serotonin are the neurotransmitters that play significant roles in the ejaculatory pathway (Fig. 14.1) [3].

L.I. Lipshultz et al. (eds.), *Management of Sexual Dysfunction in Men and Women*, DOI 10.1007/978-1-4939-3100-2_14

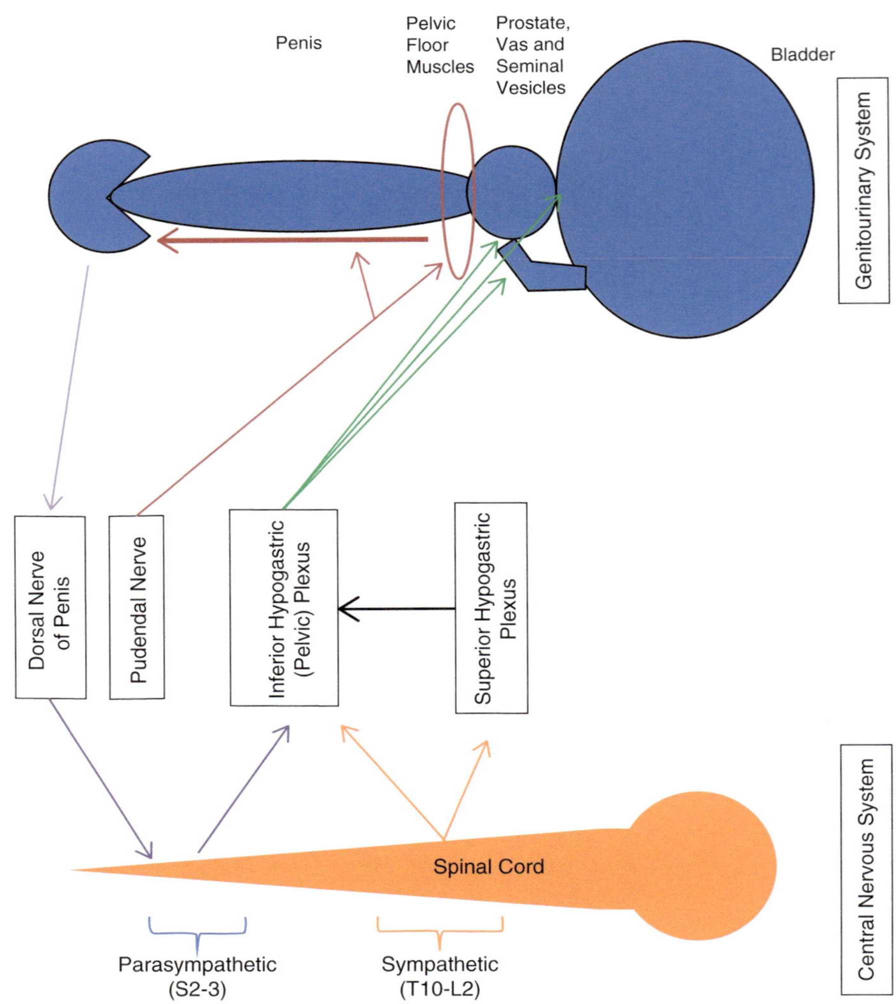

Fig. 14.1 Physiology of normal ejaculation. Sensation of the penis travels to the central nervous system. When stimulation has been sufficient, the ejaculatory reflex is initiated in the cerebral cortex, thalamus, and hypothalamus. This triggers sympathetic innervation from the spinal cords that travel to the superior hypogastric and pelvic plexuses. The hypogastric nerve allows interplay between these plexuses. During emission, sympathetics generate contraction of smooth muscles in the prostate, vas deferens, and seminal vesicles to deposit the seminal fluid in the urethra. The bladder neck is also closed to prevent retrograde ejaculation. Somatic fibers from the pudendal nerve rhythmically contract the bulbospongiosus, ischiocavernosus, as well as pelvic floor muscles to expel semen. Parasympathetic innervation regulates erections and is thought to play a role in emission [30]

14.3 Disorders of Ejaculation

The term "ejaculatory dysfunction" encompasses a number of different clinical entities, and patients may present with a spectrum of complaints. These entities include premature ejaculation, delayed ejaculation, retrograde ejaculation, anejaculation, anorgasmia, decreased volume of ejaculate, and painful ejaculation.

14.3.1 Premature Ejaculation

Premature ejaculation (PE) is the most common disorder associated with ejaculation. It is not typically caused by or associated with medical or surgical conditions. Severity of PE can be characterized by intravaginal ejaculatory latency time (IELT) defined as the time from initial vaginal penetration to ejaculation.

Numerous definitions of PE exist from multiple organizations. The American Urological Association guidelines define PE as ejaculation that occurs sooner than desired, either before or shortly after penetration, causing distress to either one or both partners [4]. The International Society for Sexual Medicine defines PE as ejaculation within approximately 1 min and the inability to delay ejaculation for all or nearly all vaginal penetrations that causes negative personal consequences. The World Health Organization's definition uses an IELT cutoff of 15 s. This 15-s cutoff is arbitrary and devoid of evidence-based literature [5].

In general, PE has three components—negative personal consequences, persistence of the symptoms over all or nearly all vaginal penetrations, and reduced IELT [5]. Negative consequences usually manifest as anxiety, distress, frustration, avoidance of sexual intercourse, and relationship angst. Clinical PE is persistent across sexual encounters, partners, and types of sexual activity. IELT is shorter than normal. The median IELT for "normal men" is 5.4 min [6]. The generally accepted pathological IELT is less than 60 s. There is, however, significant variation in the perception of what a normal IELT is. The estimated global incidence of PE is 30 %, and there is a predilection for younger males. A survey of men with self-reported PE revealed an IELT of less than 30 s on average [6].

14.3.2 Delayed Ejaculation

Anejaculation and delayed ejaculation are defined as persistent or recurrent delay or absence of ejaculation after normal sexual excitement and activity [7]. Men with normal ejaculatory function typically ejaculate within 4–10 min following vaginal penetration; intravaginal latency times in excess of 25–30 min are considered abnormal. While there are psychosocial-behavioral and cultural factors that may cause DE, the most common causes are iatrogenic. Medications that commonly induce delayed ejaculation include selective serotonin reuptake inhibitors (SSRIs), tricyclic antidepressants (TCAs), methyldopa, thiazide diuretics, phenothiazine, and benzodiazepines. Delayed ejaculation can also be due to abnormalities of the central nervous system, autonomic nervous system (primarily sympathetic), or sensory innervation of the penis (tactile stimulation). Diabetic neuropathy can decrease sensation to the penis, resulting in delayed ejaculation.

14.3.3 Anejaculation and Retrograde Ejaculation

Anejaculation is the inability to ejaculate semen and can occur with or without orgasm. Men with anorgasmic anejaculation are unable to reach orgasm and, therefore, unable to ejaculate. Failure to reach orgasm can be caused by psychological problems or can result from the side effects of certain medications including SSRIs.

With orgasmic anejaculation, men are able to orgasm, but no antegrade ejaculate is present. This entity is typically due to underlying neurological disorders (e.g., diabetes), ejaculatory duct obstruction, the use of alpha-blockers, or prior pelvic or retroperitoneal surgery that can disrupt nerves important for ejaculation. Orgasmic anejaculation can be due to abnormalities of the central or autonomic (primarily sympathetic) nervous systems, somatic innervation to the pelvic floor musculature involved in ejaculation, or sensory innervation of the penis. Diabetes mellitus can cause both neurological deficits and microvascular abnormalities that contribute to sexual dysfunction. Even in the absence of erectile dysfunction and sensory abnormalities, microvascular angiopathy can interfere with smooth muscle contraction of the vas deferens and seminal vesicles, impairing emission or causing retrograde ejaculation. Men who have undergone radical prostatectomy have anejaculation due to the absence of the seminal vesicles and truncation of the vasa deferentia.

In men who do not ejaculate, retrograde ejaculation may be the cause. With retrograde ejaculation, the ejaculate migrates retrograde into the bladder rather than down the urethra. The diagnosis of retrograde ejaculation is made by examining the first void following attempted ejaculation for sperm. Synchronous closure of the bladder neck during ejaculation is needed for normal antegrade ejaculation. A patient's surgical history may reveal the cause of retrograde ejaculation. For example, retroperitoneal lymph node dissection (RPLND), vascular surgery affecting the aorta and iliac arteries, colorectal excisions, and transurethral resection of the prostate (TURP) may all lead to either retrograde or anejaculation. TURP disrupts the bladder neck closure mechanism and causes retrograde ejaculation in the majority of men. Antegrade ejaculation may be preserved by performing a transurethral incision of the prostate (TUIP). However, TUIP can cause retrograde ejaculation in up to 45 % of men [8, 9]. In pelvic and retroperitoneal surgeries, disruption of the peripheral sympathetic innervation to the prostate, seminal vesicles, and bladder neck can be the etiology of ejaculatory dysfunction. Emission can be compromised and can occur in a retrograde fashion due to lack of bladder neck closure. Sensation to the penis, quality of erections, and sensation are typically intact. Fortunately, nerve-sparing surgery decreases the incidence of ejaculatory dysfunction [10]. The literature reports 1–40 % of men develop ejaculatory dysfunction following RPLND and 47 % following resection for low colon cancer [11].

14.3.4 Decreased Volume of Ejaculate

Some patients' chief complaint is a low-volume ejaculate. The normal range of semen ejaculate is 1.0–6.5 mL per ejaculation. The World Health Organization (2010) regards 1.5 mL as the lower limit of its reference range [12]. Etiologies and contributors to low-volume ejaculate include benign prostatic hyperplasia (BPH), medications that treat BPH, hypogonadism, ejaculatory duct obstruction, aging, and a history of prior pelvic, retroperitoneal, or bladder neck surgery. With the exception of men seeking future fertility, low-volume ejaculate is not harmful and does not have functional consequences. However, decreased volume of ejaculate can be a significant source of emotional stress, confusion, and frustration for many men and their partners.

14.3.5 Painful Ejaculation

Some patients may report pain with ejaculation. The pain may occur with ejaculation and then immediately resolve, or the pain may persist after ejaculation is complete. These symptoms may result from pelvic floor dysfunction or may be part of the chronic prostatitis/chronic pelvic pain syndrome [13].

14.3.6 Psychological Causes of Ejaculatory Dysfunction

When men with disorders of ejaculation present to their primary care providers, they often are referred to the urologist for evaluation and treatment. The initial role of the urologist is to help identify and treat pharmacological, surgical, and medical causes of ejaculatory dysfunction. As these causes are ruled out and/or when pharmacological treatment fails (see treatment section below), referral to a psychologist, psychiatrist, or other mental health specialist is indicated. The mental health provider should have familiarity with and be comfortable treating patients with sexual disorders.

14.3.7 Neurological Causes of Ejaculatory Dysfunction

If the patient's history includes any neurological abnormalities, a full neurological examination should be performed. Evaluate changes in sensation to the extremities (nociception, soft touch, proprioception) and for weakness as well. Anejaculation and delayed ejaculation can be due to abnormalities of the central or autonomic (primarily sympathetic) nervous system, somatic innervation to the pelvic floor musculature, or sensory innervation of the penis (tactile stimulation). Central nervous disorders such as multiple sclerosis can affect the brain and spinal cord at multiple and varying levels. Sexual dysfunction occurs in up to 50 % of these patients [8]. Patients can have erectile dysfunction, ejaculatory dysfunction, or both.

Patients with spinal cord injuries make up a heterogeneous group of neurological sexual dysfunction. Sensation of the penis, autonomic innervation, and somatic muscular innervation can be affected in any combination.

Diabetes mellitus can cause both neurological and microvascular abnormalities that contribute to sexual dysfunction. It commonly causes varying degrees of erectile dysfunction and can also cause ejaculatory dysfunction. In addition, diabetic neuropathy can decrease sensation to the penis.

14.4 Clinical Approach to Ejaculatory Dysfunction

A patient's medical, surgical, and sexual history is vital in the formulation of a differential diagnosis of ejaculatory dysfunction. Eliciting these histories can be difficult as men are often unaccustomed to discussing qualities of their libido, erections, and ejaculations. In North America, less than 15 % of male and female patients were asked about sexual health by medical provider in the previous year [14, 15].

The crux of the history should involve the type and degree of symptomology, frequency, age of onset, intermittency of dysfunction, and variation with partners or masturbation. The amount of self and partner bother should be clearly documented. A thorough past medical and surgical history should be elicited to help identify potential underlying causes of ejaculatory dysfunction. Specifically, it is essential to inquire about cardiovascular disease, neurological disorders, and surgical procedures with a focus on the spine, abdomen, and genitourinary tract.

A patient's religious beliefs and practices should be evaluated. Perceptions of sexual function as evil, wrong, sacrilegious, or unnatural can contribute to ejaculatory dysfunction. Also critical to the patient history are masturbation habits, frequency, and issues. Often, dysfunction with intercourse does not manifest during masturbation [16]. Patients should also be asked about their sexual practices. Does the ejaculatory dysfunction occur the same way with different partners, in different situations, at different times? Is there anxiety or concern about or during performance? Does the patient discuss sexual dysfunction openly with his partner(s)? Answers to these questions can help providers target treatments to problem areas that need to be addressed.

While the patient will not likely have details of family members with similar problems, care should be taken to discuss family history of neurological, cardiovascular, and endocrine problems.

It is critical to evaluate the current prescribed and over-the-counter medications that a patient is taking. If a patient has a history of a psychiatric disorder, it is important to determine how he is managed and by whom. Medications that can commonly induce delayed ejaculation include SSRIs, TCAs, methyldopa, thiazide diuretics, phenothiazine, and benzodiazepines. Correlate symptomology onset with timing of starting these medications (Table 14.1).

The clinician should obtain a sexual health review of systems and then tailor further questions based on positive screening questions.

Table 14.1 Medications that can induce delayed ejaculation

Medication class	Mechanism of action
Selective serotonin reuptake inhibitors (SSRIs)	Enhances serotonin at postsynaptic neurons
Tricyclic antidepressants	Similar to SSRI
Methyldopa	Blocks alpha-adrenergic receptors necessary for ejaculation
Typical antipsychotics	Blocks alpha-adrenergic receptors necessary for ejaculation
Benzodiazepines	Mechanism unknown, possibly CNS suppression

CNS Central nervous system

Issues with libido and erections should be addressed prior to disorders of ejaculation. Treating libido or erectile problems may resolve ejaculatory dysfunction. Sometimes patients will have underlying abnormalities with achieving or maintaining an erection but will perceive this as an issue with ejaculation. Some patients do not understand that rapid penile detumescence is normal following ejaculation. Patients might complain of loss of erection or difficulty maintaining an erection when premature ejaculation is actually the source of their sexual dysfunction.

A physical examination, with emphasis on the genitalia, is recommended but often does not yield much additional information as to the etiology of ejaculatory dysfunction. The penis should be examined for any abnormalities and for circumcision, which can affect penile sensation. Note the location of urethral meatus and palpate for penile plaques. Palpate the testicles and note their size, firmness, and the presence of any masses. The presence/absence of the vas deferens should be noted as this can be related to the presence/absence of accessory sex organs and other genitourinary organs. A digital rectal examination should be performed to check for palpable ejaculatory duct cysts and for prostate cancer screening when indicated.

Serum hormone profiles can be obtained to evaluate men for hypogonadism. Symptomatic hypogonadism should be screened for as well. Imaging is often low yield and should not be obtained unless there is a specific abnormality suspected based on the history or physical exam. A history of low-volume ejaculate could prompt evaluation with transrectal ultrasound to look for radiographic evidence of ejaculatory duct obstruction. Further workup and treatment of ejaculatory disorders are tailored to the disorder.

14.5 Clinical Approach to PE

PE is diagnosed based on self-reports of PE characteristics. Along with a thorough history and physical examination, the following symptomology should be discussed:

- The estimated IELT, although the patient's perception of IELT is not always representative of actual IELT.
- The duration and frequency of PE and the rate of occurrence of PE with some or all sexual encounters and partners.
- The degree to which sexual stimuli cause PE.
- The nature and frequency of sexual activity including foreplay, masturbation, and intercourse.

The clinician should also focus on sexual expectations. Patients may have expectations of sexual function that are not consistent with their physiology.

Careful attention should be paid to symptoms of erectile dysfunction, hypogonadism, and other ejaculatory dysfunction as well. The clinician should include psychological screening questions as to the quality, nature, and intimacy of the patient's relationship(s). A physical exam focusing on the penis, testicles, vas deferens, and epididymis should be performed, although there is seldom an anatomical abnormality causing PE. Laboratory and radiological testing usually is not needed for these men.

PE is categorized into four types as related to symptomology—lifelong, acquired, natural variable, and premature-like ejaculatory dysfunction. Patients with lifelong PE likely have never had a normal IELT, and PE has been a lifelong problem. If a patient developed PE at a specific point in their life, it is considered acquired PE. There is often a psychological or physiological event that induces onset of acquired PE. Patients with natural variable PE will report that their PE symptoms are intermittent and inconsistent. Variability can be associated with different partners, different sexual activities, or the use of certain drugs or alcohol. Depending on the level of bother, it may be normal to have occasional IELT times of less than one minute. Concentration on PE-associated triggers or situations is important in evaluating these patients. Premature-like ejaculatory dysfunction is described with a psychological preconception of

Table 14.2 Classifications of premature ejaculation (PE)

Type	Features
Lifelong	• PE at all or nearly all intercourse attempts • With all or nearly all women • In majority of cases within 1 min • Consistent during life • Inability to control ejaculation may be lacking (not obligatory)
Acquired	• Rapid ejaculation occurring at some point in life • Normal ejaculation before onset of premature ejaculation • Often source of problem identifiable (organic, psychological) • Inability to control ejaculation may be lacking (not obligatory)
Natural variable	• Rapid ejaculation inconsistent and irregular • Inability to control ejaculation may be lacking (not obligatory)
Premature-like ejaculatory dysfunction	• Subjective perception of rapid ejaculation • Intravaginal ejaculatory latency time in normal range • Preoccupation with imagined rapid ejaculation • Preoccupation with poor control of ejaculation • Preoccupation not accounted for by another mental disorder • Inability to control ejaculation may be lacking (not obligatory)

Adapted from [4]

PE. These patients often have normal IELT with anxiety-provoking preoccupation with sexual performance and ejaculation control (Table 14.2).

14.6 Psychological Causes of Ejaculatory Dysfunction

Once pharmacological, surgical, and medical causes of sexual dysfunction are excluded, psychological evaluation is warranted. In obtaining the patient's history, care should be taken to elucidate any anxiety the patient has toward sexual performance, intimacy, and maladapted relationships with his partner. This level of detail warrants a referral to a psychosexual therapist with specialized training in individual or couple's sexual therapy. Despite limited research, there are many described behavioral therapies to improve ejaculatory dysfunction including sexual education, anxiety reduction, masturbatory training, and stimulation training. The true effectiveness of these strategies is unknown (Fig. 14.2).

14.7 Treatment of Ejaculatory Dysfunction

Treatment of ejaculatory dysfunction should be tailored to the etiology, if known. If hypogonadism is present, treatment should be offered with exogenous testosterone or an estrogen receptor modulator if fertility is desired. Dysfunction related to medical disorders such as multiple sclerosis, diabetes mellitus, and vascular disease should be managed by treatment of the underlying disorder.

14.7.1 Treatment of Premature Ejaculation

14.7.1.1 Behavioral Therapy

Psychosexual therapy is a well-recognized treatment strategy for PE. The primary goal is to allow men to identify and monitor preorgasmic excitement and learn to either suppress orgasm or alter their physical movements to reduce stimulation. Multiple strategies have been described. The most common one is the "start-stop" technique describe by Dr. James Semans. During sexual activity, the patient should be brought to near ejaculation at which point stimulation is stopped. Once the sense of ejaculation passes stimulation is restarted. This allows a sense of control of ejaculation and can help the patient understand the sensations leading up to ejaculation. Other strategies involve delaying genital stimulation well after sexual activity has begun, trying different forms of stimulation (manual, oral), and attempts to divert the patient's thought process away from sexual stimulation. The patient should be counseled that these techniques can decrease enjoyment of sexual intercourse. These techniques should be discussed with both partners together if possible.

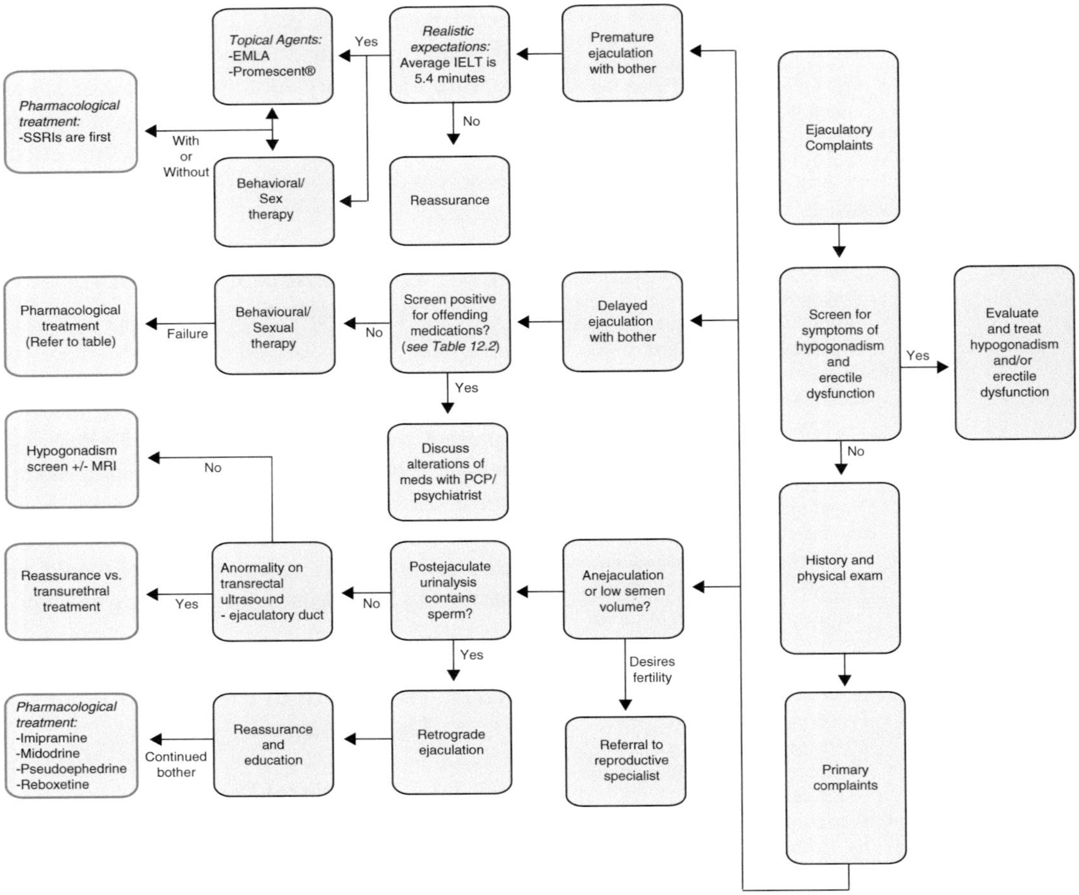

Fig. 14.2 Initial workup and management of ejaculatory dysfunction

While a clinician can discuss these PE management strategies, psychosexual therapy should be performed by a trained therapist who specializes in sexual dysfunction. There are data to support the efficacy of therapy, but it is generally recommended to utilize behavioral and pharmacological combination therapy.

14.7.1.2 Topical Treatments

Premature ejaculation can be treated with topical agents applied directly to the penis. The goal of this therapy is to decrease penile sensation to delay induction of ejaculation reflexes. The staple of these treatments is topical lidocaine or lidocaine-prilocaine (EMLA) cream. There are multiple over-the-counter agents with local anesthetic properties. Some condoms have these topical agents pre-applied. Promescent® is an over-the-counter metered lidocaine spray designed specifically for ejaculatory dysfunction. Promescent® is a eutectic spray that is absorbed significantly faster than topical creams and ointments. This minimizes anesthesia of female genitalia while preserving anesthesia of the male skin. Peer-reviewed literature for Promescent® is largely lacking, but consumer marketing has made it a popular option to try.

While these agents are typically safe and inexpensive and can be used as needed, they can negatively impact sexual intimacy and can cause penile skin irritation and delayed ejaculation or anejaculation and can decrease enjoyment of sexual intercourse due to their desensitizing qualities. These agents often causes female genital anesthesia that can decrease female enjoyment of intercourse as well. Literature on the efficacy of these agents is lacking. A double-blind clinical trial of EMLA cream demonstrated a 5.5-fold increase in IELT, but 30 % of men stopped using the agent due to its adverse effects [7]. Prilocaine has a very rare side effect of methemoglobinemia when used in high doses [17]. Promescent® lacks prilocaine, so there is no risk for methemoglobinemia.

14.7.1.3 Oral Pharmacological Treatment

Serotonin modulation is the primary means of pharmacological treatment of PE. SSRIs make up the first-line treatment of PE. Currently there is no FDA-approved pharmacotherapy to treat PE. Dapoxetine is an SSRI that was designed to treat PE and is currently approved in Europe, but not in the United States. Older SSRIs tend to be more efficacious for treating PE. Newer agents that are classified as serotonin-norepinephrine reuptake inhibitor (SNRIs) including fluvoxamine and venlafaxine are much less efficacious in treating PE. Paroxetine, fluoxetine, sertraline, and citalopram are often used off-label to treat PE. Unlike treatment for depression, which may take several weeks to months to have an effect, SSRIs prescribed for PE often are often efficacious in 1–2 weeks. To be fully effective, these medications should be given for at least 4 weeks.

Randomized controlled studies have demonstrated significant improvement in PE symptoms with SSRI treatment. Depending on the study, IELT increases two- to eightfold. Placebo increases IELT 1.5–2-fold. Paroxetine has shown a superiority over sertraline, fluoxetine, and placebo in direct comparison trials [18].

Dapoxetine is an SSRI approved in Europe for the treatment of PE and was developed specifically for PE. It is a short-acting medication that may be used on-demand, and its use shows promise [19] for effective treatment. It has a half-life of 1.5 h and reaches maximum serum concentration in 1.3 h [20]. Dapoxetine was found to increase IELT 3.5-fold in a placebo-controlled study. Patients reported better control of ejaculation and better sexual satisfaction [21]. Approximately 5 % of patients withdrew due to side effects.

The side effect profiles of SSRIs are well described and include nausea, anxiety, insomnia, anhidrosis, alterations in libido, and somnolence. Nausea is the most common side effect and is usually mild. Long-term use of SSRIs has been associated with loss of bone mineral density. Sudden cessation of SSRIs can cause acute nausea, vomiting, dizziness, headache, ataxia, drowsiness, anxiety, and insomnia. This effect can be avoided by tapering SSRIs over a 4-week period. If a patient develops withdrawal symptoms, their SSRI should be restarted and then tapered once the symptoms improve. The use of monoamine oxidase inhibitors (MAOIs) is an absolute contraindication to SSRI use due to risk of serotonin syndrome.

TCAs such as clomipramine have also been used for PE. Multiple studies have demonstrated efficacy for clomipramine; however, it has a worse side effect profile and is more dangerous in high doses than SSRIs.

Tramadol is a synthetic opioid analgesic that may be used off-label for PE. While its mechanism of action is not fully understood, it is safe and has a mild side effect profile. It can also be used in an on-demand fashion [22]. Approximately 30 % of men report improvement in IELT with the use of tramadol. Some studies have investigated the use of phosphodiesterase type 5 inhibitors (PDE5i) for the treatment of PE. If there is concurrent erectile dysfunction, it should be treated prior to treatment of PE, as PE may improve with improvement of erections. There is no role for PDE5i monotherapy to treat PE [23].

In summary, SSRIs are typically considered for first-line therapy for PE. Counseling and psychoeducation about the ejaculations should always be provided. Pharmacotherapy and psychotherapy should be used in combination to treat severe PE.

14.7.1.4 Invasive Management of PE

Intracavernosal injection therapy has been used for refractory PE. While it does not alter IELT, it delays penile detumescence that accompanies ejaculation. In theory, this allows for continued intercourse, increased sexual confidence, and partner satisfaction. Literature for this treatment is sparse, and injections should be used only after extensive patient counseling and after exhausting all other treatment options.

There are reported links between circumcision and penile sensation. The literature is overwhelmingly conflicting, and no definitive conclusions can be drawn. Premature ejaculation is not an indication to perform a circumcision, and this procedure should not be offered unless it is otherwise indicated [24].

A radical approach to PE management is operative penile denervation. There is some published literature describing microsurgical resection of selective braches of the dorsal penile nerve to treat PE [25]. In the United States and Europe, these techniques have not widely been utilized or studied. As this is not a widely accepted technique, it is not recommended to offer this option to patients.

14.7.2 Treatment of Delayed Ejaculation and Anejaculation

When presented with a complaint of delayed ejaculation, anejaculation, or retrograde ejaculation, the clinician needs to collect critical pieces of information from the patient. Ejaculatory dysfunction can often coexist with erectile dysfunction and hypogonadism. It can also be iatrogenic and caused by previous surgery or medications. It is important to determine if the patient is able to ejaculate with masturbation. Approximately 75 % of men with ejaculatory failure are actually able to ejaculate with masturbation [25, 26]. The clinician should attempt to determine whether or not the symptomology is consistent with anorgasmia, anejaculation, or both and to determine the patient's drug and alcohol use, relating substance use with timing and onset of symptoms. Excessive use of alcohol, narcotics, and stimulants can negatively impact ejaculation. Recommending that the patient decrease or stop the use of these substances if excess use is suspected is prudent, and if the patient demonstrates abuse or dependence on drug/alcohol, addiction counseling is warranted. Success with psychosocial-behavioral and cultural approaches to the treatment of DE has been reported, but to date there is only low-level anecdotal evidence in support of such an approach [27].

If medications are suspected as the cause of ejaculatory dysfunction, attempts to stop, decrease dose, or prescribe alternate medications should be made. However, most medications should be altered in consultation with the patient's primary practitioner and/or psychiatrist is involved in the decision-making. This is especially true for patients with neurological conditions or Axis I psychiatric conditions. Some SSRIs and TCAs require a taper prior to discontinuation. Withdrawal of benzodiazepines can be life threatening and should not be done in an unsupervised manner.

Pharmacological treatment for delayed ejaculation and anejaculation has been described, but currently, there are no FDA-approved medications for this disorder. However, both cabergoline and oxytocin have been used, with several case reports and small studies supporting efficacy. Oxytocin is a hormone released by the posterior pituitary gland. Most of understanding of oxytocin is in its relation to birth and lactation, but it also plays a role in ejaculation [28]. It is taken as a nasal spray at or near the moment of desired ejaculation. There is little literature that speaks to its efficacy, but there are data supporting its use [29]. Cabergoline is a dopamine receptor agonist that historically has been used to treat prolactinomas. Like oxytocin, there is little literature supporting its efficacy to treat delayed ejaculation. One study has demonstrated an increase in quality of ejaculation and a decrease in the refractory period following ejaculation [30]. These medications are generally safe to try for refractory delayed ejaculation and anejaculation. A thorough discussion of the off-label use and paucity of data supporting efficacy should

Table 14.3 Pharmacological treatment for delayed ejaculation and anejaculation

Drug	Dosage PRN	Daily
Cabergoline	ND	0.25–2 mg twice weekly
Amantadine	100–400 mg (for 2 days prior to coitus)	100–200 mg bid
Pseudoephedrine	60–120 mg (1–2 h prior to coitus)	ND
Reboxetine	ND	4–8 mg daily
Bupropion	ND	150 mg daily to bid
Buspirone	ND	5–15 mg bid
Cyproheptadine	4–12 mg (3–4 h prior to coitus)	ND
Oxytocin	24 IS intranasal during coitus	ND

ND No data
Adapted from [23]

be had with the patient prior to initiation of treatment. The theoretical mechanism of action is modification of the dopaminergic, serotonergic, or oxytocinergic neurotransmitters in the central nervous system or the adrenergic actions in the peripheral nervous system (Table 14.3).

14.7.3 Treatment of Retrograde Ejaculation

Prior to surgery, patients should be counseled about retrograde ejaculation as a potential side effect of pelvic and transurethral procedures, as it can be quite distressing to some patients. Operative techniques for reconstruction of the bladder neck are described, but literature on their efficacy is lacking [6]. If retrograde ejaculation is due to a nonsurgical cause, the initial treatment is aimed at treating the underlying condition. Patients with diabetes mellitus or multiple sclerosis should be managed by the appropriate specialty. Spinal cord injuries can take several months to stabilize, and changes in sexual function are common during this time. Pharmacotherapy directed at peripheral adrenergic modulation may have some efficacy in treating retrograde ejaculation. Imipramine, midodrine, pseudoephedrine, and reboxetine may have some benefit. There is insufficient data to fully support their efficacy, but they are generally safe medications that can be tried empirically. These medications may also benefit men with both surgical and nonsurgical retrograde ejaculation. For men who have undergone TURP, retrograde ejaculation is not treatable, and this should be discussed preoperatively.

14.7.4 Treatment of Painful Ejaculation

For men with painful ejaculation, treatment is challenging and often empirical. Alpha-blockers may be offered, but these medications carry with them a risk of decreased ejaculate volume or absence of ejaculate [31]. Pelvic floor physical therapy can be offered to treat ejaculatory pain, especially when a musculoskeletal etiology of the pain is suspected [32].

14.7.5 Treatment of Low Ejaculate Volume

Determine if the patient has normal IELT, normal sensation, and normal erections. Increased age and increased frequency of ejaculation can result in diminished semen volumes. If the patient has an acute and persistent change in ejaculate volume, a transrectal ultrasound may be obtained to evaluate for midline prostatic cysts or calcifications in the ejaculatory ducts that could lead to ejaculatory duct obstruction. If the ejaculate volumes have been persistently low, then Mullerian and Wolffian duct remnants or other anatomical malformations should be considered as causes. Transrectal ultrasound and pelvic MRI are useful imaging modalities if these are suspected, and surgical correction is required. The physician may also offer evaluation of hypogonadism. In the absence of any harmful pathology and with normal to low-normal ejaculate volume, treatment is reassurance and expectant management [2, 33, 34].

14.8 Summary

Disorders of ejaculation are prevalent and are a significant source of stress and anxiety for men and their partners. Careful history taking may reveal underlying psychosocial contributors to ejaculatory dysfunction, but iatrogenic causes (both medical and surgical) are common. SSRIs, topical anesthetics, behavioral therapy, and psychotherapy, either alone or in combination, remain the mainstays of treatment of this challenging and complex condition.

References

1. Rowland D, McMahon CG, Carmita A, Chen J, Jannini E, Waldinger MD, Ahn TY. Disorders of orgasm and ejaculation in men. J Sex Med. 2010
2. Giuliano F, Clement P. Physiology of ejaculation: an emphasis on serotonergic control. Eur Urol. 2005.
3. Giuliano F, Clement P. Neuroanatomy and physiology of ejaculation. Annu Rev Sex Res. 2005.
4. Mulhall JP. In: Wein AJ, Kavoussi LR, Novick AC, Partin AW, Peters CA, editors. Campbell-Walsh urology. 10th edn. Philadelphia: Elsevier; 2012.
5. Broderick GA. Premature ejaculation: on defining and quantifying a common male sexual dysfunction. J Sex Med. 2006.
6. McMahon CG. Management of ejaculatory dysfunction. J Intern Med. 2014.
7. Patrick DL, Althof SE, Pryor JL, Rosen R. Premature ejaculation: an observational study of men and their partners. J Sex Med. 2005.
8. Guo ZN, He SY, Zhang HL, Wu J. Multiple sclerosis and sexual dysfunction. Asian J Androl. 2012.
9. Kelly MJ, Roskamp D, Leach GE. Transurethral incision of the prostate: a preoperative and postoperative analysis of symptoms and urodynamic findings. Urology. 1989.
10. Pettus JA, Carver BS, Masterson T, Stasi J, Sheinfeld J. Preservation of ejaculation in patients undergoing nerve-sparing postchemotherapy retroperitoneal lymph node dissection for metastatic testicular cancer. Urology. 2009.
11. Phillips E, Carpenter C, Oates RD. Ejaculatory dysfunction. Urol Clin North Am. 2014.
12. World Health Organization. WHO laboratory manual for the examination and processing of human semen. Geneva: World Health Organization; 2010.
13. Trab CN, Shoskes DA. Sexual dysfunction in chronic prostatitis/chronic pelvic pain syndrome. World J Urol. 2013.
14. Althof SE, McMahon CG, Waldinger MD, Serefoglu EC. An update of the international society of sexual medicine's guidelines for the diagnosis and treatment of premature ejaculation. Sex Med. 2014.
15. Laumann EO, Paik A, Rosen RC. Sexual dysfunction in the United States: prevalence and predictors. JAMA. 1999
16. Perelman MA, Rowland DL. Retarded ejaculation. World J Urol. 2006;24(6):645–52.
17. Shamriz O, Cohen I. Methemoglobinemia induced by lidocaine-prilocaine cream. Isr Med Assoc J. 2014.
18. Waldinger MD. The neurobiological approach to premature ejaculation. Urology. 2002.
19. Buvat J, Tesfaye F, Rothman M, Rivas DA, Giuliano F. Dapoxetine for the treatment of premature ejaculation: results from a randomized, double-blind, placebo-controlled phase 3 trial in 22 countries. Eur Urol. 2009.
20. Jannini EA, Isidori AM, Aversa A, Lenzi A, Althof SE. Which is first? The controversial issue of precedence in the treatment of male sexual dysfunctions. J Sex Med. 2013.
21. Pryor JL, Althof SE, Steidle C, Rosen RC, Hellstrom WJG, Shabsigh R, Miloslavsky M, Kell S. Efficacy and tolerability of dapoxetine in treatment of premature ejaculation: an integrated analysis of two double-blind, randomised controlled trials. Lancet. 2006.
22. Salem EA, Wilson SK, Bissada NK. Tramadol HCL has promise in on-demand use to treat premature ejaculation. J Sex Med. 2008.
23. McMahon CG, McMahon CN, Leow LJ. Efficacy of type-5 phosphodiesterase inhibitors in the drug treatment of premature ejaculation: a systematic review. BJU Int. 2006;98(2):259–72.
24. Zhang SJ, Zhao YM, Zheng SG, Xiao HW. Correlation between premature ejaculation and redundant prepuce. Zhonghua Nan Ke Xue. 2006.
25. Zhang CY, Li XH, Yuan T, Zhang HF. Regional anatomy of the dorsal penile nerve and its clinical significance. Zhonghua Nan Ke Xue. 2009.
26. Rowland D, Perelman M, Althof S. Self-reported premature ejaculation and aspects of sexual functioning and satisfaction. J Sex Med. 2004.
27. Perelman MA. Delayed ejaculation. In: Binik YM, Hall KS, editors. Principles and practice of sexual therapy. New York: Guilford Press; 2014.
28. Carmichael MS, Warburton VL, Dixen J. Relationships among cardiovascular, muscular, and oxytocin responses during human sexual activity. Arch Sex Behav. 1994.

29. Veening JG, Olivier B. Intranasal administration of oxytocin: behavioral and clinical effects, a review. Neurosci Biobehav Rev. 2013.
30. Kruger TH, Haake P, Haverkamp J. Effects of acute prolactin manipulation on sexual drive and function in males. J Endocrinol. 2003.
31. Hellstrom WJ, Sikka SC. Effects of acute treatment with tamsulosin versus alfuzosin on ejaculatory function in normal volunteers. J Urol. 2006.
32. Anderson RU, Wise D, Sawyer T, Chan C. Integration of myofascial trigger point release and paradoxical relaxation training treatment of chronic pelvic pain in men. Urology. 2005.
33. Hellerstein DK, Meacham RB, Lipshultz LI. Transrectal ultrasound and partial ejaculatory duct obstruction in male infertility. Urology. 1992.
34. McMahon CG, Giuliano F, Dean J. Efficacy and safety of dapoxetine in men with premature ejaculation and concomitant erectile dysfunction treated with a phosphodiesterase type 5 inhibitor. J Sex Med. 2013.

Commentary: Clinical Evaluation and Treatment of Disorders of Ejaculation

Daniel N. Watter

Ejaculatory dysfunctions represent a common and growing problem seen in men. Scovell and Eisenberg in Chap. 13 *highlight the complexity of these conditions, showing how even with the use of contemporary technologies, our understanding of the mechanisms of these conditions is in its nascency. However, our current understanding of these conditions is nevertheless sufficient for developing effective treatment approaches using collaborative, multidisciplinary approaches. In addition to understanding the physical nature of the dysfunction, an essential part of the evaluation of men with ejaculatory disorders involves understanding the man's relationship status including the quality, nature, intimacy, and maladaptive characteristics of this relationship. Other psychological causes of ejaculatory dysfunction should be elucidated as well, including anxiety surrounding sexual performance. In the preceding chapter, Johnson and Williams comprehensively highlight both medical and psychological etiologies and approaches to ejaculatory disorders and call for a combined approach to treatment.*

In the following commentary, Watter more completely delves into the intra- and interpersonal dynamics of ejaculatory disorders, focusing on the need to address the psychological and relational distress associated with these conditions on a case-specific basis. Together, the chapter and commentary cast into stark relief how a combined treatment approach can roundly address the causes of ejaculatory dysfunction in any male. Such a treatment approach is needed regardless of a detailed understanding of the etiologies of these conditions.

The Editors

Daniel N. Watter, Ed.D
The Society for Sex Therapy and Research (SSTAR),
Morris Psychological Group, P.A., Parsippany,
NJ, USA

Commentary

For the mental health clinician, disorders of ejaculation represent a range of sexual difficulties. From the common, and often highly treatable, rapid or premature ejaculation to the less common and typically more complicated delayed ejaculation, these cases can be both interesting and challenging.

Typically, the mental health clinician will be dealing with the anxiety, frustration, and disappointment of the men and their partners experiencing such dysfunctions. Regardless of the interventions utilized to address the particulars of the ejaculatory problem, these men tend to enter treatment feeling "broken" and ineffective as sexual partners. As a result, many may have been avoiding partnered sexual opportunities for quite some time. This will likely have led to a further complicating of their situations inasmuch as they now are faced with both sexual frustrations as well as relationship tensions. In order for treatment to be successful, both the intrapersonal and the interpersonal dynamics of these sexual dysfunctions will need to be addressed.

As previously mentioned, rapid or premature ejaculation is the most commonly seen ejaculatory disorder in mental health practice. The precise definition of the disorder (as is the case with many sexual disorders) is somewhat controversial. A complete discussion of this commentary is beyond the scope of this chapter, but the reader may wish to consult the recent updates of the ISSM's guidelines for the diagnosis and treatment of premature ejaculation [1, 2]. Most clinicians would agree that when ejaculation occurs either prior to vaginal penetration or within one minute of vaginal penetration, a diagnosis of rapid or premature ejaculation can be made. However, for the mental health clinician, the intravaginal ejaculatory latency time (IELT) is often of secondary concern. The primary mental health issue is the psychological and relational distress that often results in the patient seeking treatment. These issues may be left unexplored if only pharmacological treatments are utilized.

The mental health clinician must also take into account whether the patient is experiencing lifelong or acquired rapid/premature ejaculation. In addition, it must be assessed whether this difficulty is generalized (in all situations) or situational. Treatment for those who have always had short IELT is fairly straightforward. However, treatment for those who have a history of good ejaculatory control but are now experiencing ejaculatory difficulties is typically much more challenging and complex. According to Perelman [1] and Althof [3], a combination of pharmacological and behavioral/psychotherapeutic interventions is often the treatment of choice. Clinical experience reassures that many men will also benefit from psychotherapy/behavioral interventions alone, despite some research evidence to the contrary. The disparity is due to both research sampling techniques and the difficulty in employing quantitative research methods typical of randomized clinical trials (RCT) to psychotherapeutic processes [2].

Case Example: Lifelong Rapid/ Premature Ejaculation

James was a 27-year-old married man who had been experiencing rapid/premature ejaculation since he began having sexual intercourse at 18 years old. His current wife was his second sexual partner, and he described a strong, loving, and satisfying marriage. James reported ejaculation often prior to vaginal penetration and duration of less than 2 min of intercourse as a best-case scenario. James was highly motivated to develop better ejaculatory control as this situation was becoming increasingly frustrating for both he and his wife. During the year prior to seeking treatment, James reported a great deal of sexual avoidance due to the sexual disappointment he endured.

After an initial meeting with both James and his wife, it was agreed that we would begin with a behaviorally based treatment for his ejaculatory difficulties. Given that there were no apparent underlying psychological difficulties (other than the resulting anxiety about sexual performance and relationship tensions that occurred as a result of the sexual dysfunction) and that he did not wish to utilize pharmacotherapy unless the behavioral treatment failed, James agreed to begin a trial of masturbatory retraining exercises utilizing the stop/start method [4]. These exercises were augmented by the use of male Kegel exercises. James progressed uneventfully through the masturbation retraining exercises, and then he and his wife began bridging exercises to allow James to transfer what he learned about ejaculatory control during masturbation to partnered sexual activity. Both James and his wife reported great satisfaction with the treatment outcome, as they were now able to participate in sexual intercourse for approximately 5–8 min. Gains had been maintained at 3-, 6-, and 9-month follow-up.

Case Example: Acquired Rapid/ Premature Ejaculation

Frank was a 55-year-old man who had been married for 24 years. He reported good ejaculatory control while dating his wife, as well as in the early years of marriage. After approximately 8 years of marriage, he developed ejaculatory control problems. He was started on a course of an SSRI treatment, which helped his ejaculatory latency, but he experienced side effects that necessitated discontinuation of treatment. Following cessation of pharmacotherapy, Frank reported continued improved ejaculatory control. However, approximately 4 years prior to current consultation, his ejaculatory control problems returned. Frank reported going from IELT of approximately 8–10 min to ejaculation within 30 s of vaginal penetration. Psychological assessment revealed that Frank's ejaculation difficulties (both episodes) coincided with severe marital problems. Frank described his wife as overbearing and emotionally volatile. He felt poorly equipped to deal with her emotionality and became highly anxious and avoidant of any situations that might trigger her anger.

Treatment for Frank focused less on behavioral interventions to improve IELT and primarily addressed his marital issues and need to better advocate for himself. As he became more confident in his ability to deal with his wife's emotional outbursts and less fearful of marital dissolution, his ejaculatory control improved considerably.

As was mentioned earlier, premature ejaculation is much more frequently encountered in clinical practice than is delayed ejaculation. As is the case with premature ejaculation, the precise definition and etiology of this dysfunction is controversial, and an in-depth discussion of such is beyond the scope of this chapter. For a more detailed discussion, the reader may wish to consult the recent work of Perelman and Watter [5].

For the mental health clinician, the treatment of delayed ejaculation can be quite complex, although successful use of sex therapy for many cases of non-hormonally determined DE has been reported [6]. Patients suffering from this dysfunction are often extremely frustrated and receive little satisfaction from sexual activity, most typically partnered sexual activity. Many, if not most, men complaining of delayed ejaculation are able to achieve orgasm via solo masturbation (although it may take a long time to reach ejaculation). However, achieving orgasm/ejaculation with a partner is often extremely difficult or impossible, even though they may be receiving sexual stimulation they describe as adequate and arousing. As is the case with other sexual dysfunctions, this disorder may be either lifelong or acquired and generalized or situational. Due to the limitations of the scope of this chapter, those cases of delayed ejaculation that are the result of either normal aging or SSRI induced will not be addressed.

The psychological treatment for delayed ejaculation is highly nuanced and case specific. Many men presenting with this dysfunction have a history of idiosyncratic masturbation patterns [7]. As a result, some form of masturbation retraining or reduction of masturbatory frequency is often indicated as a significant element of treatment. However, others suffering with delayed ejaculation have no such patterns, and their treatment focuses much more directly on the underlying psychological factors that may be contributing to the disorder.

Case Example: Lifelong, Situational Delayed Ejaculation

Larry was a 32-year-old male who presented for treatment of delayed ejaculation following evaluation and referral by his urologist. Larry had been able to ejaculate during solo masturbation, but it typically took him 30 min or more of vigorous masturbation in order to reach climax. While this situation was of concern to him, what prompted him to seek assistance was his wife's frustration that they would be unable to conceive since he was completely unable to reach orgasm/ejaculation via penile-vaginal intercourse. Larry further reported that he had never been able to ejaculate during intercourse in prior relationships as well. He was in otherwise good health, with no history of substance abuse, and was taking no prescribed medications.

Larry had a history of idiosyncratic masturbation. That is, he had developed a pattern of masturbating while lying on his stomach against a hard floor. He reported never being able to masturbate by hand, as he could never reach a level of arousal that would result in orgasm/ejaculation. As a result, penile-vaginal intercourse, while pleasurable, was not stimulating enough to trigger sexual climax. Larry was highly motivated to participate in treatment and course of behavioral masturbation retraining was agreed upon. Larry was encouraged to transition from masturbating prone against the floor to using his hand with lotion while sitting in a chair. After several weeks of successive approximations, he was able to achieve orgasm and ejaculation while masturbating. His wife was then brought in to the treatment to work on behavioral exercises that would assist Larry in transferring his masturbation changes to penile-vaginal intercourse. While successful, Larry reported that orgasm in the prone position was more pleasurable than his new patterns. Subsequent therapy sessions focused on the ambivalence he now experienced between what was most pleasing for him versus what was most pleasing, and preferred, by his wife.

Case Example: Situational, Acquired Delayed Ejaculation

Richard was a 36-year-old male who presented with the complaint of delayed ejaculation. Specifically, Richard reported that he was unable to ejaculate during intercourse with his wife for several years. He further reported that he was able to easily ejaculate during intercourse with her in the early years of their relationship, but in recent years orgasm/ejaculation had become impossible. Interestingly, he had no difficulty whatsoever with orgasm/ejaculation with prostitutes. Richard was in good health, took no prescribed medications, and had no history of substance abuse.

Obviously, Richard's condition was quite different from that of Larry. Richard had no physical impediments to achieving orgasm/ejaculation, as he was easily orgasmic with prostitutes. Treatment for Richard focused on the unacknowledged difficulties he has in his marital relationship and deeply felt ambivalence about intimacy, autonomy, and control. Richard's treatment took considerably longer than did Larry's, but eventually he was able to again easily reach orgasm/ejaculation with his wife. Gains were maintained on 3-, 6-, and 9-month follow-up.

As can be seen, the mental health approach to the treatment of ejaculatory disorders is varied and case specific. These disorders are often manifestations of underlying psychological difficulties that need to be evaluated and addressed in order for the man's sexual functioning to improve. In addition, considerable attention needs to be paid to the impact of delayed ejaculation on the dynamics of the interpersonal relationship, as many of these cases result from underlying psychiatric conditions related to relational difficulties. As is often the case in the treatment of male sexual dysfunction, the mental health clinician is best consulted following urologic evaluation and assessment, as the perspective of both domains can be invaluable.

References

1. Perelman MA. A new combination treatment for premature ejaculation: a sex therapist's perspective. J Sex Med. 2006;3(6):1004–12.
2. Heiman JR, Meston CM. Empirically validated treatment for sexual dysfunction. Annu Rev Sex Res. 1997;8:148–94.
3. Althof S. Treatment of premature ejaculation. In: Binik YM, Hall KSK, editors. Principles and practice of sex therapy. 5th edn. New York: Guilford Press; 2014. p. 112–37.
4. Zilbergeld B. The new male sexuality, revised edition. New York: Bantam Books; 1999.
5. Perelman MA, Watter DN. Delayed ejaculation. In: Kirana PS, Tripodi MF, Reisman Y, Porst H, editors. The efs and essm syllabus of clinical sexology. Amsterdam: Medix Publishers; 2014. p. 660–72.
6. Perelman MA. Delayed ejaculation. In: Binik YM, Hall KS, editors. Principles and practice of sexual therapy. 5th edn. Guilford Press; 2014
7. Perelman MA. Idiosyncratic masturbation patterns: a key unexplored variable in the treatment of retarded ejaculation by the practicing urologist. J Urol. 2005;173:340.

15 Evaluation and Treatment of Orgasmic Dysfunction

Christopher Yang, Tariq S. Hakky, and Rafael Carrion

15.1 Introduction

The sexual response cycle was first proposed in 1960 by Masters and Johnson [1] and revised multiple times to its current definition of four interactive phases: desire, excitation (or arousal), orgasm, and resolution [2]. The male orgasm phase of the sexual response cycle consists of the sensation of pleasure accompanied by ejaculation. The cognitive experience of pleasure during the orgasm phase is also called orgasm [3, 4]. Indeed, "orgasm" has at least 26 definitions with different meanings depending on whether it is defined by the basic scientist, the physiologist, the endocrinologist, the neuroradiologist, and the psychologist [5].

Because of the myriad definitions and usages of "orgasm," a summary of orgasmic dysfunction (OD) can be challenging. As ejaculatory dysfunction is covered in a separate chapter, we will limit the scope of this discussion primarily to the organic aspects of non-ejaculatory dysfunction of the orgasmic phase of the male sexual response cycle.

C. Yang, M.D.
North Austin Urology, Austin, TX, USA

T.S. Hakky, M.D.
Advanced Urology, Snellville, GA, USA

R. Carrion, M.D. (✉)
Department of Urology, University of South Florida, 2 Tampa General Circle, STC6, Tampa, FL 33606, USA
e-mail: rcarrion@health.usf.edu

15.2 Physiologic Control of Orgasm

While the neural, endocrine, vascular, muscular, and end-organ pathways for erection and ejaculation are well defined, the pathway that results in orgasm is poorly understood. Orgasm is a short-lived sensory manifestation that usually follows a series of physical events: contraction of accessory sexual organs and the urethral bulb and buildup and release of pressure in the distal urethra [3]. The pudendal nerve transmits the sensory stimuli resulting from the above physical events to the cerebrum, resulting in orgasm [6].

The distinction between ejaculation and orgasm is described by Newman and colleagues, who reported orgasmic sensations without input from the genitals or concomitant ejaculation [3]. Additionally, the sensation of orgasm after radical prostatectomy, which eliminates ejaculation, is well known. A similar phenomenon can be seen in patients taking alpha-blockers who experience orgasm with retrograde ejaculation.

15.2.1 Hormonal Control

The ejaculatory response is controlled by central neural pathways using serotonin and dopamine as primary neurotransmitters, with acetylcholine,

L.I. Lipshultz et al. (eds.), *Management of Sexual Dysfunction in Men and Women*, DOI 10.1007/978-1-4939-3100-2_15

nitric oxide, adrenaline, gamma-aminobutyric acid (GABA), and oxytocin playing secondary roles [6, 7]. As orgasm is normally intimately associated with ejaculation, these neurotransmitters also affect orgasm.

Oxytocin and vasopressin are also involved in sexual function. Murphy and colleagues measured oxytocin and vasopressin levels in 13 normal men during the sexual response cycle [8]. They found that vasopressin levels rise during arousal, returning to baseline levels by the time of ejaculation. Oxytocin is unchanged during arousal, rises at ejaculation, and returns to baseline levels 30 min after ejaculation. The authors do not distinguish between ejaculation and orgasm, and it can be inferred from their study design that all subjects achieved both ejaculation and orgasm at the time of increased serum oxytocin levels.

Prolactin levels rise following male orgasm, which is thought to cause the post-orgasmic refractory period [9]. Additionally, hyperprolactinemia can impair physiologic pulsatile LH release, reducing serum testosterone and leading to erectile dysfunction [10]. Despite this association with sexual function, conflicting reports exist about the association of prolactin with orgasmic dysfunction (OD). Buvat and colleagues reported 51 patients with anorgasmia, all with normal prolactin levels [11]. In contrast, Swartz and colleagues reported several men with hyperprolactinemia and isolated anorgasmia [12].

Low prolactin has also been associated with OD in middle-aged and elderly men in the European Male Aging Study, a population-based prospective study of aging in eight European centers [13]. In this study of nearly 3000 men, low prolactin levels had strong correlation with reduced enjoyment of orgasm, as measured by sexual function questionnaires.

15.3 Classification of Orgasmic Dysfunction

In 2013, the International Society for Sexual Medicine (ISSM) published its Standard Operating Procedures (SOPs) in the Disorders of Orgasm and Ejaculation [14], which provide recommendations and guidelines in the management of premature ejaculation, delayed ejaculation (DE), anejaculation, and anorgasmia. Unfortunately, the authors do not discuss anorgasmia separately from disorders of DE and anejaculation.

Indeed, the American Psychiatric Association's Diagnostic and Statistical Manual of Mental Disorders, fifth edition (DSM-V), published in 2013 no longer contains the diagnosis "male orgasmic disorder," which is found in the fourth edition. This diagnosis was changed to "delayed ejaculation," defined by the following criteria:

A. Either of the following symptoms must be experienced on almost all or all occasions (approximately 75–100 %) of partnered sexual activity (in identified situational contexts or, if generalized, in all contexts) and without the individual desiring delay:
   1. Marked delay in ejaculation
   2. Marked infrequency or absence of ejaculation
B. The symptoms in Criterion A have persisted for a minimum duration of approximately 6 months.
C. The symptoms in Criterion A cause clinically significant distress in the individual.
D. The sexual dysfunction is not better explained by a nonsexual mental disorder or as a consequence of severe relationship distress or other significant stressors and is not attributable to the effects of a substance/medication or another medical condition [15].

In defining DE, the DSM-V also contains the following discussion regarding OD:

> It is important in the history to ascertain whether the complaint concerns delayed ejaculation or the sensation of orgasm, or both. *Ejaculation occurs in the genitals, whereas the experience of orgasm is believed to be primarily subjective.* Ejaculation and orgasm usually occur together but not always. For example, a man with a normal ejaculatory pattern may complain of decreased pleasure (i.e. anhedonic ejaculation). Such a complaint would not be coded as delayed ejaculation but could be coded as other specified sexual dysfunction or unspecified sexual dysfunction. [15]

Thus, DSM-V also attempts to separate the mainly organic etiologies of DE from the psychological etiologies of OD. In the interest of accuracy, any future classification systems should separate orgasmic and ejaculatory disorders as these are now recognized as separate entities.

15.4 Evaluation of Orgasmic Dysfunction

The ISSM gives an SOP for)the diagnosis of DE, anejaculation, and anorgasmia:

> Evaluation of men presenting with DE/anejaculation should include a full medical/sexual history, a focused physical examination, determination of serum testosterone levels, and any additional investigations suggested by these findings [14].

Evaluation should focus on differentiating whether the man has ejaculatory dysfunction or OD, as ejaculatory dysfunction may have congenital, endocrine, iatrogenic, infectious, neuropathic, or psychological factors as an underlying etiology.

Additional questions to be posed concern the chronicity and conditionality of the man's OD. This determines if the OD is lifelong or acquired (occurring after a time of normal orgasmic function) and if it is generalized (occurring with every partner, stimulation, and situation) or conditional (occurring with certain partners, stimulations, and situations).

15.4.1 Pharmacologic Causes

The evaluation of the man with)OD should focus on his medications, as these are the most common cause of OD. A Micromedex® search of package inserts shows 16 discrete medications that list OD (with terminology including "orgasm disorder" or "orgasm incapacity") as an adverse) reaction in men (Table 15.1) [16]. The reported risks of these adverse reactions are low, with the majority of drug inserts citing a <10 % incidence. All of the medications listed are psychoactive drugs, with effects on serotonin, norepinephrine, and dopamine neurotransmission.

Table 15.1 Medications with package inserts listing orgasmic dysfunction for men as a potential adverse reaction

Medication	Class	Risk of adverse event (%)
Desvenlafaxine	SNRI	3
Venlafaxine	SNRI	2–5
Duloxetine	SNRI	3
Paroxetine	SSRI	3.7–10
Fluoxetine	SSRI	NA
Sertraline	SSRI	NA
Citalopram	SSRI	8
Escitalopram	SSRI	NA
Clomipramine	Tricyclic antidepressant	NA
Mirtazapine	Tetracyclic antidepressant	NA
Vilazodone	Miscellaneous antidepressant	4
Bupropion	Miscellaneous antidepressant	NA
Trazodone	Phenylpiperazine antidepressant	<1
Amisulpride	Atypical antipsychotic	NA
Risperidone	Atypical antipsychotic	NA
Ziprasidone	Atypical antipsychotic	NA

SNRI serotonin-norepinephrine reuptake inhibitor, *SSRI* selective serotonin reuptake inhibitor

More unusual reports of medication-induced orgasmic augmentation exist. McLean and colleagues reported two patients (one male, one female) successfully treated for depression with clomipramine [17]. Both noted that after starting the medication, each time they yawned, they experienced orgasm. The male patient had an intense urge to yawn without feeling tired and did not experience an increase in libido. With every yawn causing orgasm, he also experienced ejaculation and overcame his awkwardness and embarrassment by continuously wearing a condom. Discontinuation of clomipramine led to a cessation of symptoms.

Labbate reported a case of a 37-year-old patient with attention deficit disorder treated with bupropion SR [18]. He developed increased libido, increased feeling on orgasm, and rare spontaneous partial erections during the day.

After 6 weeks taking the medication, he developed a surprise second orgasm during intercourse: he had normal initial ejaculation and orgasm, followed five seconds later by a spontaneous and pleasurable second ejaculation and orgasm. This phenomenon resolved after stopping bupropion SR, returned after restarting the medication several months later, and finally resolved after stopping once again.

15.5 Treatment of Orgasmic Dysfunction

The ISSM also provides a single SOP for the treatment of DE, anejaculation, and anorgasmia:

> Treatment of DE/anejaculation should be etiology-specific and may include patient/couple psycho-education and/or psychosexual therapy, pharmacotherapy, or integrated treatment. Men/partners of reproductive age should be informed of the risk of infertility due to anejaculation following pelvic surgery and the need for sperm harvesting and assisted reproductive techniques [14].

Figure 15.1 shows a management algorithm for DE, anejaculation, and anorgasmia adapted from the ISSM SOPs that integrates diagnostic questions with the treatment of choice [6, 14]. Of note, the only recommended treatments for anorgasmia are disease-specific management for failure of emission and psychosexual therapy for inhibited male orgasm.

Men with lifelong anorgasmia may also have sexual arousal disorder. Psychosexual therapy would include masturbation training starting with self-exploration to identify pleasurable sensations. This can lead to incremental increases in arousal that leads to orgasm; these techniques can then be communicated to the man's partner.

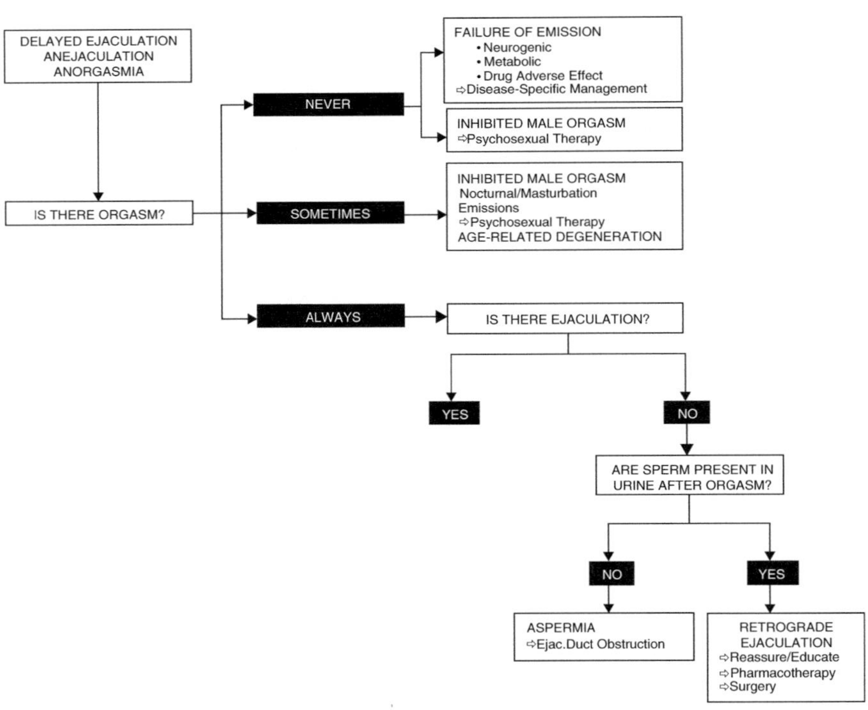

Fig. 15.1 Management algorithm for delayed ejaculation, anejaculation, and anorgasmia. *With permission from the International Society for Sexual Medicine Standard Operating Procedures*. © 2010 International Society for Sexual Medicine [6, 14]

15.5.1 Pharmacologic Treatment of Orgasmic Dysfunction

The treatment of OD with medications is limited (Tables 15.2 and 15.3). These therapies should be considered experimental, as they are not approved by regulatory agencies for the treatment of OD. Additionally, there are few large-population case series and no placebo-controlled trials showing efficacy.

15.5.1.1 Oxytocin

Ishak and colleagues reported the case of a patient with anorgasmia refractory to dopamine agonists, sex education, supportive measures, and growth hormone. The patient had resolution of OD while using 20–24 IU of intranasal oxytocin during intercourse at the point when ejaculation was desired [19]. Other studies have shown that intranasal oxytocin increases intensity of orgasm and contentment after orgasm as measured by the Arizona Sexual Experience Scale [20, 21]. However, additional research is necessary before the utility of oxytocin in the treatment of OD can be recommended.

Table 15.2 Drug therapy for anorgasmia unrelated to selective serotonin reuptake inhibitor usage

	Dosage	
Drug	As needed	Daily
Intranasal oxytocin	20–24 IU just prior to or during intercourse [19, 20]	20 IU twice daily [21]
Cabergoline		0.5 mg twice a week [22]

15.5.1.2 Cabergoline

Cabergoline is a dopamine receptor antagonist that has an inhibitory effect on prolactin secretion by the anterior pituitary. Hsieh and associates showed that of 72 anorgasmic men treated with cabergoline 0.5 mg twice a week, 50 showed improvement in orgasm. Of these, 26 men had return of normal orgasm [22]. While this is a promising series, further studies are needed to confirm the efficacy of cabergoline in anorgasmic men.

15.5.1.3 Other Treatments

Other medications may be effective in treating OD, particularly in the treatment of selective serotonin reuptake inhibitor-induced sexual dysfunction. These include amantadine, bupropion,

Table 15.3 Adjunctive drug therapy for selective serotonin reuptake inhibitor-induced sexual dysfunction

		Dosage	
Drug	Symptom	As needed	Daily
Amantadine	Anorgasmia	100–400 mg (for 2 days prior to coitus)	75–100 mg twice or three times daily
	Decreased libido		
	Erectile dysfunction		
Bupropion	Anorgasmia	75–150 mg	75 mg twice or three times daily
Buspirone	Anorgasmia	15–60 mg	5–15 mg twice daily
	Decreased libido		
	Erectile dysfunction		
Cyproheptadine	Anorgasmia	4–12 mg	On demand
	Decreased libido		
	Erectile dysfunction		
Yohimbine	Anorgasmia	5.4–10.8 mg	5.4 mg three times daily
	Decreased libido		
	Erectile dysfunction		

Used with permission from McMahon et al. [23]

buspirone, cyproheptadine, and yohimbine. These improve OD via a dopaminergic or anti-serotonergic mechanism of action. Table 15.3 lists recommended dosages for these medications. Again, these drugs are used in an off-label fashion and may require an informed consent. Additional research is necessary using appropriate placebo controls to confirm efficacy.

15.5.1.4 Acupuncture

Acupuncture is part of the practice of traditional Chinese medicine (TCM) and is a pillar of modern healthcare in China.)It continues to gain acceptance in Western medicine as an alternative therapy. TCM theory on acupuncture is based on the fact that there are approximately 2000 points on the human body connected with 12 channels or "Meridians." Normal Qi (energy) needs to flow through these channels uninterrupted throughout the body to maintain one's health. If one of these channels becomes blocked, disease or discomfort results. TCM focuses on attaining balance in the energy flow by placing needles into specific points on the Meridians. Western medicine touts acupuncture to release natural endorphins and opioids [24, 25].

TCM has been used to treat various sexual disorders; the central organ in male sexual dysfunction is the kidney. TCM holds that ejaculatory dysfunction is due to an imbalance between "yin" and "yang" along with deficiency of Qi. Today, TCM uses acupuncture alongside herbal therapy to treat male sexual dysfunction [26]. Khamba and colleagues reported subjective improvement in subjects with sexual dysfunction symptoms (including anorgasmia) due to antidepressant medication after a 12-week course of acupuncture [27]. However, controlled studies on the efficacy of acupuncture as a treatment for orgasmic dysfunction are still warranted.

15.6 Orgasmic Headache

The Headache Classification Subcommittee of the International Headache Society defines orgasmic headache as a sudden, severe ("explosive") headache that occurs at orgasm and is not attributed to another disorder such as subarachnoid hemorrhage or arterial) dissection [28]. The pathophysiology is not well understood, but orgasmic headache may be caused by segmental arterial vasospasm due to an impaired myogenic mechanism of cerebral autoregulation [29]. Others postulate that orgasmic headache is related to thunderclap headache, migraine headache, or reversible cerebral vasoconstriction syndromes [30, 31].

As orgasmic headache is a diagnosis of exclusion, other possible causes of headache should be investigated. This type of headache typically responds poorly to analgesics. Lee and colleagues reported a case of a 34-year-old man with orgasmic headache and brain magnetic resonance angiography showing severe spasm of the bilateral middle cerebral arteries. The patient was successfully treated with a course of oral nimodipine, a calcium-channel blocker [30].

15.7 Summary

Orgasmic dysfunction is a spectrum of medical conditions that can cause significant distress to the affected man as well as his partner. OD can be a separate entity from ejaculatory dysfunction, though they are often described together. Hormones including serotonin, oxytocin, and prolactin are associated with normal orgasm, and medications altering these hormone levels are known to both cause and treat disorders of orgasm. All medications available to treat OD are currently used in an off-label fashion. Acupuncture is an alternative therapy for OD that has been described, although its efficacy remains to be rigorously determined. Further research into the hormonal pathways and effective treatments of orgasmic dysfunction are warranted.

References

1. Masters WH, Johnson VE. The human female: anatomy of sexual response. Minn Med. 1960;43:31–6.
2. Levin RJ. The physiology of sexual arousal in the human female: a recreational and procreational synthesis. Arch Sex Behav. 2002;31(5):405–11.

3. Newman HF, Reiss H, Northup JD. Physical basis of emission, ejaculation, and orgasm in the male. Urology. 1982;19(4):341–50.
4. Giuliano F, Clement P. Neuroanatomy and physiology of ejaculation. Annu Rev Sex Res. 2005;16:190–216.
5. Levin RJ. An orgasm is… who defines what an orgasm is? Sex Relat Ther. 2004;19(1):101–7.
6. Rowland D, McMahon CG, Abdo C, Chen J, Jannini E, Waldinger MD, Ahn TY. Disorders of orgasm and ejaculation in men. J Sex Med. 2010;7(4 Pt 2): 1668–86.
7. Giuliano F. Neurophysiology of erection and ejaculation. J Sex Med. 2011;8 Suppl 4:310–5.
8. Murphy MR, Seckl JR, Burton S, Checkley SA, Lightman SL. Changes in oxytocin and vasopressin secretion during sexual activity in men. J Clin Endocrinol Metab. 1987;65(4):738–41.
9. Krüger THC, Haake P, Haverkamp J, Krämer M, Exton MS, Saller B, Leygraf N, Hartmann U, Schedlowski M. Effects of acute prolactin manipulation on sexual drive and function in males. J Endocrinol. 2003;179(3):357–65.
10. Buvat J. Hyperprolactinemia and sexual function in men: a short review. Int J Impot Res. 2003;15(5): 373–7.
11. Buvat J, Lemaire A, Buvat-Herbaut M, Fourlinnie JC, Racadot A, Fossati P. Hyperprolactinemia and sexual function in men. Horm Res. 1985;22(3):196–203.
12. Schwartz MF, Bauman JE, Masters WH. Hyperprolactinemia and sexual disorders in men. Biol Psychiatry. 1982;17(8):861–76.
13. Corona G, Wu FC, Rastrelli G, Lee DM, Forti G, O'Connor DB, O'Neill TW, Pendleton N, Bartfai G, Boonen S, Casanueva FF, Finn JD, Huhtaniemi IT, Kula K, Punab M, Vanderschueren D, Rutter MK, Maggi M, EMAS Study Group. Low prolactin is associated with sexual dysfunction and psychological or metabolic disturbances in middle-aged and elderly men: the European Male Aging Study (EMAS). J Sex Med. 2014;11(1):240–53.
14. McMahon CG, Jannini E, Waldinger M, Rowland D. Standard operating procedures in the disorders of orgasm and ejaculation. J Sex Med. 2013;10(1):204–29.
15. American Psychiatric Association. Diagnostic and statistical manual for mental disorders. 5th ed. Washington, DC: American Psychiatric Association; 2013.
16. Micromedix® medication, disease and toxicology management. Available from http://www.micromedexsolutions.com. Accessed 1 Feb 2014.
17. McLean JD, Forsythe RG, Kapkin IA. Unusual side effects of clomipramine associated with yawning. Can J Psychiatry. 1984;28(7):569–70.
18. Labbate LA. Bupropion-SR-induced increased libido and spontaneous orgasm. Can J Psychiatry. 1998;43(6):644–5.
19. Ishak WW, Berman DS, Peters A. Male anorgasmia treated with oxytocin. J Sex Med. 2008;5(4):1022–4.
20. MacDonald K, Feifel D. Dramatic improvement in sexual function induced by intranasal oxytocin. J Sex Med. 2012;9(5):1407–10.
21. Behnia B, Heinrichs M, Bergmann W, Jung S, Germann J, Schedlowski M, Hartmann U, Kruger THC. Differential effects of intranasal oxytocin on sexual experiences and partner interactions in couples. Horm Behav. 2014;65(3):308–18.
22. Hsieh T-C, Hollander AB, Walters RC, Lipshultz LI. 1945 Cabergoline for the treatment of male anorgasmia. J Urol. 2012;187(4):e605 (Abstract).
23. McMahon CG, Abdo C, Incrocci L, Perelman M, Rowland D, Waldinger M, Xin ZC. Disorders of orgasm and ejaculation in men. J Sex Med. 2004;1(1):58–65.
24. Brotto LA, Krychman M, Jacobson P. Eastern approaches for enhancing women's sexuality: mindfulness, acupuncture, and yoga. J Sex Med. 2008;5(12):2741–8.
25. Aydin S, Ercan M, Caşkurlu T, Taşçi AI, Karaman I, Odabaş O, Yilmaz Y, Ağargün MY, Kara H, Sevin G. Acupuncture and hypnotic suggestions in the treatment of non-organic male sexual dysfunction. Scand J Urol Nephrol. 1997;31(3):271–4.
26. Xiao Y. Treatment of functional retrograde ejaculation with acupuncture and TCM herbal drugs. J Tradit Chin Med. 2002;22(4):286–7.
27. Khamba B, Aucoin M, Lytle M, Vermani M, Maldonado A, Iorio C, Cameron C, Tsirgielis D, D'Ambrosio C, Anand L, Katzman MA. Efficacy of acupuncture treatment of sexual dysfunction secondary to antidepressants. J Altern Complement Med. 2013;19(11):862–9.
28. Headache Classification Subcommittee of the International Headache Society. The international classification of headache disorders: 2nd edition. Cephalalgia. 2004;24 Suppl 1:9–160.
29. Valença MM, Valença LP, Bordini CA, da Silva WF, Leite JP, Antunes-Rodrigues J, Speciali JG. Cerebral vasospasm and headache during sexual intercourse and masturbatory orgasms. Headache. 2004;44(3):244–8.
30. Lee JW, Ha YS, Park SC, Seo IY, Lee HS. Orgasmic headache treated with nimodipine. J Sex Med. 2013;10(7):1893–6.
31. Hu C-M, Lin Y-J, Fan Y-K, Chen S-P, Lai T-H. Isolated thunderclap headache during sex: orgasmic headache or reversible cerebral vasoconstriction syndrome? J Clin Neurosci. 2010;17(10):1349–51.

Commentary: Evaluation and Treatment of Orgasmic Dysfunction

Daniel N. Watter

Orgasmic and ejaculatory dysfunctions in men continue to be confused, often being used interchangeably. A clear distinction between orgasm and ejaculation exists, and it is clear that each process can occur independently of the other. However, orgasm and ejaculation are almost always linked in male sexual function, and therefore treatment of orgasmic and ejaculatory dysfunctions is often intertwined. Fortunately, the DSM-V now acknowledges ejaculatory disorders specifically, although male orgasmic disorders remain omitted. Furthermore, the combined, collaborative role of the physician and mental health specialist in approaching these dysfunctions is becoming clear.

The preceding chapter focuses on orgasmic dysfunction from an organic perspective, highlighting the anatomy and physiology of orgasm as well as the contemporary classification of orgasmic disorders. Discussion of the evaluation and treatment of male orgasmic dysfunction shows that while medical therapies exist, their efficacy is either limited or unclear due to a paucity of studies, and all medications currently in use are used in an off-label fashion. In the following commentary, the focus is on orgasmic anhedonia, a poorly characterized disorder that can be successfully treated using a combination of medical and psychotherapies, individualized per patient, as becomes evident in the case examples presented. Together the chapter and commentary serve as a clarion call for an interdisciplinary approach to men with orgasmic disorders, which remain incompletely understood with few medical treatment options. Combination therapy is likely to improve outcomes in afflicted men and should be considered in a patient-specific manner in all men presenting with orgasmic disorders.

The Editors

Daniel N. Watter, Ed.D.
The Society for Sex Therapy and Research (SSTAR),
Morris Psychological Group, P.A., Parsippany,
NJ, USA

Commentary

For the mental health clinician, the evaluation and treatment of orgasmic dysfunction poses several clinical challenges. From the outset, our imprecise terminology regarding sexual dysfunction may lead to some confusion regarding the disorders we are discussing. The frequent conflation of orgasm and ejaculation often leads clinicians down the wrong path regarding diagnosis and treatment. According to Waldinger [1] it is unfortunate that the DSM IV-TR [2] did not make a distinction between orgasm and ejaculation. This has been somewhat corrected in DSM-V [3] with the DSM-V substituting "delayed ejaculation" for the imprecise "male orgasmic disorder." However, the DSM-V still does not address disorders of orgasm for the male, listing only those disorders of ejaculation. For the purposes of this commentary, orgasmic dysfunction in the male refers to those cases of diminished orgasmic sensation and those often referred to as "anesthetic ejaculation" or "orgasmic anhedonia." For those looking for the mental health clinician's perspective on rapid/premature ejaculation and/or delayed ejaculation, please refer to the commentary in Chap. 12.

Little is known or written about this disorder, so the clinician has little guidance in the evaluation and treatment of this dysfunction. Given the neurological implications of orgasmic sensation, initial assessment is best performed by a physician with expertise in sexual medicine. Oftentimes, the medical evaluation is unremarkable, and the patient will then be referred for mental health evaluation and/or treatment.

The diagnosis of orgasmic disorders is further complicated by the lack of specificity of our diagnostic markers and procedures. Evaluation is based primarily on patient self-report of the intensity, or change of intensity, of orgasmic sensation. This may be associated with a reduction in volume or force of the ejaculate itself, but while related to the ejaculation process, it is the subjective cognitive/emotional experience that is the focus [4]. Obviously, the subjective nature of such report requires an extensive clinical interview in order to assess mental health status and the potential implications of such findings on the orgasmic experience. According to Perelman [5], the mental health interview would explore psychological factors such as hypoactive sexual desire disorder, depression, difficulties with sexual arousal, anxiety, fatigue, past trauma/abuse, cultural/religious views on sex, partner's sexual difficulties/concerns, and other emotionally based concerns. Sex therapy treatments may include teaching stimulation techniques to men and their partners, mindfulness techniques, yoga exercises, Kegel exercises, and challenging/realigning men's expectations of the orgasmic experience. Treatment should also emphasize enhancing greater immersion in sexual ideation/fantasy (sexual cognitions) and minimizing self-monitoring, which inhibits awareness of both subjective pleasure and physical sensation [6]. It should be clear from the above that the evaluation and treatment of orgasmic disorders in men requires a thorough examination and evaluation of a multitude of potential variables, including the possible sexual side effects of many medications, most notably the SSRIs.

As was previously noted, there is little in the psychiatric literature regarding the phenomenon of orgasmic anhedonia. Most reports are anecdotal, and many suggest that the sexual dysfunction is a symptom of a more general psychiatric/psychological condition. For example, many men who present with the complaint of orgasmic anhedonia will describe a general feeling of anhedonia as well. Typically these men are clinically depressed, experiencing significant relationship distress or some other existential crisis. When any of these situations exist, treatment of the larger symptom picture will often result in improved sexual functioning. Yet, like many "chicken and egg phenomena," it is critical to identify whether the depression is secondary to the orgasmic dysfunction or instead a precipitant to it.

In addition the mental health clinician must also be mindful of the effects this (as with any) sexual dysfunction may have on the couple's relationship. Sexual dysfunction that presents in any coupled individual will likely have an impact on their partner and their relationship. Oftentimes, couple therapy, if not the primary modality, will need to be considered to repair any damage to the relationship the sexual difficulty may have created.

Case Example

Samuel was a 39-year-old married male who was complaining of orgasmic anhedonia of 2 years of duration. Medical evaluation was unremarkable, and Samuel had no history of previous mental health treatment, psychiatric medications, or substance abuse. Samuel reported good erectile functioning, but a diminished interest in sexual activity, as well as the diminished sensation with orgasm. Samuel was highly distressed about these sexual changes, and only upon detailed questioning did it become apparent to Samuel that he had been feeling generally anhedonic and dysthymic. It was further discovered that at about the time Samuel's sexual difficulties began, his best friend from childhood passed away from an undiagnosed cardiac condition. Since that time, Samuel had become preoccupied with thoughts of his own mortality, and he found himself often thinking his own death may be around the corner. Therapy focusing on Samuel's apparent death anxiety led to substantial improvement in all symptoms, including his diminished orgasmic sensation. Couple sessions were also included toward the end of treatment in order to deal with the relationship stress that had resulted from Samuel's sexual withdrawal.

Cases of orgasmic anhedonia need to be distinguished from those cases in which a man experiences diminished orgasmic sensation as a natural consequence of the aging process. Many men do not realize that sexual functioning may change with age, and while perhaps distressing, these changes do not result from a pathological condition. However, the promise of current medical technology and the advent of medications such as sildenafil citrate have given many the notion that the sexuality of youth need never be ceded. Perelman has noted that some men will confuse their pharmaceutically enhanced erection as evidence of a greater level of sexual arousal than is actually present and will subsequently have difficulty with either a delayed, diminished, or nonexistent ejaculation and/or orgasm. In fact, the prevalence of those conditions may be increasing along with our population's age, and more and more men use medical procedures to enhance their erectile capacity and subsequently become vulnerable to diminished orgasmic disorders [7, 8].

While Kegel exercises may be somewhat helpful for many aging men, all must eventually face the reality of age-related changes in sexual function. This, in itself, may precipitate a mental health crisis for some men, and assisting them in dealing with the psychological distress some feel regarding the aging process may require therapeutic intervention, although sometimes patient education is sufficient to ameliorate the concern.

Case Example

Howard was a 57-year-old married male who complained of diminished orgasmic sensation. Medical evaluation was essentially unremarkable, but he did have a history of psychological treatment for anxiety approximately 10 years ago. Howard reported that his orgasmic changes appeared gradually, and while he still found orgasm pleasurable, it was significantly less intense than what was once the case. Howard's primary fear was that his orgasmic changes signified a diminished love and attraction for his spouse of 31 years. He reported no obvious marital stressors but was unable to ascribe his "symptoms" to any other explanation. While Howard was aware that erectile functioning might change with age (he had begun taking sildenafil citrate approximately 2 years prior), he had never heard that orgasmic intensity could change as well. While Howard was relieved that this change did not necessarily suggest an unconscious marital dissatisfaction, he was troubled by the notion that orgasmic response may never be the same as in his youth. Kegel exercises were recommended and did produce some improvements, as Howard was a diligent and compliant patient. However, the bulk of therapy consisted of assisting Howard in coming to terms with the sexual changes of aging, his anger that medical science had to "antidote" for this situation, and his anxiety regarding his own mortality. Especially helpful for Howard was McCarthy and Metz's [9] *Good Enough Sex Model*, in which the man and his partner are encouraged to become less rigid and performance-focused regarding sexual functioning and instead to develop a more flexible "sex for pleasure" orientation. Specifically, McCarthy and Metz suggest that intimacy and sex should be about acceptance, pleasure, and positive, realistic (including age-appropriate) sexual and relationship sexual expectations.

As can be seen from the above case examples, the mental health evaluation and treatment of male orgasmic disorders is varied and case-specific. For the mental health clinician, the treatment of these difficulties requires a careful assessment of underlying psychological disorders, most notably depression, anxiety, and relationship distress. As is true with all sexual dysfunctions, the mental health clinician must pay particular attention to the effect these disorders may have on the life of the couple. Rarely does the sexual dysfunction that manifests in one partner fail to have a significant effect on the patient's partner and their relationship. Often following even a "successful" resolution of the sexual difficulty, the relationship will require therapeutic attention in order to repair the damage that may have been done as a result of the sexual breakdown of the couple.

References

1. Waldinger MD. Premature ejaculation and delayed ejaculation. In: Levine SB, Risen CB, Althof SE, editors. Handbook of clinical sexuality for mental health professionals. 2nd ed. New York: Routledge; 2010. p. 267–92.
2. American Psychiatric Association. Diagnostic and statistical manual of mental disorders. 4th ed. (text rev). Washington, DC: American Psychiatric Association Press; 2000.
3. American Psychiatric Association. Diagnostic and statistical manual of mental disorders. 5th ed. Washington, DC: American Psychiatric Publishing; 2013.
4. Perelman M, McMahon C, Barada J. Evaluation and treatment of the ejaculatory disorders. In: Lue T, editor. Atlas of male sexual dysfunction. Philadelphia: Current Medicine, Inc.; 2004. p. 127–57.
5. Perelman MA. Anhedonia/PDOD: overview [Internet]. Institute for Sexual Medicine; 2010 [cited 2014 August 4]. Available from http://www.sexualmed.org
6. Perelman MA. Delayed ejaculation. In: Binik YM, Hall KS, editors. Principles and practice of sexual therapy. 5th ed. New York: Guilford Press; 2014.
7. Perelman M. Letter to the editor: regarding ejaculation: delayed and otherwise. J Androl. 2003;24(4):496.
8. Perelman MA. Delayed ejaculation. In: Binik YM, Hall KS, editors. Principles and practice of sexual therapy. 5th ed. New York: Guilford Press; 2014.
9. McCarthy B, Metz M. Men's sexual health. New York: Routledge; 2008.

16 Hypoactive Sexual Desire in Men

Yonah Krakowsky and Ethan D. Grober

16.1 Background

Low sexual desire is characterized by the absence or decrease in the frequency with which a person experiences desire for sexual activity [1]. Sexual desire can manifest as attempts to initiate sexual behavior, masturbation, erotic fantasies, sexual attraction to others, and spontaneous genital sensations of arousal [2]. The DSM V defines male hypoactive sexual desire disorder (HSDD) as persistently or recurrently deficient (or absent) sexual fantasies and desire for sexual activity that causes significant distress. This deficiency or absence of sexual desire must occur more than 75 % of the time for more than 6 months [3].

Prevalence studies looking at "normal" couples have found that up to 16 % of men report a lack of interest in sex [4]. The National Health and Social Life Survey (NHSLS) reported 14–17 % of men aged 18–44 years have low sexual desire, a rate lower than that of erectile dysfunction (ED) in the cohort. In the survey, married men were less likely to have low desire, and no association between sexual desire and ethnicity was observed [5]. The National Survey of Sexual Attitudes and Lifestyles (NATSAL), a population survey based in the United Kingdom, explored the sexual behaviors of 11,161 British men and women 16–44 years old. The most common complaint in this cohort was "lack of interest in sex" [6]. Similarly, a large Australian study investigating sexual behaviors in men ages 18–59 found 16 % of men reporting a lack of interest in sex [7]. The most commonly endorsed symptom in the Australian study was premature ejaculation, closely followed by low sexual interest. A related Swedish study revealed that of 1475 men 18–74 years old, 16 % reported low sexual desire [8]. Men 66–74 years old reported decreased interest in sex at similar rates as women, and those men with low sexual desire showed considerable comorbid sexual dysfunctions including premature ejaculation (26 %), insufficient partner lubrication (39 %), and orgasmic difficulties in the partner (24 %). An American survey using computer-assisted telephone interviews of 742 men 40–80 years old yielded "frequent lack of sexual interest" in 3.3 % of men and "periodic lack of sexual interest" in 4.8 % of men. Low sexual desire represented the third most common sexual complaint after premature ejaculation (4.7 % frequent, 7.0 % periodic) and ED (6.5 % frequent, 5.9 periodic) [9].

Clearly, large surveys of Western populations observe low sexual desire as a common symptom

Y. Krakowsky, B.Sc., M.D.
Division of Urology, Department of Surgery, University of Toronto, Toronto, ON, Canada

E.D. Grober, M.Ed., M.D. (✉)
Division of Urology, Department of Surgery, Mount Sinai and Women's College Hospital, University of Toronto, Toronto, ON, Canada
e-mail: egrober@mtsinai.on.ca

L.I. Lipshultz et al. (eds.), *Management of Sexual Dysfunction in Men and Women*, DOI 10.1007/978-1-4939-3100-2_16

in adult men across a broad age spectrum. These men may present to primary care physicians, urologists, and mental health professionals or, as often occurs, remain unevaluated. Understanding the physiology, etiology, and evaluation of these patients can empower the clinician, regardless of specialty, to feel competent in addressing hypoactive sexual desire in the male.

16.2 Physiology of Hypoactive Sexual Desire

The physiology of sexual desire involves a complex network of biochemical and psychosocial factors. The biologic basis of sexual desire in humans is still largely unknown but appears to result from an interplay between internal processes (thoughts and fantasies), neurophysiological arousal, and emotional state [10]. Much more is known about arousal (the body's anticipation of sexual activity) than the sexual desire that precedes it. Arousal leads to activation of the autonomic nervous system with parasympathetic stimulation resulting in increased blood flow to erectile tissue, as well as sympathetic nervous system activation, with a resultant increase in heart rate and muscle tone. Much less however is known about what drives sexual desire on a central level. Testosterone appears to be necessary for male sexual drive, although the relationships between testosterone and sexual desire may not be as linear as previously thought, as higher serum testosterone levels are not necessarily correlated with strong sexual desire [11]. However, studies have shown that loss of libido occurs at significant frequency in men with testosterone levels below 15 nmol/L [12].

Dopamine and prolactin both impact male sexual desire as well. Dopamine is thought to function in the mesolimbic dopaminergic pathway (the "reward pathway") to increase desire. High prolactin levels can induce reversible hypogonadism, which may contribute to decreased sexual desire. Significant increases in prolactin, as seen in patients with prolactinomas, lead to a decrease in sexual desire and worsening of erectile function, both of which can be ameliorated by administration of a dopaminergic agonist [13]. It is thought that excess prolactin decreases pulsatile LH secretion centrally, leading to decreased libido secondary to depressed testosterone secretion [14]. Dopamine directly inhibits prolactin at the level of the pituitary. In a cohort of Parkinson's patients, increasing dopamine pharmacologically was found to increase sexual desire [15], highlighting its role in low libido.

16.3 Etiology of Hypoactive Sexual Desire in Men

Many psychiatric diagnoses, medical conditions, and medications have a significant negative impact on sexual function, resulting in decreased sexual desire (Table 16.1 and Fig. 16.1). The relationship between these conditions and libido shapes the evaluation and treatment of the male patient complaining of low sexual desire. Major depression is associated with decreased sexual interest in 40 % of men [16]. Paradoxically, 9 % of men in the same study had an increase in sexual desire with the onset of depression. Due to high rates of comorbidity, evaluation of hypoactive sexual desire must include a focus on mood disorders [17]. Large studies have demonstrated a strong correlation between major depression, anxiety and somatization disorders, and hypoactive sexual desire in both men and women [18]. Both the psychiatric distress and often the pharmacological treatment can negatively impact libido. Early studies have shown loss of sexual

Table 16.1 Causes of low sex desire in men

Depression	Androgen deficiency	Stroke
Antidepressant therapy	Hyperprolactinemia	HIV
Anxiety	Thyroid disease	Heart failure
Posttraumatic stress disorder	Cushing's disease	Epilepsy
Anger	Relationship conflict	Renal failure
Aging	Iatrogenic (medications)	Coronary artery disease

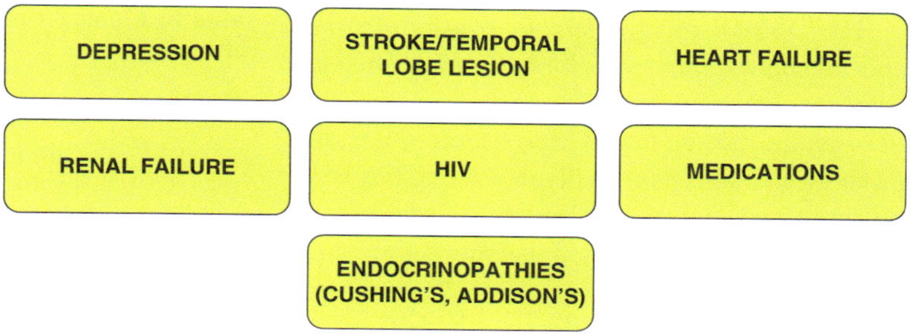

Fig. 16.1 Causes of low sex desire in men

interest in more than 70 % of patients with depressive disorders [19].

Studies have linked numerous medical conditions with decreased male sexual desire. Hypothyroidism and natural aging have been associated with decreased sexual desire in men of all ages [20]. In a Swedish study of 500 men, all 51 years old, low levels of free testosterone were associated with low sexual interest [21]. High levels of prolactin can result in both hypogonadism and hypoactive sexual desire in men. Further, the neuroleptic activity of prolactin itself may lead to depression and anxiety, compounding the effects of low androgen levels [14]. Men with prostatitis or chronic pelvic pain report less frequent sexual thoughts and desires [22]. The Global Study of Sexual Attitudes and Behaviors [23] reported a number of risk factors for low sexual desire in men including divorce, poor overall health, vascular disease, financial problems, depression, and cigarette smoking. Aging itself contributes to decreased male sexual desire, but despite this, most men in self-reported surveys have persistent mild-to-moderate interest in sex later in life [24]. A large 2007 study reported that while sexual activity does decline with age, a significant portion of men and women remain sexually active well into their ninth decade of life [25].

A significant proportion of men with HIV who initiate treatment (71 %) report some degree of sexual dysfunction after beginning their treatment, with 89 % of this sample reporting a decrease or complete loss of sexual desire as part of their overall sexual dysfunction [26].

Psychiatric medications have been associated with both hypersexuality and hyposexuality although hypoactive sexual desire is much more common than hypersexuality [27]. Tricyclic antidepressants (e.g., amitriptyline) impact libido through their anticholinergic effects [28]. Selective serotonin reuptake inhibitors (SSRIs) and serotonin-norepinephrine reuptake inhibitors (SNRIs), commonly used in treating depression, increase levels of serotonin, which may diminish sexual desire [29]. Bupropion, a non-SSRI antidepressant, causes significantly fewer sexual side effects due to its different mechanism of action [30]. Antipsychotics (e.g., haloperidol) increase prolactin levels and can cause profoundly diminished libido in many patients [31]. Atypical antipsychotics have less impact on prolactin than typical antipsychotics but may still impact sexual desire, often in a dose-dependent fashion [32]. Anticonvulsants have also been found to decrease DHEA levels, and to a lesser extent increase prolactin levels, thereby diminishing libido [33].

The interaction between partners can also strongly contribute to sexual desire. A perceived hypoactive sexual desire may be the result of different expectations between partners of a couple that is seeking counseling [34]. Anger and anxiety are two mechanisms that inhibit sexual desire and arousal [35]. Some suggest that anger and anxiety lead to performance fears, fear of pleasure, and "unconscious" fears of injury that may suppress sexual desire [36]. Many men have low sexual desire that is not clearly linked to an underlying medical or psychiatric condition. The DSM IV-TR lists *hypoactive sexual desire disorder* as a discrete diagnosis. The independent diagnosis of *hypoactive sexual desire disorder* in the DSM IV required two criteria to be met: criterion A, "persistently or recurrently deficient or absent sexual fantasies and desire for sexual activity," and criterion B, the disturbance causes "marked distress or interpersonal difficulty."

The DSM V merged *female arousal disorder* and *female hypoactive sexual disorder* into one category—*female sexual interest/arousal disorder*—and relocated *hypoactive sexual desire disorder in men* into its own diagnosis that has been renamed *male hypoactive sexual desire disorder*. The DSM V further updated its criteria to require the disorder to impact the patient 75 % of the time, to be 6 months or more in duration, and to be the cause of significant distress. Further, *substance-induced sexual dysfunction* and *sexual disorder due to a general medical condition* must be absent for the diagnosis of *male hypoactive sexual desire disorder*.

A recent study of 109 men diagnosed with *hypoactive sexual desire disorder* (according to DSM IV criteria) compared to 91 "normal" men showed no differences across age, testosterone levels, depressive symptoms, erectile function, illness, or medications. They did however differ significantly in several measures of sexual desire, supporting *hypoactive sexual desire disorder* as a valid, independent sexual disorder in men [37].

16.4 Evaluation

Assessing low sexual desire in an objective fashion is challenging. Clinicians must rely on the subjective reports of patients and couples in their initial evaluation and in assessing responses to treatment. Patients should be initially assessed with a thorough history and physical exam (Table 16.2). The history should focus on medical and sexual comorbidities, medications, and recreational drug and alcohol use. A sexual history and a concise psychiatric assessment focusing on depression/anxiety and the patient's relationships are essential. Objective assessment of sexual desire can be achieved using *The International Index of Erectile Function's* sexual desire domain [38]. The *Sexual Desire Inventory* was designed specifically to measure sexual desire and is used by some clinicians in both men and women [39]. Validated instruments exist for sexual desire assessment in women that are currently in use in clinical trials but have not been validated for men [40]. Objective assessment of sexual desire using either the IIEF or the SDI is recommended in the initial assessment of men with sexual dysfunction, as well as in assessing response to treatment.

Table 16.2 Initial workup of male with hypoactive sexual desire

History	Including history of presenting complaint, medications, medical history, urologic history, relationship history, mood disorders, sexual history
Physical	Including genital exam with testicular size, DRE
Laboratory	TSH, prolactin, testosterone

Physical exam should include a genital exam, including determination of testicular size and digital rectal exam (DRE) to assess for prostate tenderness. Signs of metabolic syndrome, liver disease, and thyroid disease should also be noted. Any abnormalities detected on history and physical should prompt the clinician to order the appropriate investigations or referrals to address the causes of low sexual desire.

Laboratory investigation should be directed toward suspected diagnoses. However, all patients should be investigated initially with evaluation of TSH, total testosterone, and prolactin levels to evaluate for the most common causes of HSD [41]. Clinicians should also obtain a baseline complete blood count (CBC), electrolytes, creatinine, and liver function tests. Luteinizing hormone (LH) and follicle-stimulating hormone (FSH) levels may also be appropriate to evaluate on a case-by-case basis.

16.5 Treatment

Patients that screen positive for depression or anxiety should receive appropriate treatment or referral. If significant relationship issues are discovered, couples' therapy should be considered. Underlying medical conditions (e.g., endocrinopathies, hypogonadism) should be treated or referred to the appropriate specialist (Fig. 16.2). Patients with abnormal TSH levels should be referred to an appropriate specialist to determine

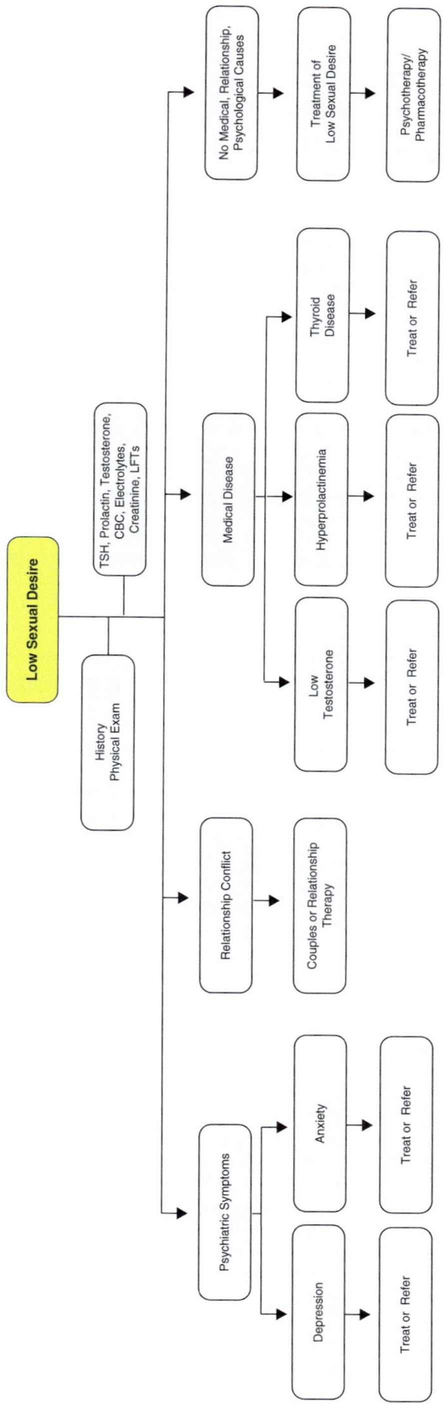

Fig. 16.2 Approach to men with low sexual desire

treatment and follow-up. Patients with elevated prolactin should undergo appropriate head imaging, additional testing, and treatment by qualified healthcare providers, and appropriate follow-up with the referring physician after the specific underlying condition is addressed should assess improvement in sexual desire. The greatest challenge is treatment of the patient with no underlying cause for low libido. There are currently no FDA-approved medications targeted to hypoactive sexual desire, with current treatment options being limited to psychotherapy and off-label pharmacotherapy.

Masters and Johnson described therapy sessions that involved bringing the couple together to discuss sexuality as but one aspect within the larger framework of a relationship [42]. Cognitive behavioral therapy (CBT) is an effective approach to low sexual desire in women but less is known about its efficacy in men [43]. CBT involves identifying negative thoughts that lead to negative feelings and dysfunctional behaviors. In the context of HSDD, CBT focuses on unrealistic expectations, partner behaviors that decrease the patient's desire in sex, and dysfunctional thoughts.

Psychotherapy has also been proposed to address men with low sexual desire and involves looking at sexual dysfunction from the perspective of unresolved, unconscious conflicts within the patient. Clinicians should familiarize themselves with therapy providers in their vicinity if they themselves aren't trained in sex therapy.

Hormone replacement is)a viable option in some men with HSDD. In hypogonadal men, exogenous testosterone can increase the frequency of fantasies, arousal, desire, ejaculation, spontaneous erections, and orgasms through coitus or masturbation [11]. In eugonadal men, however, exogenous testosterone has demonstrated no clinical benefit [44]. Testosterone supplementation using injectable formulations improved sexual interest in one study of eugonadal men but did not translate into improvement in sexual relationships [45]. Supraphysiological doses of testosterone administered to healthy volunteers as a potential male contraceptive resulted in a significant increase in psychosexual stimulation and arousal, but without changes in sexual activity or spontaneous erections [46]. Dehydroepiandrosterone (DHEA), a testosterone precursor, may benefit women with HSDD, but no benefit has been demonstrated in men using any parameter of sexual function [47].

Other options for the treatment of HSDD include neuroleptic medications. Bupropion, traditionally used for depression, anxiety, and smoking cessation, can increase desire in women via an increase in dopamine levels [48], but its effects in men with HSD are unknown. Flibanserin, a serotonin receptor agonist/antagonist, has shown some efficacy in treating HSDD in premenopausal women, but data supporting its use in men are lacking as well [49]. Gepirone is a selective serotonin receptor partial agonist that has also shown promise in treating HSDD in premenopausal women as well as men [50]. Recent reports suggest gepirone is effective in increasing sexual function in depressed men, although sexual desire didn't show the same statistically significant improvements as the other sexual domains [51].

16.6 Conclusion

Hypoactive sexual desire is a common complaint for men of all ages. By recognizing different etiologies that contribute to low libido in men, clinicians can initiate a patient-centered evaluation for men complaining of low sexual desire. A thorough history, physical exam, and appropriate laboratory investigations can identify those men with underlying medical and/or psychiatric conditions that can be addressed to improve sexual desire. Those without modifiable comorbid conditions represent a challenge to all clinicians, as male hypoactive sexual desire as a discrete diagnosis remains without targeted therapies. As the understanding of male hypoactive sexual desire evolves, more tools will become available in both assessment and treatment.

References

1. Rubio-Aurioles R. Hypoactive sexual desire on men. In: Porst H, Buvat J, The Standards Committee of the International Society for Sexual Medicine, editors. Standard practice in sexual medicine. Malden, MA: Blackwell Publishing; 2006. p. 149–57.

2. Levine SB. Hypoactive sexual desire disorder in men: basic types, causes, and treatment. Psychiatr Times. 2010;27:40–3.
3. American Psychiatric Association. Diagnostic and statistical manual of mental disorders. 5th ed. Arlington, VA: American Psychiatric Publishing; 2013.
4. Frank E, Anderson C, Rubinstein D. Frequency of sexual dysfunction in "normal" couples. N Engl J Med. 1978;299:111–5.
5. Laumann EO, Paik A, Rosen R. Sexual dysfunction in the United States: prevalence and predictors. JAMA. 1999;281:537–44.
6. Mercer CH, Fenton KA, Johnson AM, Wellings K, Macdowall W, McManus S, Nanchahal K, Erens B. Sexual function problems and help seeking behavior in Britain: national probability sample survey. BMJ. 2003;327:426–7.
7. Najman JM, Dunne MP, Boyle FM, Cook MD, Purdie DM. Sexual dysfunction in the Australian population. Aust Fam Physician. 2003;32:951–4.
8. Fugl-Meyer AR, Fugl-Meyer KS. Sexual disabilities, problems, and satisfactions in 18–74 year old Swedes. Scand J Sexol. 1999;2:79–105.
9. Laumann E, Glasser DB, Neves RCS, Moreira EDJ, GSSAB Investigators Group. A population-based survey of sexual activity, sexual problems and associated help seeking behavior patterns in mature adults in the United States of American. Int J Impot Res. 2009;21:171–8.
10. Bancroft J. Sexual desire and the brain. J Sex Marital Ther. 1988;3:11–27.
11. Isidori AM, Giannetta E, Gianfrilli D, Greco EA, Bonifacio V, Aversa A, Isidori A, Fabbri A, Lenzi A. Effects of testosterone on sexual function in men: results of a meta-analysis. Clin Endocrinol. 2005;63:381–94.
12. Zitzman M, Farber S, Nieschlang E. Association of specific symptoms and metabolic risk with serum testosterone in older men. J Clin Endocrinol Metab. 2006;91:4335–43.
13. De Rosa M, Zarrilli S, Vitale G, Di Somma C, Orio F, Tauchmanova L, Lombardi G, Colao A. Six months of treatment with cabergoline restores sexual potency in hyperprolactinemic males: an open longitudinal study monitoring nocturnal penile tumescence. J Clin Endocrinol Metab. 2004;89:621–5.
14. Buvat J. Hyperprolactinemia and sexual function in men: a short review. Int J Impot Res. 2003;15:373–7.
15. Uitti RJ, Tanner CM, Rajput AH, Goetz CG, Klawans HL, Thiessen B. Hypersexuality with antiparkinsonian therapy. Clin Neuropharmacol. 1989;12:375–83.
16. Bancroft J, Janssen E, Strong D, Carnes L, Vukadinovic Z, Long JS. The relation between mood and sexuality in heterosexual men. Arch Sex Behav. 2003;32:217–30.
17. Kennedy SH, Dickens SE, Eisfeld BS, Bagbya RM. Sexual dysfunction before antidepressant therapy in major depression. J Affect Disord. 1999;56:201–8.
18. Corona G, Petrone L, Mannucci E, Ricca V, Balercia G, Giommi R, Forti G, Maggi M. The impotent couple: low desire. Int J Androl. 2005;28:46–52.
19. Casper RC, Redmond E, Katz MM, et al. Somatic symptoms in primary affective disorders: presence and relationship to the classification of depression. Arch Gen Psychiatry. 1985;42:1098–104.
20. Meuleman E, Van Lankveld J. Hypoactive sexual desire disorder: an underestimated condition in men. Presented at University Medical Centre St Radboud and Pompekliniek, Nijmegen; 12 July 2004.
21. Nilsson P, Moller L, Solstad K. Adverse effects of psychosocial stress on gonadal function and insulin levels in middle-aged males. J Intern Med. 1995; 237:479–86.
22. Aubin S, Berger RE, Herman JR, Ciol MA. The association between sexual function, pain, and psychological adaptation of men diagnosed with chronic pelvic pain syndrome type III. J Sex Med. 2008;5:657–67.
23. Laumann EO, Nicolosi A, Glasser DB, Paik A, Ginge C, Moreira E, Wang T. Sexual problems among women and men aged 40–80 y: prevalence and correlates identified in the global study of sexual attitudes and behaviors. Int J Impot Res. 2005;17: 39–57.
24. Schiavi RC, Rehman J. Sexuality and aging. Urol Clin N Am. 1995;22:711–26.
25. Tessler Lindau S, Schumm L, Laumann E, Levinson W, O'Muircheartaigh A, Waite L. A study of sexuality and health among older adults in the United States. N Engl J Med. 2007;357:762–74.
26. Lallemand F, Salhi Y, Linard F, Giami A, Rozenbaum W. Sexual dysfunction in 156 ambulatory HIV-infected men receiving highly active antiretroviral therapy combinations with and without protease inhibitors. J Acquir Immune Defic Syndr. 2002; 30:187–90.
27. Crenshaw TL, Goldberg JP. Sexual pharmacology: drugs that affect sexual functioning. New York: W. W. Norton and Company; 1996.
28. Gutierrez MA, Stimmel GL. Management of and Counseling for psychotropic drug-induced sexual dysfunction. Pharmacotherapy. 1999;19(7):823–31. See more at http://www.pharmacytimes.com/publications/issue/2010/June2010/LossofLibido-0610#sthash.ZAXPTnWT.dpuf
29. Frye CB, Berger JE. Treatment of sexual dysfunction induced by selective serotonin-reuptake inhibitors. Am J Health Syst Pharm. 1998;55:1167–9.
30. Modell JG, Katholi CR, Modell JD, et al. Comparative sexual side effects of bupropion, fluoxetine, paroxetine, and sertraline. Clin Pharmacol Ther. 1997;61: 476–87.
31. Guthrie SK. Clinical issues associated with maintenance treatment of patients with schizophrenia. Am J Health Syst Pharm. 2002;59 Suppl 5:S19–24.
32. Segraves RT. Effects of psychotropic drugs on human erection and ejaculation. Arch Gen Psychiatry. 1989;46:275–84.
33. Reis R, Goncalves A, Sakamoto A, Ferriani R, Lara L. Altered sexual and reproductive functions in epileptic men taking carbamazepine. J Sex Med. 2013;10: 493–9.

34. Wincze JP, Carey MP. Sexual dysfunction: a guide for assessment and treatment. 2nd ed. New York: Guilford Press; 2001.
35. Bozman AW, Beck JG. Covariation of sexual desire and sexual arousal: the effects of anger and anxiety. Arch Sex Behav. 1991;20:47–60.
36. Kaplan HS. Disorders of sexual desire. New York: Brunner/Mazel; 1979.
37. DeRogatis L, Rosen R, Goldstein I, Werneburg B, Kempthorne-Rawson J, Sand M. Characterization of hypoactive sexual desire disorder (HSDD) in men. J Sex Med. 2012;9(3):812–20.
38. Rosen RC, Riley A, Wagner G, Osterloh IH, Kirkpatrick J, Mishra A. The international index of erectile function (IIEF): a multidimensional scale for assessment of erectile dysfunction. Urology. 1997;49:822–30.
39. Spector IP, Carey MP, Steinberg L. The sexual desire inventory: development, factor structure, and evidence of reliability. J Sex Marital Ther. 1996;22:175–90.
40. Clayton AH, Goldfischer ER, Goldstein I, DeRogatis L, Lewis-D'Agostino DJ, Pyke R. Validation of the decreased sexual desire screener (DSDS): a brief diagnostic instrument for generalized acquired female hypoactive sexual desire disorder (HSDD). J Sex Med. 2009;6:730–8.
41. American Association of Clinical Endocrinologist. American association of clinical endocrinologists medical guidelines for clinical practice for the evaluation and treatment of male sexual dysfunction: a couple's problem—2003 update. Endocr Pract. 2003;9:77–95.
42. Masters WH, Johnson VE. Human sexual response. Boston: Little, Brown and Co.; 1966.
43. Trudel G, Marchand A, Ravart M, et al. The effect of a cognitive-behavioral group treatment program on hypoactive sexual desire in women. Sex Relat Ther. 2001;16:145–64.
44. Morales A, Heaton JP. Hormonal erectile dysfunction. Evaluation and management. Urol Clin N Am. 2001;28:279–88.
45. O'Carroll R, Bancroft J. Testosterone therapy for low sexual interest and erectile dysfunction in men: a controlled study. Br J Psychiatry. 1984;145:146–51.
46. Bagatell CJ, Heiman JR, Matsumoto AM, Rivier JE, Bremner WJ. Metabolic and behavioral effects of high-dose exogenous testosterone in healthy men. J Clin Endocrinol Metab. 1994;79:561–7.
47. Bloch M, Meiboom H, Zaig I, Schreiber S, Abramov L. The use of dehydroepiandrosterone in the treatment of hypoactive sexual desire disorder: a report of gender differenced. Eur Neuropsychopharmacol. 2013;239(8):910–8.
48. Segraves R, Clayton A, Croft H, et al. Bupropion sustained release for the treatment of sexual desire disorder in premenopausal women. J Clin Psychopharmacol. 2004;3:339–42.
49. Goldfischer ER, Breaux J, Katz M, Kaufman J, Smith WB, Kimura T, Sand M, Pyke R. Continued efficacy and safety of flibanserin in premenopausal women with hypoactive sexual desire disorder (HSDD): results from a randomized withdrawal trial. J Sex Med. 2011;8(11):3160–72.
50. Fabre LF, Brown CS, Smith LC, Derogatis LR. Gepirone-ER treatment of hypoactive sexual desire disorder (HSDD) associated with depression in women. J Sex Med. 2011;8:1411–9.
51. Fabre L, Clayton A, Smith L, Goldstein I, Derogatis L. The effect of Gepirone-ER in the treatment of sexual dysfunction in depressed men. J Sex Med. 2012;9:821–9.

Commentary: Hypoactive Sexual Desire in Men

Eusebio Rubio-Aurioles

Hypoactive sexual desire disorder in males represents a diagnostic and therapeutic challenge to both clinicians and mental health specialists. The number of affected men is striking and highlights the need for a better understanding of decreased sexual desire in men. Diagnostically, the subjective nature of sexual desire and the absence of validated instruments to aid diagnosis specifically in men can limit accurate identification of affected men, particularly in the presence of other confounding conditions such as depression or anxiety. Thus, it is imperative that the workup thoroughly assess for conditions that can result in the patient's symptoms. The preceding chapter discusses the physiology of low sexual interest in men, as well as conditions that may predispose to decreased sexual interest. Segueing then into evaluation and treatment, Krakowsky and Grober acknowledge the diagnostic challenge inherent in identifying low sexual desire in men and discuss the role of psychotherapy, as well as limited pharmacotherapy, in the treatment of this condition.

Expanding on the discussion of the role of psychotherapy in low sexual desire in men, the following commentary focuses on the role of dual-control models in sexual function. Such models incorporate both excitatory and inhibitory factors in explaining sexual dysfunctions, providing a basis for understanding the impact of various factors and interventions. Diving more deeply into the psychological underpinnings of low sexual desire and using case vignettes, Rubio-Aurioles highlights an integrated approach to men with decreased sexual desire, marrying psycho- and pharmacotherapy.

The Editors

Eusebio Rubio-Aurioles, M.D., Ph.D.
Asociación Mexicana para la Salud Sexual, A.C.
Profesor de posgrado, Departamento de Psiquiatría y Salud Mental, Facultad de Medicina, Universidad Nacional Autónoma de México, Mexico City, Mexico

Commentary

Sexual problems in general and sexual dysfunctions in particular present a challenge to the clinician who still operates with the duality of mind-body imposed in medicine some years ago. The intertwining of factors that originated in the biological processes of the body with factors of a so-called "mental" nature is so pervasive in the reality of clinical practice that the ideal of an integral approach is an imperative when the assessment of a specific sexual problem is in order.

In the case of sexual desire, the above consideration is even more critical. Sexual desire is an elusive and mysterious experience for many people, yet it is considered one of the main motivators in life. The elusive nature of sexual desire is fairly evident for the man, who after having decided to marry the "perfect candidate" loses his desire for sexual interaction with her with absolutely no clue as to why his desire remains vivid, but not for his wife.

The problems surrounding sexual desire for clinicians begin with the diagnosis of the condition. "Low libido," "hypoactive sexual desire disorder," and "lack of interest in sex" are terms used to describe this clinical problem [1]. Libido refers to the Freudian construct of drive, and its use, although generalized, does not give honor to the original ideas of what libido [2] was supposed to be.[1] Hypoactive sexual desire makes reference to the inclusion in the 1980s [2] of the condition initially called inhibited sexual desire and then modified to hypoactive sexual desire disorder in the classification of mental disorders. The problem with these terms is that they refer to a condition that actually excludes most of the patients presenting with the complaint of low or absent sexual desire due to depression, hormonal problems, and relationship issues that should not be present for a diagnosis of hypoactive sexual desire disorder to be made. Another problem is that the term "desire" is not always understood or interpreted uniformly; the term "sexual interest" has been suggested in its stead [3]. In my opinion, the use of the term "low sexual desire/interest" facilitates the frame of mind needed in the clinical setting to address this condition [4].

The Psychological Factors in Low Sexual Desire

In the last several years, a number of models have been proposed to explain variations in sexual desire/interest. Several of these models can be grouped under the term "dual-control models," which serve to synthesize activating and inhibiting components involved in sexual desire.

Helen Kaplan [5], who devoted considerable time and effort to conceptualize sexual desire problems as a distinct sexual dysfunction, organized factors that produce the experience of lust as sexual incentives and sexual suppressors or inhibitors, both of a physiological and a psychological nature. Among the psychological inhibitors of desire Kaplan enumerates are partner unattractive, negative thoughts, anti-fantasies, negative emotions, and stress and anger. Some time later, John Bancroft [6] proposed a model named the dual-control model that is supported by psychosocial research where inhibitory processes are considered "active processes." These inhibitory processes serve either functional purposes, such as the inhibition of sexual activity when there is real danger or threat, or dysfunctional ones, such as situations in which there is only perceived danger or when the individual has a "high inhibitory tone." Michael Perelman organized these ideas in a model called the Sexual Tipping Point (TM) Model [7]. The model proposes that a balance between pro and con factors results in activation or deactivation of the sexual experience; the lack or deficit in desire/interest would be the result of the predominance of inhibitory processes over excitatory ones (Fig. 16.3).

[1] Just as an example, see the definition of libido in a psychoanalytical online resource: Libido: the psychosexual energy originating in the id. Libido is the electric current of the mechanism of personality. It powers all psychological operations, invests desires, and undergoes ready displacement. It is the basic fuel of the self. Because it is of a relatively fixed quantity, like gasoline in a tank, it obeys laws of psychical "economy" in that a surplus in one system means a loss somewhere else. It can be either free or bound.

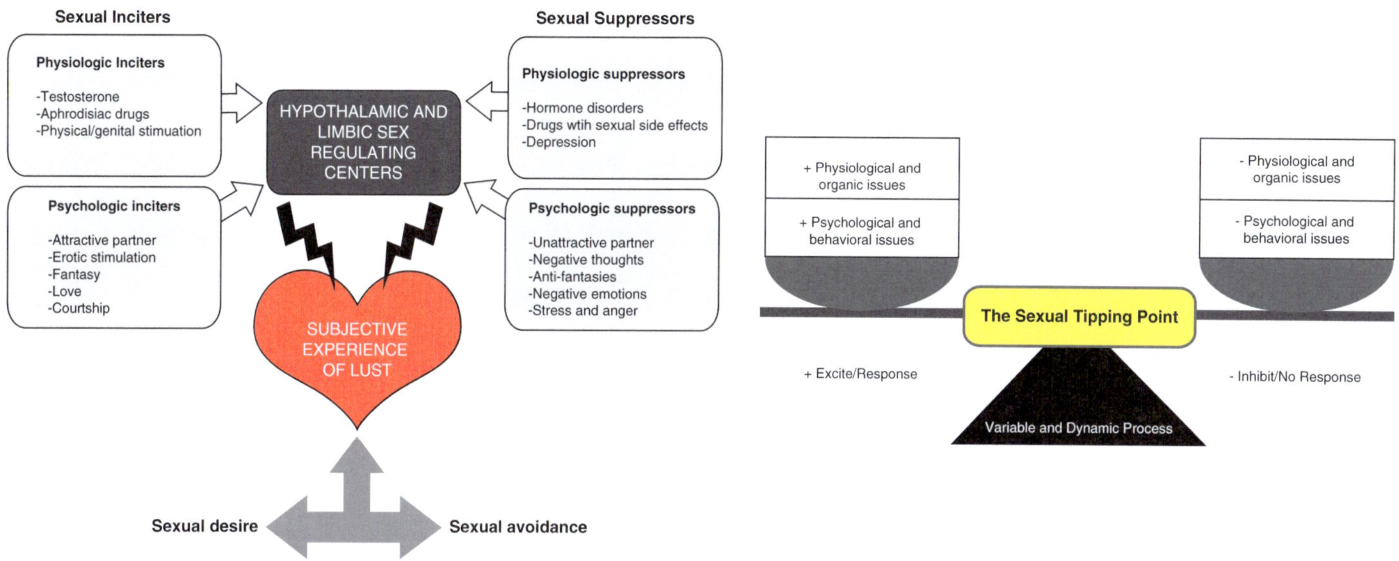

Fig. 16.3 Representation of two models that consider factor pro-desire and anti-desire to the *left* after Helen Kaplan and to the *right* the Sexual Tipping Point from Michael Perelman [1, 2]

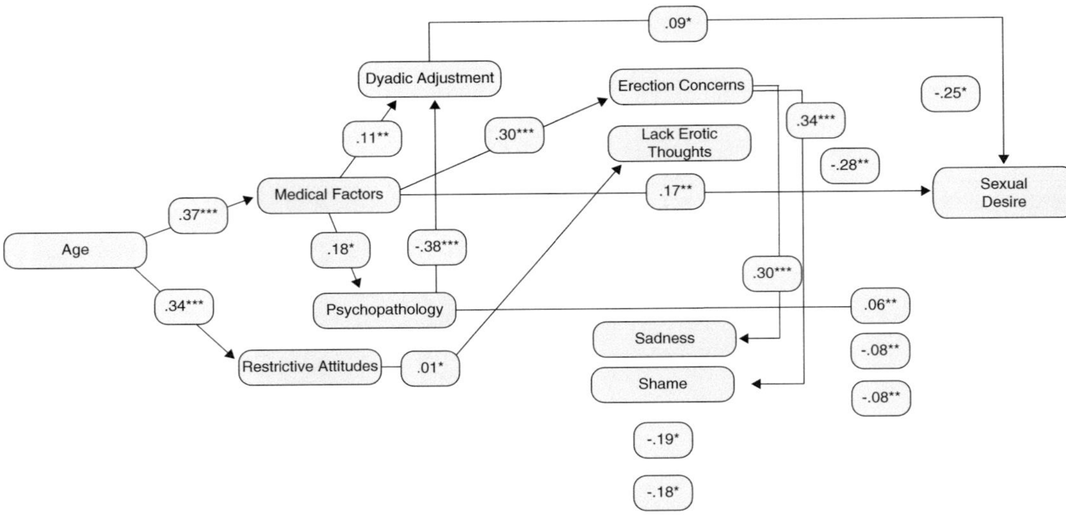

Fig. 16.4 Path analysis of causal directions between predictors and sexual desire in men (standardized regression coefficient β), $N = 205$ [10]

Several of these ideas have been tested empirically. Bozman and Beck [8, 9] studied the effects of anger and anxiety on sexual desire and sexual arousal and found that these emotional states reduce sexual desire. More recently, Carvalho and Nobre [10] tested an integrative model of biopsychosocial determinants of men's sexual desire using sophisticated statistical techniques (path analysis) to assess the relationships between several psychological variables and the level of sexual desire. Their investigation supports the previous elaborations offered by clinicians and researchers but shows that for some of the variables traditionally related to low sexual desire, such as dyadic adjustment, the effect is not as important as, for instance, the lack of erotic thoughts and erectile concerns (Fig. 16.4).

Psychological Etiologies in Low Sexual Desire of Men

Krakowsky and Grober have presented the array of possible etiological processes in detail in the preceding chapter. Psychological or mental processes are often involved when a man complains of low sexual desire. Figure 16.5 presents an algorithm for diagnosis and shows the processes where psychological considerations are critical, although the psychological impact of the condition is almost always present, regardless of the etiological process (Fig. 16.5).

Case Examples

The following clinical vignettes present typical situations where the psychological factors are predominant in men seeking consultation for low sexual desire/interest.

Depression, Anxiety, and Chronic Stress

David, 44 years of age, was an executive from a big accounting firm. He recently lost his job after a large illegal transaction was discovered; he has been looking for a new position for 10 months unsuccessfully. He explains that his wife, who is a successful public relations manager in a big pharma company, told him that the situation in their intimacy is no longer acceptable and that either he finds a solution for his lack of interest in sexual intimacy or they were going to divorce. He accepts that his desire and interest in sexual

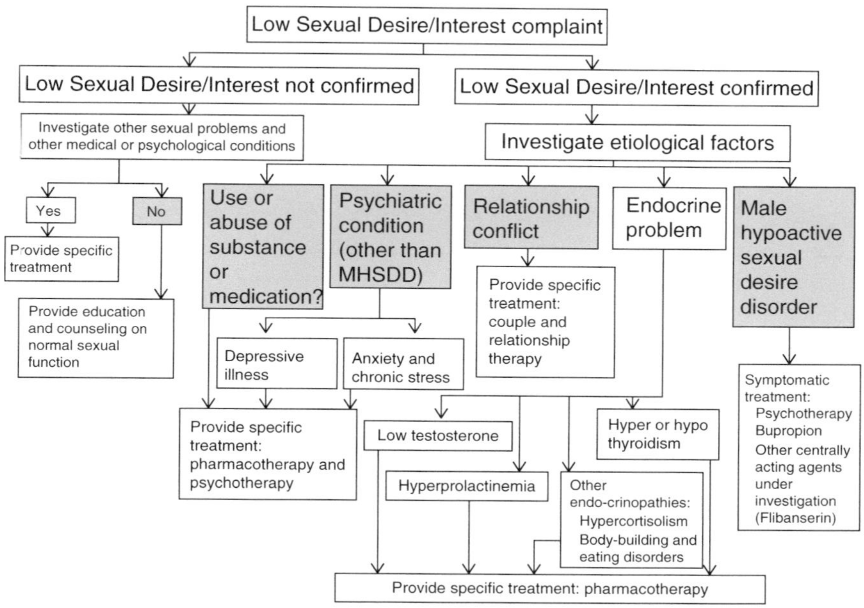

Fig. 16.5 Diagnostic algorithm for men with low sexual desire/interest. Highlighted in *gray* are processes identified with mental health MHSDD = male hypoactive sexual desire disorder. Modified from [4]

activity has disappeared and indicates that no other sexual partners exist and that he has been faithful during the 10 years of marriage which he considers otherwise very good. David considers himself to be in good health, with no medical history of relevance. His erectile function is normal according to the SHIM questionnaire. Basic laboratory studies including testosterone, prolactin, and TSH are normal.

Depression can impair sexual desire, as it is one of the frequent symptoms that accompany this medical condition. Depressive illness can be easily identified with two questions [11]; a "no" response to these two questions makes it highly unlikely for the man to have a depression:

- During the past month, have you often been bothered by feeling down, depressed, or helpless?
- During the past month, have you often been bothered by little interest or pleasure in doing things?

If the initial clinical impression of depressive illness is confirmed, proper treatment and consideration of referral to a mental health specialist is in order.

The impact of depression in the health of the relationship is clear in this example. The partner of a man with low desire feels rejection, and this can be the beginning of a new problem as the relationship deteriorates. Usually, healthy partners are direct in their communication and frequently request their male partners with low desire to address the issue directly.

Treatment of depression represents still another challenge, as most antidepressants have a negative impact on sexual desire. However, to treat the depressive illness is critical for the recovery of health; a clear explanation of the next steps during treatment is helpful and much better if the partner is present in the consultation.

Relationship Conflict

Jose, 50 years of age, is a successful entrepreneur that runs a construction company that was started by him 20 years ago. His first marriage lasted 15 years and ended because of multiple disagreements regarding the time Jose devoted to family and work. Three years ago he initiated a new relationship with a young and attractive woman who treated him very well and after a year moved in with Jose, who lived alone before that. As the couple stared their cohabitation, his desire for sexual interaction started to diminish. As the relationship progressed, her economic demands increased. In addition, significant arguments revolving the amount of money allotted to the first wife by the divorce agreement and requests to help her family have been pervasive. Jose recognizes the beauty and initial attraction and would like to find ways to repair his current relationship as he considers a second failure impossible to bear. There has been no sexual interaction during the last 6 months. Jose masturbates when she is not around with no problems and with fantasies of different women. Basic laboratory studies, including testosterone, prolactin, and TSH levels, are normal.

Many men experience difficulties with their sexual desire when the environment in the relationship turns hostile. Identifying the conflict in a relationship is easy when this is explicit, but sometimes this is not the case.

Conflict with the sexual partner is a long recognized etiology of secondary and selective (specific to the partner) low sexual desire [12]. Conflict in relationships is easy to identify if the right questions are asked. Sometimes asking directly about the quality of the relationship will provide enough information. The questions presented below can provide good clinical information about the quality of the relationship. Although they were developed in a research setting, these questions provide good guidance on what to investigate when a couple is being evaluated [13]:

- Do you and your partner agree or disagree on displays of affection?
- Do you often think about getting a divorce or separation or ending your current relationship?
- In general, would you say that everything is fine between you and your partner?
- Do you confide in your partner?
- Do you ever regret getting married (or living together)?
- How many times do you and your partner calmly discuss something?
- How many times do you and your partner work together in something?
- Circle the number that best corresponds to your level of happiness as a couple (rate between 1 and 7, 7 being perfectly happy).

Male Hypoactive Sexual Desire Disorder

Victor is a 35-year-old professor at a recognized university. He has been dedicated to his career and academic advance, and his efforts have culminated in international recognition and a good number of publications. Three years ago he decided to start a formal relationship with a former student, who is now a promising professor at the same university. They decided to marry 2 years ago. He and his partner, who presents herself to the consultation, consider their marriage as very good with the exception of the almost nonexistent sexual life. Victor had a depressive episode when he was 17 years old after the passing of his mother; he recognizes the depressive illness and gives assurance during the consultation that he is not depressed now. When sexual interaction occurs, it is highly pleasurable for both, with no problems with the erection, lubrication, and easiness of orgasm and ejaculation control. Basic laboratory studies, including testosterone, prolactin, and TSH, are normal.

Low sexual desire, in the absence of medical and psychosocial factors that could otherwise explain it, is referred to as male hypoactive sexual desire disorder. A recent report characterized these men [14], who have been shown to have differences in the pattern of activation in response to sexual stimuli [15].

Identifying these patients is essential in directing therapeutic interventions more efficiently.

Treatment Approaches for the Psychological Factors in Low Sexual Desire

Treatment of Low Sexual Desire Secondary to Depressive Illness and/or Anxiety Disorder

Major depression is associated with decreased sexual interest in >40 % of men [16]. Treatment of depression should include the use of pharmacotherapy. While many of the medications used to treat depression impact sexual function, antidepressants that have less impact on sexual function include mirtazapine, bupropion, and the serotonin-norepinephrine reuptake inhibitors venlafaxine and duloxetine [17, 18]. There is ample evidence that the combination of pharmaco- and psychotherapy improves the efficacy of the treatment of depression [19]; therefore, such combinations should be provided whenever possible.

Several anxiety disorders might be related to low sexual desire, among them: posttraumatic stress disorder, acute stress disorder, and generalized anxiety disorder. Identification and proper treatment of these conditions might be critical for the management of low sexual desire [20].

Treatment of Low Sexual Desire Secondary to Relationship Conflict

Conflict and relationship distress may cause low sexual desire; when this factor is encountered, the patient and his partner should be referred to couple/relationship therapy (sometimes called marital therapy), a specialized form of psychotherapy that has proven efficacy in addressing couple distress [21]. Although reports on the application of couple therapy to low sexual desire are still anecdotal [22], clinical experience suggests this approach is sensible and effective. Sometimes, troubled relationships benefit from relatively simple interventions. Straightforward, small changes in couple dynamics can improve partner interaction for some couples, and such "treatment" can be performed in the primary care setting. Examples include the use of open communication on sexual issues with an open and honest approach, more time dedicated to physical intimacy and to talking about intimacy issues and sharing of feelings [23]. Severe conflict should be referred to a specialized professional.

Treatment of Male Hypoactive Sexual Desire Disorder

There are two possible approaches to thetreatment of male hypoactive sexual desire disorder: pharmacological approaches and psychotherapeutic approaches. Regarding pharmacological approaches, there are no effective symptomatic treatments as there are for other sexual dysfunctions such as erectile dysfunction (i.e., phosphodiesterase type 5 inhibitors). Bupropion, an antidepressant that affects reuptake of dopamine and norepinephrine [24], has been studied and has shown a modest effect on women [25, 26]. Flibanserin, an agonist/antagonist of serotonin receptors, has shown efficacy in treating hypoactive sexual desire disorder (HSDD) in premenopausal women in several studies [27]. Although no reports of its efficacy in men with HSDD exist, flibanserin has the potential for possible benefit. Current experience is only in research settings as flibanserin has not yet been approved in any country.

Specific psychotherapeutic interventions for hypoactive sexual desire disorder have the following components [17]: affectual awareness that strives to identify positive and negative emotions related to sexual interaction and desire; insight and understanding, where a framework to understand the problem is offered to the patient; cognitive and systemic therapy, when individual psychological causes are addressed and interaction factors are addressed and corrected; and, finally, behavioral intervention, where a number of strategies are utilized to gradually overcome obstacles to sexual interaction.

Psychosexual therapy has developed approaches to treat hypoactive sexual desire in men, combining the classical interventions designed by Masters and Johnson [28] with more integrated psychodynamic and systemic interventions developed by Helen Kaplan in her classical approach to psychosexual therapy [6]. In short, these procedures involve the use of prescribed sequences of progressively more integrated and complex sexual behaviors for the patient to engage with his partner (or during self-stimulation with structured fantasies) and a variety of psychotherapeutic interventions including interpretation, confrontation, and restructuring of the couple interaction to address the more unconscious processes that are considered to block the experience of sexual desire.

Conclusion

Low sexual desire is a common complaint that has several etiologies. Investigating all levels of possible causality is critical for success in clinical management of this condition. The psychological factors are highly prevalent, and the clinician addressing this important area of health with patients should include an integrated and holistic approach to adequately evaluate and treat men with low sexual desire.

References

1. Chalquist C. A glossary of Freudian terms: http://www.terrapsych.com/freud.html, consulted on 21 Dec 2014.
2. American Psychiatric Association. Diagnostic and statistical manual of mental disorders (DSM.III). 3rd ed. American Psychiatric Association; 1980.
3. Fugl-Meyer KS, Lewis RW, Corona G, Hayes RD, Laumann EO, Moreira ED, Rellini AH, Segraves T. Definitions, classification, and epidemiology of sexual dysfunction. In: Montorsi F, Basson R, Adaikan G, Becher E, Clayton A, Giuliano F, Khoury S, Sharlip I, editors. Sexual medicine sexual dysfunctions in men and women: 3rd international consultation on sexual medicine. Paris: Health Publication Ltd; 2010. p. 41–117.
4. Rubio-Aurioles E, Bivalacqua TJ. Standard operational procedures for low sexual desire in men. J Sex Med. 2013;10:94–107.
5. Kaplan HS. The sexual desire disorders: dysfunctional regulation of sexual motivation. New York: Brunner/Mazel; 1995.
6. Bancroft J. Central inhibition of sexual response in the male: a theoretical perspective. Neurosci Biobehav Rev. 1999;23:763–84.
7. Perelman MA. The sexual tipping point: a model to conceptualize etiology, diagnosis and combination treatment of female and male sexual dysfunction. J Sex Med. 2006;3(1 suppl):52. Abstract 121.
8. Bosman AW, Beck JG. Covariation of sexual desire and sexual arousal: the effects of anger and anxiety. Arch Sex Behav. 1991;20(1):47–60.
9. Beck JG. Bosman AW. Gender differences in sexual desire: the effects of anger and anxiety. Arch Sex Behav. 1995;24(6):47–60.
10. Carvalho J, Nobre P. Biopsychosocial determinants of men's sexual desire: testing an integrative model. J Sex Med. 2011;8:754–763.
11. Whooley M, Avins A, Miranda J, Browner W. Case finding instruments for depression: two questions are as good as many. J Gen Intern Med. 1997;12:439–45.
12. Levine SB. Hypoactive sexual desire disorder in men: basic types, causes, and treatment. Psychiatr Times. 2010;27:40–3.
13. Begin C, Sabourin M, Bovin E. Frénetté. Paradis. The couple—Part 1—Couple distress factors associated with evaluating the spousal relationship. In: Quebec Longitudinal Study of Child Development (QLSCD 1998–2002) from birth to 29 months, vol 2, issue 11. Québec: Institut de la statistique du Québec; 2002.
14. DeRogatis L, Rosen RC, Goldstein I, Werneburg B, Kempthorne-Rawson J, and Sand M. Characterization of hypoactive sexual desire disorder (HSDD) in men. J Sex Med. 2012;9:812–20.
15. Stoléru S, Redouté J, Costes N, Lavenne F, Le Barsb D, Dechaud H, Forest MG, Pugeat M, Cinotti L, Pujol JF. Brain processing of visual sexual stimuli in men with hypoactive sexual desire disorder. Psychiatry Res. 2003;124:67–86.
16. Pridal CG, Lopiccolo J. Multi-element treatment of desire disorders: integration of cognitive, behavioral, and systemic therapy. In: Leiblum SR, Rosen RC, editors. Principles and practice of sex therapy. 3rd ed. New York: The Guilford Press; 2000.
17. Clayton A, Keller A, McGarvey E. Burden of phase-specific sexual dysfunction with SSRIs. J Affect Disord. 2006;91:27–32.
18. Clayton A, Kornstein S, Prakash A, Mallinckrodt C, Wohlreich M. Changes in sexual functioning associated with duloxetine, escitalopram, and placebo in the treatment of patients with major depressive disorder. J Sex Med. 2007;4:917–29.
19. Cuijpers P, van Straten A, Hollon SD, Andersson G. The contribution of active medication to combined treatments of psychotherapy and pharmacotherapy for adult depression: a meta-analysis. Acta Psychiatr Scand. 2010;121:415–23.
20. Corretti G, Baldi I. The relationship between anxiety disorders and sexual dysfunction. Psychiatr Times. 2007;24:1–7.

21. Klann N, Hahlweg K, Baucom DH, Kroeger C. The effectiveness of couple therapy in Germany: a replication study. J Marital Fam Ther. 2011;37:200–8.
22. Gehring D. Couple therapy for low sexual desire: a systemic approach. J Sex Marital Ther. 2003;29: 25–38.
23. Rosen RC. Psychogenic erectile dysfunction. Classification and management. Urol Clin N Am. 2001;28:269–78.
24. Ferris RM, Cooper BR, Maxwell RA. Studies of bupropion's mechanism of antidepressant activity. J Clin Psychiatry. 1983;44:74–8.
25. Segraves RT, Croft H, Kavoussi R, Ascher JA, Batey SR, Foster VJ, Bolden-Watson C, Metz A. Bupropion sustained release (SR) for the treatment of hypoactive sexual desire disorder (HSDD) in nondepressed women. J Sex Marital Ther. 2001;27:303–16.
26. Segraves RT, Clayton A, Croft H, Wolf A, Warnock J. Bupropion sustained release for the treatment of hypoactive sexual desire disorder in premenopausal women. J Clin Psychopharmacol. 2004;24: 339–42.
27. Goldfischer ER, Breaux J, Katz M, Kaufman J, Smith WB, Kimura T, Sand M, Pyke R. Continued efficacy and safety of flibanserin in premenopausal women with hypoactive sexual desire disorder (HSDD): results from a randomized withdrawal trial. J Sex Med. 2011;8:3160–70.
28. Masters WH, Johnson V. Human sexual inadequacy. Boston: Little Brown; 1970.

Pelvic Floor Physical Therapy in the Treatment of Sexual Dysfunctions

17

Amy Stein

Sexual dysfunction and the pelvic pain that typically accompanies it can profoundly affect the lives of the many men and women who suffer from these disorders. This is a prevalent issue: In a study of 112 women with genital pain, 78 of them—67.8 % ($p<0.0001$)—suffered some form of female sexual dysfunction (FSD). The most prevalent form of FSD, affecting 58 of the 78, or 74.3 %, was dyspareunia [1]. Similarly, in a study of men with pelvic pain, 88.3 % suffered pelvic floor myalgia and pelvic floor dysfunction [2]. The consequences for these individuals can be far reaching. Loving relationships are strained, and the individual's sense of self-worth as a fully functioning human and sexual being can be severely impaired. Yet this is an issue that rarely gets attention from either clinicians or the public at large.

Perhaps even more significantly, little consideration is given to the musculoskeletal impairments that commonly cause sexual dysfunction and pelvic pain. Rather, when we do think about sexual dysfunction, we typically mean yeast, urinary tract, and sexually transmitted infections, and when we think about sexual inactivity, we typically refer to a decreased sexual response. While sexual inactivity and infections certainly contribute to pelvic pain and sexual dysfunction, we often forget about the underlying joints, bones, and muscles of the pelvis as potential generators of pain or weakness. As a result, when laboratory tests and other diagnostic procedures reveal neither disease nor infection, patients' symptoms are too often written off as purely psychogenic. Yet their pain and dysfunction persist.

In the absence of a clear medical cause, it is likely that these patients are suffering from pelvic floor musculoskeletal dysfunction—PFD. The potential causes of such dysfunction can reach as far back as childhood and may result from such insults as abdominopelvic surgery, trauma, parturition, or bony misalignment. PFD may also appear insidiously such as with endometriosis or scoliosis. Whatever the original cause, patients with PFD who present with musculoskeletal dysfunction and who have not found relief from their symptoms through traditional medical means are perfect candidates for pelvic floor physical therapy.

Pelvic floor physical therapy is the practice of a growing number of physical therapists. Extensively schooled in the body's musculoskeletal and neuromuscular systems, these physical therapists have often pursued specialized post-graduate study in musculoskeletal dysfunctions of the pelvic floor. They are uniquely suited to diagnose and treat patients whose pelvic dysfunction may stem from disorders of the pelvic floor muscles and surrounding structures. Although the

A. Stein, D.PT., BCB-PMD, IF (✉)
Beyond Basics Physical Therapy, LLC,
110 E 42nd St Suite #1504, New York,
NY 10017, USA
e-mail: amy@beyondbasicspt.com

L.I. Lipshultz et al. (eds.), *Management of Sexual Dysfunction in Men and Women*, DOI 10.1007/978-1-4939-3100-2_17

dysfunction may manifest as a complex of impairments, these can be categorized as due to either (1) pelvic floor muscle underactivity or weakness with no pain and no muscle shortening/tightness, resulting in decreased sexual response, prolapse, or leakage, or (2) pelvic floor muscle overactivity with or without pain but with concomitant muscle and tissue shortening and possible trigger points. Some patients may suffer both categories of dysfunction.

17.1 Anatomy

The pelvic floor muscles and fascia) surround the urethra, anorectal region, and genitals (Figs. 17.1 and 17.2). They assist with voluntary sphincteric control and sexual arousal and performance [3]. Dysfunction of the neuromuscular system can negatively affect bowel, bladder, and sexual function [4] and can contribute to abdominopelvic pain and possible peripheral or central sensitization [5]. The muscles and fascia also function structurally to support the abdominopelvic organs and to assist in lumbo-pelvic stability (Figs. 17.3 and 17.4). Pelvic floor muscles are 80 % slow-twitch (type I) skeletal fibers and 20 % fast-twitch (type II) skeletal fibers [6].

The skeletal structures surrounding the pelvic floor help to keep the entire musculoskeletal and neuromuscular system in alignment [3].

17.2 Common Symptoms

Both men and women may present with a variety of subjective complaints, and both may be treated by pelvic floor physical therapists. Men with pelvic pain and sexual dysfunction typically complain of pain in the testicles, groin, rectum, tip of the penis, and abdomen. They may also complain of inability to achieve an erection, premature ejaculation, and/or post-ejaculatory pain [7]. Often these symptoms are misdiagnosed or confused with prostatitis.

Women typically complain of symptoms ranging from vulvar burning, pain in the clitoris, introital dyspareunia, pain in the introitus, pain deep within the vagina to pelvic pain. In both male and female patients suffering from pelvic floor weakness, the first of the two categories of dysfunction, decreased sexual response (i.e., difficulty reaching climax or orgasm), may be an additional complaint.

Both men and women may also complain of symptoms not related to sexual function—for example, urinary or fecal incontinence and/or urinary and/or bowel frequency, urgency, the sensation of incomplete emptying, or constipation.

17.3 Evaluation

A physical therapist or healthcare provider specializing in pelvic floor issues typically performs a manual examination to evaluate the muscles, tissues, and nerves of the pelvic floor. The aim is to gauge pelvic nerve involvement and to identify muscles and fascial tissue that may be either shortened, tender when palpated, and weak or lengthened with diminished tissue elasticity, making it difficult to support the pelvic contents or to achieve a positive sexual response.

The evaluation will also include a medical history and a pain diary in which the patient notes increases or decreases in pain; instances of bladder, bowel, and sexual dysfunction; and previous treatments and whether they helped or worsened the condition. The patient's gait patterns, posture, alignment, joint mobility, range of motion, and strength levels are all evaluated, as all may affect the dysfunction.

To assess the patient's musculoskeletal system, the practitioner will also evaluate for any physiological and biomechanical changes in the pelvis, trunk, lower extremities, and pelvic floor muscles, probing for overactive, underactive, and/or shortened muscles, increased or decreased sensation, skin and tissue changes, and pain patterns. These conditions may be caused by myofascial trigger points, altered nerve sensitivity, and/or increased fascial/connective tissue restrictions [6, 8, 9].

In women, trigger points in the urogenital triangle and pubococcygeus muscle may result in superficial introital pain and pain at the vestibule

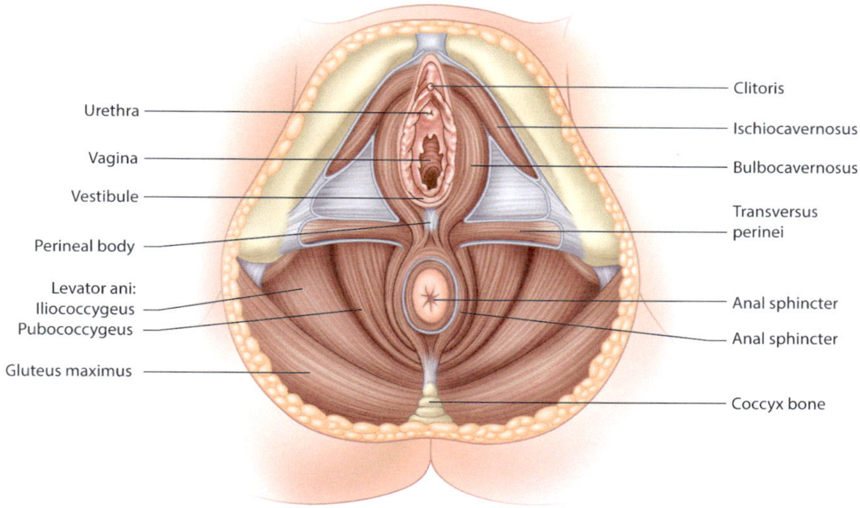

Fig. 17.1 Female pelvic floor anatomy

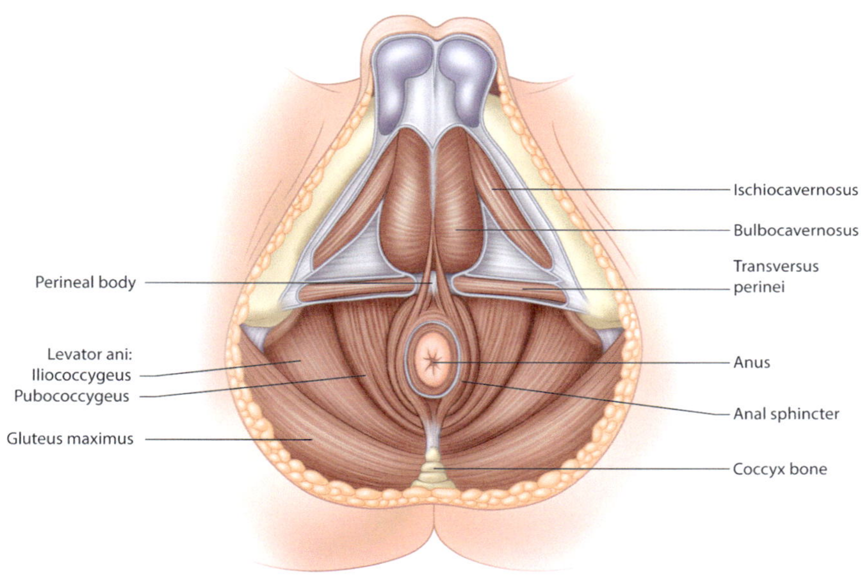

Fig. 17.2 Male pelvic floor anatomy

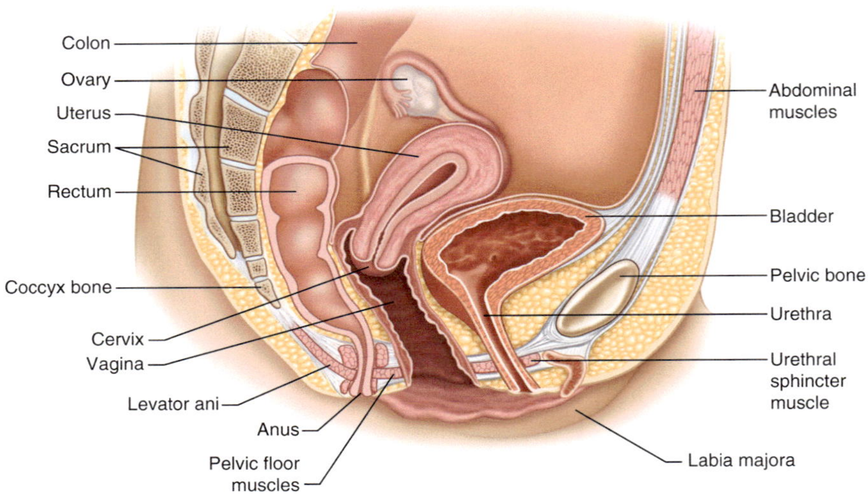

Fig. 17.3 Female urogenital system (midsagittal section)

Fig. 17.4 Male urogenital system (midsagittal section)

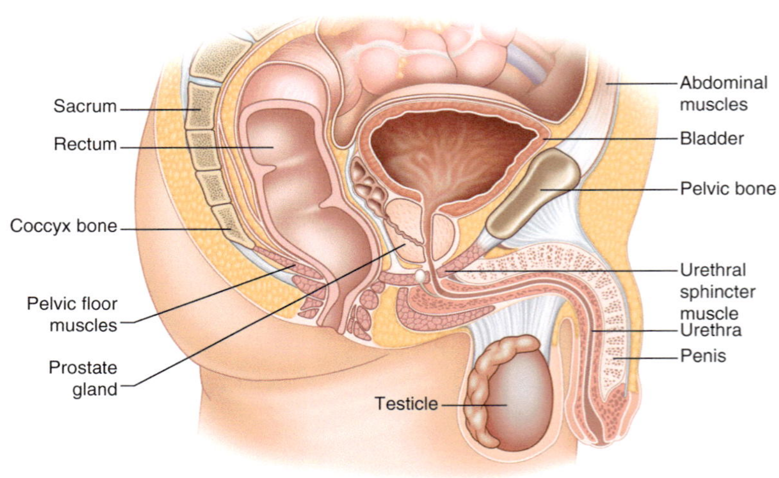

(see Fig. 17.2). Trigger points in the deep levator ani, obturator internus, coccygeus, and piriformis muscles, however, can cause deep, penetrating pain [6]. Trigger points in either area can result in postorgasmic and post-ejaculatory pain. Neville et al. [10] found that women with chronic pelvic and genital pain presented with significantly more abnormal muscle findings than pain-free women.

Specific nerves that innervate the genital and pelvic region—the pudendal, the posterior and lateral femoral cutaneous, iliohypogastric, ilioinguinal, levator ani, and genitofemoral nerves—should be evaluated for unfavorable neural tension, which may result in hyposensitivity, dysesthesia, or hyperalgesia, and for changes in neurodynamics that could result in underactive muscles and weakness, or in overactive muscles and increased pain [11, 12]. Either condition may result from connective tissue restrictions in and around the pelvic floor and genital region or around nerves and can leave the pelvic floor muscle dysfunctional [8]. In addition, nerve irritation or injury may be a result of such biomechanical abnormalities as foraminal narrowing, scarring of a nerve canal, or myofascial trigger points. Patients may describe the resulting muscle tension and/or neuropathic pain as burning, itching, tingling, cold, sharp, and shooting pain or, in the case of decreased sexual response, as weakness and incontinence [6, 8, 13]. The variety of responses is just one reason why it is so important to assess the body from head to toe to discover all impairments that could be affecting a patient's symptoms and function.

17.4 Treatment

Physical therapy for pelvic floor and sexual dysfunction will of course be based on what the therapist has found in the examination and evaluation process. The therapist's arsenal includes neural and visceral mobilization and mobilization of connective tissue, internal and external myofascial trigger point release [6], pelvic and core mobilization and stabilization, and such modalities as biofeedback and electrical stimulation [14]. All of these practices reduce tender points and decrease tissue restrictions while also strengthening and stabilizing any weakened muscles or joints; they therefore apply primarily to dysfunctions in the category of pelvic floor weakness and are aimed at restoring the proper length of the pelvic floor muscles and tissues and at reducing neural tension and sexual dysfunction [8, 15–17].

Where such events as scarring from endometriosis, prostatectomy, vaginal childbirth with perineal laceration or episiotomy, or caesarean section have caused abdominal and pelvic scarring, the goal of physical therapy is to enable the structures of the pelvis to move more freely and to increase blood circulation; the therapist therefore applies manual techniques to loosen areas of restriction. Internal and external massage can reduce the amount of tension and restrictions in the sensitive structures of the abdomen and pelvis and thereby alleviate pain.

Many category-one patients—those evaluated for pelvic floor weakness—may present with underactive pelvic floor muscles unable to support the pelvic organs and assist in sphincteric control. They are unable or less able to contract the pelvic floor muscles, which can result in incontinence and decreased sexual response. The lack of support may also make the patient feel heaviness and discomfort in the pelvic area, which worsens over the course of the day. In these cases, the physical therapist will guide the patient in ways to strengthen the pelvic core while maintaining proper bodily alignment to ensure that the pelvic muscles are in their optimal positions for proper functioning.

For category-two patients—both males and females with pelvic and/or sexual dysfunction—physical examination typically shows pelvic floor muscles and tissues that are overly tight or have gone into spasm. In this case, the physical therapist may choose manually to correct any bony misalignments, then stretch, and lengthen the muscles out of spasm and tightness [18, 19]. The American Urological Association (AUA) guidelines for the management of this kind of pelvic pain recommend manual physical therapy by clinicians appropriately trained in treating pelvic floor overactivity, and they suggest that patients avoid such improper pelvic floor strengthening exercises such as Kegels [20].

In addition to their manual skills, pelvic floor physical therapists have at their disposal a number of effective tools for treating patients' pain and dysfunction. Among them is biofeedback, a highly effective technique for "teaching" patients how to relax and contract the muscles of the pelvic floor. Electrodes are placed either at the rectal opening or inside the vagina or anus and are connected to a computer; the computer translates patients' responses into graphic measurements on the computer screen so patients are able to view their own pelvic floor muscle activity in real time. As the physical therapist guides the patient through relaxation and strengthening techniques, the patient can thus "see" how his or her pelvic floor muscles function and how the techniques affect that function and their own pain levels. It is a form of reeducation of the muscles that helps category-two patients coordinate and down-train overactive muscles [8] or category-one patients to coordinate, uptrain, and strengthen the pelvic floor muscles [21–23].

In addition, in extreme cases of pelvic floor weakness, such as those caused by a neurological pathology like multiple sclerosis or by postsurgical weakness, a physical therapist might use neuromuscular stimulation (NMES) to help the patient gain muscle strength. Using a setup similar to that of biofeedback, NMES works by sending electricity directly to the muscles of the pelvic floor. The electrical stimulation causes the muscle fibers of the pelvic floor to contract; this assists in gradually strengthening the pelvic floor to allow for greater muscle function.

Adding a home program that is specific to the objective findings from the pelvic floor, physical therapy evaluation is also essential to the patient's recovery, as is monitoring of the home treatment plan. For example, for women who are experiencing painful penetration secondary to tight vaginal muscles and tissues, a physical therapist might teach the patient to use dilators or a massage wand in her home program as a way to stretch the vaginal tissues or to address trigger points and so tolerate her partner's penis or other sexual activity. This will require the monitoring and supervision of the treating physical therapist to ensure proper guidance of the home program.

The pelvis is an extremely complex area of the human body in which a lot can go wrong. When treating individuals who suffer from chronic pain and sexual dysfunction, it is therefore essential to consider all of the systems of the body in the process of evaluation and diagnosis, including the musculoskeletal system. Where traditional methods have failed, physical therapists addressing that system—and attending to the patient's mental state as well—have helped alleviate the suffering of numerous patients and have advanced their rehabilitation [15, 16, 24, 25]. It is important for the patient and the prescribing healthcare provider to understand that "flare-ups" are not unusual and that pelvic floor rehabilitation is not usually a quick fix. With persistence and proper guidance, however, such rehabilitation can be extremely effective for patients suffering from pelvic floor and sexual dysfunction.

References

1. Verit FF, Verit A, Yeni E. The prevalence of sexual dysfunction and associated risk factors in women with chronic pelvic pain: a cross-sectional study. Arch Gynecol Obstet. 2006;274(5):297–302.
2. Schmidt R. Male pelvic pain syndrome. J Urol. 1999;161:903–8.
3. Irion JM, Irion GL. Women's health in physical therapy. Philadelphia: Lippincott Williams and Wilkins; 2010.
4. Haylen BT, de Ridder D, Freeman RM, et al. An International urogynecological association (IUGA)/international continence society (ICS) joint report on the terminology for female pelvic floor dysfunction. Neurourol Urodyn. 2010;29(1):4–20. doi:10.1002/nau.20798.
5. Hilton S, Vandyken C. The puzzle of pelvic pain – a rehabilitation framework for balancing tissue dysfunction and central sensitization. I: Pain physiology and evaluation for the physical therapist. J Womens Health Phys Ther. 2011;35:103–11.
6. Simons DG, Travell JG. Myofascial origins of low back pain. 3. Pelvic and lower extremity muscles. Postgrad Med. 1983;73(2):99–105. 2.
7. Anderson, et al. Integration of myofascial trigger point release and paradoxical relaxation training treatment of chronic pelvic pain in men. J Urol. 2005;174:155–60.
8. FitzGerald MP, Kotarinos R. Rehabilitation of the short pelvic floor. I: Background and patient evaluation. Int

Urogynecol J Pelvic Floor Dysfunct. 2003;14(4):261–8 (Epub 2003 Aug 2. Review).
9. Montenegro ML, Mateus-Vasconcelos EC, Rosa e Silva JC, Nogueira AA, Dos Reis FJ, Poli Neto OB. Importance of pelvic muscle tenderness evaluation in women with chronic pelvic pain. Pain Med. 2010;11(2):224–8.
10. Neville CE, Fitzgerald CM, Mallinson T, Badillo S, Hynes C, Tu F. A preliminary report of musculoskeletal dysfunction in female chronic pelvic pain: a blinded study of examination findings. J Bodyw Mov Ther. 2012;16(1):50–6.
11. Darnis B, Robert R, Labat JJ, Riant T, Gaudin C, Hamel A, Hamel O. Perineal pain and inferior cluneal nerves: anatomy and surgery. Surg Radiol Anat. 2008;30(3):177–83.
12. Jamieson DJ, Steege JF. The prevalence of dysmenorrheal, dyspareunia, pelvic pain and irritable bowel syndrome in primary care practices. Obstet Gynecol. 1996;87(1):55–8.
13. Weiss J, Prendergast S. Screening for musculoskeletal causes of pelvic pain. Clin Obstet Gynecol. 2003;46:773–82.
14. Hartmann E. The perceived effectiveness of physical therapy treatment on women complaining of chronic vulvar pain and diagnosed with either vulvar vestibulitis syndrome or dysesthetic vulvodynia. J Women's Health Phy Ther, APTA. 2001;25:13–8.
15. Prendergast SA, Weiss JM. Screening for musculoskeletal causes of pelvic pain. Clin Obstet Gynecol. 2003;46(4):773–82.
16. FitzGerald MP, Payne CK, Lukacz ES, et al. Randomized multicenter clinical trial of myofascial physical therapy in women with interstitial cystitis/painful bladder syndrome and pelvic floor tenderness. J Urol. 2012;187(6):2113–8.
17. FitzGerald MP, Anderson RU, Potts J, et al. Randomized multicenter feasibility trial of myofascial physical therapy for the treatment of urological chronic pelvic pain syndromes. J Urol. 2009;182(2):570–80.
18. Oyama IA, Rejba A, Lukban JC, Fletcher E, Kellogg-Spadt S, Holzberg AS, Whitmore KE. Modified Thiele massage as therapeutic intervention for female patients with interstitial cystitis and high-tone pelvic floor dysfunction. Urology. 2004;64(5):862–5.
19. Weiss JM. Pelvic floor myofascial trigger points: Manual therapy for interstitial cystitis and the urgency-frequency syndrome. J Urol. 2001;166:2226–31.
20. Winters JC, Dmochowski RR, Goldman HB, et al. Urodynamic studies in adults: AUA/SUFU guideline. J Urol. 2012;188 Suppl 6:2464–72.
21. Glazer HI, Rodke G, Swencionis C, Hertz R, Young AW. Treatment of vulvar vestibulitis syndrome with electromyographic biofeedback of pelvic floor musculature. J Reprod Med. 1995;40(4):283–90.
22. Glazer HI, Jantos M, Hartmann EH, Swencionis C. Vulvodynia and asymptomatic women. J Reprod Med. 1998;43(11):959–62.
23. McKay E, Kaufman RH, Doctor U, Berkova Z, Glazer H, Redko V. Treating vulvar vestibulitis with electromyographic biofeedback of pelvic floor musculature. J Reprod Med. 2001;46(4):337–42.
24. Ree ML, Nygaard I, Bø K. Muscular fatigue in the pelvic floor muscles after strenuous physical activity. Acta Obstet Gynecol Scand. 2007;86(7):870–6.
25. Gyang A, Hartman M, Lamvu G. Musculoskeletal causes of chronic pelvic pain: what a gynecologist should know. Obstet Gynecol. 2013;121(3):645–50.

Additional Reading

Baker P. Contemporary Management of Chronic Pelvic Pain. 1993;20(4):719–42.

Bergeron S, Lord MJ. The integration of pelvi-perineal reeducation and cognitive-behavioral therapy in the multidisciplinary treatment of the sexual pain disorders. Br Assoc Sex Relationship Ther. 2003;18:135–41.

King R, et al. Increasing orgasm and decreasing dyspareunia by a manual physical therapy technique. Medscape Gen Med. 2004;6(4):47.

Nygaard et al. Prevalence of symptomatic pelvic floor disorders in US women. JAMA. 2008;300(11):1312.

Schultz et al. Women's sexual pain and its management. J Sex Med. 2005;2:302.

Part II

Sexual Dysfunction in the Female

18 The Female Sexual Response: Anatomy and Physiology of Sexual Desire, Arousal, and Orgasm in Women

Johannes Bitzer

The anatomy and physiology of the female sexual response comprises the structural and functional elements of the female external genitalia, the physiological changes occurring during the sexual response cycle, and the endocrine and neurobiological regulation of this response.

18.1 The Female External Genitalia, the Vulva

The external genitalia are composed of the mons pubis, the labia majora, the labia minora, Bartholin's glands, the Skene's glands, minor vestibule glands, the clitoris, the vulvar vestibule, the perineum, and the urethral and anal openings, collectively representing the vulva (Fig. 18.1) [1–3].

The *mons pubis* consists of fatty tissue that covers the pubic bone. During puberty, it becomes covered with hair. The mons pubis contains oil-secreting (sebaceous) glands that release substances that are involved in sexual attraction (pheromones).

The *labia majora* ("big lips") are two marked folds of skin that extend from the mons pubis downward and backward to merge with the skin of the perineum. The major function of the labia majora is protection of the softer tissues of the vulva. Unlike the inner structures of the vulva, the labia majora contain many pubic hairs that help to protect the rest of the vulva from mechanical stress and friction.

The *labia minora* are "small lips" that lie inside the labia majora and surround the openings to the urethra and vagina. The labia minora can be very small or up to 2 in. wide. They are covered with hairless skin and contain very little adipose tissue. Blood flowing through the many capillaries in the connective tissue layer gives the labia minora their pinkish color. During sexual stimulation, the small blood vessels become engorged with blood, causing the labia minora to swell and become more sensitive to stimulation. At their anterior end, the labia minora meet at the clitoral hood, or prepuce, where they envelope the lateral sides of the clitoris. From the clitoral hood, the labia minora extend inferiorly toward the anus, where they gradually decrease in size before merging with the skin of the perineum. Many sebaceous glands are also present in the connective tissue and extend to the surface of the labia minora via ducts.

The *vulvar vestibule* surrounds the opening of the vagina. It extends from Hart's line on the medial aspect of the labia minora to the hymen. The vestibule is covered by a nonkeratinized squamous endothelium and contains many nerve fibers and the ostia of the Bartholin's glands,

J. Bitzer, M.D. (✉)
Department Obstetrics and Gynecology,
University Hospital Basel, Switzerland
e-mail: JBitzer@uhbs.ch; Johannes.Bitzer@usb.ch

L.I. Lipshultz et al. (eds.), *Management of Sexual Dysfunction in Men and Women*, DOI 10.1007/978-1-4939-3100-2_18

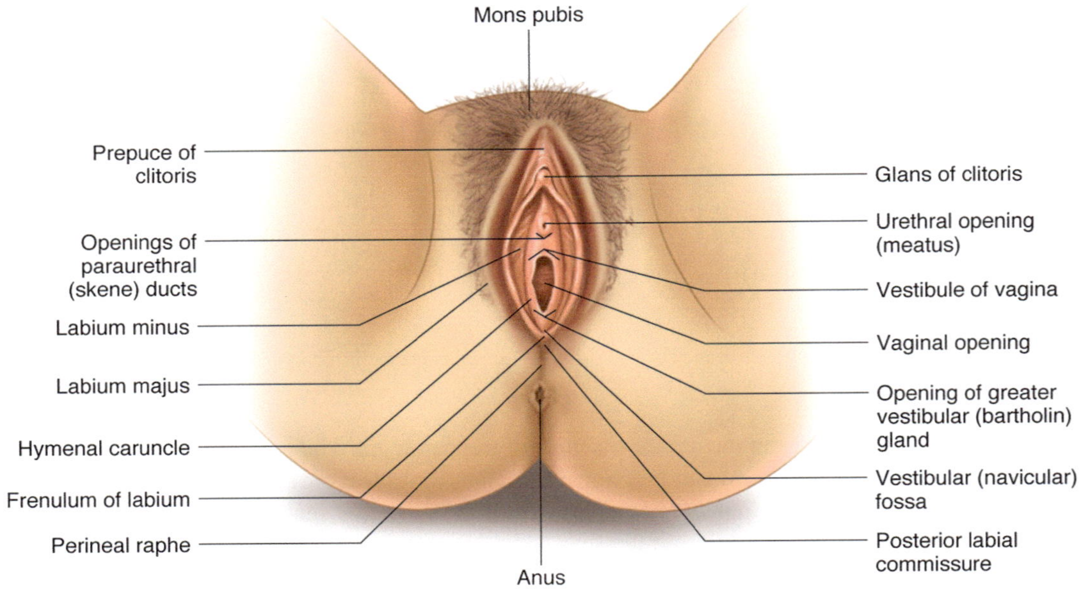

Fig. 18.1 The female external genitalia

Skene's glands (the female prostate), and the minor vestibule glands—all of which are androgen-dependent mucin-secreting glands. The tissues below the skin include the vestibular bulbs, which contain erectile tissue and are part of or the internal portion of the clitoris (see below).

The Bartholin's glands are androgen-dependent mucin-secreting glands that are responsible for lubrication during arousal. These glands are innervated by the autonomic nervous system and the ostia of the gland are at the 4 and 8 o'clock positions of the vulvar vestibule.

The Skene's glands are androgen-dependent glands that are embryologic equivalents to the male prostate. The Skene's glands surround the urethra and, combined with the clitoral crura, make up the anatomic suture known as the G-spot. The ostia of the Skene's glands are adjacent to the urethral meatus [4, 5].

18.2 Clitoris

The *clitoris* can be subdivided into several parts: clitoral hood, glans clitoris, clitoral body, clitoral crurae (Fig. 18.2).

18.2.1 Clitoral Hood

The clitoral hood projects at the front of the labial commissure, where the edges of the labia majora meet at the base of the pubic mound; it forms as part of the external folds of the labia minora and covers the glans and external shaft. There is considerable variation in how much of the glans protrudes from the hood and how much is covered by it, ranging from completely covered to fully exposed, and tissue of the labia minora also encircles the base of the glans.

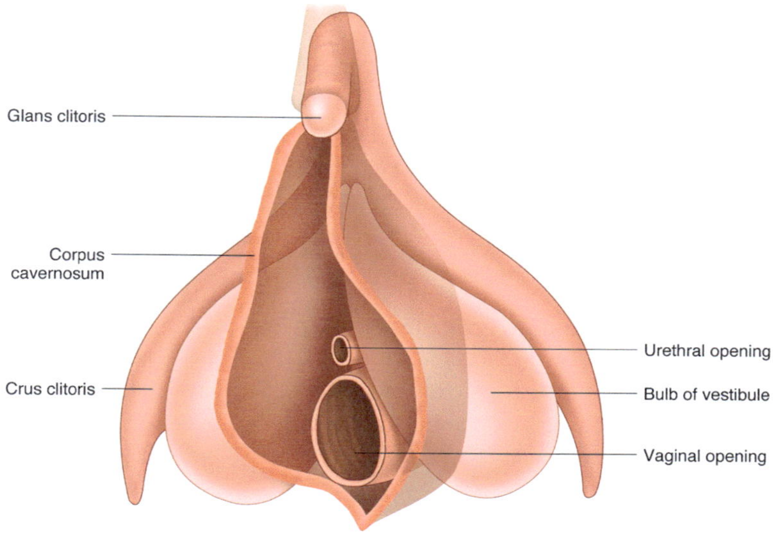

Fig. 18.2 The clitoris

18.2.2 The Glans Clitoris

The glans forms the pointed tip of the clitoris extending outward from the body and beyond the prepuce that covers the rest of the clitoris. It consists of a midline shaft lying in the medial sagittal plane about 2–4 cm long and 1–2 cm wide.

18.2.3 The Clitoral Body

The clitoral body forms a wishbone-shaped structure containing the corpora cavernosa—a pair of sponge-like aggregations of erectile tissue that contain most of the blood in the clitoris during clitoral erection. Arterial inflow includes the dorsal and clitoral cavernosal arteries, which arise from the iliohypogastric pudendal bed. The autonomic efferent motor innervation arises from the cavernosal nerve of the clitoris arising from the pelvic and hypogastric plexus.

Under the surface of the skin, two legs of erectile tissue known as the clitoral crura fan out to support the exterior structures of the clitoris and attach to the underlying tissues. Associated are the urethral sponge, perineal sponge, a network of nerves and blood vessels, and the suspensory ligament of the clitoris, muscles, and the pelvic floor.

Innervation of the clitoris is mainly supplied by the dorsal nerve, a branch of the paired pudendal nerve (left and right), which carries sensory and motor signals to the perineum of both women and men. There may be additional innervation of the clitoris from the genitofemoral nerve as well as the ilioinguinal nerve. Other structures involved in the autonomic innervation of the clitoris are cavernous nerves originating from the vaginal nervous plexus and traveling at the 5 and 7 o'clock positions along the urethra. The genitofemoral nerve supplies the labia majora with sensory fibers. The mons and labia majora contain sensory fibers from the ilioinguinal nerve.

18.2.4 Vestibular or Clitoral Bulbs

The *vestibular bulbs*, also known as the *clitoral bulbs*, are aggregations of erectile tissue that are an internal part of the clitoris. They can also be found throughout the vestibule—next to the clitoral body, clitoral crura, urethra, urethral sponge, and vagina. Thousands of touch and pressure-sensitive nerve endings are found throughout the clitoris. Nerve endings in the clitoral body and glans are sensitive to direct external touch and pressure, while the nerve endings of the crus are sensitive to stimulation from within the vagina.

18.3 The Vagina

The vagina links the vulvar structures to the inner genitalia (Fig. 18.3).

The vagina has three layers: the internal mucosal layer, the intermediate muscularis layer, and the external adventitial layer.

18.3.1 The Internal Mucosal Layer

The vaginal mucosa has folds, or rugae, and is composed of the epithelium and the lamina propria. The vaginal epithelium is nonkeratinized stratified squamous epithelium. There are no glands, so there is no mucin secretion. The lamina propria of the vaginal mucosa contains many elastic fibers as well as a dense network of blood and lymphatic vessels and nerves. Transudate from these blood vessels, combined with cervical mucus, provides lubrication during sexual arousal and intercourse.

18.3.2 The Muscularis

The vaginal muscularis layer consists of autonomically innervated smooth muscle fibers arranged into outer longitudinal and inner circular layers.

18.3.3 The Adventitia

The adventitia is rich in collagen and elastin, provides structural support to the vagina, and allows for expansion of the vagina during intercourse and childbirth. Surrounding the adventitia are three sets of powerful pelvic striated muscles: (a) the ischiocavernosus and bulbocavernosus, which are the most superficial layer, (b) the transverse perinei providing intermediate support, and (c) the levator ani forming the deeper layer of the pelvic diaphragm across the anterior of the pelvis. The largest medial portion is the pubococcygeus and puborectalis.

18.3.4 The Grafenberg Spot: G-Spot

In 1950, the German gynecologist Ernst Gräfenberg first, published his work on "the role of the urethra in female orgasms" and hypothesized that an erogenous zone might be located on

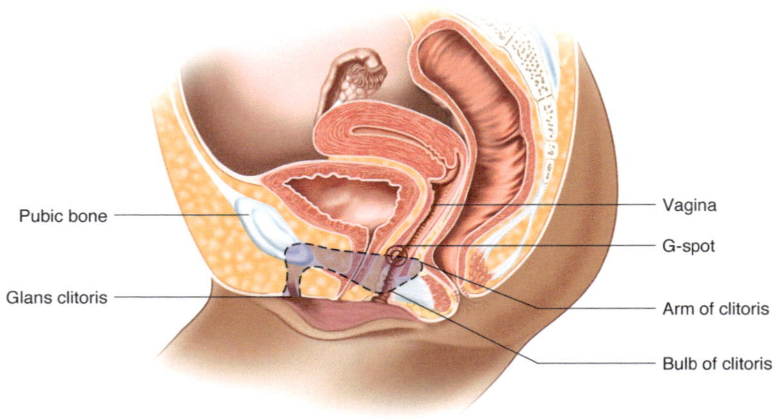

Fig. 18.3 The vagina relative to other components of the female reproductive tract

the anterior wall of the vagina, along the course of the urethra (Fig. 18.3) [6]. Stimulation of this area would lead to discharge of fluid from the Skene's gland ostia, which some have consequently considered female ejaculation. There is one case report in which, during orgasm, this area was being "pressed downwards against the finger like a small cystocele" protruding into the vaginal canal. In reference to this anecdotal observation, Addiego [7] described this area as the "G-spot" in 1981, and ever since, especially after publication of the book *The G-Spot and Other Recent Discoveries About Human Sexuality* by three American sexologists a year later [8, 9], public interest has grown around this topic. Taking into account the controversy about the separate existence of this anatomical site, the G-spot may at this moment be considered an excitable area along the entire length of the urethra running along the anterior vaginal wall.

18.3.5 Halban's Fascia

Halban's fascia is the space ,between the trigone of the bladder and the anterior part of the vaginal wall. It is filled with mesenchymal lamina, a fibroelastic sheet composed of collagen, elastic and muscular fibers with a rich blood supply, and a nerve supply containing Krause bodies or pseudo-corpuscular nerve endings. On stimulation, this space becomes vasocongested and creates an erotic pleasurable response.

18.3.6 Innervation of the Vagina

Autonomic efferent innervation to the, upper two thirds of the vagina is through the uterovaginal plexus, which contains both sympathetic and parasympathetic fibers. Sympathetic efferent fibers from the lumbar splanchnic nerves travel first through the superior hypogastric plexus, then through the bilateral hypogastric nerves to reach the inferior hypogastric plexuses, and finally the uterovaginal plexus. Parasympathetic efferent input to the uterovaginal plexus is from the pelvic splanchnic nerves. Nerves from the uterovaginal plexus travel within the uterosacral and cardinal ligaments to supply the proximal two thirds of the vagina. Autonomic efferent innervation to the lower vagina is carried through the pudendal nerve (S2, 3, 4), which reaches the perineum through Alcock's canal.

Autonomic afferent fibers from the upper vagina travel through the pelvic splanchnic nerves to sacral spinal cord segments, whereas autonomic afferents from the lower vagina leave the sacral spinal cord through the pudendal nerve. Somatic sensation exists primarily in the distal one third of the vagina and is also carried by the pudendal nerve to the sacral spinal cord [3].

18.3.7 The Physiology of the Female Sexual Response Cycle

By observing sex workers under laboratory ,conditions, Masters and Johnson were able to describe visible changes in the genital organs during sexual encounters, which led them to define a linear model of the human sexual response, applicable to both genders. Their model still serves as a basic description of physical changes during sex and has served as the blueprint from which further knowledge about the anatomy and physiology of the female sexual response has been accumulated [10, 11].

They differentiate four phases with typical characteristics: (1) excitement, (2) plateau, (3) orgasmic, and (4) resolution [12].

18.3.7.1 Excitement Phase

The *excitement phase* (also known as the *arousal* or *initial excitement phase*) results in an increase in heart and breathing rates and a rise in ,blood pressure. Vasocongestion of the skin, commonly referred to as the sex flush, will occur in approximately 50–75 % of females. During this sex flush, pinkish spots develop under the breasts and then spread to the breasts, torso, face, hands, soles of the feet, and possibly over the entire body. Vasocongestion is also responsible for the darkening of the clitoris and the walls of the vagina during sexual arousal (Fig. 18.4a, b). The sex flush typically disappears soon after

a

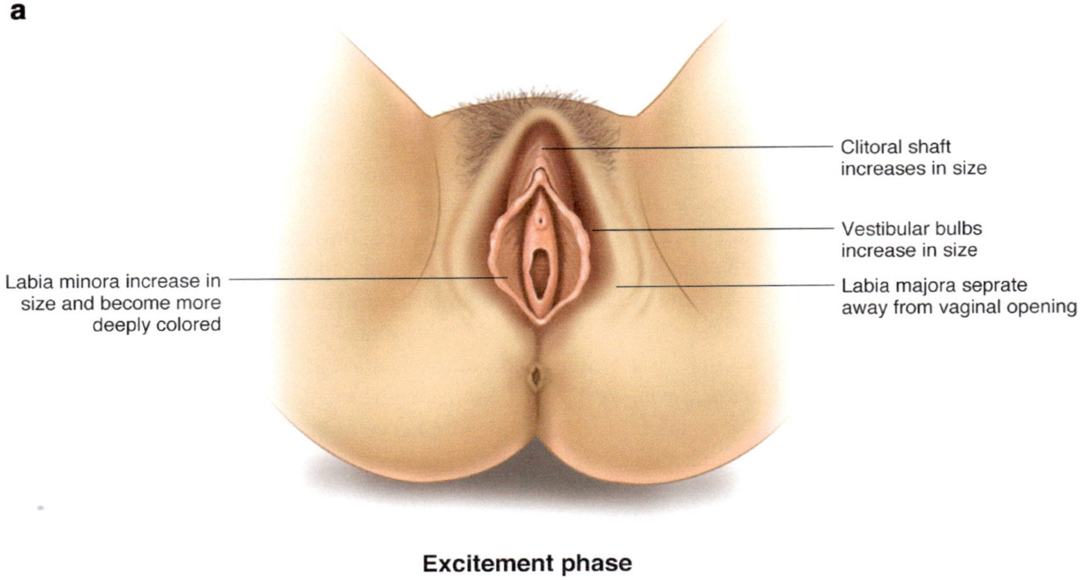

b

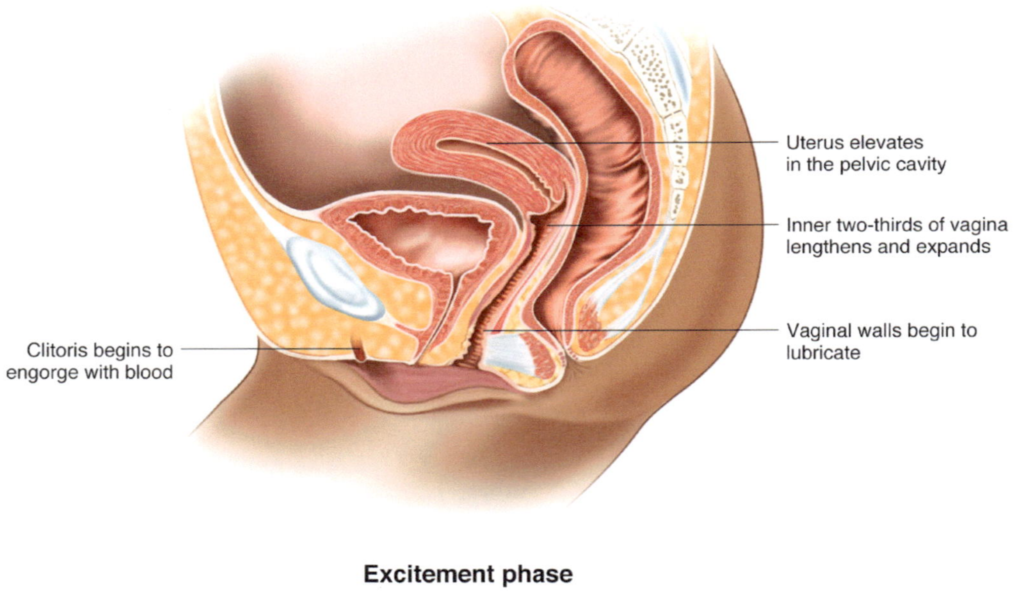

Fig. 18.4 (**a**, **b**) Physical changes during the excitement phase of the sexual cycle (Modified from Clayton AH. Sexual function and dysfunction in women. Psychiatric Clinics of North America 2003;26:673–682 [13])

orgasm occurs, but this may take up to 2 h and sometimes results in simultaneous intense sweating. An increase in muscle tone (myotonia) of the levator ani muscles occurring voluntarily and involuntarily begins during this phase. Also, the external anal sphincter may contract upon contact (or later during orgasm without contact).

In females, the excitement phase can last from several minutes to several hours. The onset of vasocongestion is due to an increase in vaginal blood flow and can be measured by plethysmography, which provides information about the basal vaginal pulse amplitude. Vasocongestion during the excitement phase results in swelling of the woman's clitoris, labia minora, and vagina. On sexual arousal, the blood supply to the vaginal epithelium is rapidly increased by parasympathetic inputs from S2 to S4, and at the same time, the venous drainage is probably reduced, resulting in vasocongestion.

The increased blood flow to the genitals is activated by the VIPergic innervation of the large vessels supplying the epithelium and possibly aided by calcitonin gene regulating peptide (CGRP) enhanced permeability of the capillary tufts. This allows serum to leak out of blood vessels through the vaginal mucosa, and this transudate acts as a lubricant during intercourse. Neuropeptide Y (NPY), a known vasoconstrictor, may be involved in constricting the venous drainage. There appears to be very little nitric oxide synthase (NOS) in the blood vessels of the premenopausal vagina and none in the postmenopausal. During the excitement phase, the androgen-dependent glands of the vulvar vestibule (Bartholin's, Skene's) secret mucin to act as a lubricant at the introitus. In addition to the vascular changes during the excitement phase, the pubococcygeus muscle surrounding the vaginal opening tightens and the uterus elevates and increases in size. Meanwhile, the breasts increase slightly in size and nipples become hardened and erect.

18.3.7.2 Plateau Phase

The plateau stage in females represents a continuation ,of the changes that occur during the excitement phase. The glans clitoris becomes extremely sensitive and withdraws slightly under the clitoral hood, and the vestibular glands produce further lubrication (Fig. 18.5a, b). The tissues of the outer third of the vagina swell, and the pubococcygeus muscle tightens, reducing the diameter of the vaginal opening [12].

18.3.7.3 Orgasmic Phase

Orgasm is the conclusion of the plateau phase, ,and it is accompanied by quick cycles of lower pelvic muscle contraction (Fig. 18.6a, b). Between arousal and orgasm, there is an increase in vaginal luminal pressure. The smooth muscle layers contain a great variety of classical and peptidergic transmitters including serotonin (5HT), norepinephrine, acetylcholine, dopamine, vasoactive intestinal peptide (VIP), NPY, gastrin-releasing peptide (GRP), thyrotropin-releasing hormone (TRH), CGRP, somatostatin, substance P, oxytocin, cholecystokinin (CCK), and relaxin, but the exact function of each neurotransmitter in sexual response is unknown.

A series of pelvic, clonic, striated muscle contractions occur at approximately 0.8 s intervals which gradually get longer and the contractions weaker. They can last for 5–60 s. These contractions are concomitant with the subjective feeling of orgasm. Voluntary contractions of the pelvic striated muscles do not give a feeling of intense pleasure but are often used to enhance arousal. During sexual arousal and up to orgasm, individual uterine contractions may occur, while during orgasm a series of uterine contractions occurs, mediated by the sympathetic nervous system via the hypogastric nerve. Orgasms are often associated with other involuntary actions, including vocalizations and muscular spasms in other areas of the body, and a generally euphoric sensation. Heart rate is increased even further during this phase of sexual arousal.

18.3.7.4 Resolution Phase

The *resolution phase* occurs after orgasm and allows the muscles to relax, blood pressure to drop, and ,the body to slow down from its excited state. The refractory period, which is part of the resolution phase, is the period during which a man is unable to orgasm again. While less common, women can also experience a refractory period, although according to Masters and Johnson, women have the ability to orgasm again very quickly as long as they have effective stimulation. They are, as a result, able to have multiple orgasms in a relatively short period of time. Though generally reported that women do not experience a refractory period and thus can experience an additional orgasm, or multiple orgasms, soon after the first, for some women, the clitoris is very sensitive after climax, making additional stimulation initially painful. After the initial orgasm, subsequent orgasms for women may also be stronger or more pleasurable as the stimulation accumulates.

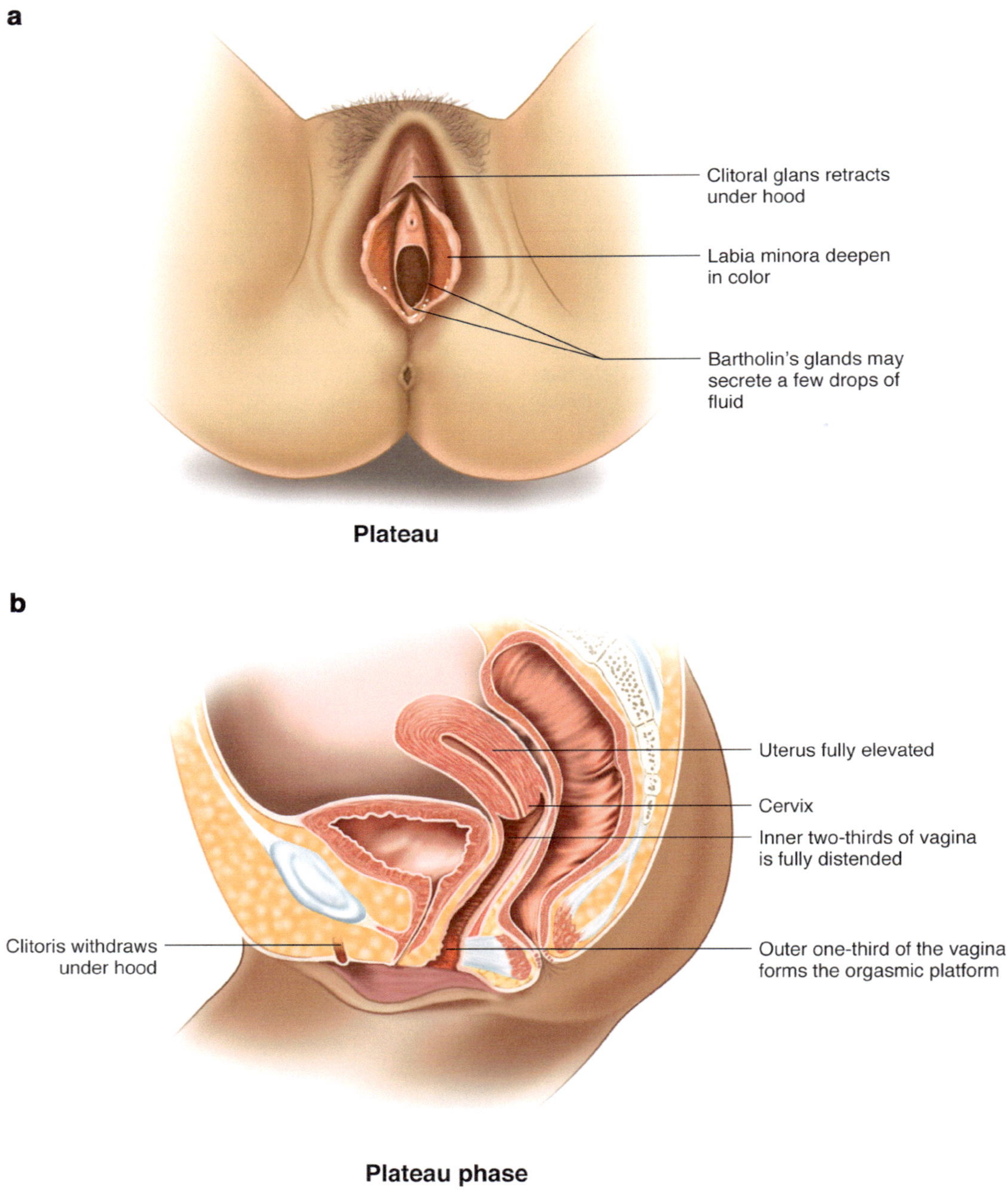

Fig. 18.5 (**a**, **b**) Physical changes during the plateau phase of the sexual cycle

This model of the anatomy and physiology of the female sexual response is helpful in understanding and studying the different processes as if they were separate entities, facilitating observation and analysis. The model, however, has two major limitations:

(a) The different phases described do not always occur in linearly, with some phases not occurring, overlapping with others, or having missing elements.
(b) This model is a strictly objective physiological description not accounting for the subjec-

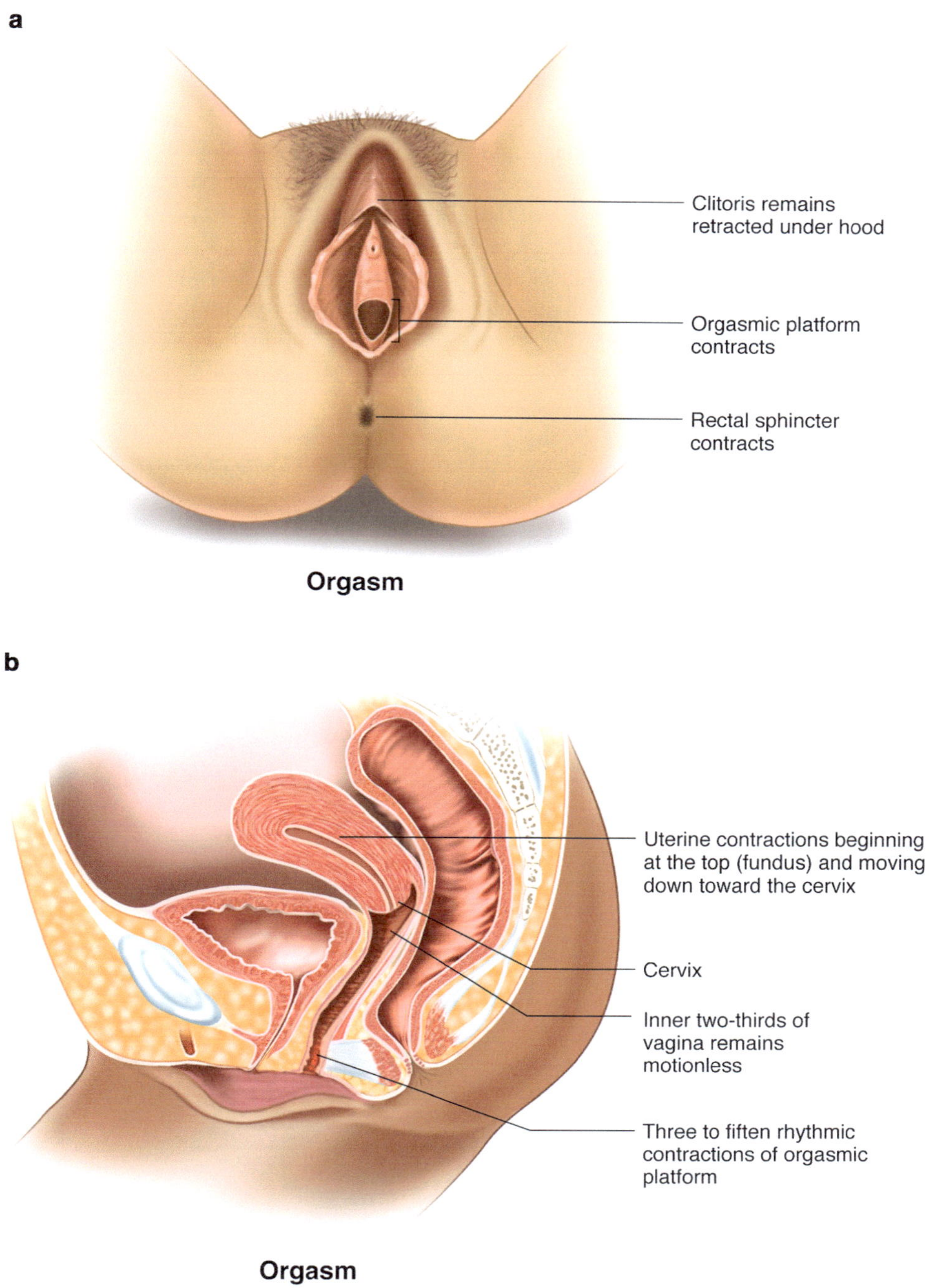

Fig. 18.6 (**a**, **b**) Physical changes during the orgasmic phase of the sexual cycle

tive experience and the cognitive, emotional, and behavioral dimensions of the female sexual response.

The first broadening of the Masters and Johnson model was the introduction of sexual desire as the first phase of the female sexual response by Helen Singer Kaplan [14]. Desire has since become one of the most enigmatic and interesting phenomena in sexuality because of the inability to directly observe it. Other models have tried to describe the motivational and behavioral characteristics of the sexual response cycle, taking into account the nonlinearity of the female sexual response, pointing to a more circular model of positive and negative feedback and interaction between stimuli and motivational states [15]. One of the latest models has been constructed around the three categories: wanting, liking, and satiety [16].

18.3.7.5 The Endocrine and Neurobiological Regulation of the Female Sexual Response

Animal and human studies have contributed ,to our knowledge, which is best summarized in what has been called the Dual Control System.

The Dual Control System identifies the human sexual response as a dynamic result of the interaction between excitatory processes and inhibitory processes (Sexual Wanting and Sexual Inhibition). This Dual System response is present and active in the regulation of the peripheral response (see above) and also functional in the central regulation.

Regulation of the Peripheral Response

The above-described peripheral response is regulated, and modified according to the setting resulting from interactions between:

(a) Gonadal steroids [17]
(b) Autonomic nervous system
(c) Neurotransmitters
(d) Amino acids

All these systems interact with each other and upregulate or downregulate the peripheral response (Fig. 18.7) [18, 19, [22]].

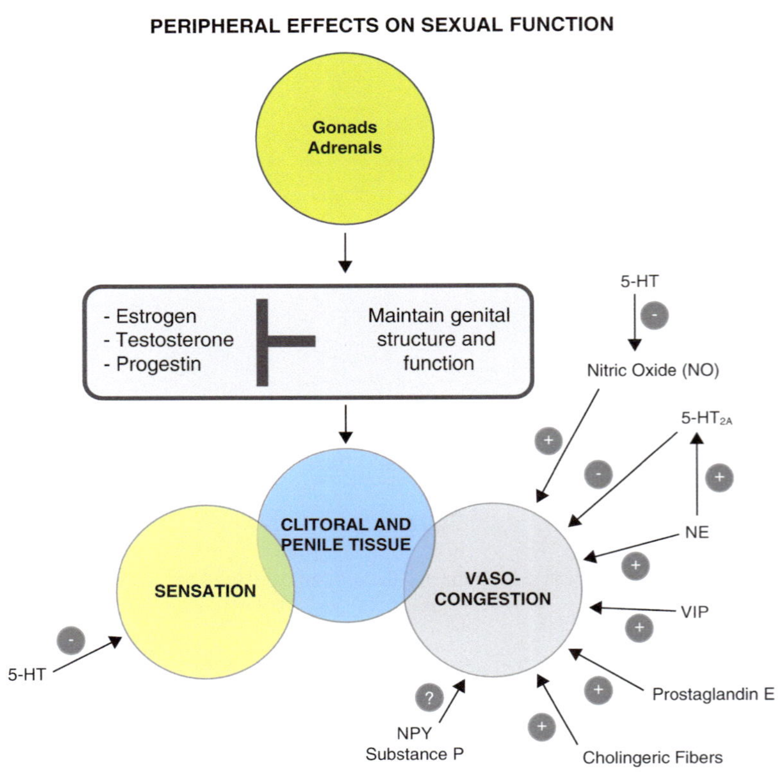

Fig. 18.7 Regulatory factors affecting sexual function (Modified from Clayton AH. Sexual function and dysfunction in women. Psychiatric Clinics of North America 2003;26:673–682 [13])

18.4 Regulatory Factors Affecting Sexual Function

18.4.1 Estrogens

Estradiol, and to a minor degree estriol, plays an important role in maintaining the ability of the vulvovaginal unit to respond to sexual stimuli and in enhancing the response through the following actions:

(a) Estrogens stimulate the proliferation of the vaginal mucosal epithelium. This increase leads to the formation of superficial cells. Glycogen, stored in the epithelial cells, reaches maximal levels at ovulation, after which time the glycogen-rich superficial layer of epithelium is shed. Breakdown of the glycogen by bacteria in the vagina produces lactic acid, causing the vaginal environment to have an acid pH of about 3. This inhibits growth of other bacteria, bacterial pathogens, and fungus. It also limits the time during which sperm can survive in the vagina. This effect on the epithelium is thus important in maintaining the healthy ecosystem of the vagina and directly and indirectly maintaining the peripheral response.

(b) Besides the important effect on the vaginal epithelium, estrogens maintain collagen tissue and stromal cells in the vagina. This effect provides stability and elasticity of the vagina during intercourse.

(c) Estrogens have a stimulating effect on the smooth muscle in the muscularis layer of the vagina. This effect leads to a partial thickening of the muscularis, which is probably enhanced by testosterone.

(d) Estrogens increase the pelvic nerve innervated blood flow in the small vessels of the vagina and maintain the ability of the epithelium to transudate. This effect is mediated by VIP and neuronal and endothelial NOS in the vagina [17].

18.4.2 Testosterone

The role of testosterone in the peripheral sexual response is less well investigated. It seems, however, that testosterone is an important cofactor for the estrogen action and may increase vaginal blood flow. In addition, the Bartholin's glands, Skene's glands, and minor vestibular glands are testosterone-dependent, mucin-secreting glands that are essential for lubrication of the introitus. Lastly, testosterone may also lead to relaxation of the smooth muscle in the muscularis layer.

18.4.3 Progesterone

The role of progesterone in the sexual response has not yet been elucidated. It is assumed that progesterone exerts a protective effect on neurons, which would be nonspecific and not directly related to the peripheral sexual response.

18.4.4 Receptors in the Vagina

It is important to note that effects of steroids depend on the presence of steroid receptors in the vagina. These receptors can be up- and downregulated and can thus modify the response to hormones. Receptors for estrogen, testosterone, and progesterone have been found in the vaginal tissues. Their differential action during the menstrual cycle and during different phases of the reproductive life of a woman remains to be investigated.

18.5 Amino Acids, Neuropeptides, and Tissue Activators

Besides the action on their receptors, sex steroids act via the autonomic nervous system, inducing either neuronal changes and/or the secretion of amino acids and neuropeptides that can be found in various vaginal tissues. VIP is an important vasodilator together with NOS, while other neuropeptides have a more vasoconstrictive action (NPY, norepinephrine, CGRP) [18]. Local prostaglandin production relaxes small blood vessels and increases blood flow.

18.6 Autonomic Nervous System

Activation of the autonomic nervous system is part of the preparation of the body for sexual activity. During this preparation, sympathetic nervous system transmitters such as epinephrine play an important role by increasing heart rate and breathing intensity, but the parasympathetic nervous system also acts via vasodilation of vessels in the genital organs. Activation of the sympathetic system facilitates genital blood flow not alone but in the context of appropriate sexual stimulation.

While norepinephrine exerts a stimulatory effect, serotonin and 5HT have an inhibitory effect on sensation and vasocongestion.

18.6.1 Central Nervous Regulation

The peripheral response regulation of the sexual response is best understood in the context of excitatory and inhibitory pathways [16, 19, 20].

18.6.1.1 Excitatory Pathways and Processes

Sexual stimuli can be principally perceived via two pathways. The first pathway is fast and transmits sexual signals (visual, tactile, auditory) to parts of limbic system including the ventral striatum (which includes the nucleus accumbens), the amygdala, the anterior cingulate cortex (ACC), and the orbitofrontal cortex (OFC). The second pathway is slower and closer to consciousness, relying on the prefrontal cortex and linking to the hippocampus as part of the explicit memory system. The regulation of these excitatory pathways is affected by gonadal steroids and neurotransmitters (Fig. 18.8) [21].

18.6.1.2 Gonadal Steroids

It has been shown that estrogens have central excitatory effects. While no specific centers are involved, estrogens appear to provide a priming effect by genomic and non-genomic effects on different parts of the mesolimbic system. The effect can best be described as facilitating arousability and responsiveness.

Testosterone has been shown in animal and human studies to have an "initiating" or "sex wanting" effect. Although the importance of testosterone for healthy women's desire and arousability is still controversial, there is now evidence that lack of testosterone in specific clinical

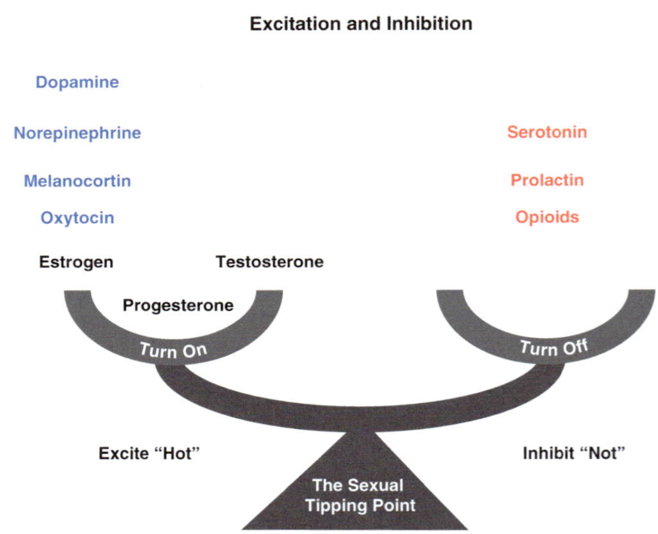

Fig. 18.8 Regulation of excitation and inhibition in the context of the sexual response—the "Sexual Tipping Point"

conditions such as after bilateral ovariectomy or in the setting of premature ovarian failure increases the risk for female sexual dysfunction and that replacement therapy has a therapeutic effect. This includes also women around and after natural menopause.

18.6.1.3 Neurotransmitters

Studies in animals have shown that sexual desire is stimulated by excitatory neurochemical mechanisms in the brain involving the following regions and neurotransmitters [22]:

(a) The mesolimbic system and nucleus accumbens are involved in the dopamine pathway critical for sexual incentive motivation.
(b) The hypothalamus and the limbic system are involved in the oxytocin and melanocortin pathway mediating sexual attraction.
(c) Ascending noradrenaline pathways acting in hypothalamic, limbic, and cortical regions to augment sexual arousal.

18.7 Inhibitory Pathways and Processes

The inhibitory pathway, like the excitatory pathway, also involves brain structures, hormones, and neurotransmitters.

18.7.1 Brain Structures

The brain structures involved in sexual inhibition seem to include hyperactivity in the prefrontal cortex, increased activity in ventral prefrontal and dorsal parietal areas, and decreased activity in the middle cingulate cortex [22].

18.7.2 Hormones

Whereas gonadal steroids serve the purpose of reproduction and thus act as "turn on" substances, lowering of these hormones by other neuroendocrine mechanisms and hormones can have an inhibitory effect on sexual desire. Prolactin appears to be an inhibitory signal; whether this is an indirect effect via suppression of ovarian steroids, or a direct effect on receptors in the brain is not yet clear.

18.7.3 Neurotransmitters

The main inhibitory neurotransmitters are serotonin and to a certain extent opioids, which mediate the state of receptor saturation. Endogenous opioids represent important biological molecules involved in female sexual response and enforce a strong reward signal followed by a prolonged period of relaxation.

In summary, the anatomy and physiology of the female sexual response is characterized by a complex interaction of peripheral genital organs and neuroendocrine and neurobiological centers of processing sexual stimuli and directing responses along neuroendocrine, neurovascular, and neuromotor pathways which are still under investigation.

References

1. Farage MA, Maibach HI. The vulva: anatomy, physiology, and pathology. London: CRC Press; 2006.
2. Constance Marjorie Ridley, Neill SM, Lewis FM. Ridley's the vulva. Chichester: Wiley-Blackwell; 2009.
3. Schiebler TH, Korf H-W. Anatomie: Histologie, Entwicklungsgeschichte, makroskopische und mikroskopische Anatomie, Topographie. New York: Springer; 2007.
4. Jannini EA, Simonelli C, Lenzi A. Sexological approach to ejaculatory dysfunction. Int J Androl. 2002;25(6):317–23.
5. Jannini EA, Simonelli C, Lenzi A. Disorders of ejaculation. J Endocrinol Invest. 2002;25(11):1006–19.
6. Grafenberg E. The role of the urethra in female orgasm. Int J Sexol. 1950;3:145–8.
7. Addiego F. Female ejaculation: a case study. J Sex Res. 1981;17:1–13.
8. Whipple B, Perry JD, Ladas AK. The G spot and other recent discoveries about human sexuality. New York: Holt, Rinehart, and Winston; 1982.
9. Ostrzenski A. G-spot anatomy: a new discovery. J Sex Med. 2012;9:1355–9.
10. Masters WH, Johnson VE. Human sexual inadequacy. Toronto: Bantam Books; 1970.

11. Levin RJ. Critically revising aspects of the human sexual response cycle of Masters and Johnson: correcting errors and suggesting modifications. Sex Relat Ther. 2008;23(4):393–9.
12. Masters WH, Johnson V. Human sexual response. Boston: Little, Brown, and Co.; 1966.
13. Clayton AH. Sexual function and dysfunction in women. Psychiatr Clin N Am. 2003;26:673–82.
14. Kaplan HS. The new sex therapy: active treatment of sexual dysfunctions. New York: Brunner/Mazel, Publishers, Inc.; 1974.
15. Basson R. The female sexual response: a different model. J Sex Marital Ther. 2000;26:51–65.
16. Pfaus JG, Scepkowski LA. The biologic basis for libido. Curr Sex Health Rep. 2005;2:95–100.
17. Traish A, Kim NN. Modulation of female genital sexual arousal by sex steroid hormones. In: Goldstein I, Meston CM, Davis SR, Traish AM, editors. Women's sexual function and dysfunction. Study, diagnosis and treatment. London: Taylor and Francis; 2006. p. 181–92.
18. Giraldi A, Levin RJ. Vascular physiology of female sexual function. In: Goldstein I, Meston CM, Davis SR, Traish AM, editors. Women's sexual function and dysfunction. Study, diagnosis and treatment. London: Taylor and Francis; 2006. p. 174–80.
19. Clayton AH, Hamilton DV. Female sexual dysfunction. Psychiatr Clin N Am. 2010;2:323–38.
20. Clayton AH. Epidemiology and neurobiology of female sexual dysfunction. J Sex Med. 2007;4 Suppl 4:260–8.
21. Janssen E. The psychophysiology of sex. Bloomington: Indiana Press, Kinsey Institute; 2000.
22. Georgiadis JR, Kringelbach ML, Pfaus JG. Sex for fun: a synthesis of human and animal neurobiology. Nat Rev Urol. 2012;9:486–98.

Diagnosis of Female Sexual Dysfunction

19

Richard Balon and Terri L. Woodard

19.1 Introduction

Diagnosis is important for many reasons. It helps clinicians name what they observe and communicate their observations with others. The process of generating a differential diagnosis also allows them to sharpen their observations and to be able to describe and classify them more precisely. Diagnosis also helps patients: first, they may feel more assured when the clinician is able to name their malady, which increases their confidence that the provider understands and knows what he/she is doing, and, second, it enables them to seek and acquire more information about their condition themselves. Last but not least, diagnosis is the starting point and cornerstone of the treatment process.

So, what is a diagnosis? It is a short "scientific" description for taxonomic classification and/or process of deciding the nature of a diseased condition by examination of symptoms. It can also be described as a careful examination and analysis of facts in an attempt to understand and explain something or a decision made based on such observation. In psychiatry and in many other medical specialties, diagnosis is derived from a composition of symptoms (or signs) that delineate a disorder (which implies disordered function), rather than a disease of known etiology.

Diagnosis should strive for a high degree of validity and reliability. Robins and Guze [1] outlined a method for achieving validity in psychiatric illness that consists of five phases: (1) clinical description, (2) laboratory study, (3) exclusion of other disorders, (4) follow-up study, and (5) family study. Others [2, 3] added further criteria, such as physical and neurological factors discussed by Feighner [2] and antecedent validators (familial aggregation, premorbid personality, precipitating factors), concurrent validators (e.g., psychological testing), and predictive validators (diagnostic consistency over time, rates of relapse and recovery, and response to treatment) proposed by Kendler [3]. The issue of reliability has been addressed during the creation of Diagnostic and Statistical Manual of Mental Disorders, Third Edition [4], and diagnostic interviews based on the criteria published in this manual. Most of the diagnoses listed in DSM-III were found to be fairly reliable in studies using structured interviews and other approaches.

There are various classification systems for diseases and disorders; however, two of the

R. Balon, M.D. (✉)
Department of Psychiatry,
Tolan Park Building 3rd floor, 3901 Chrysler Service Dr., Detroit, MI 48201, USA
e-mail: rbalon@wayne.edu

T.L. Woodard, M.D.
Department of Gynecologic Oncology and Reproductive Medicine, MD Anderson, Houston, TX, USA

L.I. Lipshultz et al. (eds.), *Management of Sexual Dysfunction in Men and Women*, DOI 10.1007/978-1-4939-3100-2_19

systems most commonly used to diagnose and classify sexual dysfunctions are the International Classification of Diseases and Related Health Problems (ICD) and the Diagnostic and Statistical Manual of Mental Disorders (DSM). The ICD is published by the World Health Organization (WHO) and is the global health information standard for mortality and morbidity statistics as well as the diagnostic classification standard for all clinical and research purposes (ICD information sheet). Its Tenth Revision (ICD-10) is currently in use; however, the ICD-11 is anticipated to be finalized and released in 2017. The DSM is published by the American Psychiatric Association and was developed to provide standard criteria for the classification of mental disorders. Its Fifth Edition (DSM-5) was published in 2013 and contained extensive revisions [5].

The ICD-10 classifies sexual dysfunction based on the sexual response cycle, similar to the previous edition of the DSM (DSM-IV) [6]. However, the ICD-10 places emphasis on sexual dysfunction not being caused by an organic disorder or disease, while the DSM-IV had provisions for sexual dysfunction due to a general medical condition and substance-induced sexual dysfunction. ICD-10 diagnoses that are specifically applicable to the area of female sexual dysfunction (FSD) are listed in Table 19.1.

The intent of the newly revised DSM-5 was to refocus on the validity of diagnosis in all areas, including sexual dysfunctions. One major paradigm change was that the linear sexual response cycle was abandoned as a guiding concept in diagnosing sexual dysfunctions, based on research that questions the validity of the linear model of sexual response in women [7, 8]. The diagnoses of sexual dysfunctions in the DSM-5 are now listed alphabetically instead of according to the phase of sexual response cycle. In addition, gender-specific diagnoses were added, duration of dysfunction for at least 6 months became a required criterion, and two new female sexual dysfunction diagnoses—Female Sexual Interest/Arousal Disorder (FSIAD) and Genito-Pelvic Pain/Penetration Disorder (GPPPD)—were created through the merging of the former DSM-IV diagnoses of Female Hypoactive Sexual Desire Disorder with Female Sexual Arousal Disorder and Dyspareunia with Vaginismus, respectively. Sexual Aversion Disorder was discarded, because of a lack of empirical support for the diagnosis. The diagnosis of sexual dysfunction due to a general medical was also discarded. DSM-5 diagnoses applicable to the area of female sexual dysfunction are listed in Table 19.2. In addition, Table 19.3 compares the DSM-IV and DSM-5 symptomatology/changes of female gender-specific diagnoses.

Only time and more research will reveal whether the changes introduced in the DSM-5 are progressive, meaningful, and clinically relevant. It is noteworthy that even with the newly sparked interest in the validity of diagnosis of sexual dysfunction, none of the diagnostic systems adhere to the principles outlined by Robins

Table 19.1 ICD-10 classification of sexual dysfunction

Lack or loss of sexual desire (frigidity and hypoactive sexual desire disorder)
Sexual aversion and lack of sexual enjoyment (sexual anhedonia)
Failure of genital response (female sexual arousal disorder)
Orgasmic dysfunction (inhibited orgasm in female, psychogenic anorgasmy)
Nonorganic vaginismus (psychogenic vaginismus)
Nonorganic dyspareunia (psychogenic dyspareunia)
Excessive sexual drive (nymphomania)
Other sexual dysfunction not caused by organic disorder or diseases
Unspecified sexual dysfunction not causes by organic disorder or disease

ICD International classification of diseases and related health problems

Table 19.2 DSM-5 classification of female sexual dysfunction

Female orgasmic disorder (FOD)
Female sexual interest/arousal disorder
Genito-pelvic pain/penetration disorder
Substance/medication-induced sexual dysfunction (in women)
Other specified sexual dysfunction
Unspecified sexual dysfunction

DSM Diagnostic and statistical manual of mental disorders

Table 19.3 Comparison of DSM-IV and DSM-5 criterion A (symptomatology) of gender-specific female sexual dysfunctions

DSM-IV diagnosis	DSM-IV criterion A	DSM-5 diagnosis	DSM-5 criterion A
Hypoactive sexual desire disorder (both male and female)	Persistently or recurrently deficient (or absent) sexual fantasies and desire for sexual activity. The judgment of deficiency or absence is made by the clinician, taking into account factors that affect sexual functioning such as age and the context of person's life	*Female sexual interest/arousal disorder*	Lack of or significantly reduced sexual interest/arousal, as manifested by at least three of the following: 1. Absent/reduced interest in sexual activity 2. Absent/reduced sexual/erotic thoughts or fantasies 3. No/reduced initiation of sexual activity and typically unreceptive to a partner's attempts to initiate 4. Absent/reduced sexual excitement/pleasure during sexual activity in almost all or all (approximately 75–100 %) sexual encounters (in identified situational contexts, or, if generalized, in all contexts) 5. Absent/reduced sexual interest/arousal in response to any internal or external sexual/erotic cues (e.g., written, verbal, visual) 6. Absent/reduced genital or nongenital sensations during sexual activity in almost all or all (approximately 75–100 %) sexual encounters (in identified situational contexts or, if generalized, in all contexts)
Female sexual arousal disorder	Persistent or recurrent inability to attain, or maintain until completion of the sexual activity, and adequate lubrication-swelling response to sexual excitement		
Female orgasmic disorder	Persistent or recurrent delay in, or absence of, orgasm following a normal sexual excitement phase. Women exhibit wide variability in the type or intensity of stimulation that triggers orgasm. The diagnosis of female orgasmic disorder should be based on the clinician's judgment that the woman's orgasmic capacity is less than would be reasonable for her age, sexual experience, and the adequacy of sexual stimulation she receives	*Female orgasmic disorder*	Presence of either of the following symptoms and experienced on almost all or all (approximately 75–100 %) sexual encounters (in identified situational contexts or, if generalized, in all contexts) 1. Marked delay in, marked infrequency of, or absence of orgasm 2. Markedly reduced intensity of orgasmic sensations

(continued)

Table 19.3 (continued)

DSM-IV diagnosis	DSM-IV criterion A	DSM-5 diagnosis	DSM-5 criterion A
Dyspareunia	Recurrent or persistent genital pain associated with sexual intercourse in either male or female	*Genito-pelvic pain/penetration disorder*	Persistent or recurrent difficulties with one (or more) of the following: 1. Vaginal penetration during intercourse 2. Marked vulvovaginal or pelvic pain during vaginal intercourse or penetration attempts 3. Marked fear or anxiety about vulvovaginal or pelvic pain in anticipation of, during, or as a result of vaginal penetration 4. Marked tensing or tightening of the pelvic floor muscles during attempted vaginal penetration
Vaginismus	Recurrent or persistent involuntary spasm of the musculature of the outer third of the vagina that interferes with sexual intercourse		
Sexual aversion disorder	Persistent or recurrent extreme aversion to, and avoidance of, all (or almost all) genital sexual contact with a sexual partner		

DSM Diagnostic and statistical manual of mental disorders

and Guze [3], Feighner [4], and Kendler [5]. Some of the new changes in the DSM-5 have been vigorously criticized as confusing and have not been accepted by all experts [9]. In fact, there are some who have questioned the true existence of female sexual dysfunction disorders and feel that women's sexual concerns have been excessively medicalized, partially due to pressure from the pharmaceutical industry.

It is essential to distinguish between relatively more common "sexual problems" and true diagnosable sexual dysfunction disorders. Sexual problems are transient disturbances or disruptions in sexual functioning which may arise due to temporary stressors, relationship problems, and/or other conditions that have a short duration (less than 6 months). We will focus on the diagnosis of female sexual dysfunction disorders using the DSM-5 criteria as a descriptive framework for describing and assessing FSD.

19.2 Female Sexual Dysfunction in the DSM-5

The three female gender-specific DSM-5 [5] sexual dysfunction diagnoses—FSIAD, FOD and GPPPD—have their specific symptomatologies summarized in Criterion A of each diagnosis and share the same three criteria B, C, and D (see Table 19.4). For all three diagnoses, it should be specified whether the distress over the symptoms is mild, moderate, or severe and whether the dysfunction is lifelong (ever since the woman became sexually active) or acquired (the dysfunction started after a period of relatively normal sexual functioning).

The DSM-5 recognizes that 'sexual response has a requisite biological underpinning, yet is usually experienced in an intrapersonal, interpersonal, and cultural context.' Thus, sexual func-

Table 19.4 DSM-5 criterions B, C, and D

Criteria B	Persisted for a minimum duration of approximately 6 months
Criteria C	Symptoms in criterion A cause clinically significant distress in the individual (based on the clinician's judgment)
Criteria D	Should not be better explained by a nonsexual mental disorder or as a consequence of severe relationship distress (e.g., partner violence) or other significant stressor and is not attributable to the effects of a substance/medication or another medical condition

DSM Diagnostic and statistical manual of mental disorders

tion involves a complex interaction among biological, sociocultural, and psychological factors. Accordingly, the DSM-5 recommends that a number of associated features "be considered during the assessment of sexual dysfunction, given that they may be relevant to etiology and/or treatment and that they may contribute, to varying degrees, across individuals:

(1) Partner factors (such as partner's sexual problems and partner's health status)
(2) Relationship factors (including poor communication, discrepancies between partners in desire for sexual activity)
(3) Individual vulnerability factors (e.g., poor body image, a history of sexual or emotional abuse), psychiatric comorbidity (i.e., depression, anxiety), or stressors (such as job loss, bereavement)
(4) Cultural or religious factors (including sociocultural mores with regard to sexual activity and behavior, negative attitudes toward sexuality)
(5) Medical factors relevant to prognosis, course, or treatment [5, p. 423]"

In many clinical contexts, the precise etiology of a sexual problem is uncertain. However, a sexual dysfunction diagnosis requires ruling out problems that are better explained by a nonsexual mental disorder, the effect of a substance, or a medical condition or by severe relationship distress, partner violence, or other stressors [5, p. 423]. The DSM-5 also specifically states that if the sexual dysfunction is attributable to another medical condition, the individual does not receive a psychiatric diagnosis; yet it stops short of proposing that sexual dysfunction disorders be categorized as exclusively psychiatric diagnoses.

In spite of the complexity of female sexual dysfunction disorders, the descriptive framework is a concept that can be useful to psychiatry as well as other related disciplines where women often present with sexual health concerns, such as obstetrics and gynecology and urology. Using this framework, a provider can assess symptoms and identify possible etiologic factors.

19.2.1 Specific FSD Diagnoses

19.2.1.1 Female Orgasmic Disorder

The diagnosis of female orgasmic disorder (FOD) requires the presence of (1) a marked delay in, marked infrequency of, or absence of orgasm and/or (2) a markedly reduced intensity of orgasmic sensations. These symptoms should be experienced on all or almost all (approximately 75–100 %) occasions of sexual activity. FOD specifiers should identify whether the dysfunction is generalized (occurs under all circumstances) or situational (i.e., only with certain types of stimulation, situations or partners). It should also be specified if a woman has never experienced an orgasm under any situation.

19.2.1.2 Female Sexual Interest/Arousal Disorder

The diagnosis of Female Sexual Interest/Arousal Disorder (FSIAD) is characterized by a lack of or significantly reduced sexual interest/arousal. It must be manifested by at least three of the following (in any combination): (1) absent/reduced interest in sexual activity, (2) absent/reduced sexual/erotic thoughts or fantasies, (3) no or reduced initiation of sexual activity and being unreceptive to a partner's attempts to initiate sex, (4) absent or reduced sexual excitement/pleasure during sex in all or almost all (approximately

75–100 %) of sexual encounters, (5) absent or reduced sexual interest/arousal in response to any internal or external sexual/erotic cues (e.g., verbal, visual), and (6) absent or reduced genital or nongenital sensations during sexual activity in almost all or all (approximately 75–100 %) of sexual encounters.

FSIAD replaces the diagnoses of Hypoactive Sexual Desire Disorder and Female Sexual Arousal Disorder as defined in the DSM-IV. These two diagnoses were combined based on data suggesting that desire and arousal are not separate entities and that women do not reliably distinguish between desire and arousal. However, many critics have argued that the new diagnostic criteria exclude a significant number of women with low desire and arousal. While there is general agreement that considerable overlap exists when comparing symptoms between these two constructs, differences between the tails of the normal distribution curve describing those with FSIAD would also be clearly evident.

Unlike Female Sexual Arousal Disorder as defined in the DSM-IV [6], a lack of adequate swelling-lubrication response is no longer specifically required, but it is subsumed under (6)—absent or reduced genital sensations. The change is based on data that physiological measures of genital response do not differentiate women who report sexual arousal concerns from those who do not; therefore, the DSM-5 states that the "self-report of reduced or absent genital or nongenital sensations is sufficient" [5, p. 434]. FSIAD specifiers should identify whether the dysfunction is generalized or situational.

19.2.2 Genito-Pelvic Pain/Penetration Disorder

The diagnosis of Genito-Pelvic Pain/Penetration Disorder (GPPPD) requires persistent or recurrent difficulties with one or more of (1) vaginal penetration during intercourse; (2) marked vulvovaginal or pelvic pain during intercourse or penetration attempts; (3) marked fear of anxiety about vulvovaginal or pelvic pain in anticipation of, during, or as a result of vaginal penetration; and (4) marked tensing or tightening of the pelvic floor muscles during attempted vaginal penetration.

GPPPD replaces the diagnoses of dyspareunia and vaginismus from the DSM-IV, based on research that suggests that the two conditions have a great degree of overlap and cannot be reliably differentiated.

19.2.3 Substance/Medication-Induced Sexual Dysfunction

A non-gender-specific FSD diagnosis of *Substance/Medication-Induced Sexual Dysfunction* requires presence of significant disturbance in sexual function with the evidence (based on history, physical examination, or laboratory findings) that the dysfunction developed during or soon after substance intoxication or withdrawal or after exposure to a medication and that the involved substance or medication is capable of producing the dysfunction. The dysfunction should not occur during delirium. It should be specified whether the onset was during intoxication, during withdrawal, or after medication use and whether the distress is mild, moderate, or severe.

19.3 Factors Contributing to FSD

There are numerous "etiological" factors that may contribute to FSD, and all should be considered during diagnosis. There are normative changes in sexual functioning that occur in women during menopause, pregnancy, parturition, and breastfeeding that may lead to the development of a sexual dysfunction [10]. Factors such as age, lower levels of education, lower socioeconomic class, poor physical and emotional health, and a history of sexual abuse have all been associated with FSD. Several recent review articles [11–14] reviewed possible biologic factors underlying sexual dysfunction (psychological and relational factors have been discussed previously):

(a) Anatomical: pelvic floor injury, pelvic floor spasm, vulvovaginal atrophy.
(b) Endocrine: adrenal failure, diabetes mellitus, hypothalamo-pituitary-ovarian dysfunction, hyperprolactinemia, hypothyroidism, chronic hormonal contraceptive use, liver failure, premature ovarian failure.
(c) Genetic: there is some evidence of a strong influence of genetic factors on vulnerability to sexual dysfunction in women.
(d) Neurogenic: multiple sclerosis, Parkinsonism, peripheral neuropathy, spinal cord injury, stroke, upper motor neuron injury.
(e) Pharmacological and substances of abuse: use of medications (e.g., SSRIs, antiestrogens, antiandrogens, antihistamines, antipsychotics, antihypertensives, metronidazole, alcohol, opioids, sedatives)—this is classified under the Substance/Medication-Induced Sexual Dysfunction.
(f) Vascular: atherosclerosis, trauma, stroke.
(g) Other: arthritis, cancer, chronic kidney disease, chronic pain, endometriosis, fibromyalgia, lichen sclerosis, lupus, pelvic inflammatory disease, rheumatic disease, and smoking.

19.4 Establishing the Diagnosis of FSD

There are significant barriers to the identification and diagnosis of FSD. As Jha and Thakar [11] point out, women do not always directly voice complaints of sexual dysfunction, but may present with more covert symptoms such as pelvic pain, distress about menses, general dissatisfaction with a contraceptive precaution, or distaste for genital area or for sexual activity at the time of genital examination. Physicians and others may be reluctant to discuss sexual activity and sexual history for various reasons (lack of training, lack of practice, being embarrassed or fearing that patient may be embarrassed, male gender, and others [11]). Nevertheless, evaluation of sexual functioning should be part of any comprehensive evaluation by any healthcare professional regardless of profession of origin.

Proper evaluation [15, 16] of sexual function/dysfunction consists of several components, as indicated:

(1) The clinical interview, including a complete history and review of systems
(2) The physical examination, including a pelvic examination
(3) Laboratory testing (when indicated by clinical findings)
(4) Psychometric assessments (such as validates questionnaires and scales)

The clinical interview is the primary and most important source of information, and a variety of methods have been described elsewhere [17]. Derogatis and Balon [16] proposed a matrix of three sequential levels: Level 1 determines why the patient is seeing the clinician and what has prompted the visit and clarifies whether the patient currently has or has previously complained of sexual dysfunction. Her partner's input can be quite helpful at this level. Level 2 focuses on the character and nature of the patient's sexual dysfunction (FOD, FSIAD, GPPPD). If the woman complains of more than one dysfunction, effort should be made to identify which is the primary one. It also should be determined whether the dysfunction is transient, fluctuating, permanent, generalized, or situational. At this level, one may use the diagnostic algorithm based on DSM-5 outlined by Latif and Diamond [13]. This algorithm progresses from asking the patient about sexual interest to questions about sexual arousal, orgasm, and sexual pain. Level 3 seeks to establish the etiology of the patient's sexual dysfunction (e.g., atherosclerosis, depression, endometriosis, infection, marital discord).

Questions about sexual functioning should be direct and specific. Vague questioning such as "How is your sex life?" should be avoided, as it may generate ambiguous answers such as "OK." The interview should be semi structured, yet tailored to the individual patient. The questions should be asked in a respectful yet serious manner [16]. One may use questions modeled on the DSM-5 criteria of FSDs to arrive to a preliminary diagnosis of a specific FSD.

The history should include a sexual history (including details about first sexual experimentation, intercourse, masturbation), reproductive history, status of current sexual relationship, sociocultural and personal beliefs about sexuality, and history of sexual trauma [13]. A detailed medical and surgical history as well as information about substance abuse (including smoking) and medications (including over the counter, herbal, and contraceptives [13]) should be elicited.

The clinical interview should be followed by a complete physical examination which includes a pelvic examination [13]. The pelvic examination is especially important for women with possible GPPPD. There are several physiologic measures of sexual function that could potentially help determine organic factors underlying the diagnosis of sexual dysfunction [13]. These include vaginal photoplethysmography (a measure of genital blood flow) and measurements of vaginal lubrication, volume, pressure, and compliance [13]. There are many other tests and measures that could be used (e.g., measuring the bulbocavernosus reflex, electromyograms of pelvic muscle floors, electrovaginograms), but most of these methods are "invasive, poorly defined, and lack standardization, validity, and reliability" and thus have little value in establishing a diagnosis [13]. Currently, such testing cannot be routinely recommended and should be reserved for use in investigational protocols.

Laboratory tests should be ordered based on clinical information and suspicion of underlying pathology. Laboratory tests are rarely definitive in determining the etiology of FSD, but they may help rule out biological factors and conditions [16]. Diagnostic testing that may be considered includes plasma estradiol, total testosterone, free testosterone, sex hormone-binding globulin, thyroid-stimulating hormone, and prolactin. Other assays such as a lipid profile, dehydroepiandrosterone, glycosylated hemoglobin A1C, thyroid panel, luteinizing hormone, follicle-stimulating hormone, and complete blood count may be warranted based on clinical findings.

There are a number of validated questionnaires and scales that are available for psychometric assessment of various aspects of female sexual functioning. These include the Derogatis Interview for Sexual Functioning (DSIF/DSIF-SR) [18], which has gender-specific versions; the Female Sexual Function Index [19]; the Profile of Female Sexual Functioning (PFSF) [20], which also has a brief form (B-PFSF) [21]; the Sexual Function Questionnaire [22]; the Sexual Interest and Desire Inventory (SIDI) [23]; the Female Sexual Distress Scale (FSDS) [24]; and the Shor Personal Experience Questionnaire (SPEQ) [25] (see Table 19.5). Their usefulness, validity, and reliability have been summarized by Derogatis [15] and Derogatis and Balon [16]. It is important to emphasize that none of these instruments are diagnostic tools. They should be used as an additional source of information that is integrated with information obtained by the clinical interview, physical examination, and other testing. Giraldi and colleagues [26] note that there is a serious lack of standardized, internationally (culturally) acceptable tools that are truly validated in the general population that can be used to assess FSD in women with or without a partner, independent of the partner's gender. Nevertheless, Clegg et al. [27] strongly recommend including FSD questionnaires/scales as part of the clinician's routine encounters with female patients. According to them, these instruments have several important roles, including serving as an assessment tool to detect FSD and diagnose a particular disorder [27, p. 161], identifying and assessing distress and patient satisfaction/problems, and measuring treatment-induced change. However, it is important to note that no specific questionnaire/tool has been developed in response to the new diagnostic concepts introduced in the DSM-5.

Table 19.5 Selected validated questionnaires and scales

Instrument	Domain	Questions	Gender	Interview/Self-report
Derogatis interview for sexual functioning (DISF/DISF-SR)	Cognition/fantasy, drive/relationship, arousal, behavior/experience, orgasm, total score	25	Female and male	Both
Profile of female sexual functioning (PFSF)	Desire, arousal, orgasm, pleasure, concerns, responsiveness, self-image	37	Female	Self-report
Sexual function questionnaire	Desire, arousal-sensation, arousal-lubrication, enjoyment, orgasm, dyspareunia, partner relationship, total score	26	Female	Self-report
Female sexual function index (FSFI)	Desire, arousal, lubrication, orgasm, satisfaction, pain	19	Female	Self-report
Sexual interest and desire inventory (SIDI)	Overall total score	13	Female	Clinical interview
Female sexual distress scale (FSDS)	Sexually related personal distress, revised version added desire item	12 (revised: 13)	Female	Self-report
Short personal experience questionnaire (SPEQ)	Feelings for partner, sexual responsivity, sexual frequency, libido, distress/dyspareunia, partner problems	9	Female	Self-report

19.5 Conclusion

The diagnosis of FSD is complex, complicated, and continuously emerging. The new DSM-5 [5] and, hopefully, the next revision of the ICD introduce simpler, though untested classification systems that facilitate valid and reliable diagnosis of female sexual function disorders. At present, data obtained from the clinical interview, physical examination, targeted laboratory testing, and, possibly, psychometric assessment should be used in conjunction with the DSM-5 diagnostic criteria as a descriptive framework to establish diagnosis and etiology, of sexual dysfunction disorders in women.

References

1. Robins E, Guze SB. Establishment of diagnostic validity in psychiatric illness: its application to schizophrenia. Am J Psychiatry. 1970;126:983–7.
2. Feigner JP. Nosology of primary affective disorders and application to clinical practice. Acta Psychiatr Scand Suppl. 1981;290:29–41.
3. Kendler KS. The nosologic validity of paranoia (simple delusional disorder): a review. Arch Gen Psychiatry. 1980;37:699–706.
4. American Psychiatric Association. Diagnostic and statistical manual of mental disorders. 3rd ed. Washington, DC: American Psychiatric Association; 1980.
5. American Psychiatric Association. Diagnostic and statistical manual of mental disorders. 5th ed. Arlington, VA: American Psychiatric Association; 2013.
6. American Psychiatric Association. Diagnostic and statistical manual of mental disorders. 4th ed. Washington, DC: American Psychiatric Association; 1994.
7. Basson R. The female sexual response: a different model. J Sex Marital Ther. 2000;26:51–65.
8. Giraldi A, Kristensen E, Sand M. Endorsement of models describing sexual response of men and women with sexual partner: an online survey in a population sample of Danish adults ages 20–65 years. J Sex Med. 2015;12:116–28.
9. Balon R, Clayton AH. Female sexual interest/arousal disorder: a diagnosis out of thin air. Arch Sex Behav. 2014;43:1227–9.
10. Hayes R, Dennerstein L. The impact of aging on sexual function and sexual dysfunction in women: a review of population-based studies. J Sex Med. 2005;2:317–30.
11. Jha S, Thakar R. Female sexual dysfunction. Eur J Obstet Gynecol Reprod Biol. 2010;153:117–23.
12. Tsai TF, Yeh CH, Hwang TIS. Female sexual dysfunction: physiology, epidemiology, classification, evaluation and treatment. Urol Sci. 2011;22:7–13.

13. Latif EZ, Diamond MP. Arriving at the diagnosis of female sexual dysfunction. Fertil Steril. 2013;100:898–904.
14. Chen HC, Lin YC, Chiu LH, Chu YH, Ruan FF, Liu WM, Wand PH. Female sexual dysfunction: definition, classification, and debates. Taiwan J Obstet Gynecol. 2013;52:3–7.
15. Derogatis L. Clinical and research evaluations of sexual dysfunctions. Adv Psychosom Med. 2008;29:7–22.
16. Derogatis LR, Balon R. Clinical evaluation of sexual dysfunctions. In: Balon R, Segraves RT, editors. Clinical manual of sexual disorders. Arlington, VA: American Psychiatric Publishing, Inc; 2009. p. 23–57.
17. Althof SE, Rosen RC, Perelman MA, Rubio-Aurioles E. Standard operating procedures for taking sexual history. J Sex Med. 2013;10:26–35.
18. Derogatis LR. The Derogatis interview for sexual functioning (DISF/DISF-SR): an introductory report. J Sex Marital Ther. 1997;23:291–304.
19. Rosen R, Brown C, Heiman J, Leiblum S, Meston C, Shabsigh R, Fergusson D, D'Agostino D. The female sexual function index (FSFI): a multidimensional self-report instrument for the assessment of female sexual function. J Sex Marital Ther. 2000;26:191–208.
20. McHorney CA, Rust J, Golombok S, Davis S, Bouchard C, Rodenberg C, Derogatis LR. Profile of female sexual function: a patient-based, international psychometric instrument for the assessment of the hypoactive sexual desire in oophorectomized women. Menopause. 2004;11:1–10.
21. Rust J, Derogatis LR, Rodenberg C, Koochaki P, Schmidt C, Golombek S. Development and validation of a new screening tool for hypoactive sexual desire disorder: the brief profile of female sexual function (B-PFSF). Gynecol Endocrinol. 2007;23:638–44.
22. Quirk FH, Heiman J, Rosen RC, Laan E, Smith MD, Boolel M. Development of a sexual function questionnaire for clinical trials of female sexual function. J Womens Health Gend Based Med. 2002;11:277–85.
23. Clayton AH, Segraves RT, Leiblum S, Basson R, Pyke R, Cotton D, Lewis-D'Agostino D, Evans KR, Sills TL, Wunderlich G. Reliability and validity of the sexual interest and desire inventory-female (SIDI-F), a scale designed to measure severity of female hypoactive sexual desire disorder. J Sex Marital Ther. 2006;32:115–35.
24. Derogatis LR, Rosen RC, Leiblum S, Burnett A, Heiman J. The female sexual distress scale (FSDS): initial validation of a standardized scale for the assessment of sexually related personal distress in women. J Sex Marital Ther. 2002;28:317–30.
25. Dennerstein L, Lehert P, Dudley E. Short scale to measure female sexuality: adapted from McCoy female sexuality questionnaire. J Sex Marital Ther. 2001;27:339–52.
26. Giraldi A, Rellini A, Pfaus JG, Bitzer J, Laan E, Jannini EA, Fugl-Meyer AR. Questionnaires for assessment of female sexual dysfunction: a review and proposal for a standardized screener. J Sex Med. 2011;8:2681–706.
27. Clegg M, Towner A, Wylie K. Should questionnaires of female sexual dysfunction be used in routine clinical practice? Maturitas. 2012;72:160–4.

The Epidemiology and Diagnosis of Hypoactive Sexual Desire Disorder and Causes of HSDD: Situational, Depression, Drugs, Chronic Illnesses, and Hormonal Depletion

20

Sharon J. Parish and Steven R. Hahn

20.1 Introduction and Definition

Diminished sexual desire that causes personal distress, the defining symptom of hypoactive sexual desire disorder (HSDD), is a relatively common but commonly undiagnosed problem that significantly affects 8.9 % of US women between the ages of 18 and 44, 12.3 % of women ages 45–64, and 7.4 % of women over 65 [1]. In the past decade, substantial research has emerged on the epidemiology and natural history of HSDD, its impact on women and their partners, and approaches to detection and diagnosis, motivated partly in pursuit of effective treatment. This chapter will describe the epidemiology and impact of HSDD, discuss causes and factors, and present strategies for screening and diagnosis of this important condition.

S.J. Parish, M.D. (✉)
Weill Cornell Medical College, New York, NY, USA

Westchester Division, New York Presbyterian Hospital, 21 Bloomingdale Rd, White Plains, NY 10605, USA
e-mail: shp9079@mail.cornell.edu

S.R. Hahn, M.D., F.A.C.P.
Albert Einstein College of Medicine, Bronx, NY, USA

20.1.1 Definition of HSDD: DSM-IV-TR vs. DSM-5

HSDD is defined in the *Diagnostic and Statistical Manual of Mental Disorders, Fourth Edition* (DSM-IV), as persistent deficient sexual fantasies and desire for sexual activity that causes marked distress or interpersonal difficulty and is not better accounted for by another psychiatric disorder or due exclusively to the direct effect of a substance, medication, or general medical condition [2]. In the fifth edition of the *Diagnostic and Statistical Manual of Mental Disorders,* published in May 2013, desire and arousal disorders have been merged into a singular category entitled female sexual interest/arousal disorder (FSIAD) [3]. However, clinicians have utilized DSM-IV-TR criteria for several decades and have no research data or real clinical experience applying DSM-5 criteria to female sexual dysfunctions. Therefore, the discussion in this chapter is based on the long-standing DSM-IV-TR criteria.

The main differences between the DSM-IV-TR and DSM-5 are the merger of desire and arousal into the single female sexual interest/arousal disorder; the rating of disorders as mild, moderate, and severe; the requirement that the disorder be present for at least 6 months during the majority (>75 %) of encounters; and that it causes significant distress in the individual. Both schemas include the specifiers, indicating

L.I. Lipshultz et al. (eds.), *Management of Sexual Dysfunction in Men and Women*, DOI 10.1007/978-1-4939-3100-2_20

whether the disorder is lifelong (no prior history of normal functioning) or acquired (previous normal function) and whether it is generalized (all partners, activities, situations, forms of sexual expression) or situational (certain partners, situations, practices). When the disorder is situational, the woman may continue to masturbate or have partners outside the primary relationship but has decreased interest in her primary partner.

Women with HSDD usually do not initiate sexual activity and participate only reluctantly when their partners initiate sex. Sexual activity is often infrequent. Standards for frequency and degree of sexual desire do not exist; therefore, the diagnosis of this disorder is mainly based on clinical judgment, evaluating the individual's characteristics, her interpersonal situation, the life stage and circumstances, and sociocultural factors.

20.1.1.1 Further Defining HSDD

In the DSM-IV-TR schema, HSDD is also subtyped as due to psychological or combined factors or "due to a medical condition" or a substance. HSDD is usually not diagnosed when the sexual dysfunction is due exclusively to another psychiatric disorder such as major depressive disorder, unless the decreased desire predated depression or is "a focus of independent clinical attention" [2].

The American Urological Association (AUA) has added an absence of sexual thoughts and a lack of desire in response to sexual stimulation (responsive desire) to the DSM-IV-TR definition. A further modification is the specification that the decrease in interest in sex must exceed that normally observed with increasing age and with the duration of sexual relationships [4]. Currently, the ICD-10 system used worldwide classifies sexual dysfunctions under *behavioral syndromes associated with physiological disturbances and physical factors* (F52 for female sexual dysfunction) and states that "Sexual dysfunction covers the various ways in which an individual is unable to participate in a sexual relationship as he or she would wish" [5]. HSDD is defined as a lack or loss of sexual desire that is the principal problem and is not secondary to other sexual difficulties, such as dyspareunia.

20.1.2 Models of Female Sexual Response

Female sexual dysfunction has been classified in the DSM based on the traditional human sexual response cycle which, when first described by Masters and Johnson [6], consisted of four phases: excitement, plateau, orgasm, and resolution. Kaplan [7] and Lief [8] modified this model by adding a desire phase and eliminating the plateau and resolution phases resulting in the linear three-phase model: desire, arousal, and orgasm. Basson and others argue that the three phases are more circular than linear [9]. Women may experience arousal, orgasm, and satisfying sexual experiences without initially, or ever, having desire for sex as a distinct experience. Women may be motivated to engage in sexual activity for many reasons besides desire for sexual activity per se including desire for intimacy or to communicate affection for a partner. Accordingly, sexually stimulating physical intimacy, initiated in response to one of these motives, may lead to arousal and only subsequently to what has been called "responsive desire" [4]. In a cross-sectional nonclinical cohort of 573 Danish women, approximately one-third of the study population endorsed each of the three models (Masters and Johnson, Kaplan, Basson) and 12.5 % none of the models; women who endorsed the cyclical Basson model or none of the models were more likely to have sexual dysfunction and distress ($P=0.01$) [10].

20.2 Epidemiology

West et al. assessed 1944 nonpregnant women ages 30–70 in steady relationships for 3 months or longer. The prevalence of low sexual desire was 36.2 %, and the prevalence of distressing low sexual desire was 8.3 % [11]. The prevalence of low sexual desire increased with age and was higher in surgically menopausal women regardless of their current age or their age at the time of surgery. The highest rate of low sexual desire with distress was observed in young, surgically menopausal women (19.8 %).

Another study by Hayes et al. in women ages 20–70 also found that the proportion of women with low desire increased with age, but the increase was counterbalanced by a decrease in the proportion of women with distress about low sexual desire; as a result, the prevalence of distressing low sexual desire was relatively constant with age, ranging from 6 to 13 % in Europe and 12–19 % in the USA [12].

20.2.1 The PRESIDE Study and HSDD Registry

In the widely cited study, the Prevalence of Female Sexual Problems Associated with Distress and Determinants of Treatment Seeking (PRESIDE), desire, arousal, and orgasm problems in a large population-based survey of adult US women (n=31,581) were evaluated [1]. A response of "never" or "rarely" to the single question, "How often do you desire to engage in sexual activity?" was used to define a problem with desire, and the Female Sexual Distress Scale (FSDS) [13] was used to define distress (score of at least 15 out of a possible 48 points). The combination of low desire plus an FSDS score of 15 or higher was used as the self-report survey-based indicator of decreased sexual desire with distress. Low desire was reported in 37.7 % (age-adjusted estimate) of subjects and was the most common sexual problem reported, and distressing low desire affected 10 % of US women. Low sexual desire with distress occurred with a second distressing sexual problem in fewer than 5 %, and 2.3 % had all three distressing problems.

The HSDD Registry for Women is a multicenter, longitudinal study of women with HSDD which enrolled 1500 women with clinically diagnosed HSDD between 2008 and 2010. Half (50.2 %) of 426 premenopausal women also had arousal problems and 43.5 % reported lubrication problems, while 58 % of 174 sexually active postmenopausal women had arousal and 56.9 % had lubrication problems [14].

20.2.2 Impact of Low Desire on Quality of Life

Women with distressing low sexual desire have lower health-related quality of life. In the National Health and Social Life Survey (NHSLS), women with desire, arousal, and sexual pain problems had lower physical and emotional satisfaction with their partners and lower general happiness than women without sexual problems [15]. In the WISHeS study of postmenopausal US women, distressing low sexual desire was associated with lower health-related quality of life in seven out of eight domains of functioning including physical function, general health, vitality, social functioning, emotional role functioning, and mental health [16]. Women with low desire were more likely to be dissatisfied with their sex life, their partner, or their marriage and experienced more negative emotional states including frustrations, hopelessness, anger, poor self-esteem, and loss of femininity [16].

20.3 Factors Associated with Distressing Low Desire

20.3.1 Partners and Life Situation

In the PRESIDE study, life situation and social status had a significant relationship with the prevalence of distressing low sexual desire [17]. Caucasian women were more likely than African-American women to have HSDD. Working, midlife, married, and partnered women were more likely to have distressing low sexual desire. When marital status and availability of a sexual partner were considered together, single women with a sexual partner were at lowest risk for distressing sexual desire.

20.3.2 Menopause, General Health, and Psychiatric Disorders

In the WISHeS study, postmenopausal women, especially young women with surgical menopause, were more likely to have distressing low sexual desire than cycling premenopausal women [16]. In PRESIDE, while self-reported distressing low sexual desire was not associated with current hormone use in postmenopausal women, perceived overall health status, thyroid disease, and urinary incontinence showed significant associations with this sexual problem [17]. Depression, based on positive response to either of the two screening questions about depressed mood or anhedonia or the current use of antidepressants, and anxiety substantially increased the likelihood of distressing low sexual desire. In the HSDD Registry for Women study, one-third of premenopausal women met criteria for depression and also reported lower sexual function and relationship quality [18].

20.3.3 Antidepressant and Other Medications and Substances

Although the determination about whether the loss of desire is primarily due to depression alone may be challenging, treatment may clarify the importance of comorbid HSDD. Most antidepressants are associated with both orgasm and desire disorders, afflicting at least one-third of more users [19]. Therefore, treatment of depression with medication may substitute one cause of sexual dysfunction for another. However, in the HSDD Registry for Women study, women inadequately treated for depression had more severe sexual dysfunction as compared to women whose depression was in remission [18]. Bupropion appears to have significantly less sexual dysfunction compared to selective serotonin reuptake inhibitors (SSRIs) and selective serotonin and norepinephrine uptake inhibitors (SNRIs) [20]. The use of antidepressants and other medications as well as drugs and alcohol should be included in the evaluation of all female sexual dysfunctions. Medications such as β-blockers, oral steroids, H2 blockers, and antidepressants have been reported to be associated with changes in sexual desire.

20.4 Psychophysiological Models of HSDD

The interrelationship between psychosocial and physiological factors and causes of HSDD is complex; Bancroft, Perelman, Pfaus, and others have offered the following elaborative concepts [21].

20.4.1 Dual Control of Sexual Interest and Response

Sexual response is the result of an interaction between sexual excitatory and inhibitory influences that may act independently. HSDD may be the result of insufficient excitatory processes or increased inhibition of sexual interest or response. Inhibition of sexual interest or responsiveness may be an adaptive response to relationship difficulties or life circumstances that serves to help avoid risky, distressing, or threatening sexual situations and behavior [22].

20.4.2 Central Nervous System and HSDD

Sexually excitatory processes include central pathways in the limbic system and hypothalamus utilizing neurotransmitters such as dopamine, oxytocin, melanocortin, and norepinephrine. Sexual inhibitory processes include neurotransmitter systems such as the opioid, endocannabinoid, and serotonergic systems [23] (Table 20.1). Studies using functional brain scanning have demonstrated distinguishable patterns of brain activity during erotic compared to non-erotic experiences in women, and patterns also differ between pre- and postmenopausal women [24]. Specific differences in processing arousing stimuli and/or retrieval of past erotic experiences were reported in women with HSDD, who appeared to pay more attention to monitoring their own responses when compared with women without sexual dysfunction.

20.4.3 Intra- and Interpersonal Psychosocial and Cultural Influences

Understanding the intra- and interpersonal psychosocial and cultural components that contribute to a woman's sexual dysfunction is a critical aspect of the diagnostic process [25]. Her beliefs and in particular her erotic thoughts and her inhibition of them (conscious and/or unconscious) will play a role in critical feedback in facilitating or inhibiting her desire in much the same dualistic manner as the biological factors discussed above. Furthermore, a woman's sexual dysfunction may be due to or exacerbated by her partner's sexual problems [26]. Decreased desire, erectile dysfunction, and premature or delayed ejaculation in male partners may produce frustration with sexual activity that leads to a decrease in sexual desire [27]. Assessment of HSDD should include the patient and partner's sexual practices, frequency of sexual activity, and discrepancies in desire for sex, as well as communication between partners [28]. However, not all discrepancies in frequency preference reflect the presence of HSDD, as other relationship issues may be causing such disparity. In fact, sexual dissatisfaction with a partner or dissatisfaction about any other aspect of the relationship may contribute to sexual problems [29]. Women who only experience decreased desire regarding their partner, but have sexual fantasies or desire for other sexual activities, do not have generalized HSDD; they have a desire problem that is specific to their relationship. A common relationship difficulty that underlies HSDD is an unresolved conflict that leads to covert anger, buried resentment, and unconscious alienation [30]. A past history of sexual trauma is also

Table 20.1 Decreased sexual desire screener (DSDS)

	No	Yes
1. In the past, was your level of sexual desire or interest good and satisfying to you?		
2. Has there been a decrease in your level of sexual desire or interest?		
3. Are you bothered by your decreased level of sexual desire or interest?		
4. Would you like your level of sexual desire or interest to increase?		
5. Please circle all the factors that you feel may be contributing to your current decrease in sexual desire or interest:		
A. An operation, depression, injuries, or other medical condition		
B. Medications, drugs, or alcohol you are currently taking		
C. Pregnancy, recent childbirth, menopausal symptoms		
D. Other sexual issues you may be having (pain, decreased arousal or orgasm)		
E. Your partner's sexual problems		
F. Dissatisfaction with your relationship or partner		
G. Stress or fatigue		
The patient qualifies for the diagnosis of generalized, acquired HSDD if • She answers "YES" to all of questions 1–4, and your review confirms "NO" to all of the factors in question 5. *The patient MAY qualify for the diagnosis of generalized, acquired HSDD if* • She answers "YES" to all of questions 1–4 and "YES" to any of the factors in question 5; clinical judgment is required to determine if the answers to question 5 indicate a primary diagnosis other than generalized, acquired HSDD. Co-morbid conditions such as arousal or orgasmic disorder do not rule out a concurrent diagnosis of HSDD. *The patient does NOT qualify for the diagnosis of generalized, acquired HSDD if* • She answers "NO" to any of the questions 1–4		

Clayton et al. J Sex Med 2009;6:730–738

associated with chronic and intermittent desire disorders [31] that are strongly influenced by the individual's comfort with safety and intimacy in a relationship.

20.4.4 Hormonal Influences on HSDD

Hormonal abnormalities that can influence desire include hyperprolactinemia, thyroid dysfunction, and androgen deficiency caused by panhypopituitarism, oophorectomy, or adrenalectomy. Following bilateral oophorectomy, testosterone levels decrease by approximately 50 %, and many women report impaired sexual functioning [32]. The age-related decline in androgens parallels a midlife increase in HSDD, and naturally postmenopausal women have higher rates of low desire in comparison to premenopausal women [33, 34]. Overall, testosterone levels are variably associated with distressing low desire [35]. Several studies of postmenopausal women reported a positive correlation between free testosterone levels and self-reported desire [36, 37]. However, in two other population studies, testosterone levels were not correlated with sexual function, and no single testosterone level was predictive of sexual function [38, 39]. In a recent cross-sectional study of 560 pre- and postmenopausal women, free testosterone and androstenedione, measured by mass spectrometry, significantly correlated with sexual desire; but no correlations were observed between the primary androgen metabolite androsterone glucuronide (ADT-G) and sexual desire [40].

Testosterone's variable association with desire disorders may be based in part on genetic differences in the responsiveness of androgen receptors to testosterone [41]. Also, assays for testosterone levels have not been designed to assess the lower levels found in women and measure testosterone produced in target cells [42].

Decreasing estrogen levels in postmenopausal women result in vulvovaginal mucosal changes, decreased lubrication, dyspareunia, and impaired arousal and may secondarily affect desire [43]. Oral hormonal contraceptives and oral menopausal hormone therapy decrease testosterone production and increases sex hormone-binding globulin (SHBG), thereby decreasing free testosterone and sometimes sexual interest [44]. Increases in SHBG due to hormonal contraception may persist for years, even after termination of oral contraceptive (OC) use [45]. The effect of OCs on sexual functioning is varied. In some studies, the use of OCs is associated with sexual problems including decreased interest in sexual activity and sexual arousal [46]. OC use has also been associated with vestibulodynia or vulvar vestibulitis and inflammation of the vulvar vestibule, as well as an increase in sexual pain [47, 48]. A recent study demonstrated that women who developed vulvar vestibulitis on combined hormonal contraceptives were more likely to have longer CAG repeat lengths in the androgen receptor (AR) gene on the X chromosome than women who did not develop vestibulodynia on the same OCs; the authors postulated that this difference in the impact of OC use on the occurrence of vestibular inflammation is due to decreased free testosterone combined with an "inefficient AR that predisposes women to vestibular pain" [49]. Overall, results regarding the effects of OCs on sexual functioning are mixed, with studies showing increased, decreased, and no change in sexual desire [50, 51]. OC use may improve sexual function by diminishing fear of pregnancy, improving personal appearance (e.g., acne), and decreasing menstrual irregularity and dysmenorrhea. However, in patients in whom OC use may be contributing to decreased interest, arousal, and vestibular pain, alternative forms of contraception (e.g., IUD) should be discussed.

20.5 Diagnosis of HSDD

The diagnosis of generalized HSDD requires establishing a history of few or absent sexual fantasies and/or spontaneous or responsive desire for sexual activity that is associated with personal distress and/or interpersonal difficulties and not limited to a specific situation or relationship and not better explained by a medical or nonsexual psychiatric disorder or the use of medications or substances. Distressing low desire may be characterized by low initiation and frequency or the lack of receptivity to sexual activity. The diagnosis of *acquired HSDD* requires establishing that the low desire was preceded by a period of normal sexual desire.

20.5.1 Decreased Sexual Desire Screener

Clinicians commonly face an array of barriers when engaging in sexual history taking and the clinical evaluation of sexual problems. Such barriers include discomfort with the topic, time constraints, lack of knowledge about evaluating and managing HSDD and other sexual problems, perceived lack of treatment options, and lack of training in communication skills. Self-administered questionnaires can assist in overcoming some of these roadblocks to effective sexual medicine care.

The Decreased Sexual Desire Screener (DSDS) is a validated, self-report questionnaire that can assist clinicians in making an accurate diagnosis of generalized, acquired HSDD [52] (Fig. 20.1). The first four yes/no questions establish the presence of an acquired decrease in sexual desire that is distressing and that the patient wishes to increase. The fifth question presents an array of causes or exacerbating factors related to lessened desire. Patients who endorse all four need a clinical assessment to confirm their responses and determine the extent to which any of the items reported in question 5 are contributing to decreased desire.

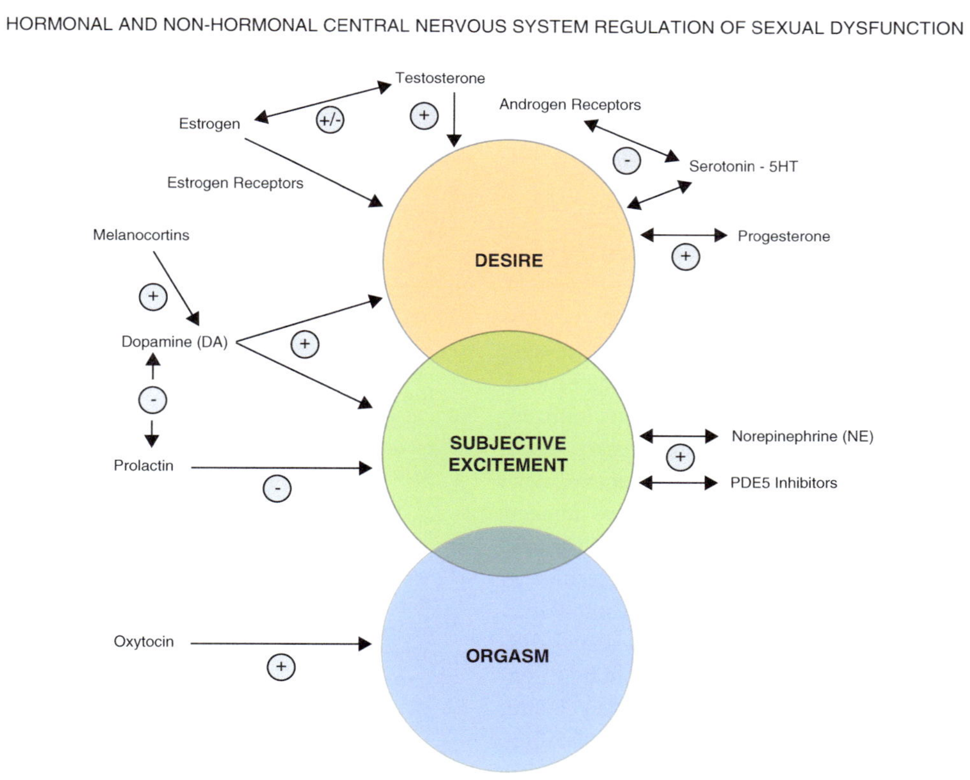

Fig. 20.1 Hormonal and nonhormonal central nervous system regulation of sexual function. Modified from Clayton, AH. Sexual function and dysfunction in women. Psychiatric Clinics of North America 2003;26:673–682. [53]

20.5.2 Other Questionnaires

While the DSDS is based on the diagnostic criteria for HSDD, other screening tools for female sexual dysfunction have been developed that are more dimensional and less specific to HSDD. The female sexual function index (FSFI)© is a 19-item, brief, multidimensional self-report instrument that assesses key dimensions of sexual function in women, including desire, subjective arousal, lubrication, orgasm, satisfaction, and pain. It has been validated in several patient samples, reliably discriminates between sexually disordered and healthy women, and is appropriate for clinical use [54]. The questionnaire, scoring appendix, and computation table for the domain sub-scores and the total score are available at www.fsfiquestionnaire.com. The maximum score is 36, with a cutoff of <26.5 indicating sexual dysfunction. The Female Sexual Distress Scale (FSDS)© and the revised version (FSDS-R)© are validated questionnaires that contain 12 and 13 items which assess distress about sexual problems; the FSDS-R has an additional question about the impact of low desire [55].

20.6 Conclusion

Distressing low sexual desire in women is a common complaint, affecting 7–12 % of women. While low desire increases with age, distress decreases; therefore, the prevalence of distressing low desire is relatively similar across age groups. Young, surgically menopausal (oophorectomized) women are more likely to be distressed about diminished desire than naturally menopausal women. HSDD has significant negative impacts on relationship satisfaction, quality of life, and overall happiness. HSDD should be classified as lifelong or acquired and generalized or situational, and it should be distinguished from sexual dysfunctions which can be better explained by a general medical condition, a nonsexual psychiatric disorder, or the use of a substance or medication. HSDD is described dynamically as an imbalance in the relationship of sexual excitatory and inhibitory processes which are independent of one another and determine sexual response. Inhibitory factors include life situation and relationship factors, personal sexual beliefs and related behaviors, and biological factors, including comorbid medical and mental disorders, medications, and substance use. Given the patient and clinician barriers related to addressing sexual problems, self-report questionnaires can help to facilitate the interview, detection, and identification process.

References

1. Shifren JL, Monz BU, Russo PA, Segreti A, Johannes CB. Sexual problems and distress in United States women: prevalence and correlates. Obstet Gynecol. 2008;112(5):970–8.
2. Diagnostic and statistical manual for mental disorders. 4th ed. rev.: DSM-IV-R. Washington, DC: American Psychiatric Association; 2003.
3. Diagnostic and statistical manual of mental disorders. 5th ed. Arlington, VA: American Psychiatric Association; 2013.
4. Basson R, Leiblum S, Brotto L, et al. Definitions of women's sexual dysfunction reconsidered: advocating expansion and revision. J Psychosom Obstet Gynaecol. 2003;24(4):221–9.
5. World Health Organization: international statistical classification of diseases and related health problems. 10th Revision, Edition 2010 (4th ed. ICD-10). Geneva: WHO Press, World Health Association; 2011.
6. Master WH, Johnson VE. Human sexual response. Boston, MA: Little Brown, Co.; 1966.
7. Kaplan HS. Hypoactive sexual desire. J Sex Marital Ther. 1977;3(1):3–9.
8. Leif HI. Inhibited sexual desire. Med Aspects Hum Sex. 1977;7:94–5.
9. Basson R. Women's sexual function and dysfunction: current uncertainties, future directions. Int J Impot Res. 2008;20(5):466–78.
10. Giraldi A, Kristensen E, Sand M. Endorsement of models describing sexual response of men and women with a sexual partner: an online survey in a population sample of Danish adults ages 20–65 years. J Sex Med. 2015;12(1):116–28. doi:10.1111/jsm.12720. Epub 2014 Nov 3.
11. West SL, D'Aloisio AA, Agans RP, Kalsbeek WD, Borisov NN, Thorp JM. Prevalence of low sexual desire and hypoactive sexual desire disorder in a nationally representative sample of US women. Arch Intern Med. 2008;168(13):1441–9.
12. Hayes RD, Dennerstein L, Bennett CM, Koochaki PE, Leiblum SR, Graziottin A. Relationship between hypoactive sexual desire disorder and aging. Fertil Steril. 2007;87(1):107–12.
13. Derogatis LR, Rosen R, Leiblum S, Burnett A, Heiman J. The female sexual distress scale (FSDS):

initial validation of a standardized scale for assessment of sexually related personal distress in women. J Sex Marital Ther. 2002;28(4):317–30.

14. Maserejian NN, Shifren J, Parish SJ, Segraves RT, Huang L, Rosen RC. Sexual arousal and lubrication problems in women with clinically diagnosed hypoactive sexual desire disorder: preliminary findings from the hypoactive sexual desire disorder registry for women. J Sex Marital Ther. 2012;38(1):41–62.
15. Laumann EO, Paik A, Rosen RC. Sexual dysfunction in the United States: prevalence and predictors. JAMA. 1999;281(6):537–44.
16. Leiblum SR, Koochaki PE, Rodenberg CA, Barton IP, Rosen RC. Hypoactive sexual desire disorder in postmenopausal women: US results from the women's international study of health and sexuality (WISHeS). Menopause. 2006;13(1):46–56.
17. Rosen RC, Shifren JL, Monz BU, Odom DM, Russo PA, Johannes CB. Correlates of sexually related personal distress in women with low sexual desire. J Sex Med. 2009;6(6):1549–60.
18. Clayton AH, Maserejian NN, Connor MK, Huang L, Heiman JR, Rosen RC. Depression in premenopausal women with HSDD: baseline findings from the HSDD registry for women. Psychosom Med. 2012;74(3):305–11.
19. Clayton AH. Female sexual dysfunction related to depression and antidepressant medications. Curr Womens Health Rep. 2002;2(3):182–7.
20. Clayton AH, Balon R. The impact of mental illness and psychotropic medications on sexual functioning: the evidence and management. J Sex Med. 2009;6(5):1200–11.
21. Pfaus JG. Pathways of sexual desire. J Sex Med. 2009;6:1506–33.
22. Bancroft J, Graham CA, Janssen E, Sanders SA. The dual control model: current status and future directions. J Sex Res. 2009;46(2):121–42.
23. Pfaus JG. Pathways of sexual desire. J Sex Med. 2009;6(6):1506–33.
24. Jeong GW, Park K, Youn G, et al. Assessment of cerebrocortical regions associated with sexual arousal in premenopausal and menopausal women by using BOLD-based functional MRI. J Sex Med. 2005; 2(5):645–51.
25. Perelman MA. The sexual tipping point: a mind/body model for sexual medicine. J Sex Med. 2009;6: 629–32.
26. Dunn KM, Croft PR, Hackett GI. Satisfaction in the sex life of a general population sample. J Sex Marital Ther. 2000;26(2):141–51.
27. Fisher W, Rosen R, Eardley I, Sand M, Goldstein I. Sexual experience of female partners of men with erectile dysfunction: the female experience of men's attitudes to life events and sexuality (FEMALES) study. J Sex Med. 2005;2(5):675–84.
28. Litzinger S, Gordon KC. Exploring relationships among communication, sexual satisfaction, and marital satisfaction. J Sex Marital Ther. 2005;31(5): 409–24.
29. Witting K, Santtila P, Varjonen M, et al. Female sexual dysfunction, sexual distress, and compatibility with partner. J Sex Med. 2008;5(11):2587–99.
30. Metz ME, Epstein N. Assessing the role of relationship conflict in sexual dysfunction. J Sex Marital Ther. 2002;28(2):139–64.
31. Rellini AH, Ing AD, Meston CM. Implicit and explicit cognitive sexual processes in survivors of childhood sexual abuse. J Sex Med. 2011;8(11):3098–107. doi:10.1111/j.1743-6109.2011.02356.x. Epub 2011 Jun 16.
32. Shifren JL, Braunstein GD, Simon JA, Casson PR, Buster JE, Redmond GP, et al. Transdermal testosterone treatment in women with impaired sexual function after oopherectomy. N Engl J Med. 2000;343:682–8.
33. Davison SL, Bell R, Donath S, Montalto JG, Davis SR. Androgen levels in adult females: changes with age, menopause, and oophorectomy. J Clin Endocrinol Metab. 2005;90(7):3847–53.
34. Davis SR. Androgen use for low sexual desire in midlife women. Menopause. 2013;20(7):795–7.
35. Bancroft J. Sexual effects of androgens in women: some theoretical considerations. Fertil Steril. 2002;77 Suppl 4:S55–9.
36. Bachmann GA, Leiblum SR. Sexuality in sexagenarian women. Maturitas. 1991;13(1):43–50.
37. Santoro N, Torrens J, Crawford S, et al. Correlates of circulating androgens in mid-life women: the study of women's health across the nation. J Clin Endocrinol Metab. 2005;90(8):4836–45.
38. Davis SR, Davison SL, Donath S, Bell RJ. Circulating androgen levels and self-reported sexual function in women. JAMA. 2005;294(1):91–6.
39. Gerber JR, Johnson JV, Bunn JY, O'Brien SL. A longitudinal study of the effects of free testosterone and other psychosocial variables on sexual function during the natural traverse of menopause. Fertil Steril. 2005;83(3):643–8.
40. Wåhlin-Jacobsen S, Pedersen AT, Kristensen E, Laessøe NC, Lundqvist M, Cohen AS, et al. Is there a correlation between androgens and sexual desire in women? J Sex Med. 2015;12(2):358–73. doi:10.1111/jsm.12774. Epub 2014 Dec 5.
41. Dennerstein L, Hayes R. Confronting the challenges: epidemiological study of female sexual dysfunction and the menopause. J Sex Med. 2005;2 Suppl 3:118–32.
42. Wierman ME, Basson R, Davis SR, et al. Androgen therapy in women: an endocrine society clinical practice guideline. J Clin Endocrinol Metab. 2006; 91(10):3697–710.
43. Basson R. Sexual desire and arousal disorders in women. N Engl J Med. 2006;354:1497–506.
44. Graham CA, Bancroft J, Doll HA, Greco T, Tanner A. Does oral contraceptive-induced reduction in free testosterone adversely affect the sexuality or mood of women? Psychoneuroendocrinology. 2007;32(3):246–55.
45. Panzer C, Wise S, Fantini G, et al. Impact of oral contraceptives on sex hormone-binding globulin and androgen levels: a retrospective study in women with sexual dysfunction. J Sex Med. 2006;3(1):104–13.

46. Caruso S, Agnello C, Intelisano G, Farina M, Di ML, Cianci A. Sexual behavior of women taking low-dose oral contraceptive containing 15 microg ethinylestradiol/60 microg gestodene. Contraception. 2004;69(3):237–40.
47. Bohm-Starke N, Johannesson U, Hilliges M, Rylander E, Torebjork E. Decreased mechanical pain threshold in the vestibular mucosa of women using oral contraceptives: a contributing factor in vulvar vestibulitis? J Reprod Med. 2004;49(11):888–92.
48. Goldstein AT, Burrows L. Vulvodynia. J Sex Med. 2008;5(1):5–14; quiz 15. doi:10.1111/j.1743-6109.2007.00679.x.
49. Goldstein AT, Belkin ZR, Krapf JM, Song W, Khera M, Jutrzonka SL, Kim NN, Burrows LJ, Goldstein I. Polymorphisms of the androgen receptor gene and hormonal contraceptive induced provoked vestibulodynia. J Sex Med. 2014;11(11):2764–71. doi:10.1111/jsm.12668. Epub 2014 Sep 4.
50. Davis AR, Castano PM. Oral contraceptives and libido in women. Annu Rev Sex Res. 2004;15:297–320.
51. Stuckey BG. Female sexual function and dysfunction in the reproductive years: the influence of endogenous and exogenous sex hormones. J Sex Med. 2008;5(10):2282–90.
52. Clayton AH, Goldfischer ER, Goldstein I, Derogatis L, Lewis-D'Agostino DJ, Pyke R. Validation of the decreased sexual desire screener (DSDS): a brief diagnostic instrument for generalized acquired female hypoactive sexual desire disorder (HSDD). J Sex Med. 2009;6:730–8.
53. Clayton AH. Sexual function and dysfunction in women. Psychiatr Clin N Am. 2003;26:673–82.
54. Rosen R, Brown C, Heiman J, Leiblum S, Meston C, Shabsigh R, et al. The female sexual function index (FSFI): a multidimensional self-report instrument for the assessment of female sexual function. J Sex Marital Ther. 2000;26:191–208.
55. DeRogatis L, Clayton A, Lewis-D'Agostino D, Wunderlich G, Fu Y. Validation of the female sexual distress scale-revised for assessing distress in women with hypoactive sexual desire disorder. J Sex Med. 2008;5(2):357–64. Epub 2007 Nov 27.

Management of Hypoactive Sexual Desire Disorder (HSDD)

21

Jill M. Krapf, John E. Buster, and Andrew T. Goldstein

21.1 Introduction

Low sexual desire is the most common of the female sexual dysfunctions, with about 10 % of premenopausal women and up to 52 % of postmenopausal women reporting reduced sexual desire [1, 2]. When low desire leads to personal distress and is not related to a psychological disorder, medication, or medical condition, it meets the criteria for diagnosis of hypoactive sexual desire disorder (HSDD) (DSM-IV 2000) [3]. In the fifth edition of the *Diagnostic and Statistical Manual of Mental Disorders* (DSM), female sexual desire and arousal disorders were combined to form one disorder, sexual interest/arousal disorder (SIAD) (DSM-5) [4]. Female sexual interest/arousal disorder (FSIAD) is characterized by reduced interest in sexual activity, reduced fantasies or thoughts about sex, reduced initiation and/or non-receptivity to partner's attempts to initiate, reduced sexual pleasure, reduced response to erotic cues, and reduced genital or nongenital sensations during sexual encounters. The decision to combine HSDD and arousal disorder into one diagnosis raised concerns about the accuracy of the diagnosis and how this could affect treatment approaches for women with decreased sexual desire.

HSDD can be linked to situational circumstances, such as dysfunctional interpersonal relationships, or it can be caused by physiologic causes. Often these physiologic causes are iatrogenic, such as decreased androgen levels resulting from oral contraceptive pills or elevated serotonin levels caused by some antidepressants. In older women, HSDD is usually caused by a decline in androgen levels as a result of ovarian failure or following oophorectomy. A transdermal testosterone patch (Intrinsa®) is approved in Europe and Australia based on clinical trials demonstrating efficacy in treatment of HSDD. Unfortunately, as of March 2015 (when this chapter was written), there are no medications approved by the US Food and Drug Administration (FDA), for the treatment of HSDD or FSIAD. However, there are medications in clinical development for the treatment of HSDD/FSIAD. It is the hope of the authors that one or more of these medications will prove to be efficacious and safe for the treatment of HSDD. As such, one goal of this chapter will be to discuss medications currently being studied for HSDD and the biologic mechanism on which they are based.

J.M. Krapf, M.D.
Department of Obstetrics and Gynecology, George Washington University School of Medicine, Washington, DC, USA

J.E. Buster, M.D.
Division of Reproductive Endocrinology and Infertility, Women and Infants Hospital, Providence, RI, USA

A.T. Goldstein, M.D., FACOG, IF (✉)
The George Washington University School of Medicine, 3 Washington Circle NW, Suite 205, Washington, DC 20027, USA
e-mail: obstetrics@yahoo.com

L.I. Lipshultz et al. (eds.), *Management of Sexual Dysfunction in Men and Women*, DOI 10.1007/978-1-4939-3100-2_21

21.2 Physiologic Mechanisms of Sexual Desire

Sexual desire (libido) is modulated by the interactions of both sex steroids and neurotransmitters [5]. Although the exact central neuroendocrine mechanisms remain undiscovered, several areas of the brain including the hypothalamus and the amygdala appear important in sexual desire [6]. There are both excitatory and inhibitory factors that can influence sexual desire. Excitatory factors (neurotransmitters and hormones) include testosterone, melanocortin, oxytocin, dopamine, and norepinephrine [7]. Inhibitory factors include serotonin, prolactin, and endogenous opioids. It has been hypothesized that if the excitatory hormone and neurotransmitter levels are high, then sexual behavior is "tipped" in the direction of sexual desire and vice versa [5, 7]. This balance between excitation and inhibition is best described by Perelman's sexual tipping point model [7].

21.3 Psychosocial Considerations

Normal female sexual desire often requires a safe environment, self-esteem, and an attractive and available partner. Situational HSDD, such as that which occurs with a dysfunctional relationship, external stressors, or loss of a partner, is a common cause of low desire [8]. Situational HSDD from adverse life events, particularly in younger women, can be managed with reassurance or relationship counseling. Sometimes a new and attractive partner is all that is needed. It is important that this issue be acknowledged and placed in context while the life events right themselves. Depression and other major psychiatric conditions can be serious or even life threatening [9, 10]. These disorders need to be identified and managed by a skilled psychiatrist or sex therapist. In situations where sexual desire is a chronic, long-term problem, more intensive psychotherapy may be necessary.

21.4 Management of Contributing Factors

Although psychological conditions, certain medications, and general medical conditions may cause or contribute to low sexual desire, a diagnosis of HSDD does not technically apply in these cases based upon the DSM definition. A list of conditions and medications associated with decreased sexual desire is presented in Table 21.1. Treatment generally involves managing these inciting factors or discontinuing and replacing offending medications. Patients should be counseled on the sexual side effects with a new diagnosis or initiating therapy that affects sexual function.

Low desire may be seen in the context of major depression, as well as a result of medications commonly used to treat depression. Antidepressants, particularly selective serotonin reuptake inhibitors (SSRIs), are associated with decreased sexual desire in a dose-dependent fashion [10]. It may be necessary to adjust dosage levels or replace the medication to decrease sexual side effects. Mirtazapine and bupropion have

Table 21.1 Common contributing factors to low sexual desire

Psychological
Depression
Medications
Antidepressants (selective serotonin reuptake inhibitors)
Oral contraceptives
Oral estrogens
Glucocorticoids
Chemotherapy
Aromatase inhibitors
General medical conditions
Diabetes
Hypertension
Obesity
Hypopituitarism
Breast cancer
Premature ovarian failure

the lowest rates of associated sexual dysfunction. Mirtazapine, the first noradrenergic and specific serotonergic antidepressant, has fewer sexual side effects than sertraline [11, 12]. Bupropion, a noradrenaline and dopamine reuptake inhibitor, has a low risk of sexual dysfunction, likely related to its limited effect on serotonergic neurotransmission [13, 14].

Oral contraceptives inhibit the mid-cycle surge of testosterone and can be a cause of HSDD in younger women [15]. Some progestins in oral contraceptives also potentiate depression and mood disorders, contributing to decreased sexual desire [16]. Discontinuing combined oral contraceptives and replacing with a long-acting reversible contraceptive option may be warranted. Premature ovarian failure may also be a cause of low sexual desire in younger women [17]. Pelvic floor surgery with musculoskeletal dysfunctions may impair sexual desire through fear of pain or perception of physical deformity. Endometriosis and pelvic adhesions can lead to severe dyspareunia and decreased sexual desire, resulting in an aversion to sex.

In postmenopausal women, oral estrogens commonly used in hormone replacement therapy increase SHBG and bind circulating testosterone, impairing testosterone action and decreasing its effects. Loss of testosterone effect can be a complicating factor in women with HSDD taking oral estrogens. Transdermal estrogens, in contrast, do not affect SHBG in the same manner [16]. Atrophic vaginitis commonly leads to dyspareunia, sexual aversion, and loss of sexual desire.

Decreased sexual desire can result from inadequate treatment or poor control of chronic diseases such as diabetes, hypertension, obesity, hypopituitarism, or breast cancer. Women afflicted with panhypopituitarism and adrenal insufficiency frequently suffer from HSDD [18]. Glucocorticoids suppress adrenal androgen production and may therefore be associated with low desire. Because they induce atrophy of the zona reticularis of the adrenal gland, the androgen suppression can be permanent in women who have been on long-term therapy [19].

Treatment of gynecologic cancer may also result in decreased desire. Pelvic radiation may induce premature ovarian failure, leading to decreased androgens. In treatment of breast cancer, chemotherapy and administration of antiestrogens, such as tamoxifen and aromatase inhibitors, may cause decreased sexual desire [20].

21.5 Role of Androgens in HSDD

In women, approximately half of testosterone is derived from the ovaries and adrenal glands, with the remaining half arising from precursors such as androstenedione and dehydroepiandrosterone (DHEA) through peripheral conversion. About 99 % of circulating testosterone is bound to sex hormone-binding globulin (SHBG). During the reproductive years, testosterone secretion originates from the theca cells of the dominant ovarian follicle. A mid-cycle rise in testosterone occurs in conjunction with the luteinizing hormone (LH) surge and is directly linked to increased mid-cycle sexual desire, which occurs during the reproductive years but is lost after menopause [21, 22]. As women age, there is a slow and progressive decline in serum testosterone due to decreased ovarian and adrenal function [23]. The levels of prohormones such as DHEA-S and DHEA also fall with increasing age [24]. In addition, SHBG increases after menopause, especially in women treated with oral estrogen therapy, leading to decreased free testosterone [25, 26]. Unlike natural menopause, bilateral oophorectomy is associated with a 40–50 % decrease in serum testosterone levels [23].

21.6 Testosterone Therapy for HSDD

There is abundant research demonstrating that testosterone increases sexual desire and well-being in postmenopausal women with HSDD. Based upon this evidence, the transdermal testosterone patch is approved for treatment of women with HSDD in Europe and Australia. However, in the United States, the FDA has yet to approve a testosterone product for treating HSDD in women. There are many androgen and testosterone products under investigation, compounded preparations, and FDA-approved medications for men, which are commonly prescribed off label for women. Many of these alternative testosterone products are currently in phase 1 and 2 clinical trials.

21.6.1 Oral Testosterone

Methyltestosterone is available in doses of 1.25 or 2.5 mg per day and is usually prescribed in combination with conjugated estrogens (0.625 mg/day or 1.25 mg/day) as Estratest® (Solvay). The use of methyltestosterone is also associated with significant decreases in high-density lipoprotein (HDL) cholesterol and increased total cholesterol/HDL ratio, but a significant decrease in triglycerides. There are limited data but some high-quality, prospective, randomized clinical trial data exist on this treatment approach [27].

Micronized testosterone is available in custom formulations from compounding pharmacies, with oral or sublingual administration, and has been prescribed empirically. Micronized testosterone is generally not well absorbed orally. A buccal formulation (Striant) is FDA approved for use in men. In addition, custom-compounded sublingual and buccal formulations are available, but they have not been evaluated in clinical trials [28].

DHEA is a prohormone (converted to testosterone in vivo) available as an over-the-counter supplement in 25 or 50 mg tablets. Of the nine published randomized trials of oral DHEA for low sexual function in postmenopausal women, three showed a positive effect and the others failed to show a benefit. Although vaginally administered DHEA may improve vaginal atrophy with possible benefit in sexual function, oral DHEA does not have demonstrated efficacy in the treatment of HSDD [29].

21.6.2 Testosterone Matrix Patches

Transdermal testosterone delivered by matrix patch (Intrinsa®, Procter and Gamble) has been the most extensively studied formulation in women with HSDD. There are now seven randomized blinded, clinical trials involving the testosterone matrix patch involving nearly 3000 postmenopausal women with HSDD [30–36]. In the first four trials, the subjects were all women who had undergone oophorectomy [30–33]. Doses of 150 ug/day, 300 ug/day, or 450 ug/day were studied. These dose ranges approximated the lower and upper limits of endogenous testosterone production in premenopausal women.

All trials demonstrated dose-related, significant increases in sexual desire with testosterone patches versus placebo when the dose was maintained at 300 ug/day or greater. At 300 ug/day, the first five trials all demonstrated consistent increases in sexual desire and decreases in distress related to lack of sexual interest with few adverse effects. Interestingly, no treatment effect was seen with the 150 or the 450 ug/day dose, raising the possibility of a dose-response curve for testosterone. Side effects in these first five 24-week trials were minimal and included minor and reversible patch site irritation and hirsutism. A 300 ug/day testosterone matrix patch for women (Intrinsa®) was approved by the European Medicines Agency, the European Union's equivalent of the US Food and Drug Administration, in 2006. Matrix patches for women, however, are still not available in the United States [37], and it was withdrawn from the European market because of poor sales.

Several alternatives for transdermal testosterone delivery are used off label for women with HSDD. Androderm® and Testoderm® are testosterone matrix patches FDA approved for use in men. These patches deliver supraphysiologic doses in women, which can lead to unwanted androgenic side effects. Some clinicians prescribe these products off label for women by cutting them down to size 1/5th to 1/10th doses. There is extensive information available on this product in men but not women [38].

21.6.3 Transdermal Testosterone Preparations

AndroGel® and Testim® are testosterone transdermal gels that are FDA approved in the United States for use in men. They are sometimes used off label in women by reducing the amount applied to about 1/5th to 1/10th doses. However, testosterone delivery is imprecise, and blood testosterone levels are needed to dose these preparations safely. There is extensive information available on this product in men but not women [39].

Testosterone in pluronic lecithin organogel (PLO) gel for transdermal administration may be compounded to treat women with HSDD. PLO gel testosterone is available in 10 cc syringes or small pumps, both of which deliver consistent dosing. One widely used regimen is testosterone in PLO gel, 32 mg/cc dosed at 1 cc given in the evening. The gel can be applied to the wrists, lower abdomen, thighs, or backs of the knees. These custom preparations require the monitoring of blood testosterone levels to be administered safely. Patients should be monitored clinically and with testosterone levels to document therapeutic delivery and to avoid supraphysiologic dosing. Even though compounded testosterone creams are among the most widely used androgen treatments of HSDD in women, there is only anecdotal information on this practice.

21.6.4 Testosterone Implants and Injectable Formulations

Custom-compounded testosterone pellets are also available for off-label use in women with HSDD. Testosterone implants of 25–100 mg can be purchased from compounding pharmacies. They are inserted subcutaneously with a trocar though a small incision using local anesthesia. The most common dose is 50 mg and the implants remain effective for 4–6 months. Implantation should be guided by monitoring testosterone levels [40].

Intramuscular testosterone injection products are approved for use in men. Testosterone can be injected in a slow-release form as a testosterone ester (cypionate, propionate, and enanthate). Doses are 25–50 mg every 2–4 weeks. In both open and blinded clinical trials, this agent is highly effective for treatment of HSDD, but this treatment requires frequent dosing and testosterone levels are not consistent [41, 42].

21.6.5 Intravaginal Dehydroepiandrosterone

Although oral preparations of dehydroepiandrosterone (DHEA) have not shown consistent benefit, intravaginal administration of DHEA positively affects vulvovaginal atrophy (VVA) as well as HSDD [43, 44]. In a multicenter randomized double-blind placebo-controlled trial of 218 postmenopausal women with VVA, intravaginal DHEA (prasterone) cream inserted nightly for 12 weeks increased sexual desire, arousal, organism, and dyspareunia in a time- and dose-dependent fashion [44]. Daily administration of intravaginal DHEA also significantly improved vaginal atrophy at 2 weeks, with minimal changes in serum estradiol or testosterone levels [45].

21.6.6 Intranasal Testosterone (TBS-2)

A low-dose nasal testosterone gel, TBS-2, has been investigated in women with female orgasmic disorder (FOD), as well as HSDD. In a randomized, parallel group study of 16 women with HSDD, women received five doses of TBS-2 or a testosterone patch for three consecutive days. Women receiving intranasal TBS-2 showed a significant increase in sexual arousal and sensuality as assessed by validated subjective arousal questionnaires compared to women who received the testosterone patch at both 30 min and 4.5 h after administration [46]. Although this medication has been primarily studied in FOD, it also holds promise in treatment of HSDD.

21.6.7 Testosterone with Phosphodiesterase Type 5 Inhibitor (T+PDE5i) and Testosterone with 5-Hydroxytryptamine$_{1A}$ Receptor Agonist (T+5-HT$_{1A}$ra)

Single doses of 0.5 mg sublingual testosterone have been shown to increase the sensitivity of the brain to sexual cues. However, in many women, particularly those with HSDD, the effects of testosterone alone may not be sufficient for achieving necessary levels of arousal and desire for sexual activity. While proposed etiologies of HSDD are widely varied, two prominent understandings of HSDD have emerged. The first describes HSDD as the result of an insensitive brain system for sexual cues, and the second assigns responsibility to overactive sexual inhibitory mechanisms [47, 48]. Thus, due to the divergent nature of these etiologies, two therapies are under development.

In a 2012 study conducted by Emotional Brain LLC in the Netherlands, women diagnosed with HSDD were divided into categories of high or low sensitivity to sexual stimuli by testing their preconscious attentional bias for sexual cues using a masked version of an emotional Stroop test. Participants were instructed to name the color of the masked words as quickly as possible and the length of time to vocal response was recorded. Thirty-two unambiguous neutral words from one category (furniture; examples are "chair" and "table") and 32 unambiguous erotic words (examples are "penis," "coitus," and "vagina") were presented to the participants. The differences between the mean reaction times of the erotic and the neutral words were used to categorize participants as having either "high sensitivity to sexual cues" (reaction time to neutral words<erotic words) and "low sensitivity to sexual cues" (reaction time to neutral words>erotic words) [48].

For women with low sensitivity, efforts were aimed at increasing sensitivity to sexual cues. Sexual stimulation causes the release of nitric oxide (NO) from nerves and endothelium, resulting in an increase in cyclic guanosine monophosphate (cGMP). The rise in cGMP is key in the relaxation of smooth muscle for the engorgement of erectile tissue. Phosphodiesterases (PDE5s) hydrolyze cGMP, and consequently PDE5 inhibitors (PDE5i's) prolong the action of vasodilation. In order for PDE5i's to act on vasodilation, central stimulation must be present. Thus, testosterone, which increases the brain's response to sexual cues, combined with PDE5i, aimed to enhance genital sexual response, was coupled in a coinciding time-delay manner and tested in a double-blind, placebo-controlled crossover study with 56 women with HSDD [48].

Women were treated with testosterone 0.5 mg and PDE5i (sildenafil 50 mg) (T+PDE5i) 4 h prior to sexual activity. Participants were permitted to use the medication up to 14 times during a 4-week period with a minimum of 48 h between doses. Women taking the T+PDE5i for 4 weeks had an improved physiological and subjective sexual response as measured by institutional psychophysiological lab standards and by at-home evaluations as compared with women taking placebo. More specifically, participants on T+PDE5i showed increased preconscious attention for sexual cues as well as statistically significant increases in subjective sexual function, such as genital arousal and desire. Additionally, participants who were found to have low sensitivity to sexual cues demonstrated much greater benefit from T+PDE5i therapy than women assessed as having high sensitivity to sexual clues who did not have an increase in intensity or satisfaction of sexual events [48, 49].

In addition to being assigned to treatments of T+PDE5i and placebo for 4 weeks each, women in the trial were given 4 weeks of testosterone with 5-hydroxytryptamine$_{1A}$ receptor agonist (T+5-HT$_{1A}$ra). The T+5-HT$_{1A}$ra treatment was aimed at addressing overactive sexual inhibition processes. Serotonin or 5-hydroxytryptamine (5HT$_{1A}$) is neurotransmitter important for mediating inhibitory mechanisms localized to the prefrontal cortex (PFC). As the PFC is an important regulator of inhibition and as 5HT$_{1A}$ is a critical neurotransmitter in the PFC, it was hypothesized that acute treatment with a 5HT$_{1A}$ receptor agonist (5HT$_{1A}$ra) could limit the effects of 5HT$_{1A}$, thereby decreasing inhibition of sexual response. After acute administration, 5HT$_{1A}$ra binds to somatodendritic autoreceptors of the raphe nuclei in the midbrain. The hyperpolarizing effect of activated 5-HT1A autoreceptors decreases both serotonergic firing activity and inhibition of serotonin release from the presynaptic terminal thereby reducing serotonin levels in the PFC. In a similar fashion to the T+PDE5i treatment, T+5-HT$_1$Ara was designed to act maximally 3–6 h after administration [50].

In participants considered to have high inhibition, taking T+5-HT_{1A}ra showed statistically significant increases in sexual satisfaction, desire, genital arousal and sexual function, and vaginal pulse amplitude (VPA) as compared with placebo. In contrast, the low-inhibition group did not show statistically significant changes in these areas. Furthermore, the low-inhibition group showed much greater improvement on these measures with treatment of T+PDE5i [50]. Therefore, as hypothesized, the low-sensitivity group responded best to T+PDE5i, while the high-sensitivity group showed the greatest improvements with the T+5-HT_{1A}ra. Pharmacokinetic studies of the combined T (0.5 mg)+PDE5i showed that maximum concentration of serum total testosterone (mean C_{max} 7.84 ± 3.69 ng/mL) was reached in 0.201 ± 0.043 h (time to maximum concentration, T_{max}) and the half-life of testosterone ($T_{1/2}$) was 0.598 ± 0.08 h. Given the relatively low T_{max} and short $T_{1/2}$, it is unlikely that these levels will produce any androgen-related side effects [51].

21.6.8 Safety of Testosterone Therapy

Consensus reports from the Endocrine Society and the North American Menopause Society have been cautionary regarding testosterone therapy in women [52, 53]. There are 60 years of publications and FDA transcripts examining the safety of testosterone administered to women [54–60]. FDA safety concerns focus mainly on cardiovascular and breast cancer risk in lieu of the Heart Estrogen Replacement Study and the Women's Health Initiative Study. None of the studies report serious adverse effects due to transdermal or implanted testosterone in physiologic doses, even with doses that produce moderately supraphysiologic levels of testosterone [54, 60]. Hirsutism and acne are the major adverse reactions, which are dose related and generally reversible with discontinuation of medication. Not only does the literature not support an increased breast cancer risk with testosterone therapy, data may even indicate a beneficial role of testosterone in breast protection. Safety data from controlled studies spanning up to 2 years, as well as observational data from women receiving testosterone with postmenopausal hormone therapy regimens and testosterone-treated female-to-male transsexuals, provide much reassurance.

21.7 Non-testosterone Drugs in Development

21.7.1 Flibanserin

Flibanserin is a nonhormonal therapy that acts on the brain to increase sexual desire. While the exact mechanism of action is not clearly understood, flibanserin is a 5-HT1A agonist and 5-HT2A antagonist. In addition, flibanserin binds with moderate affinity to 5-HT2B, 5-HT2C, and dopamine D4 receptors [61]. This mixed interaction of flibanserin with serotonin and dopamine receptors is thought to inhibit sexually inhibitory serotonergic effects, while promoting dopaminergic effects that are associated with an excitatory impact on sexual function. In addition, serotonin exerts an inhibitory influence over adrenergic tone, and decreased serotonin levels can elevate norepinephrine, which is also known to stimulate sexual function and excitement. It has been suggested that the combined mechanisms of action of flibanserin normalize CNS neurotransmitter levels, enhancing sexual desire.

Flibanserin has been studied in three large phase 3 randomized, placebo-controlled trials [62–64] in which 3548 HSDD patients were treated—2310 with flibanserin and 1238 with placebo. Efficacy endpoints included the number of satisfying sexual events (SSEs) measured by daily electronic diary entries and scores on the desire domain of the female sexual function index (FSFI). In addition, the trials used a revised version of the FSDS (FSDS-R) that included an additional question (Item 13) to specifically assess distress due to low sexual desire. After 24 weeks of treatment with flibanserin administered in a single daily dose at bedtime of 100 mg, statistically and clinically significant improvement relative to placebo was seen in the number of

SSEs, level of sexual desire measured by the FSFI desire domain, and reduction of distress related to low sexual desire measured by FSDS-R item 13. The rate of serious adverse events (SAEs) in the flibanserin groups was ≤0.9 % and no SAE was considered related to treatment. The most common adverse events (AEs) reported by patients were dizziness, nausea, fatigue, and somnolence with frequencies of 9–12 % in the women taking flibanserin [62–64].

21.7.2 Bremelanotide

Bremelanotide (BMT) is a cyclic melanocortin peptide that acts as a melanocortin receptor 4 (MCR4) agonist. Though it was originally designed for sunless tanning, the synthetic analog of melanocyte-stimulating hormone (MSH), which activates the melanocortin receptors MC3R and MCR4 in the central nervous system, was found to increase sexual arousal and desire. During phase 2 trials, BMT administered intranasally showed promising results for the treatment of HSDD and FSIAD; however, reports of elevated blood pressures halted the trial [65].

In a phase 2B trial, BMT was reformulated as a lower dose, subcutaneous injection to measure efficacy for HSDD and/or FSAD treatment in premenopausal women. In a 4-week at-home trial, 1.75 mg BMT showed statistically significant improvements as compared with placebo in five measures of FSD: number of satisfying sexual events per month, total and sexual domain scores on the FSFI, and total and desire domain scores on the FSDS. BMT was associated with minimal and transient increases in blood pressure (~3 mmHg) that were limited to the first four hours after administration. Protocol-defined blood pressure withdrawal criteria were not met at higher frequency in BMT-treated subjects than in those taking placebo. Further studies on BMT dosing have suggested optimal increases in arousal, desire, and satisfaction with sexual events with 1.25 and 1.75 mg subcutaneous injections. At these doses, adverse events included nausea (22 % and 24 %, respectively), placebo 3 %; flushing (14 % and 17 %, respectively), placebo 0 %; and headache (9 % and 14 %, respectively), placebo 3 % [18, 19]. MC3R and MCR4 receptors are involved in many physiological systems and there may be theoretical risks of activating these receptors [65]. The long-term effects of BMT are unknown.

21.7.3 Bupropion with Trazodone

Although certain antidepressants may contribute to HSDD, restoring the balance of dopamine, serotonin, and norepinephrine may play a role in regulation sexual inhibition and exhibition. S1 Biopharma is investigating the combination of bupropion and trazodone for treatment of HSDD in phase 2a clinical trials, although no data is currently available.

21.8 Conclusion

Low sexual desire in women has many causes and contributing factors. Treatment should focus on identifying and addressing these conditions. While HSDD may be related to situational factors in young women, medications such as oral contraceptives and antidepressants are also common causes. HSDD in postmenopausal women is likely due to androgen deficiency. Testosterone therapy is the mainstay of treatment for these women, but most preparations are investigational or given off label, despite a reassuring safety and efficacy profile. There are a number of drugs currently in phase 2 and 3 clinical trials that show promise in treatment of HSDD. Continued research and long-term safety data are likely necessary to obtain FDA approval of a medication for the treatment of HSDD.

References

1. Rosen RC, Shifren JL, Monz BU, Odom DM, Russo PA, Johannes CB. Correlates of sexually related personal distress in women with low sexual desire. J Sex Med. 2009;6:1549–60.
2. West S, D'Aloisio A, Agans R, Kalsbeck W, Borisov N, Thorp JM. Prevalence of low sexual desire and

hypoactive sexual desire disorder in a nationally representative sample of US women. Arch Intern Med. 2008;168:1441–9.
3. American Psychiatric Association. Diagnostic and statistical manual of mental disorders. 4th ed, text revision. Washington, DC: American Psychiatric Press; 2000.
4. American Psychiatric Association. Diagnostic and statistical manual of mental disorders. 5th ed, text revision. Washington, DC: American Psychiatric Press; 2013.
5. Simons J, Carey M. Prevalence of sexual dysfunctions. Arch Sex Behav. 2001;30(2):177–219.
6. Kingsberg S, Rezaee R. Hypoactive sexual desire in women [review]. Menopause. 2013;20(12):1284–300.
7. Perelman M. The sexual tipping point: a mind/model for sexual medicine. J Sex Med. 2009;6:629–32.
8. Graziottin A. Iatrogenic and post-traumatic female sexual disorder. Standard practice in sexual medicine. Oxford: Blackwell; 2006.
9. Zemishlany Z, Weizman A. The impact of mental illness on sexual dysfunction. Adv Psychosom Med. 2008;29:89–106.
10. Kennedy SH, Rizvi S. Sexual dysfunction, depression and the impact of antidepressants. J Clin Psychopharmacol. 2009;29:157–64.
11. Behnke K, Søgaard J, Martin S, Bäuml J, Ravindran AV, Ågren H, Vester-Blokland ED. Mirtazapine orally disintegrating tablet versus sertraline: a prospective onset of action study. J Clin Psychopharmacol. 2003; 23:358–64.
12. Saiz-Ruiz J, et al. Assessment of sexual functioning in depressed patients treated with mirtazapine: a naturalistic 6-month study. Hum Psychopharmacol Clin Exp. 2005;20(6):435–40.
13. Coleman CC, et al. A placebo-controlled comparison of the effects on sexual functioning of bupropion sustained release and fluoxetine. Clin Ther. 2001;23(7): 1040–58.
14. Serretti A, Chiesa A. Treatment-emergent sexual dysfunction related to antidepressants: a meta-analysis. J Clin Psychopharmacol. 2009;29(3):259–66.
15. Davis AR, Castaño PM. Oral contraceptives and libido in women. Annu Rev Sex Res. 2004;15:297–320.
16. Serin IS, Ozcelik B, Basbuğ M, Aygen E, Kula M, Erez R. Long-term effects of continuous oral and transdermal estrogen replacement therapy on sex hormone binding globulin and free testosterone levels. Eur J Obstet Gynecol Reprod Biol. 2001;99(2):222–5.
17. van der Stege JG, et al. Decreased androgen concentrations and diminished general and sexual well-being in women with premature ovarian failure. Menopause. 2008;15(1):23–31.
18. Basson R. Female sexual dysfunction in hypopituitarism. Lancet. 2007;370(9589):737. author reply 737–8.
19. Abraham GE. Ovarian and adrenal contribution to peripheral androgens during the menstrual cycle. J Clin Endocrinol Metab. 1974;39(2):340–6.
20. Krychman ML, Katz A. Breast cancer and sexuality: multi-modal treatment options. J Sex Med. 2012; 9(1):5–13.
21. Guay A, Munarriz R, Jacobson J, et al. Serum androgen levels in healthy premenopausal women with and without sexual dysfunction: Part A. Serum androgen levels in women aged 20–49 years with no complaints of sexual dysfunction. Int J Impot Res. 2004;16:112–20.
22. Haselton MG, Mortezaie M, Pillsworth EG, Bleske-Reschek A, Fredrick DA. Ovulatory shifts in human female ornamentation: near ovulation, women dress to impress. Horm Behav. 2007;51(1):40–5.
23. Davidson SL, Bell R, Donath S, Montalto JG, Davis SR. Androgen levels in adult females: changes with age, menopause, and oophorectomy. J Clin Endocrinol Metab. 2005;90:3847–53.
24. Labrie F, Belanger A, Cusan L, et al. Marked decline in serum concentrations of adrenal C19 sex steroid precursors and conjugated androgen metabolites during aging. J Clin Endocrinol Metab. 1997;82: 2396–402.
25. Burger HG, Dudley EC, Cui J, et al. A prospective longitudinal study of serum testosterone, dehydroepiandrosterone sulfate, and sex hormone-binding globulin levels through the menopausal transition. J Clin Endocrinol Metab. 2000;85:2832–8.
26. McTiernan A, Wu L, Barnabei VM, WHI Investigators, et al. Relation of demographic factors, menstrual history, reproduction and medication use to sex hormone levels in postmenopausal women. Breast Cancer Res Treat. 2008;108:217–31.
27. Lobo RA, Rosen RC, Yang HM, Block B, Van Der Hoop RG. Comparative effects of oral esterified estrogens with and without methyltestosterone on endocrine profiles and dimensions of sexual function in postmenopausal women with hypoactive sexual desire. Fertil Steril 2003;79(6):1341–52. (Level I).
28. Slater CC, Souter I, Zhang C, Guan C, Stanczyk FZ, Mishell DR. Pharmacokinetics of testosterone after percutaneous gel or buccal administration. Fertil Steril. 2001;76(1):32–7.
29. Panjari M, Davis SR. DHEA for postmenopausal women: a review of evidence. Maturitas. 2010;66(2): 172–9.
30. Shifren JL, Braunstein GD, Simon JA, et al. Transdermal testosterone treatment in women with impaired sexual function after oophorectomy. N Engl J Med. 2000;343:682–8.
31. Buster JE, Kingsberg SA, Aguirre O, et al. Testosterone patch for low sexual desire in surgically menopausal women: a randomized trial. Obstet Gynecol. 2005;105(5Ptl):944–52. (Level 1).
32. Simon J, Braunstein G, Nachtigall L, et al. Testosterone patch increases sexual activity and desire in surgically menopausal women with hypoactive sexual desire disorder. J Clin Endocrinol Metab. 2005;90(9):5226–33. (Level 1).
33. Braunstein GD, Sundwall DA, Katz M, et al. Safety and efficacy of a testosterone patch for the treatment of hypoactive sexual desire disorder in surgically menopausal women: a randomized, placebo-controlled trial. Arch Intern Med. 2005;165(14): 1571–2. (Level 1).

34. Davis SR, van der Mooren MJ, van Lunsen RH, et al. Efficacy and safety of a testosterone patch for the treatment of hypoactive sexual desire disorder in surgically menopausal women: a randomized, placebo-controlled trial. Menopause. 2006;(3):387–96. (Level 1).
35. Shifren JL, Davis SR, Moreau M, et al. Testosterone patch for the treatment of hypoactive sexual desire disorder in naturally menopausal women: results from the INTIMATE NM1 Study. Menopause. 2006;13(5):770–9. (Level 1).
36. Davis SR, Moreau M, Kroll R, et al. Testosterone for low libido in postmenopausal women not taking estrogen. N Engl J Med. 2008;359(19):2005–17. (Level 1).
37. Seibel M. Men, women and testosterone: why did the FDA fail Intrinsa? Sex Reprod Menopause. 2005;1:1–2.
38. Kronawitter D, Gooren L, Zoliver H, Oppelt P, Beckmann M, Dittrich R. Effects of transdermal testosterone or oral dydrogesterone on hypoactive sexual desire disorder in transsexual women: results of a pilot study. Eur J Endocrinol. 2009;161:363–8. [Epub ahead of print] (Level 2).
39. Nathorst-Böös J, Flöter A, Jarkander-Rolff M, Carlström K, Schoultz B. Treatment with percutaneous testosterone gel in postmenopausal women with decreased libido-effects on sexuality and psychological general well-being. Maturitas. 2006;53(1):11–8. [Epub 2005 Sept 23]. (Level II-A).
40. Davis SR, McCloud P, Strauss BJ, Burger H. Testosterone enhances estradiol's effects on postmenopausal bone density and sexuality. Maturitas. 1995;21(3):227–36. (Level I).
41. Sherwin BB, Gelfand MM, Brender W. Androgen enhances sexual motivation in females: a prospective, crossover study of sex steroid administration in the surgical menopause. Psychosom Med. 1985;47(4):339–51. (Level I).
42. Sherwin BB, Gelfand MM. The role of androgen in the maintenance of sexual functioning in oophorectomized women. Psychosom Med. 1987;49(4):397–409. (Level I).
43. Panjari M, Davis SR. Vaginal DHEA to treat menopause related atrophy: a review of the evidence. Maturitas. 2011;70(1):22–5.
44. Labrie F, Archer D, Bouchard C, Fortier M, et al. Effect of intravaginal dehydroepiandrosterone (prasterone) on libido and sexual dysfunction in postmenopausal women. Menopause. 2009;15(5):923–31.
45. Labrie F, Archer D, Bouchard C, Fortier M, Cusan L, Gomez J, Girard G, Baron M, Ayotte N, Moreau M, et al. Intravaginal dehydroepiandrosterone (prasterone), a highly efficient treatment of dyspareunia. Climacteric. 2011;14:282–8.
46. van Gorsel H, Laan E, Tkachenko N, et al. Pharmacokinetics and pharmacodynamic efficacy of testosterone intranasal gel in women with hypoactive sexual desire disorder and anorgasmia. Poster presented at International Society for the Study of Women's Sexual Health Annual Meeting (ISSWSH), Jerusalem, 19–22 Feb 2012.
47. Bloemers J, van Rooij K, Poels S, Goldstein I, Everaerd W, Koppeschaar H, Chivers M, Gerritsen J, van Ham D, Olivier B, et al. Toward personalized sexual medicine (part 1): integrating the "dual control model" into differential drug treatments for hypoactive sexual desire disorder and female sexual arousal disorder. J Sex Med. 2013;10(3):791–809.
48. Poels S, Bloemers J, van Rooij K, Goldstein I, Gerritsen J, van Ham D, van Mameren F, Chivers M, Everaerd W, Koppeschaar H, et al. Toward personalized sexual medicine (part 2): testosterone combined with a PDE5 inhibitor increases sexual satisfaction in women with HSDD and FSAD, and a low sensitive system for sexual cues. J Sex Med. 2013;10(3):810–23.
49. Poels S, Bloemers J, van Rooij K, Koppeschaar H, Olivier B, Tuiten A. Two novel combined drug treatments for women with hypoactive sexual desire disorder. Pharmacol Biochem Behav. 2014;121:71–9.
50. van Rooij K, Poels S, Bloemers J, et al. Toward personalized sexual medicine (part 3): testosterone combined with a Serotonin1A receptor agonist increases sexual satisfaction in women with HSDD and FSAD, and dysfunctional activation of sexual inhibitory mechanisms. J Sex Med. 2013;10(3):824–37.
51. van Rooij K, Leede L, Frijlink HW, Bloemers J, Poels S, Koppeschaar H, Olivier B, Tuiten A. Pharmacokinetics of a prototype formulation of sublingual testosterone and a buspirone tablet, versus an advanced combination tablet of testosterone and buspirone in healthy premenopausal women. Drugs R D. 2014;14:125–32.
52. Wierman ME, Basson R, Davis SR, Khosia S, Miller KK, Rosner W. Androgen therapy in women: an Endocrine Society Clinical Practice guideline. J Clin Endocrinol Metab. 2006;91(10):3697–710. Epub 2006 Oct 3.
53. North American Menopause Society. The role of testosterone therapy in postmenopausal women: position statement of The North American Menopause Society. Menopause. 2005;12(5):496–511. Epub 2005 Sept 1.
54. Shufelt CL, Braunstein GD. Safety of testosterone use in women. Maturitas. 2009;63(1):63–6. Epub 2009 Feb 27.
55. Shufelt CL, Braunstein GD. Testosterone and the breast. Menopause Int. 2008;14(3):117–22.
56. Traish A, Guay AT, Spark RF, Testosterone Therapy in Women Study Group. Are the Endocrine Society's Clinical Practice guidelines on androgen therapy in women misguided? A commentary. J Sex Med. 2007;4(5):1223–34. discussion 1234–5.
57. Hubayter Z, Simon JA. Testosterone therapy for sexual dysfunction in postmenopausal women. Climacteric. 2008;11(3):181–91.
58. Kingsberg SA, Simon JA, Goldstein I. The current outlook for testosterone in the management of hypoactive sexual desire disorder in postmenopausal women. J Sex Med. 2008;5 Suppl 4:182–93.
59. Braunstein GD. The Endocrine Society Clinical Practice guideline and The North American Menopause Society position statement on androgen

therapy in women: another one of Yogi's forks. J Clin Endocrinol Metab. 2007;92(11):4091–3.
60. van Staa TP, Sprafka JM. Study of adverse outcomes in women using testosterone therapy. Maturitas. 2009;62(1):76–80. Epub 2008 Dec 24.
61. Thorp Jr J, Palacios S, Symons J, Simon J, Barbour K. Improving prospects for treating hypoactive sexual desire disorder (HSDD): development status of flibanserin. BJOG. 2014;121(11):1328–31.
62. Thorp J, Simon J, Dattani D, Taylor L, Kimura T, Garcia Jr M, Lesko L, Pyke R, DAISY Trial Investigators. Treatment of hypoactive sexual desire disorder in premenopausal women: efficacy of flibanserin in the DAISY study. J Sex Med. 2012; 9(3):793–804.
63. Derogatis LR, Komer L, Katz M, Moreau M, Kimura T, Garcia Jr M, Wunderlich G, Pyke R, VIOLET Trial Investigators. Treatment of hypoactive sexual desire disorder in premenopausal women: efficacy of flibanserin in the VIOLET Study. J Sex Med. 2012;9(4): 1074–85.
64. Katz M, DeRogatis LR, Ackerman R, Hedges P, Lesko L, Garcia Jr M, Sand M, BEGONIA Trial Investigators. Efficacy of flibanserin in women with hypoactive sexual desire disorder: results from the BEGONIA trial. J Sex Med. 2013;10(7):1807–15.
65. Portman DJ, Edelson J, Jordan R, et al. Bremelanotide for hypoactive sexual desire disorder: analyses from a phase 2B dose-ranging study. Obstet Gynecol. 2014;123 Suppl 1:31S.

Commentary: Management of Hypoactive Sexual Desire Disorder (HSDD)

Marianne Brandon

Hypoactive sexual desire disorder (HSDD), now part of the controversial new DSM-5 condition termed female sexual interest/arousal disorder (FSIAD), is one of the most common yet vexing female sexual dysfunctions to treat. This is due in part to the nuanced complexity of the interplay between physical and psychological factors that contribute to desire, as well as to our imperfect understanding of all etiologies of this condition. Given this complexity and multifactorial nature, HSDD/FSIAD represents a prototype condition benefiting from a biopsychosocial approach merging medical with psychotherapeutic treatments.

In the preceding chapter, Krapf, Goldstein, and Buster outline the known physiology of sexual desire, highlighting the excitatory and inhibitory neurotransmitters and brain regions essential in determining sexual desire. Discussing the known causes of low desire, including medications and medical conditions, the authors then segue into a discussion of the prominent role of androgens in sexual desire, providing a detailed discussion of current and upcoming treatment options for low desire. In the following complementary commentary, the broader approach to FSIAD is outlined, with a clear perspective on the rationale behind how and why obtaining a detailed sexual history is so critical to appropriate and complete treatment of this condition. How to merge medical and psychotherapies is then outlined, so that the reader develops a comprehensive overview of how to approach FSIAD.

Marianne Brandon, Ph.D.
Wellminds Wellbodies, LLC, Annapolis, MD, USA

Commentary

Drs. Kraph, Buster, and Goldstein offered an excellent and thorough review of the physiologic management of hypoactive sexual desire disorder in women. As they indicated, the assessment and treatment of psychosocial etiologies are equally important in the care of patients with desire concerns. Indeed, it was Dr. Goldstein himself who introduced the biopsychosocial model to me many years ago as I embarked on my specialization in sex therapy. This commentary will summarize an approach to assessing and treating the psychosocial aspects of desire disorders in women.

Most sexual medicine professionals would likely agree that desire disorders are among the most difficult to treat—largely due to the complex and often subtle psychological, relationship, and contextual dynamics that can interfere with libido. In spite of these challenges, surveys suggest that the majority of men and women consider sexual intimacy to be a vital aspect of a romantic relationship [1], and sexual satisfaction correlates with relationship satisfaction and life satisfaction [2]. As such, the experience of low desire can be extremely upsetting for a woman and/or her partner. In fact, fully one-third of women with low desire express distress about their lack of sexual interest [3]. Many of the women with low desire that I have worked with ruminate about this problem daily, feel tremendous guilt about depriving their partner of a critical aspect of intimacy, worry that their partner will leave or have an affair because of a lack of intimacy, and/or miss what was once a profound intimate experience making them feel vital, alive, and connected to their partner. However, it can also be the case that a woman's distress about her low desire is the result of her partner's negative reactions and she herself is not bothered by her lack of interest.

The diagnostic criteria for low desire in women have recently been modified from hypoactive sexual desire disorder (HSDD) as defined in the DSM-IV-TR [4] to the current DSM-5 classification of female sexual interest/arousal disorder (FSIAD) [5]. This recent modification is not without significant controversy. How to diagnosis low desire and even whether or not to regard low desire as a diagnosis in women [6] will likely remain contentious issues in the field of sexual medicine for some time. Indeed, female sexual medicine is a relatively new field, with still many unanswered questions. For example, recent research suggests that asexuality, or the absence of sexual attraction, may be normative for a subset of the population [7]. More research is clearly needed to clarify this hypothesis.

Currently, the diagnostic criteria for FSAID must include symptoms in at least three of the following categories: reduced interest in sexual activity, reduced fantasies or thoughts about sex, reduced initiation and/or non-receptivity to partner's attempts to initiate, reduced sexual pleasure, reduced response to erotic cues, and reduced genital or nongenital sensations during sexual encounters. These symptoms must persist for a minimum of 6 months, cause a woman significant distress, and not be attributable to a mental disorder, medication, or substance abuse. Diagnosis also requires specification of whether the disorder is lifelong or acquired and generalized or specific to a situation and severity is rated as mild, moderate, or severe.

The assessment of low desire can be challenging for many reasons, not the least of which is a disturbing lack of training opportunities for physicians [8]. Time constraints, limitations on insurance reimbursement, and the potential awkwardness of discussing a patient's intimacy concerns may also inhibit practitioners in assessing FSAID [9]. There are a variety of reliable and valid questionnaires that can assist in this process, including: the sexual interest and desire inventory-female (SIDI-F) [10], the decreased sexual desire screener (DSDS) [11], the female sexual distress scale-revised (FSDS-R) [12], and the female sexual function index (FSFI) [13].

Three principles may be considered the foundation for taking a sexual history: using a patient-centered approach, offering evidence-based diagnostic and treatment recommendations, and using a unified management approach for treatment [9]. Adherence to these basic principles ensures that the patient feels understood and receives state-of-the-art medical care. Desire concerns may cut to the core of her identity, as lovemaking is when she is most vulnerable and exposed. Thus, issues relating to her sexuality may be among the most difficult topics she will discuss with a medical professional in her lifetime.

In taking a sexual history, it is of course essential to maintain cultural and religious sensitivity, as well as to avoid an assumption of heterosexuality. It is also necessary to remain aware of your voice tone and other nonverbal cues that communicate information. As much as she is seeking relief for her symptoms, a patient may be acutely aware of your reactions and adjust her responses accordingly. A woman may thus not offer all necessary information during the initial assessment period, and instead, her story may unfold over multiple appointments. Indeed, she may not be ready to acknowledge to herself, or verbalize to another, information that is critical in understanding her low desire. For example, perhaps she is having an affair, or she is disgusted by the way her genitals changed following a traumatic childbirth, but she is too ashamed to admit this. Acute sensitivity when responding to her concerns is necessary.

A sexual history provides the practitioner with information to answer three critical questions: whether or not the patient has a disorder, what underlying organic and psychogenic factors contribute to the disorder, and whether or not the patient should be treated [14]. The sexual tipping point [15] is one comprehensive guide for evaluating the role that multiple biopsychosocial influences may have on the etiology of a woman's low desire. This model conceptualizes low desire as being impacted by physiological, organic, psychosocial, and cultures issues. Thus, a woman's psychological and medical health, the quality of her romantic and sexual relationship, and issues relating to the context of her life are all given consideration.

It is useful to ask a woman her understanding of her low libido and what, if any, treatment she has previously attempted. However, be prepared to probe her responses further. For example, it is not unusual for a patient to initially state, "Everything is perfect in my relationship except for my lack of desire," only to verbalize upon further exploration that significant challenges involving such essential dynamics as power, trust, physical attraction, sexual technique, communication, or respect do exist but are difficult for her to articulate. The context of her current life is also relevant, including her stress level, sexual dysfunction in her partner, and parenting or eldercare responsibilities that can all interfere with her desire to make love. Historical issues relating to her sexual debut [16] or past trauma [17] can also impact her current experience of desire. In sum, sex drive can be a sensitive barometer of balance in just about any aspect of a woman's life.

A thorough assessment enables a practitioner to determine whether or not treatment is indicated and, relatedly, which treatments to recommend. The biopsychosocial model of care necessitates that a woman's psychological and biological treatment needs are all attended to. This is essential regardless of the etiology of a patient's low desire. Ultimately, physiological etiologies have psychological ramifications, just as psychological issues eventually impact a woman's biology [9, 18].

The initial phase of treatment may include education about FSAID, including a conversation about the differences between spontaneous and responsive sexual desire [19]. Specifically, it is considered non-dysfunctional for some women to feel open and responsive to a partner's advances without ever feeling the spontaneous desire for sex. Prepare the patient that she will function as an active member of her treatment team, which will likely include a medical professional and sex therapist. Discussing the relatively high rates of sexual dysfunction and dissatisfaction in the general population [20] may help her feel less alone.

It will be helpful to have a list of qualified therapists as referral sources that you can offer your patient at this time. Even if your patient does not meet the diagnostic criteria for a sexual dysfunction, she may be struggling with her own or her partner's expectations about her sexual function, and thus it is likely that a psychotherapy referral will be helpful. On this list you can include the organizations offering sex therapist referrals: the American Association of Sex Educators, Counselors, and Therapists (www.AASECT.org), the Society for Sex Therapy and Research (www.SSTARnet.org), and the International Society for the Study of Women's Sexual Health (www.ISSWSH.org). You may also identify local therapist referral sources by contacting your state psychological association.

Therapists approach the treatment of low desire in women from a variety of perspectives. A focus on the development and cultivation of sexual excitatory mechanisms to support libido is generally more beneficial than attempting to decrease the inhibitory mechanisms making sex less appealing for her [21]. Evidence-based practice includes the development of mindfulness skills [22], therapy groups that focus on communication skills training, sensate focus, fantasy training, intimacy exercises and education [23, 24], and/or an intersystems model addressing familiar and intergenerational influences to low desire [25, 26]. Therapists will make decisions regarding whether individual therapy, couple therapy, or both are necessary. Patients may report that their progress in reaching their treatment goals is variable, in part because the desire disorders exhibit a strong placebo response [27] and in part because, as previously described, the etiologies of desire disorders can be so complex and multi-determined.

In sum, low desire concerns in women are classic mind-body phenomenon, requiring an integrated biopsychosocial treatment approach [28]. Communication among members of the treatment team is strongly encouraged, as it will help to ensure that the patient's unique needs are being addressed. For further training opportunities in female sexual medicine, please see the International Society for the Study of Women's Sexual Health (www.ISSWSH.org).

References

1. Leiblum SR. Clinical perspectives on and treatment for sexual desire disorders. In: Leiblum SR, editor. Treating sexual desire disorders. New York: The Guilford Press; 2010.
2. Davison SL, Bell RJ, LaChina, M. The relationship between self-reported sexual satisfaction and general well-being in women. J Sex Med. 2009;6:2690–7.
3. Rosen RC, Shifren JL, Monz BU, Odom DM, Russo PA, Johannes CB. Correlates of sexually related personal distress in women with low sexual desire. J Sex Med. 2009;6:1549–60.
4. American Psychiatric Association. Diagnostic and statistical manual of mental disorders. 4th ed. Washington, DC: American Psychiatric Association; 2000.
5. American Psychiatric Association. Diagnostic and statistical manual of mental disorders. 5th ed. Washington, DC: American Psychiatric Association; 2013.
6. Teifer L, Hall M. A skeptical view of desire norms and disorders promotes clinical success. In: Leiblum SR, editor. Treating sexual desire disorders: a clinical casebook. New York: The Guilford Press; 2010.
7. Brotto LA, Yule MA, Gorzalka BB. Asexuality: an extreme variant of sexual desire disorder? J Sex Med. 2015;13(3):646–60.
8. Parish S, Clayton A. Sexual medicine education: review and commentary. J Sex Med. 2007;4:259–67.
9. Althof SA, Rosen RC, Perelman MA, Rubio-Aurioles E. Standard operating procedures for taking a sexual history. J Sex Med. 2013;10:26–35.
10. Clayton A, Seagraves RT, Leublum S, Basson R, Pyke R, Cotton D, Lewis-D'Asostino D, Evans KR, Sills TL, Wunderlich GR. Reliability and validity of the sexual interest and desire inventory-female (SIDI-F), a scale designed to measure severity of female hypoactive sexual desire disorder. J Sex Marital Ther. 2006;32:115–35.
11. Clayton A, Goldfischer E, Goldstein I, Derogatis L, Lewis-D'Agostino D, Pyke R. Validation of the decreased sexual desire screener (DSDS): a brief diagnostic instrument for generalized acquired female hypoactive sexual desire disorder (HSDD). J Sex Med. 2009;6:730–8.
12. Derogatis L, Clayton A, Lewis-D'Agostino D, Wunderlich G, Fu Y. Validation of the female sexual distress scale-revised for assessing distress in women with hypoactive sexual desire disorder. J Sex Med. 2008;5:357–64.
13. Rosen R, Brown C, Heiman J, Leiblum S, Meston C, Shabsigh R, Ferguson D, D'Agostino R Jr. The female sexual function index (FSFI): a multidimensional self-report instrument for the assessment of female sexual function. J Sex Marital Ther. 2000;26:191–208.
14. Perelman M. Psychosocial history. Women's sexual function and dysfunction: study, diagnosis, and treatment. London: CRC Press; 2005.
15. Perelman M. The sexual tipping point: a mind/body model for sexual medicine. J Sex Med. 2009;6(3): 629–32.
16. Rapsey CM. Age, quality, and context of first sex: associations with sexual difficulties. J Sex Med. 2014;11(12):2873–81.

17. Yehuda R, Lehrner A, Rosenbaum TY. PTSD and sexual dysfunction in men and women. J Sex Med. 2015;12:1107–19.
18. Perelman M. Female sexual dysfunction and the central nervous system. J Sex Med. 2007;4(4):257–9.
19. Basson R, Brotto LA, Laan E, Redmond G, Utian WH. Assessment and management of women's sexual dysfunctions: problematic desire and arousal. J Sex Med. 2005;2(3):291–300.
20. Laumann EO, Paik A, Rosen RC. Sexual dysfunction in the United States. J Am Med Assoc. 1999;281:537–44.
21. Janssen E, Bancroft J. The dual control model: the role of sexual inhibition and excitation in arousal and behavior. In: Janssen E, editor. The psychophysiology of sex. Bloomington, IN: Indiana University Press; 2007.
22. Brotto L, Woo JT. Cognitive-behavioral and mindfulness-based therapy for low sexual desire. In: Leiblum SR, editor. Treating sexual desire disorders. New York: The Guilford Press; 2010.
23. ter Kuile MM, Both S, van Lankveld JJDM. Cognitive behavioral therapy for sexual dysfunctions in women. Psychiatr Clin N Am. 2010;33:595–610.
24. Trudel G, Marchand A, Ravart M, Aubin, S Turgeon L, Fortier P. The effect of a cognitive-behavioral group treatment program on hypoactive sexual desire in women. Sex Relat Ther. 2010;16(2):145–64.
25. Weeks GR, Hertlein KM, Gamdescia N. The treatment of hypoactive sexual desire disorder. J Fam Psychother 2009;20:129–49.
26. Weeks G, Gamdescia N. Definition, etiology, and treatment of absent/low desire in women. In: Hertlein KM, Weeks GR, Gambescia N, editors. Systemic sex therapy. New York: Routledge; 2015.
27. Bradford A, Meston C. Placebo response in the treatment of women's sexual dysfunctions. J Sex Marital Ther. 2009;35:164–81.
28. Perelman M. Clinical application of CNS-acting agents in FSD. J Sex Med. 2007;4(4):280–90.

Diagnosis and Management of Female Sexual Arousal Disorder

22

Seth D. Cohen and Irwin Goldstein

22.1 Introduction

Women have more sexual health concerns in general than men, and women with sexual health problems have significant impairment of their life quality [1]. Ironically, the study, diagnosis, and treatment of women with sexual health concerns are limited. Following Masters and Johnson's groundbreaking work in the early 1970s, there was a flurry of scientific inquiry into the etiology and treatment of female sexual dysfunction [2]. With the introduction of an oral treatment for erectile dysfunction, sildenafil, a second wave of scientific enthusiasm regarding female sexual dysfunction evolved. Now with the support from various medical and surgical societies like the International Society for Sexual Medicine (ISSM) and the International Society for the Study of Women's Sexual Health (ISSWSH), new treatment models are being studied and utilized to treat female sexual problems.

Although female sexual arousal disorder (FSAD) is prevalent, it is often not well defined or understood. The current definition of FSAD discussed below is based on the *Diagnostic and Statistical Manual of Mental Disorders, Fourth Edition Revised* (DSM-IV-TR), which includes a requirement that the woman has concomitant distress. According to the DSM-IV, the diagnostic criteria to define sexual arousal disorder are (1) persistent or recurrent inability to attain, or to maintain until completion of the sexual activity, an adequate lubrication-swelling response of sexual excitement, (2) the disturbance causes marked distress or interpersonal difficulty, and (3) the sexual dysfunction is not better accounted for by another axis I disorder (except another sexual dysfunction) and is not due exclusively to the direct physiological effects of a substance (e.g., a drug of abuse, a medication) or a general medical condition [1, 3, 4]. Oftentimes medications such as selective serotonin reuptake inhibitors (SSRIs) can lead to such sexual dysfunctions including arousal and desire dysfunction. Thus, the DSM definition of arousal disorder may be limited in its ability to appropriately classify some of these patients.

It is worth noting that FSAD is rarely a solitary diagnosis. Since hypoactive sexual desire disorder (HSDD) is frequently diagnosed in these patients, a new disorder was proposed for the DSM-5: sexual interest/arousal disorder [5].

The term sexual arousal has been labeled in a variety of ways [6, 7]. Some authors discuss sexual arousal as if it is synonymous with genital arousal; however, it, and possibly orgasm,

Commentary by Annamaria Giraldi, M.D., Ph.D., F.E.C.S.M.

S.D. Cohen, M.D., M.P.H.
Advanced Urological Care, New York, NY, USA

I. Goldstein, M.D. (✉)
San Diego Sexual Medicine, San Diego, CA, USA
e-mail: dr.irwingoldstein@comcast.net

L.I. Lipshultz et al. (eds.), *Management of Sexual Dysfunction in Men and Women*, DOI 10.1007/978-1-4939-3100-2_22

involves (1) information processing of relevant stimuli, (2) arousal in a general sense, (3) incentive motivation, and (4) genital response [3]. Desire may be experienced once sexual stimuli have triggered arousal. Arousal and desire co-occur and reinforce each other. Women's subjective arousal may be minimally influenced by genital congestion. Some experts in the field of women's sexual health feel that women do not assess their experience of arousal to any large extent from genital sensations; this appears to be especially so at low and moderate levels of arousal. Genital engorgement becomes more important for women at higher levels of arousal [2]. An absence of desire any time during the sexual experience designates disorder. Arousal disorder subtypes are proposed that separate an absence of subjective arousal from all types of sexual stimulation, from an absence of subjective arousal when the only stimulus is genital [3].

Most current research on sexual arousal in women assumes that the lack of sexual arousal is due to a lack of excitation, with little attempt to differentiate between inhibited sexual desire and lack of desire [8]. According to Bancroft and Jensen's research on the central nervous system's response to sexual excitement, it is the balance between excitatory and inhibitory systems that determines whether sexual arousal occurs [9, 10]. In addition, the authors postulate that individuals vary in their propensity for both sexual excitation and inhibition. The voluntary inhibition of sexual response can be seen as an adaptive trait, as a means for an individual to avoid risks that would be associated with a given situation. However, for some, sexual inhibition can be uncontrollably elevated, resulting in significant stress and bother as in cases of persistent genital arousal disorder [1].

The cause of FSAD is multifactorial and may include psychological problems such as depression or anxiety disorders, relationship conflicts, partner performance and technique problems, issues relating to prior abuse, medical illness, medications, menopause, stress, or gynecological problems that make sexual activity uncomfortable.

22.2 Etiology

Maintaining sexual health during menopause is a challenge because the progressive decline in sex hormones interacts with the aging process. The biological changes in hormone levels, specifically the decrease in estrogen in menopausal women, and the vaginal changes that ensue as a result can significantly affect arousal. Menopause occurs when the ovaries stop producing estrogen, the hormone that controls the reproductive cycle. Anything that damages the ovaries or blocks estrogen effects can cause premature menopause. This includes chemotherapy in the setting of malignancy or surgery to remove the ovaries; in these cases, early menopause is a side effect [11]. Vaginal atrophy and dryness associated with low estrogen levels can cause arousal to take longer or be harder to achieve. Often the first noticeable change associated with menopause is reduced vaginal lubrication during arousal, as less estrogen results in reduced blood circulation to the vulva, clitoris, and vagina [12]. Lastly, psychological and contextual factors have a significant influence on organic components of sexual arousal.

22.3 Assessment

During the evaluation of women with FSAD, common symptoms range from low interest in sex, decreased arousal and orgasmic capabilities, and diminished genital sensation and blood flow during sexual stimulation as well as pain due to lack of lubrication. When assessing these patients, it is important to address any predisposing factors that can exacerbate or alleviate symptoms. If the patient is in a current sexual relationship, both partners need to be evaluated to understand the aforementioned factors. A multidisciplinary approach is recommended to achieve an optimal outcome. Especially for lifelong sexual dysfunctions like FSAD, developmental sexual abuse and past relationships, as part of the past history, are also very relevant. Lastly, assessing comorbidities that may contribute to the woman's sexual dysfunction is germane to tailoring an appropriate treatment regimen.

The assessment of female genital arousal is generally considered difficult in comparison with that of men [13]. Arousal and arousal problems are best assessed using a biopsychosocial approach exploring predisposing, precipitating, and maintaining factors with the woman [1]. Levin pointed out that the relationship between vaginal lubrication and sexual arousal is uncertain [14]. Although lubrication does usually increase during sexual arousal, it may not be maintained, especially after a lengthy period of stimulation. Because measuring vaginal lubrication or swelling can be difficult, studies dating back to the 1970s investigating genital response in women have mainly assessed pulse amplitude in the vaginal wall (VPA), using vaginal photoplethysmography [15, 16]. Although reproducible increases in VPA occurred in response to erotic stimuli, subjective sexual arousal was low or nonexistent [17].

Vaginal Doppler ultrasound (US) has been used to assess blood flow changes within vaginal and clitoral tissues. Huang et al. studied blood flow improvement within vaginal tissues after application of local estrogen [18]. The authors used color Doppler flow imaging to observe the flow spectrum of the genitourinary tract in 78 cases of postmenopausal females on local estrogen. The Doppler parameters included the vaginal wall, urethra resistance index (RI), and systolic/diastolic ratios [19].

There is no consensus on recommended routine laboratory tests for the evaluation of women with sexual arousal concerns. Blood testing should be dictated by clinical suspicion based on the history and physical examination. If appropriate, the clinician may assess multiple androgen and estrogen values including total testosterone, free testosterone, sex hormone-binding globulin (SHBG), dihydrotestosterone (DHT), estradiol, and progesterone. Pituitary function may be measured using luteinizing hormone (LH), follicle-stimulating hormone (FSH), and prolactin levels. Thyroid-stimulating hormone (TSH) should be measured to exclude subclinical thyroid disease.

22.4 Treatment

FSAD is a complex problem with multiple overlapping etiologies. Thus, there are many treatment options with the optimal therapy depending on the etiology of the problem. Available therapeutic options include adjustment of medications, counseling, treatment of depression or anxiety, stress and fatigue reduction, sex therapy, devices, and hormone replacement therapy.

22.5 Hormone Supplementation

There is some evidence pointing to the effect of estradiol on sexual arousability in women [19, 20]. Overall, data suggest that topical or systemic estrogen supplementation is effective and may improve vaginal lubrication and decrease vaginal dryness and irritation. Dennerstein et al. investigated the effects of estrogen and progesterone on female sexual behavior in 49 women who had undergone hysterectomy and bilateral salpingo-oophorectomy in a double-blind placebo-controlled crossover study. Over a 12-month period, each woman received 3 months each of ethinyl estradiol, 50 μg/day; levonorgestrel, 250 μg/day; a combination of the two (Nordiol); and placebo. Significant differences between medications were found with regard to sexual desire, enjoyment, and orgasmic frequency. The most beneficial effects, in terms of improvement in arousal, occurred with use of ethinyl estradiol [17].

Although no androgen therapies are currently approved by the Food and Drug Administration for FSAD, they are being used "off label" in clinical practice. Androgens play an important role in healthy female sexual function, especially in stimulating sexual interest and in maintaining desire. Androgens are also vital for the health and maintenance of vaginal tissues including the vulva, vestibule, and vagina. Thus, many sexual medicine providers use off-label testosterone supplementation to improve FSAD symptoms.

There are multiple reasons why women can have low androgen levels, with the most common being age (menopause), a history of oophorectomy, and the use of oral contraceptives. Symptoms of androgen deficiency include absent or greatly diminished arousal, sexual motivation and/or desire, and persistent unexplainable fatigue or lack of energy. Although there are no androgen preparations that have been specifically approved by the FDA for the treatment of androgen deficiency in women, androgen therapy has been used off label to treat low arousal, low libido, and sexual dysfunction in women for over 40 years.

Although there are sparse data on the role of testosterone in female arousal, there appears to be a considerable positive response to androgens [21]. Historically, androgens were identified predominantly with male sexual function, contributing to a lack of recognition of the effects of androgens in women. Androgens, including testosterone, are necessary not only for reproductive function and hormonal balance in women but represent important precursors for the biosynthesis of estrogens. We know that androgens have multiple biochemical effects in the body including, but not limited to, sexual desire, bone density, muscle mass and strength, mood, energy, and psychological well-being. However, sex steroid hormone actions are quite complex and involve critical enzymes and critical hormone receptors that also determine tissue exposure, tissue sensitivity, and tissue responsiveness.

Systemic testosterone can be administered via transdermal application or intramuscular injection or with a subcutaneous pellet. The dose for any systemic testosterone given to women is at one-tenth the dose administered to men. When checking laboratory values, it is important to keep women's free testosterone in a range of 0.6–0.8 ng/dl. It is important to discuss with the patient the strategy of serial blood testing to address safety concerns during treatment including any side effects from androgen supplementation.

22.6 Nonhormonal Supplementation

Sexual motivation is encouraged, sustained, and ended by a number of central nervous system neurotransmitter and receptor changes induced, in part, by the action of the central neurotransmitter dopamine. The activation of dopamine receptors may be a key intermediary in the stimulation of incentive sexual motivation and sexual reward. These neurotransmitters and receptor changes in turn activate central sexual arousal and desire. Contemporary animal research reveals that dopamine neurotransmitter systems may play a critical intermediary role in the central regulation of sexual arousal and excitation, mood, and incentive-related sexual behavior. Nonhormonal neuropeptides like oxytocin and prolactin have also been utilized in this clinical setting with good success [6].

Vasoactive agents including phosphodiesterase inhibitors (PDEi's) have been investigated in several studies for treatment of FSAD. In a small proportion of the studies, women with FSAD endorsed a beneficial effect on arousal, while in most of the studies, vasoactive agents had no effect when compared with placebo. Smaller studies in populations with other medical conditions have shown more consistent effects. As such, PDEi's may be beneficial in specific groups of women with FSAD (for review, see [4]) [22].

Bupropion, which is a noradrenaline and dopamine reuptake inhibitor with nicotinic antagonist properties originally marketed as an antidepressant, may have a beneficial effect on women with sexual arousal disorder [6, 21]. In one placebo-controlled trial [21], bupropion produced an increase in desire and frequency of sexual activity when compared with placebo. Segraves et al. [6] investigated the role of sustained release bupropion in a randomized, double-blind, placebo-controlled, multiple-site escalating-dose 112-day trial. Outcomes were measured by investigator-rating and self-administered questionnaires. The changes in sexual functioning questionnaire (CSFQ) indicated that bupropion had significant effects on increasing measures of sexual arousal, orgasm, and sexual satisfaction. Traditional antidepressant dosing starts at 150 mg twice a day; however, low-dose bupropion at 75 mg twice a day can achieve an optimal improvement in sexual arousal potential.

Other dopamine agonists used are cabergoline administered at 0.5 mg up to three times per week and ropinirole 0.25 mg administered daily [23]. Oxytocin lozenges, linked to improved arousal and desire, are administered at 250 IU sublingually 30 min to 1 h before sexual activity. Research with oxytocin has shown marked improvement in a number of components of sexual function, including arousal and orgasm. Lastly, amphetamine salts including dextroamphetamine/amphetamine (Adderall) and other drugs used to treat attention deficit disorder have been increasingly useful in helping women to concentrate and thus improving arousal [23, 24].

Lastly, flibanserin and bremelanotide, two drugs in development, may show promise for the future of FSAD treatments. Flibanserin is a nonhormonal treatment for premenopausal women with HSDD [25, 26]. Flibanserin is a 5-HT1A receptor agonist and 5-HT2A receptor antagonist that was initially investigated as an antidepressant [27, 28]. Preclinical evidence suggested that flibanserin targets the above receptors preferentially in selective brain areas, restores a balance between inhibitory and excitatory effects, and may show benefit in the treatment of FSAD [29, 30].

Bremelanotide is a drug under development for female sexual dysfunction, hemorrhagic shock, and reperfusion injury. It functions by activating the melanocortin receptors MC1R and MC4R, to modulate inflammation and limit ischemia [31]. Bremelanotide was originally tested for intranasal administration in treating female sexual dysfunction, but this application was temporarily discontinued in 2008 after concerns were raised over adverse side effects including elevated blood pressure. As of December 2014, the company is conducting a human phase 3 study using a subcutaneous drug delivery system that appears to have little effect on blood pressure [32].

22.7 Conclusion

In a comprehensive textbook on couple's sexual health, it is important and appropriate to have a detailed chapter on the biologically focused management of FSAD. Increasing numbers of clinicians will manage women with these types of sexual health concerns since more and more women will expect such management. In addition, those clinicians who want to maximize overall women's healthcare delivery will increasingly engage in the management of women's sexual health concerns, in addition to the traditional focus on continence and urological conditions. In the future, it will become increasingly more difficult for female urologists and urogynecologists not to provide at least first-line sexual healthcare to women. Non-pharmacological treatments of FSAD have also been introduced and studied and include mindfulness training, couple therapy with focus on adequate sexual stimulation, and the use of lubricants.

The basic premise of biologically focused management of FSAD is that the normal physiologic processes regulating sexual arousal are altered by biologic pathology. How each specific medical condition modulates female arousal requires additional clinical and basic science investigation. If the biologic basis of the arousal disorder can be diagnosed by history and physical examination and laboratory testing, management outcome may be successfully directed to the source of pathophysiology. Of the many challenges facing healthcare professionals today, the first is to improve the ability to accurately diagnose women with sexual health concerns and the second is to ensure that women receive the best evidence-based available management options.

References

1. Laumann EO, Paik A, Rosen RC. Sexual dysfunction in the United States: prevalence and predictors. JAMA. 1999;281(6):537–44.
2. Masters WH, Johnson VE. Human sexual response. Toronto: Bantam Books; 1966.
3. APA. Summary of practice-relevant changes to the DSM-IV-TR; 2000.
4. http://www.icd10data.com/ICD10CM/Codes/F01-F99/F50-F59/F52-/F52.22
5. Graham CA. The DSM diagnostic criteria for female sexual arousal disorder. Arch Sex Behav. 2009;39(2):240–55.
6. Bancroft J. The endocrinology of sexual arousal. J Endocrinol. 2005;186:411–27.
7. Singer B. Conceptualizing sexual arousal and attraction. J Sex Res. 1984;20:230–40.

8. Graham CA, Sanders SA, Milhausen RR, McBride KR. Turning on and turning off: a focus group study of the factors that affect women's sexual arousal. Arch Sex Behav. 2004;33(6):527–38.
9. Bancroft J. Central inhibition of sexual response in the male: a theoretical perspective. Neurosci Biobehav Rev. 1999;23:763–84.
10. Bancroft J, Janssen E. The dual control model of male sexual response: a theoretical approach to centrally mediated erectile dysfunction. Neurosci Biobehav Rev. 2000;24:571–9.
11. Bober SL, Recklitis CJ, Bakan J, Garber JE, Patenaude AF. Addressing sexual dysfunction after risk-reducing salpingo-oophorectomy: effects of a brief, psychosexual intervention. J Sex Med. 2015;12(1):189–97.
12. Nappi RE, Martini E, Martella S, Capuano F, Bosoni D, Giacomini S, Beraghi M, Spinillo A. Maintaining sexuality in menopause. Post Reprod Health. 2014; 20(1):22–9.
13. Bartlik B, Goldberg J. Female sexual arousal disorder. In: Leiblum SR, Rosen RC, editors. Principles and practice of sex therapy. 3rd ed. New York: Guilford; 2000. p. 85–117.
14. Levin RJ. The ins and outs of vaginal lubrication. Sex Relat Ther. 2003;18:509–13.
15. Laan E, Everaerd W. Determinants of female sexual arousal: psychophysiological theory and data. Annu Rev Sex Res. 1995;6:32–76.
16. Sintchak G, Geer JH. A vaginal photoplethysmograph system. Psychophysiology. 1975;12:113–15.
17. Everaerd W, Laan E, Both S, van der Velde J. Female sexuality. In: Szuchman L, Muscarella F, editors. Psychological perspectives on human sexuality. New York: Wiley; 2000. p. 108–22.
18. Huang FH, Zhang XL, Xiao LP, Xu YY, Zhang YZ. Study of blood flow improvement of topical application of estrogen on low genitourinary tract and its safety. Zhonghua Yi Xue Za Zhi. 2012; 92(39):2778–80.
19. Dennerstein L, Burrows GD, Wood C, Hyman G. Hormones and sexuality: effect of estrogen and progestogen. Obstet Gynecol. 1980;56:316–22.
20. Sherwin BB. The impact of different doses of estrogen and progestin on mood and sexual behavior in postmenopausal women. J Clin Endocrinol Metab. 1991;72:336–43.
21. Woodis CB, McLendon AN, Muzyk AJ. Testosterone supplementation for hypoactive sexual desire disorder in women. Pharmacotherapy. 2012;32(1):38–53. doi:10.1002/PHAR.1004.
22. Chivers ML, Rosen RC. Phosphodiesterase type 5 inhibitors and female sexual response: faulty protocols or paradigms? J Sex Med. 2010;7(2 Pt 2): 858–72.
23. Afonso VM, Mueller D, Stewart J, Pfaus JG. Amphetamine pretreatment facilitates appetitive sexual behaviors in the female rat. Psychopharmacology (Berl). 2009;205(1):35–43.
24. Afonso VM, Bablekis V, Pfaus JG. Sensory mediation of female-male mounting in the rat: II. Role of tactile and conspecific cues. Physiol Behav. 2006;87(5):863–9. Epub 2006 Feb 20.
25. Borsini F, Evans K, Jason K, Rohde F, Alexander B, Pollentier S. Pharmacology of flibanserin. CNS Drug Rev. 2002;8(2):117–42.
26. Jolly E, Clayton A, Thorp J, Lewis-D'Agostino D, Wunderlich G, Lesko L. Design of phase III pivotal trials of flibanserin in female hypoactive sexual desire disorder (HSDD). Sexologies. 2008;17 Suppl 1:S133–4.
27. D'Aquila P, Monleon S, Borsini F, Brain P, Willner P. Anti-anhedonic actions of the novel serotonergic agent flibanserin, a potential rapidly-acting antidepressant. Eur J Pharmacol. 1997;340(2–3):121–32.
28. Invernizzi RW, Sacchetti G, Parini S, Acconcia S, Samanin R. Flibanserin, a potential antidepressant drug, lowers 5-HT and raises dopamine and noradrenaline in the rat prefrontal cortex dialysate: role of 5-HT1A receptors. Br J Pharmacol. 2003;139(7): 1281–8.
29. Pfaus JG. Pathways of sexual desire. J Sex Med. 2009;6(6):1506–33.
30. Allers K, Dremencov E, Ceci A, et al. Acute and repeated flibanserin administration in female rats modulates monoamines differentially across brain areas: a microdialysis study. J Sex Med. 2010;7(5):1757–67.
31. Bremelanotide for organ protection and related indications, Palatin Technologies fact sheet. Retrieved 18 Jan 2009.
32. Palatin announces start of Bremelanotide Phase 3 program for female sexual dysfunction. PR Newswire. Retrieved 17 Feb 2015.

Commentary: Diagnosis and Management of Female Sexual Arousal Disorder

Annamaria Giraldi

The definition of female sexual arousal disorder (FSAD) attempts to coalesce physical and psychological aspects of the condition, although the current definition primarily focuses on the physical manifestations of arousal. However, approaching FSAD objectively requires an understanding of both the physical and psychological characteristics that can impact sexual desire and arousal. In the preceding chapter, Cohen and Goldstein describe the physical findings and symptoms of FSAD, providing an in-depth perspective on diagnosis and treatment. In progressing through the etiologies of FSAD, the authors focus on physical causes of the condition, and although they touch on relationship issues as a consideration during assessment of affected women and indicate the negative impacts of psychotropic medications, the "tangible" aspects of the condition are hewed to closely.

In the following commentary, this perspective is expanded with a thought-provoking discussion of the meaning and individual nature of arousal in women. More importantly, a discussion of broad etiologic categories of female sexual arousal which include strictly psychological, strictly genital, and combined causes is highlighted. The distinctions between these etiologies are critical and undoubtedly impact treatment approaches; one can certainly imagine that treatment for arousal disorder stemming from psychological causes can differ significantly from that arising from physical causes. It is essential that clinicians and mental health professionals who treat women with FSAD consider these distinctions and approach these women accordingly so as to maximize the potential for treatment success.

The Editors

Annamaria Giraldi, M.D., Ph.D., F.E.C.S.M.
Sexological Clinic, Psychiatric Center Copenhagen,
Institute of Clinical Medicine, University of
Copenhagen, Copenhagen, Denmark

Commentary

In the previous chapter, the definition and clinical treatment of female sexual arousal disorder (FSAD) were described. When thinking about FSAD, one should ask what women really mean when they talk about arousal. In the DSM-IV-TR and ICD-10, the diagnostic criteria for FSAD focus on the physical responses of the genitals, as increased blood flow results in tumescence of the genitals and vaginal lubrication, which is highly influenced by age, vascular response, and neurologic and endocrine state [1–4]. So, is it only the physical genital response that women describe when they refer to sexual arousal? Some women may describe the physical genital response, whereas others may talk about being "turned on" and "feeling excited" and describe a more subjective picture not necessarily focused on the genitals. Interestingly, the DSM-III-R described arousal as either an impaired genital response or lack of a subjective sense of sexual excitement [5], with the latter portion of the definition excluded in the DSM-IV. Consequently, most recent epidemiological studies have focused on the physical genital response in assessing the prevalence of arousal problems, showing a steep increase with age and menopause attributable to hormonal and vascular changes [6].

Janssen and colleagues state that arousal can be described by two components in which the mind's processing of sexual stimuli is of importance: (1) conscious and unconscious processing leading to an automatic genital response and (2) a cognitive process appraising the sexual content of the stimulus [7, 8]. Based on these observations, FSAD can be described as both a diminished genital response and/or a lack of appraisal of the response in the genitalia and absence of a reaction to sexual stimuli.

In 2003, Basson et al. suggested a new classification of FSAD including (1) genital sexual arousal disorder, with a focus on the genital response; (2) subjective arousal disorder, with a focus on the woman having absent or diminished feelings of sexual arousal (excitement or pleasure), even though the genital response is intact; and (3) combined sexual arousal disorder including difficulties in both genital and subjective arousal [9]. These definitions encompass a broad group of women. Genital FSAD would embrace women with a clear genital impairment such as postmenopausal women and women with adverse effects stemming from antihormonal treatment after breast cancer or after radiation therapy or surgery involving the pelvic floor. The subjective FSAD would include women that might have problems with recognizing, processing, or appraising their genital response, consequently with a lack of subjective excitement, and the combined definition would encompass women with problems in both domains. However, the suggested classifications were not incorporated into any broadly applied diagnostic systems. Instead, in the recent changes in the DSM-5, a new disorder was created, female sexual interest/arousal disorder (FSAID) [1, 4], which has led to significant debate [10–12]. One of the major drawbacks of the FSAID definition is that women with a predominantly genital arousal disorder, such as that resulting from antihormonal treatment or pelvic radiation therapy, but with intact desire (spontaneous or receptive) would not be diagnosed with FSAID despite their problem stemming from a lack of arousal.

There is evidence that, especially for women, genital sexual arousal responses do not always coincide with the subjective experience of being aroused and "turned on" and that the women's experience may be based more on the interpretation of the situation than on the genital response [13, 14]. Thus, for some women, the objective and subjective aspects of arousal do not coincide. As such, are arousal problems in women without any evident impairment of genital response due to an inability to identify sexual cues from their genitals as suggested by Barlow et al. and not a lack of genital response [15]? There is likely more than one answer—some women may have a genital impairment, whereas others may have normal genital response but do not recognize it as they are more focused on the lack of subjective arousal. Alternatively, some women may not receive sufficient sexual stimuli or do not fully perceive the stimuli they receive.

In the post-phosphodiesterase 5 inhibitor (PDE5i) era, several studies have investigated the possible beneficial effect of PDE5i's for women with FSAD alone or combined with desire or orgasmic disorders [16]. The majority of these studies showed that while PDE5i's increase both vaginal and clitoral blood flow along with vaginal lubrication, they do not, in a majority of the studies, improve female sexual function significantly when compared with placebo. This may reflect the fact that most studies evaluated premenopausal women, in whom the genital response is unlikely to be impaired, and the complaints were better accounted for by a "subjective FSAD" or the fact that even though the women had an increased genital arousal, whether or not they perceived it, it did not alter their phenomenological or subjective sense of arousal. For them, unlike many men using the same drugs, increased vasocongestion did not correlate with an increased sense of erotic arousal.

So what are the clinical and research implications? First, we need to specify what we mean when we talk about FSAD, both as researchers and clinicians. Is it objective or subjective arousal or a combination? Different disciplines may focus on different aspects of FSAD, which will have implications for how we approach the problem and which questions we apply to research, diagnosis, and defining individualized treatments. An ongoing debate about the definition of FSAD is necessary, not only to clarify the diagnostic criteria, which will help identify affected women, but ultimately to benefit all the women who are candidates for treatment and who are currently overlooked. With our female patients, we need to explore how women define arousal and how they individually interpret it.

A better understanding of FSAD will also have implications for treatment choice. Some studies have shown beneficial effects of PDE5i's in women where it is more likely that there is a biologically determined genital component of dysfunction, such as women with spinal cord injury (for a review, see [16]) or the many postmenopausal women in whom estrogen treatment relieves the symptoms of genital FSAD [16–18]. On the other hand, women with subjective FSAD may benefit from approaches that help focus the woman's attention on an increased genital response. The studies from Brotto have shown that mindfulness training that focuses on recognizing what is happening in the body found a positive effect on self-assessed genital wetness despite little or no change in actual physiological arousal and a marginally significant improvement in subjective and self-reported physical arousal during an erotic stimulus [19]. Other studies have shown that distraction is associated with lower levels of genital arousal [20]. An interesting new pharmacological concept is to develop pharmacological treatment that enhances both the genital response using a PDE5i and the sensitivity to recognize the sexual cue from the genitals using testosterone, as described by Poels et al. [21]. Both the pharmacological as well as the psychotherapeutic treatments need to be further investigated to better define efficacy and the group of patients who may benefit from these approaches.

In conclusion, arousal is not just arousal and may be perceived differently by individual women, clinicians, and researchers. Furthermore, the definitions of arousal disorders have changed with every new version of the DSM, with the focus shifting between genital and subjective aspects. Our continued clinical and research experiences continuously drive the development of a better understanding of pathologic mechanisms and subsequent treatment modalities, integrating medical and psychotherapeutic approaches.

References

1. American Psychiatric Association. Diagnostic and statistical manual of mental disorders. DSM-III-R. 3rd ed. Washington, DC: American Psychiatric Press; 1987.
2. Giraldi A, et al. Female sexual arousal disorders: review. J Sex Med. 2013;10(1):58–73.
3. World Health Organisation. International statistical classification of diseases and health related problems (ICD-10); 1992.
4. Diagnostic and statistical manual of mental disorders. DSM-5. 5th ed. Washington, DC: American Psychiatric Publishing; 2015.

5. American Psychiatric Association. Diagnostic and statistical manual of mental disorders. DSM-IV-TR. 4th ed. Washington, DC: American Psychiatric Press; 2000.
6. Hayes R, Dennerstein L. The impact of aging on sexual function and sexual dysfunction in women: a review of population-based studies. J Sex Med. 2005;2(3):317–30.
7. Janssen E, et al. Automatic processes and the appraisal of sexual stimuli: toward an information processing model of sexual arousal. J Sex Res. 2000;37(1):8–23.
8. Spiering M, Everaerd W, Janssen E. Priming the sexual system: implicit versus explicit activation. J Sex Res. 2003;40(2):134–45.
9. Basson R, et al. Definitions of women's sexual dysfunction reconsidered: advocating expansion and revision. J Psychosom Obstet Gynaecol. 2003;24(4):221–9.
10. Graham CA, Brotto LA, Zucker KJ. Response to Balon and Clayton (2014): female sexual interest/arousal disorder is a diagnosis more on firm ground than thin air. Arch Sex Behav. 2014;43(7):1231–4.
11. DeRogatis LR, et al. Should sexual desire and arousal disorders in women be merged? Arch Sex Behav. 2011;40(2):217–9.
12. Clayton AH, et al. Intended or unintended consequences? The likely implications of raising the bar for sexual dysfunction diagnosis in the proposed DSM-V revisions: 2. For women with loss of subjective sexual arousal. J Sex Med. 2012;9(8):2040–6.
13. Laan E, van Driel EM, van Lunsen RH. Genital responsiveness in healthy women with and without sexual arousal disorder. J Sex Med. 2008;5(6):1424–35.
14. Chivers ML, et al. A sex difference in the specificity of sexual arousal. Psychol Sci. 2004;15(11):736–44.
15. Barlow DH. Causes of sexual dysfunction: the role of anxiety and cognitive interference. J Consult Clin Psychol. 1986;54(2):140–8.
16. Chivers ML, Rosen RC. Phosphodiesterase type 5 inhibitors and female sexual response: faulty protocols or paradigms? J Sex Med. 2010;7(2 Pt 2):858–72.
17. Suckling J, Lethaby A, Kennedy R. Local oestrogen for vaginal atrophy in postmenopausal women. Cochrane Database Syst Rev 2003;4:CD001500.
18. Basson R. Pharmacotherapy for women's sexual dysfunction. Expert Opin Pharmacother. 2009;10(10):1631–48.
19. Brotto LA, Basson R, Luria M. A mindfulness-based group psychoeducational intervention targeting sexual arousal disorder in women. J Sex Med. 2008;5(7):1646–59.
20. Salemink E, van Lankveld JJ. The effects of increasing neutral distraction on sexual responding of women with and without sexual problems. Arch Sex Behav. 2006;35(2):179–90.
21. Poels S, et al. Toward personalized sexual medicine (part 2): testosterone combined with a PDE5 inhibitor increases sexual satisfaction in women with HSDD and FSAD, and a low sensitive system for sexual cues. J Sex Med. 2013;10(3):810–23.

Diagnosis and Management of Female Orgasmic Disorder

23

Seth D. Cohen and Irwin Goldstein

23.1 Introduction

Orgasm is a sensation of intense pleasure creating an altered consciousness state accompanied by pelvic striated circumvaginal musculature and uterine contractions that induces a state of well-being and contentment [1]. Women's orgasms can be prompted by erotic stimulation of a variety of genital and nongenital sites. The clitoris and vagina are the most common sites, although stimulation of the periurethral tissues (G-spot), breast/nipple, mental imagery, or fantasy may also induce orgasm [2]. Female orgasms can be achieved with mechanical stimulation of the vagina alone, with direct stimulation of the external clitoris or using a combination of both maneuvers.

To date, no definitive orgasm triggers exist. Initial studies looking to define brain anatomy during orgasm used brain imaging techniques including positron emission tomography (PET) coupled with magnetic resonance imaging (MRI) [3, 4]. Increased activation at orgasm, compared to pre-orgasm arousal, has been observed in the paraventricular nucleus (PVN) of the hypothalamus, periaqueductal gray area of the midbrain, hippocampus, and cerebellum [5].

Orgasm can occur in response to imagery in the absence of physical stimulation. A study to determine whether the subjective report of imagery-induced orgasm is accompanied by physiological and perceptual events that are characteristic of genitally stimulated orgasm included women who claimed that they could experience orgasm using imagery alone [5]. Orgasm from self-induced imagery or genital self-stimulation resulted in significant increases in systolic blood pressure, heart rate, pupil diameter, pain detection threshold, and pain tolerance threshold over resting control conditions [1]. These findings provide evidence that orgasm from self-induced imagery and genital self-stimulation can result in significant sympathetic activation and increases in pain thresholds. Additional studies comparing brain regions activated by orgasm with those activated during sexual arousal without orgasm are needed to determine which brain regions are specifically responsible for triggering orgasm in women.

Some women, however, do not reach orgasm despite having different partners and using different modes of stimulation [6]. These women are the focus of this chapter.

S.D. Cohen, M.D., M.P.H.
Advanced Urological Care, New York, NY, USA

I. Goldstein, M.D. (✉)
San Diego Sexual Medicine, San Diego, CA, USA
e-mail: dr.irwingoldstein@comcast.net

L.I. Lipshultz et al. (eds.), *Management of Sexual Dysfunction in Men and Women*, DOI 10.1007/978-1-4939-3100-2_23

23.2 Female Orgasmic Disorder

Several definitions of female orgasmic disorders (FOD) have been proposed. The Diagnostic and Statistical Manual of Mental Disorders, 4th Edition, Text Revision (DSM-IV-TR) defines female orgasmic disorder as a persistent or recurrent delay in, or absence of, orgasm following normal sexual excitement that causes marked distress [7]. An international classification committee sponsored by the American Urological Association defined FOD as either a lack of orgasm, markedly diminished intensity of orgasmic sensations, or marked delay of orgasm from any kind of stimulation, despite the self-report of high sexual arousal/excitement [8]. Central for all definitions of female orgasmic disorder, including the recent DSM 5, is a difficulty in achieving orgasm, substantially decreased intensity of orgasm, or both [9]. As for the diagnosis of FOD, one or both of the following should be present 75–100 % of the time: absence, infrequency, or delay of orgasm and/or reduced intensity of said orgasm.

Currently, epidemiologic data on the potential impact of orgasmic disorders on interpersonal relationships and quality of life are relatively scant. Classic descriptions of FOD have observed a prevalence of 22–24 % in the general adult female population and 26–28 % in females 20–40 years old [10]. Molina et al. [11] surveyed a sample of women from Mexico City using an online questionnaire. Women between 18 and 40 years old were selected, and the orgasm domain from the Female Sexual Function Index was used to identify FOD, with a prevalence of 18 % observed. Univariate and multivariate analyses examined the relationship between potential risk factors and sexual function. Univariate analysis identified younger age, lower degree of education, single marital status, and dissatisfaction with the thickness and/or size of partner's penis as significant variables related to FOD [7]. Fugl-Meyer et al. compared female sexual dysfunction and personal distress, looking more specifically at associations with sociodemographics and level of sexual well-being. The subjects were a nationally representative sample of sexually active Swedish women ($n = 1056$) 18–65 years old who participated in a combined structured interview/questionnaire investigation. The authors concluded that three factors—sexual desire, orgasm, and genital function—were powerful classifiers of the level of sexual well-being [2].

Findings from the National Social and Health Life Survey suggest that FOD is the second most frequently reported sexual problem in women [12]. In this random sample of women, 24 % reported a lack of orgasm in the past year for at least several months. Although these data are supported by other studies, a precise estimate of the incidence of orgasmic disorder in women is difficult to determine given the lack of well-controlled studies.

23.3 Etiology

While the etiology of FOD remains uncertain, literature has identified multiple risk factors related to FOD including psychological, physiological, sociodemographic, hereditary, and comorbid medical conditions. Vascular disease, chronic diseases, diabetes, multiple sclerosis, spinal cord injury, and pelvic conditions can all exacerbate symptoms of FOD. In addition, medications such as selective serotonin reuptake inhibitors (SSRIs), antipsychotics, mood stabilizers, cardiovascular medications, chemotherapy agents, and antihypertensives can all negatively impact orgasmic potential. SSRIs, most commonly used as antidepressants, are well known to have a negative impact on orgasmic function, with approximately 31–57 % of women taking SSRIs reporting delay or inhibition of orgasm [13, 14].

Multiple psychological conditions can interfere with a woman's ability to reach orgasm. Such conditions include, but are not limited to, anxiety, depression, attention deficit disorder, body image disorders, sexual abuse, and negative religious views on sex [15]. Because multiple factors can affect orgasmic potential, it is important to assess each patient using a biopsychosocial approach (Fig. 23.1). Lastly, there is some early evidence supporting a genetic influence on the ability to reach orgasm, with an estimated heritability variation of 34 % for difficulty reaching orgasm

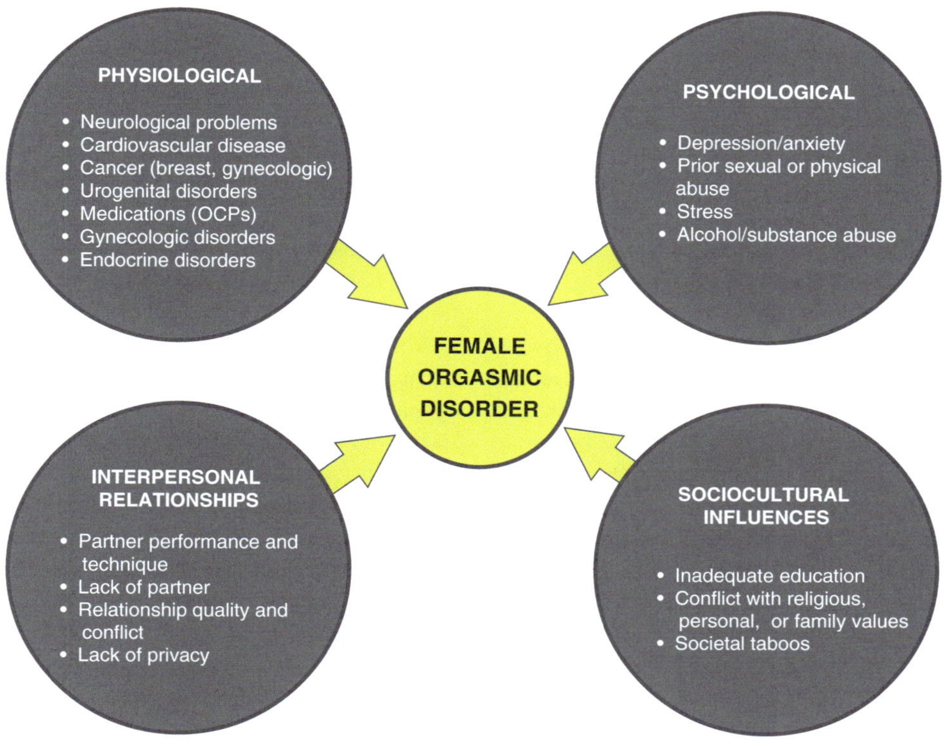

Fig. 23.1 Evaluation and treatment of female orgasmic disorder. Modified from Parish SJ. From whence comes HSDD? J Fam Pract. 2009 Jul;58(7 Suppl Hypoactive):S16–21 [16]

during sexual intercourse and 45 % for difficulty reaching orgasm with masturbation [17].

23.4 Assessment

An important concept in the assessment and treatment of FOD is the relatively common occurrence of other concurrent sexual dysfunctions [18]. It is estimated that among women with FOD, 31 % also reported difficulties with sexual arousal, 18 % with lubrication, 14 % with desire, 12 % with pain, and 0.9 % with vaginismus [19]. Because of this high level of comorbidity, it is often hard to determine risk factors and treatment regimens tailored specifically to FOD. It also means that most women will present with a complex combination of sexual dysfunctions, requiring a comprehensive assessment that takes into consideration other relevant biopsychosocial factors [15].

It is important to rule out insufficient and/or inadequate stimulation before assigning an FOD diagnosis. For example, case studies and quantitative empirical studies have indicated that women in relationships in which male partners have erectile dysfunction and/or premature ejaculation are likely to experience difficulties with reaching orgasm. The orgasm problem may have started as a lack of adequate stimulation, although a careful assessment is needed to identify whether other maintenance factors have developed with time [17].

Despite the fact that female urologists and urogynecologists are in a unique position to understand the anatomy and physiology of the genitalia and pelvic floor, sexual medicine issues are often highly complex and are generally secondary to interrelated psychological, physiological, and relationship issues intertwined with distinct couple dynamics. Thus, a thorough medical history is vital in the assessment of

FOD. In most cases, women with sexual health concerns should consider undergoing concomitant psychological and physical therapy assessment and management by an appropriately trained specialist [20].

23.5 Psychosocial/Sexual Assessment/History

The clinician should screen all patients for obvious psychopathology that can impact the treatment algorithm for FOD (Fig. 23.1). The presence of current or previously treated psychiatric symptoms should be assessed, as these symptoms may be related to the sexual disorder. Having this information will help guide the clinician in defining goals and boundaries for the patient.

23.6 Physical Examination

The physical examination for a woman with orgasmic concerns should be tailored to the individual patient. If a woman with orgasmic problems is under the age of 50 and has sexual pain, a careful physical examination should evaluate for the presence of hormonally mediated vestibulodypnia vs. neuroproliferative vestibulodynia [21, 22]. Similar orgasmic complaints in a woman over 50 years of age should assess for the presence of vaginal atrophy with dryness, loss of rugae, mucosal thinning, pale hue, and lack of shiny vaginal secretions, all indications of a menopausal hormonal status.

Patient consent to examination is particularly important. It is vital that the patient is aware of the purpose of the exam and understands that she has the final authority to terminate the physical examination, to ask questions, to have control over who is in attendance, and to understand the extent of the assessment. Inclusion of the sexual partner, with permission of the patient, is advantageous and provides needed patient support. Allowing the patient to observe any pathology via digital photography is often therapeutic, allowing, for the first time in many cases, an illustration and connection of a detected physical abnormality with the sexual health problem. If a genital sexual pain history exists, the patient should point with her finger to the location/s of the discomfort during the physical examination.

Normal function of the pelvic floor musculature is essential in maintaining appropriate sexual function. Both "low-tone pelvic floor dysfunction" and "high-tone pelvic floor muscle dysfunction" can be closely associated with women's sexual health concerns [23]. Hypotonus of the pelvic floor muscles, secondary to childbirth, trauma, and/or aging, is related to urinary incontinence during orgasm, vaginal laxity, and/or thrusting dyspareunia secondary to pelvic organ prolapse. Hypertonus of the pelvic floor secondary to childbirth, postural stressors, micro-trauma, infection, adhesions, and surgical trauma can contribute to symptoms of urinary retention, reduced force of stream, dysuria, urgency, penetrative dyspareunia, and/or vaginismus.

23.7 Laboratory Testing

There is no consensus on recommended routine laboratory tests for the evaluation of women with sexual orgasmic health concerns. Blood testing should be dictated by clinical suspicion, particularly based on the results of the history and physical examination. If appropriate, the clinician may assess serum hormone levels including total testosterone, free testosterone, sex hormone-binding globulin (SHBG), dihydrotestosterone (DHT), estradiol, and progesterone. Pituitary function may be measured by obtaining luteinizing hormone (LH), follicle-stimulating hormone (FSH), and prolactin levels. Thyroid stimulating hormone (TSH) should be measured to exclude subclinical thyroid disease [24, 25].

23.8 Diagnosis

The diagnosis of female orgasmic dysfunction should be based on the clinician's judgment that the woman's orgasmic capacity is less than would be reasonable for her age, sexual experience, and the adequacy of sexual stimulation she receives [1]. Studies of women diagnosed with FOD note a high percentage, and these women are also diagnosed with concomitant female sexual arousal disorder. Regarding women who can achieve orgasm during masturbation or during intercourse with manual stimulation but not during intercourse alone, the clinical consensus is that those women do not meet criteria for diagnosis of FOD [1].

23.9 Treatment

23.9.1 Cognitive and Behavioral Techniques

In cases where orgasm problems are acquired or manifest themselves only during partnered sex, the partner should be involved in the assessment and treatment or at least included in the communication training related to sexual problems.

The treatment of anorgasmia has been approached from many different perspectives including psychoanalytic, cognitive behavioral, and pharmacological, but substantial research is available only for cognitive behavioral therapies [26]. Cognitive behavioral therapy for anorgasmia focuses on promoting changes in attitudes and sexually relevant thoughts, decreasing anxiety, and increasing orgasmic ability and satisfaction. Behavioral exercises traditionally prescribed to induce these changes include directed masturbation (DM), sensate focus (SF), and systematic desensitization [1]. Sex education, communication skills training, and Kegel exercises are also often included in cognitive behavioral treatment programs for anorgasmia [1].

Among the different cognitive and behavioral techniques, directed masturbation (DM) training is the approach that is strongly recommended with Grade A evidentiary support by the Consensus of the International Society for Sexual Medicine [27]. DM training is a behavioral technique, consisting of 4–16 weekly therapy sessions of graded exposure to genital stimulation. This can include role-playing orgasm response, use of sexual fantasy, and/or vibrators to facilitate heightened arousal and orgasm [17]. It is highly effective based on findings in the literature; of the eight randomized controlled trials that compared DM with no treatment, only one study failed to show efficacy for the active treatment arm [28]. The success rates for DM in women with primary anorgasmia are high: 60–90 % of the women become orgasmic with masturbation and 33–85 % will become orgasmic with a partner-involved sexual activity. Some studies have shown significant results after four sessions of 30 min, while other studies demonstrated that beneficial effects extended up to 2 months after the end of therapy [29, 30].

Anxiety can cause significant disturbance that disrupts the processing of erotic pleasure by causing the woman to focus instead on lack of performance, embarrassment, and/or guilt. As originally described by Masters and Johnson, sensate focus (SF) is an anxiety-reducing technique that involves a stepwise sequence of body touching maneuvers, moving from nonsexual to increasingly sexual touching of a partner's body [31]. Initial assessments of this approach showed promising results [29], but later studies have not demonstrated sustained, significant benefit at follow-up [30]. However, across all comparison-controlled studies, DM plus SF has proven to be more effective than DM alone [32].

23.9.2 Hormone Supplementation

Although no androgen therapies are currently approved by the Food and Drug Administration (FDA) for FOD, several are used in clinical practice. Androgens play an important role in healthy female sexual function, especially in stimulating sexual interest and in maintaining desire. Androgens are also vital for the health and maintenance of vaginal tissues including the vulva, vestibule, and vagina. A number of studies have shown that different types of androgen treatments can have beneficial effects on FOD. In one study of 300 women who received bilateral salpingo-oophorectomy and hysterectomy, a 300 mg of testosterone patch showed improvements in FOD symptoms [33]. In another study, 10 mg of testosterone gel showed similar positive effects on orgasm improvement in women [34].

23.9.3 Nonhormonal Supplementation

Currently there are no FDA-approved nonhormonal medications for treatment of FOD. However, there are medications used in an off-label fashion that have shown promising results when used in properly selected patients.

23.10 PDE-5 Inhibitors

Among the numerous strategies proposed for managing sexual dysfunction associated with SSRI treatment, phosphodiesterase type 5 inhibitors (PDE5is) have the best data to support broad-based and clinically meaningful treatment efficacy [35]. One randomized controlled study evaluated the efficacy of sildenafil for sexual dysfunction associated with selective and nonselective serotonin reuptake inhibitors in women [36]. The authors were able to show beneficial effects of PDE5is in the setting of adverse side effects of SSRI use on orgasm. Another study with no control groups observed similar positive effects of PDE5is for FOD induced by antidepressants [37]. Further research on the efficacy of PDE5is on orgasmic function is needed to better define the effects on female orgasmic improvement.

Bupropion, which is a noradrenaline and dopamine reuptake inhibitor with nicotinic antagonist properties originally marketed as an antidepressant, may have a beneficial effect on woman with FOD [38, 39]. In a placebo-controlled trial [38], the changes in sexual functioning questionnaire indicated that bupropion had significant effects on increasing measures of sexual arousal, orgasm completion, and sexual satisfaction. Traditional bupropion dosing starts at 150 mg twice a day, although low-dose bupropion at 75 mg twice a day can achieve an optimal improvement in sexual arousal potential as well.

Other dopaminergic medications used in the treatment of orgasmic dysfunction include cabergoline, administered at 0.5 mg up to three times per week, and ropinirole 0.25 mg administered daily, both of which can improve orgasmic potential [35]. Oxytocin lozenges, linked to improved arousal, desire, and orgasm, are administered at 250 IU sublingually 30 min to one hour before sexual activity. Research with oxytocin has shown marked improvement in a number of components of sexual function, including libido and orgasm [40]. Amphetamines such as dextroamphetamine and other drugs used to treat attention deficit disorder have been useful in helping women concentrate and thus improve orgasmic potential and intensity [41]. All these treatments have been trialed on small numbers of patients with no control groups, and larger, more definitive studies are needed to truly define the effects.

23.11 Conclusion

Sexual problems are widespread in society and are influenced by both health-related and psychosocial factors. The role of the latter implies that stress-inducing events, due to either individual or social sources, can affect sexual functioning in both men and women. Due to the high level of comorbidity with other sexual disorders, most women will present with a complex combination of problems, requiring a comprehensive assessment that takes into consideration the known correlates of FOD.

In the assessment and treatment of FOD, a thorough biopsychosocial history should be taken including assessing adequacy, variety, and amount of preferred sexual stimulation, specifically inquiring about known psychosocial, cognitive/affective, and relationship factors found to be related to FOD. The diagnosis of female orgasmic disorder should be based on the clinician's judgment that the woman's orgasmic capacity is less than would be reasonable for her age, sexual experience, and the adequacy of sexual stimulation she receives. A medical history including the use of medications known to interfere with orgasmic function is recommended.

The treatment of anorgasmia has been approached from cognitive behavioral therapy and pharmacological perspectives, but substantial empirical outcome research is available only for cognitive behavioral treatment methods. Treatment of FOD should include directed masturbation, which has shown well-established efficacy in several different treatment formats with sensate focus as a useful adjunct. A thorough understanding of the risks and benefits of hormonal and nonhormonal treatments should be discussed with the patient before initiation.

References

1. Meston CM, Hull E, Levin RJ, Sipski M. Disorders of orgasm in women. J Sex Med. 2004;1(1):66–8.
2. Levin RJ. The mechanisms of human female sexual arousal. Ann Rev Sex Res. 1992;3:1–48.
3. Whipple B, Komisaruk BR. Brain (PET) responses to vaginal-cervical self-stimulation in women with complete spinal cord injury: preliminary findings. J Sex Marital Ther. 2002;28:79–86.
4. Komisaruk BR, Whipple B, Crawford A, Grimes S, Kalnin AJ, Mosier K, Liu WC, Harkness B. Brain activity (fMRI and PET) during orgasm in women, in response to vaginocervical self-stimulation. Abst Soc Neurosci. 2002;841:17.
5. Whipple B, Ogden G, Komisaruk BR. Physiological correlates of imagery-induced orgasm in women. Arch Sex Behav. 1992;21(2):121–33.
6. Jannini EA, Whipple B, Kingsberg SA, Buisson O, Foldès P, Vardi Y. Who's afraid of the G-spot? J Sex Med. 2010;7:25–34.
7. American Psychiatric Association. Diagnostic and statistical manual of mental disorders. 4th ed. Arlington, VA: American Psychiatric Association; 1994.
8. Basson R, Leiblum S, Brotto L, Derogatis L, Fourcroy J, Fugl-Meyer K, Graziottin A, Heiman JR, Laan E, Meston C, Schover L, van Lankveld J, Schultz WW. Definitions of women's sexual dysfunction reconsidered: advocating expansion and revision. J Psychosom Obstet Gynaecol. 2003;24:221–9.
9. American Psychiatric Association. Diagnostic and statistical manual of mental disorders. 5th ed. Arlington, VA: American Psychiatric Association; 2013. p. 429–32.
10. Laumann EO, Paik A, Rosen RC. Sexual dysfunction in the United States: prevalence and predictors. JAMA. 1999;281:537–44.
11. Villeda Sandoval CI, Calao-Pérez M, Enríquez González AB, Gonzalez-Cuenca E, Ibarra-Saavedra R, Sotomayor M, Castillejos Molina RA. Orgasmic dysfunction: prevalence and risk factors from cohort of young females in Mexico. J Sex Med. 2014; 11(6):1505–11.
12. Laumann EO, Gagnon JH, Michael RT, Michaels S. The social organization of sexuality: sexual practices in the United States. Chicago: University of Chicago Press; 1994.
13. Montejo-Gonzalez AL, Llorca G, Izquierdo JA, Ledesma A, Bousono M, Calcedo A, Carrasco JL, Ciudad J, Daniel E, Dela Gandara J, Derecho J, Franco M, Gomez MJ, Macias JA, Martin T, Perez V, Sanchez JM, Sanchez S, Vicens E. SSRI induced sexual dysfunction: fluoxetine, paroxetine, sertraline, and fluvoxamine in a prospective, multicenter, and descriptive clinical study of 344 patients. J Sex Marital Ther. 1997;23:176–94.
14. Clayton AH, Balon R. The impact of mental illness and psychotropic medications on sexual functioning: the evidence and management. J Sex Med. 2009;6:1200–11.
15. Laan E, Rellini AH, Barnes TJ. Standard operating procedures for female orgasmic disorder: consensus of the international society for sexual medicine. J Sex Med. 2013;10(1):74–82.
16. Parish SJ. From whence comes HSDD? J Fam Pract. 2009;58(Suppl 7 Hypoactive):S16–21.
17. Dunn KM, Cherkas LF, Spector TD. Genetic influences on variation in female orgasmic function: a twin study. Biol Lett. 2005;1:260–3.
18. Segraves KB, Segraves RT. Hypoactive sexual desire disorder: prevalence and comorbidity in 906 subjects. J Sex Marital Ther. 1991;17:55–8.
19. Nobre PJ, Pinto-Gouveia J, Gomes FA. Prevalence and comorbidity of sexual dysfunctions in a Portuguese clinical sample. J Sex Marital Ther. 2006;32:173–82.
20. Levine SB. The first principle of clinical sexuality. J Sex Med. 2007;4(4 Pt 1):853–4.
21. Landry T, Bergeron S. How young does vulvo-vaginal pain begin? Prevalence and characteristics of dyspareunia in adolescents. J Sex Med. 2009;6:927–35.
22. Goldstein AT, Burrows L. Vulvodynia. J Sex Med. 2008;5:5–14.
23. Rosenbaum TY. Pelvic floor involvement in male and female sexual dysfunction and the role of pelvic floor rehabilitation in treatment: a literature review. J Sex Med. 2007;4(1):4–13.
24. Pasquali D, Maiorino MI, Renzullo A, Bellastella G, Accardo G, Esposito D, Barbato F, Esposito K. Female sexual dysfunction in women with thyroid disorders. J Endocrinol Invest. 2013;36(9):729–33. doi:10.3275/8933 (Epub 2013 Apr 12).
25. Ishak WW, Bokarius A, Jeffrey JK, Davis MC, Bakhta Y. Disorders of orgasm in women: a literature review of etiology and current treatments. J Sex Med. 2010;7(10):3254–68.
26. Fugl-Meyer KS, Oberg K, Lundberg PO, Lewin B, Fugl-Meyer A. On orgasm, sexual techniques, and erotic perceptions in 18- to 74-year-old Swedish women. J Sex Med. 2006;3:56–68.
27. Whipple B. Report of the international consensus development conference on female sexual dysfunction: definitions and classifications. J Urol. 2000;163: 888–93.
28. Ter Kuile MM, Both S, van Lankveld JJDM. Sexual dysfunctions in women. In: Sturmey P, Hersen M, editors. Handbook of evidence-based practice in clinical psychology. Volume II: Adult disorders. New York: Wiley.

29. Heinrich AG. The effect of group and self-directed behavioral-education treatment of primary orgasmic dysfunction in females treated without their partners. Ph.D. dissertation, University of Colorado, Boulder, CO; 1976.
30. Heiman JR. Psychologic treatments for female sexual dysfunction: are they effective and do we need them? Arch Sex Behav. 2002;31:445–50.
31. Masters W, Johnson V. Human sexual inadequacy. Boston: Little Brown; 1970.
32. Heiman JR, Meston CM. Empirically validated treatment for sexual dysfunction. Annu Rev Sex Res. 1997;8:148–94.
33. Braunstein GD, Sundwall DA, Katz M, Shifren JL, Buster JE, Simon JA, Bachman G, Aguirre OA, Lucas JD, Rodenberg C, Buch A, Watts NB. Safety and efficacy of a testosterone patch for the treatment of hypoactive sexual desire disorder in surgically menopausal women: a randomized, placebo-controlled trial. Arch Intern Med. 2005;165:1582–9.
34. Davis SR, Moreau M, Kroll R, Bouchard C, Panay N, Gass M, Braunstein GD, Hirschberg AL, Rodenberg C, Pack S, Koch H, Moufarege A, Studd J. Testosterone for low libido in postmenopausal women not taking estrogen. N Engl J Med. 2008;359:2005–17.
35. Rudkin L, Taylor MJ, Hawton K. Strategies for managing sexual dysfunction induced by antidepressant medication. Cochrane Database Syst Rev. 2013;5, CD003382. doi:10.1002/14651858.CD003382.pub3.
36. Nurnberg HG, Hensley PL, Heiman JR, Croft HA, Debattista C, Paine S. Sildenafil treatment of women with antidepressant associated sexual dysfunction: a randomized controlled trial. JAMA. 2008;300: 395–404.
37. Nurnberg HG, Hensley PL, Lauriello J, Parker LM, Keith SJ. Sildenafil for women patients with antidepressant-induced sexual dysfunction. Psychiatr Serv. 1999;50:1076–8.
38. Clayton AH, Warnock JK, Kornstein SG, et al. A placebo-controlled trial of bupropion SR as an antidote for selective serotonin reuptake inhibitor-induced sexual dysfunction. J Clin Psychiatry. 2004;65:62–7.
39. Segraves RT, Clayton A, Croft H, Wolf A, Warnock J. Bupropion sustained release for the treatment of hypoactive sexual desire disorder in premenopausal women. J Clin Psychopharmacol. 2004;24:339–42.
40. MacDonald K, Feifel D. Dramatic improvement in sexual function induced by intranasal oxytocin. J Sex Med. 2012;9:1407–10.
41. Winland C, Haycox C, Bolton JL. Methamphetamine enhances sexual behavior in female rats. Pharmacol Biochem Behav. 2011;98(4):575–82.

Commentary: Diagnosis and Management of Female Orgasmic Disorder

Annamaria Giraldi

Progress in sexual medicine has led to an improved understanding of female orgasm, with current work being able to discern areas of the brain activated and suppressed during experience of this phenomenon. Other seminal work has defined some of the factors that facilitate orgasm, yet a complete understanding of female orgasm eludes medical science. Twenty-first century science primarily attempts to deconstruct orgasm into its individual parts and demonstrate its physiologic basis. While crucial to a thorough understanding of orgasm, such a piecemeal approach often misses the holistic perspective that needs to be considered when looking at orgasm as a whole. Similarly, the etiologies of female orgasmic disorder (FOD) are incompletely understood, leading to treatments with incomplete efficacy.

In the preceding chapter, Cohen and Goldstein provide a comprehensive overview of FOD, from epidemiology to a thorough discussion of treatment options, including cognitive behavioral approaches as well as pharmacotherapy. At the end of the chapter, the reader is left with an excellent understanding of what the current state of the art in the approach to FOD provides, which is significant. In the following commentary, a broader perspective on what orgasm is and what it means to women and their male partners is considered, uniting the approach to orgasmic disorders with a perspective on the meaning of orgasm.

The Editors

Annamaria Giraldi, M.D., Ph.D., F.E.C.S.M.
Sexological Clinic, Psychiatric Center Copenhagen, Institute of Clinical Medicine, University of Copenhagen, Copenhagen, Denmark

Commentary

In 1966 Masters and Johnson, in their landmark book *Human Sexual Response*, described the human female orgasm as a "psychophysiologic experience occurring within, and made meaningful by, a context of psychosocial influence" and as a "drive of biologic-behavioral origin deeply integrated into the condition of human existence" [1]. Orgasm has also been described as "a sensation of intense pleasure accompanied by an alteration in consciousness, contraction of the genitourinary musculature, and in some cases involuntary vocalization" [2].

Humans are one of few species (the others are chimpanzees, bonobos, and dolphins) who have heterosexual activity when the female partner is not in estrus [3], meaning that sexual activity has a recreational purpose in addition to its reproductive purpose. Sex represents an intimate bond with the partner and creates physical pleasure, which for many is an important aspect of sexual satisfaction [4].

It has been claimed that the woman's orgasm plays a role in facilitating sperm transportation into the uterus. However, this hypothesis is not supported by the literature [5], and there is agreement that orgasm is not essential for fertility or achievement of pregnancy (for a review, see [6]). Focus has also been placed on the pleasure of orgasm, and studies have shown that prolactin and oxytocin peak during orgasm, leading to an overall sense of well-being. It has been speculated that the major effect of prolactin is sexual satiety. However, the capability of women to have multiple orgasms, despite a low postorgasmic prolactin level, contradicts this hypothesis (for a review, see [6]). The role of oxytocin has historically attracted a lot of attention. Oxytocin may be involved in the feeling of well-being, improved social intentions and trust, affiliative behavior, and fear reduction [7, 8], all effects that may facilitate bonding with the sexual partner and a desire for further sexual activity and orgasm. In a study by Behnia et al., intranasal oxytocin resulted in women feeling more relaxed and a subgroup of women expressed better ability to share sexual desire and empathize with their partners compared with the placebo group [9]. Hence, an important function of the female orgasm is related to the dynamic with the partner. In a study by Salisbury et al., men and women were interviewed about their beliefs, experiences, and concerns regarding female orgasm in heterosexual relationships. The women expressed that orgasm was a "bonus," but for some of them, the most important component of sex was intimacy with their partners, not reaching orgasm every time. However, they also expressed that the female orgasm was important for the male partner's ego and sense of himself as a competent lover, being "able to give her an orgasm." Male partners expressed that he would become distressed if the female partner did not reach orgasm, given that male partners worried about their female partners' pleasure. Furthermore, the men felt that the female partners' orgasms were extremely sexually satisfying and important for the men's sexual pleasure and that it was important that the female partners be communicated when they did not reach orgasm [10]. These findings emphasize the dynamic within the couple; orgasm is satisfying for the individual woman but also has a direct positive impact on the male partner's sexuality and pleasure.

The physical and emotional well-being, as well as dyadic importance related to orgasms, explains why many women with orgasmic disorders express significant distress related to their condition. In a study by Kingsberg et al., 92 % of women with difficulties in reaching orgasm were bothered to some degree by the condition. Sixty-eight percent claimed they were very or extremely bothered, and 46 % described feeling frustrated [11], indicating that even though intimacy is important for women, lack of orgasm is a distressing condition.

The ability to reach orgasm may be influenced by many biopsychosocial factors (for a review, see [12]). Interestingly, studies have indicated that in addition to the effects of hormonal imbalances, medical conditions, and pharmacological treatments (i.e., with psychotropic medications) on women's orgasmic function, genetic factors influence the ability of women to reach orgasm, both during intercourse and when masturbating [13, 14]. However, social factors are also important.

In a large epidemiological study, Fugl-Meyer et al. observed that good orgasmic function was predicted by a relatively early age at first orgasm, a relatively greater repertoire of sexual techniques used, especially oral or manual caress by the partner, being relatively easily sexually aroused, and achievement of orgasm during vaginal intercourse [15]. Other studies have shown that relationship distress is correlated to orgasmic dysfunction, while marital satisfaction [16], happiness, and stability have been found to positively correlate with being able to reach orgasm.

Thus, the observations made 50 years ago by Masters and Johnson that the female orgasm is a "psychophysiologic experience occurring within, and made meaningful by, a context of psychosocial influence" and as a "drive of biologic-behavioral origin deeply integrated into the condition of human existence" [1] still prove to be valid. In the search for sexual health for both men and women, it is important to educate women and their partners about the female orgasm and how a woman's orgasm is influenced by biology, her relationships, an open-minded attitude toward women's sexuality, and the importance of sufficient stimulation as a part of pleasurable sex. Women as well as their male partners will benefit from a better understanding of the woman's orgasm, contributing to a mutual enjoyment of a satisfying sexual life.

References

1. Masters WH, Johnson VE. The female orgasm. In: Masters WH, Johnson VE, editors. Human sexual response. 1st edn. London: J&A Churchill LTD; 1966. p. 127–40.
2. Meston CM, et al. Disorders of orgasm in women. Review. J. Sex. Med. 2004;1:66–8.
3. Clayton AH, Hamilton DV. Female orgasmic disorder. In: Balon R, Segraves RT, editors. Clinical manual of sexual disorders. 1st edn. Arlington: American Psychiatric Publishing; 2009. p. 251–71.
4. Pascoal PM, Narciso IS, Pereira NM. What is sexual satisfaction? Thematic analysis of lay people's definitions. J Sex Res. 2014;51(1):22–30.
5. Levin RJ. The human female orgasm: a critical evaluation of its proposed reproductive functions. Sex Rel Ther. 2012;26:1–14.
6. Levin RJ. The pharmacology of the human female orgasm – its biological and physiological backgrounds. Pharmacol Biochem Behav. 2014;121:62–70.
7. Feldman R. Oxytocin and social affiliation in humans. Horm Behav. 2012;61(3):380–91.
8. Ishak WW, Kahloon M, Fakhry H. Oxytocin role in enhancing well-being: a literature review. J Affect Disord. 2011;130(1–2):1–9.
9. Behnia B, et al. Differential effects of intranasal oxytocin on sexual experiences and partner interactions in couples. Horm Behav. 2014;65(3):308–18.
10. Salisbury CM, Fisher WA. "Did you come?" A qualitative exploration of gender differences in beliefs, experiences, and concerns regarding female orgasm occurrence during heterosexual sexual interactions. J Sex Res. 2014;51(6):616–31.
11. Kingsberg SA, et al. Characterization of orgasmic difficulties by women: focus group evaluation. J Sex Med. 2013;10(9):2242–50.
12. Rellini AH, Clifton J. Female orgasmic disorder. Adv Psychosom Med. 2011;31:35–56.
13. Burri A, Spector T, Rahman Q. A discordant monozygotic twin approach to testing environmental influences on sexual dysfunction in women. Arch Sex Behav. 2013;42(6):961–72.
14. Dunn KM, Cherkas LF, Spector TD. Genetic influences on variation in female orgasmic function: a twin study. Biol Lett. 2005;1(3):260–63.
15. Fugl-Meyer KS, et al. On orgasm, sexual techniques, and erotic perceptions in 18- to 74-year-old Swedish women. J Sex Med. 2006;3(1):56–68.
16. Mah K, Binik YM. The nature of human orgasm: a critical review of major trends. Clin Psychol Rev. 2001;21(6):823–56.

Vaginismus: When Genito-Pelvic Pain/Penetration Disorder Makes Intercourse Seem Impossible

24

Samara Perez, Claudia Brown, and Yitzchak M. Binik

24.1 Patient Profile

My husband and I waited until we were married to have sex. To our disappointment, our wedding night was not the magical, lovemaking night we had envisioned. I had told him about my fear of intercourse, and he said we could take it slow. I enjoyed it when he touched and kissed me, and we decided to try to gradually work up to intercourse. When we did try, I became very tense and afraid and my legs would snap shut, and my arms would push him away. I went to the gynecologist who could not examine me and told me "to relax." We have been trying to have intercourse for three years without success and are getting worried because we really want to start a family.

The above presenting description is quite typical for vaginismus. The primary motive for consultation is often the desire to start a family and/or to save the relationship. The woman has often avoided having a gynecological exam. In addition to not being able to experience intercourse, the woman may experience the following symptoms: fear and anxiety about penetration, marked tensing or tightening of the pelvic floor muscles, as well as marked vulvar pain, either in anticipation of, during, or as a result of vaginal penetration attempts (e.g., finger, tampon) [1–10]. The pain is often described as a sharp pain or a burning sensation around the opening and inside of the vagina. Women often refer to this tensing as some sort of "blockage" or "wall" that prevents penetration. Women with vaginismus may also report that their anatomy is not normal or that they feel defective, e.g., "they are too small inside" or "[that] it doesn't fit" [10] and may experience shame and disgust regarding their genitals [11–16].

24.2 Definition and Nosology

As of 2013, the term[1] vaginismus no longer appears in the Diagnostic and Statistical Manual of Mental Disorders (Fifth Edition, DSM-5) [17].

S. Perez, Ph.D.(c) (✉) • Y.M. Binik, Ph.D.
Department of Psychology, McGill University, 1205 Dr. Penfield Avenue, Montreal, QC, Canada H3A 1B1
e-mail: samara.perez@mail.mcgill.ca

C. Brown, M.Sc., P.T.
Faculty of Medicine, School of Physical and Occupational Therapy, McGill University, Montreal, QC, Canada

Physiotherapie Polyclinique Cabrini, UroSanté, Montreal, QC, Canada

[1] Vaginismus is still listed in International Classification of Diseases (ICD-10). The ICD classification is currently under revision, and the ICD-11 is due to appear in 2017.

L.I. Lipshultz et al. (eds.), *Management of Sexual Dysfunction in Men and Women*, DOI 10.1007/978-1-4939-3100-2_24

In the DSM-5, vaginismus and dyspareunia were combined into one disorder called Genito-pelvic pain/penetration disorder (GPPPD) [17]. This change occurred for several reasons [2, 8, 18–27]. First, the defining feature required for diagnosis of vaginismus in previous DSMs [28, 29] and other classifications [30] was the presence of vaginal muscle spasm.[2] Research, however, has failed to prove the presence of muscle spasm as a valid or reliable diagnostic criterion [2, 27, 31, 32]. In fact, the assessment of vaginal muscle spasm by a healthcare professional is often impossible on the first visit, due to the woman's fear and avoidance, as she may be unable or unwilling to undergo to an internal vaginal examination [18, 33]. Second, diagnosis based solely on vaginal spasm [28, 29, 34] fails to consider the key elements of fear of penetration, anxiety, and pain, which are important components of this condition [2, 18, 35]. Third, several studies have shown that the similarities between dyspareunia/provoked vestibulodynia (PVD) and vaginismus outweigh the differences, making the diagnostic differentiation "difficult or nearly impossible" [1, 2, 6, 8, 9, 16, 27, 35, 36].

The current DSM-5 diagnostic criteria for GPPPD are persistent or recurrent difficulties with one (or more) of the following: (1) vaginal penetration during intercourse, (2) marked vulvovaginal or pelvic pain during vaginal intercourse or penetration attempts, (3) marked fear or anxiety about vaginal or pelvic pain in anticipation of, during, or as a result of vaginal penetration, and (4) marked tensing or tightening of the pelvic floor muscles during attempted vaginal penetration. To be diagnosed with GPPPD, at least one of the symptoms in criteria 1–4 must be present for at least 6 months and needs to cause significant clinical distress. Finally, the symptoms in criteria 1–4 cannot be better accounted for by a nonsexual mental disorder or as a consequence of severe relationship distress (e.g., partner violence) or other significant stressors and are not attributable to the effects of a substance/medication or another medical condition [17]. The diagnosis requires the specifications, *lifelong* (woman who has never been able to have penetration) or *acquired* (woman who has previously been able to have penetration and currently is unable) and *generalized* (to all types of vaginal penetrations, e.g., vaginal intercourse, tampons, medical examinations) or *situational* (only to one specific situation, namely, vaginal penetration during sexual intercourse) [17]. It is important to note that the term "lifelong" GPPPD does not imply that this condition will never resolve, but that the condition has been present since the woman's first attempt at penetration.

Some experts have argued that this new nosology may do a disservice to those women who would have previously been diagnosed with *lifelong vaginismus* [1, 21] because they are a distinct category. Other experts reason that women with lifelong vaginismus are better included in the new category of GPPPD, as GPPPD is based on a spectrum of symptoms which covary and include fear, anxiety, pelvic muscle tension and pain during intercourse—all of which have an impact on their inability to have vaginal penetration [37]. The nosology debate is far from over [21, 26, 37], and it will certainly take some time before consensus is reached in the research and clinical domains.

Irrespective of the nosological debate, there exists a group of women who have never been able to achieve vaginal penetration during attempted intercourse despite their expressed wish to do so. This chapter deals with these women [2, 38]. We will outline the etiology, assessment, and treatment for this group of women, who for the purpose of this chapter will be referred to as suffering from vaginismus. A case study will be used to illustrate an interdisciplinary approach to treatment using therapist-aided exposure combined with psychotherapy.

24.3 Prevalence and Etiology

There are wildly differing prevalence estimates for vaginismus, with population estimates ranging from 0.5 to 9 % [39–42] and other estimates

[2] Vagin*ismus* implies spasm of the vagina as *ismus* denotes spasm or contraction.

ranging from 7 to 76 % in specialist and clinical settings [43–48]. This large variation is likely a result of different sampling methods and methods of assessment (e.g., questions about spasm, penetration, pain), the overlap in previous definitions of vaginismus and dyspareunia, and perhaps cultural perception. Irrespective of the variation in prevalence estimates, gynecologists and specialists in sexual dysfunction all receive frequent referrals of women who cannot experience vaginal penetration.

Currently, the cause(s) of vaginismus remains unknown [8, 27, 49, 50]. Although vaginismus has been linked with psychogenic etiological factors such as conservative religious upbringing, abstinence until marriage, negative sexual attitudes, ignorance, and lack of sexual education and experience [38, 51], the few available high-quality studies do not support these associations [8, 50, 52, 53]. Other hypothesized but unsubstantiated etiological factors include the occurrence of dysfunctional couple/marital relationships and sexual/physical abuse or trauma [54, 55].

One proposed theoretical explanation for the development of vaginismus follows the fear-avoidance model for phobias and pain [1]: the woman is apprehensive and fears pain during vaginal penetration. During her first attempt at penetration (often experienced with a tampon), the woman's pelvic floor musculature contracts involuntarily, serving as a protective mechanism to occlude the vaginal entrance and prevent the feared penetration. If the woman tries to have penetration in spite of this muscle contraction or tension, she may indeed experience pain, from the compression on the vaginal entrance caused by the contraction. This pain increases her anxiety with respect to her next attempt at penetration, and a vicious cycle of pain, fear, anxiety, catastrophizing negative thoughts, and muscle tension is established. The increased fear and anxiety can lead to avoidance, as discussed by ter Kuile and Reissing in their fear-avoidance model of vaginismus [1]. This etiological mechanism has not been confirmed empirically, but is nonetheless a useful heuristic for the clinician and for future research. It remains unclear, however, whether these women avoid penetration (sex, gynecological exams, or other) in order to diminish their anxiety level similar to individuals suffering from a specific phobia or in response to their pain experience or both. However, women with dyspareunia typically do not avoid penetration to the same degree as women suffering from vaginismus [35].

24.4 Assessment and Diagnosis

The assessment of a woman with vaginismus requires *sensitivity—to a woman who is experiencing pain/fear that is entrenched in emotionally charged and intimate behaviors* [1, 56] and *patience*—to spend the time needed for the woman to be heard, which serve as a basis for a successful clinician–patient relationship. It is possible that the woman has previously consulted with other medical professionals who may have claimed that the problem could not be real or suggested that the pain was "in her head" [57, 58]. It is important to reassure the woman that she is not alone in suffering from vaginismus, that she did well to consult, and that effective treatment options do exist. For some, it is important that the disorder be named (i.e., introducing the terms vaginismus and GPPPD), as she may wish to subsequently consult online and/or with other professionals.

A detailed overview of how to successfully assess and diagnose female sexual dysfunction more broadly and the information one needs to obtain from a thorough clinical interview, physical examination, laboratory testing, and psychometric tools are outlined in Chapter 19. The relevant and specific components to consider for the assessment and diagnosis of vaginismus are outlined below.

24.4.1 Medical Screening

When a woman with vaginismus decides to seek professional help, she will likely first consult a general practitioner or gynecologist [59]. Although a medical screening may help to rule out conditions that can explain the woman's difficulties with penetration (see Table 25.1), a physical cause for the inability to have vaginal penetration will rarely be found. Specifically, there are a few conditions such as congenital anomalies of the hymen (e.g., imperforate hymen, hymen semilunaris altus, septate hymen) or vaginal agenesis that can directly prevent vaginal penetration. In addition, it is helpful for the clinician to perform a moist cotton swab test of the vulvar vestibule to assess whether there is pain since the comorbidity of vaginismus and PVD is very high [2, 18, 27]. Almost all women can undergo at least a partial pelvic examination if treated with encouragement, patience, and instructions for relaxation through deep breathing. This may take some time, but in and of itself it can be highly therapeutic for the woman with vaginismus and can instill a sense of hope for further recovery. A suggested list of recommendations [58, 60] for the clinician to consider prior to and during the examination of a woman with vaginismus are outlined in Table 24.1. Because of the intense fear and anxiety that some women with vaginismus experience with respect to vaginal penetration, it may sometimes be advisable to delay the examination to be performed on a subsequent visit [60].

Table 24.1 Reccomendations for the pelvic/gynecological examination of a woman with vaginismus

Before the examination:
• While she is dressed, explain to the woman step-by-step what you will do during the examination
• Give her control by reassuring her that you will stop immediately at any time during the examination
• Tell her she can ask questions at any point
• Explain that the vaginal entrance has the potential to expand
• Using a mirror, show the woman her genitals, and show areas that could be touched without pain
If she agrees to be examined:
• Be gentle and encourage her to breathe deeply
• Begin with flat pressure on the surface of the vulva
• Proceed with light pressure between the labia, and then gently move the lubricated and gloved index finger in an anteroposterior direction
• Ask the woman to squeeze and let go (contract and relax her pelvic floor muscles) prior to digital insertion
• Digital insertion should be done slowly with liberal use of lubricant
A pediatric speculum can be used, but do not attempt a speculum examination if a manual exam is not possible

24.4.2 Pelvic Floor Examination

An external pelvic examination may reveal the presence of protective reactions, which can range from complete refusal by the woman to assume the lithotomy position, to verbal expressions of anxiety, retraction of the pelvis, closing of the legs, facial grimacing, or crying [33]. Protective reactions may also include pelvic floor hypertonicity or an involuntary pelvic floor muscle contraction. This contraction can often be palpated externally, with compression of the soft tissue that lies inferior to the symphysis pubis and medial to the ischiopubic rami and ischial tuberosities. The hypertonic pelvic floor will demonstrate an increased resistance to palpatory compression of this tissue. If internal palpation is possible, pelvic floor hypertonicity may present as an increased resistance to passive stretch at the introitus. Assessment thus includes the degree to which the introitus may be "opened" (i.e., is it possible to fully insert the digit past the vaginal vestibule and into the vagina, to insert two digits, and to open the digits in the horizontal plane) and an evaluation of muscle tone, contractility, and post-contractile relaxation of the pelvic floor musculature. Some women who cannot tolerate vaginal palpation may be able to tolerate anal palpation, which may be done to identify the same muscular attributes and the presence of protective reactions.

24.4.3 Psychosocial and Sexual History

Understanding the woman's psychosocial status (e.g., age, religion, and culture are particularly relevant) and sexual history can help with the evaluation and treatment [60, 61]. This includes inquiring about current and past partner relationships (e.g., duration, commitment), relevant factors in the woman's developmental history such as physical, sexual, and/or emotional abuse (past and present), sexual self-esteem, and sexual orientation. The woman's sexual education (e.g., formal vs. informal, family beliefs about sex, rules about sex), knowledge, and awareness of vaginal anatomy (e.g., has she discovered her own anatomy) are also important focus areas that need to be assessed [60, 61]. The assessment also creates an opportunity to begin unpacking the cognitions (e.g., "no partner wants me"), emotions (e.g., fear, anxiety, sadness, anger, frustration, disgust, inadequacy, embarrassment, guilt), and behaviors (e.g., avoidance of dating, sexual activities) underlying the presenting problem. A detailed understanding of the woman's "self-talk" during any attempted sexual activity will provide important information which can be used during treatment to reduce anxiety and correct misinformation, e.g., "nothing will go in there that doesn't hurt."

24.5 Treatment

Historically, there has been much debate surrounding the of choice for vaginismus [8]. In the mid-nineteenth century, surgical interventions that included removal of the hymen, the incision of the vaginal orifice, and subsequent dilation were recommended [62, 63]. This practice was reconsidered when it became apparent that gradual vaginal dilation was effective [27, 64]. Throughout the twentieth century and until today, different variants of psychotherapy, (e.g., psychoanalysis, couple therapy) and pharmacotherapy [e.g., local anesthetics, anxiolytic medications, botulinum toxin (i.e., botox)] were often recommended [63, 65, 66]. Masters and Johnson pioneered the use of behaviorally oriented sex therapy with the couple that included sex education and practicing insertion with the use of graded dilators [67]. This became the primary treatment method after 1970 and was deemed highly successful [8, 27, 67]. Recently, there is increasing use of pelvic floor physiotherapy, which applies in vivo Masters and Johnson-type dilation, with the addition of biofeedback and manual techniques [10, 68–72]. Despite this history and the fact that many of these treatments continue to be used, there was limited empirical evidence that these interventions were efficacious [8, 73, 74].

In 2006, Masters and Johnson-type treatment for vaginismus was rigorously evaluated for the first time using a randomized controlled trial (RCT) comparing a cognitive behavioral group therapy to a cognitive behavioral bibliotherapy and a wait-list control [53]. The treatment included vaginal dilation techniques, sex education, relaxation, and sensate focus exercises given in group therapy format or in the form of educational literature. Three months posttreatment, 18 % of women in the treatment groups (14 % group therapy; 9 % bibliotherapy) reported successful penile–vaginal intercourse, while none of the women in the wait-list control group reported successful intercourse. There was a significant treatment effect, but this effect was significantly lower than the high success rates previously reported by Masters and Johnson and others [67, 75–77].

Following the publication of new literature reconceptualizing vaginismus as a phobic disorder related to an intense fear of vaginal penetration [1, 53, 78, 79], ter Kuile et al. applied to vaginismus the highly effective in vivo gradual exposure and response prevention method used to treat phobias. In a recent RCT, they found that therapist-aided exposure for a hierarchy of fear-inducing vaginal penetration objects was highly effective in decreasing penetration fears and avoidance behaviors for women with lifelong vaginismus [1]. Impressively, 89 % (31/35) of women in the treatment group reported having had sexual intercourse post-treatment compared with 11 % of women (4/35) in the control group [78]. In 90 % of the successfully treated women, penetrative vaginal intercourse was possible within the first two weeks of treatment.

The treatment procedure used by ter Kuile et al. in this study may be outlined as follows [78, 79]: Prior to the first meeting, the woman has been physically examined by a gynecologist/physician, and physical conditions that prevent the possibility of penetration are ruled out. During an introductory hour-long session, the woman and her partner meet with the therapist (an experienced female psychologist–sexologist or gynecologist), and the treatment rationale and procedure are explained. The woman is asked to create her own, personalized hierarchical fear ladder[3] consisting of all vaginal penetration situations from the least to the most fearful. She rates each of these situations on a scale of 0 = no fear at all up to 100 = maximum fear possible. The partner is asked to measure the circumference of his erect penis, so that the last dilator to be used before intercourse is of at least this circumference.

This is followed by one to three *therapist-aided exposure sessions* (on average 150 min each) in a room equipped with gynecological stirrups. The treatment consists of step-by-step in vivo practice as the woman works up her way up her fear ladder by gradually inserting progressively larger objects into her vagina, thereby exposing herself to more fear-inducing situations (e.g., self-insertion of one finger, a tampon, partner inserts two fingers, movement of his fingers, graduated phallic insertion devices, i.e., dilators), with the ultimate goal of successfully experiencing intercourse at home. During these sessions, the therapist encourages the woman to carry out the penetration in the office/hospital, and she is then asked to practice at home. It is important that the woman's partner takes an active part in treatment by being present during the therapist-aided exposure sessions and by taking part during the home exercises. As this is an intensive week of treatment, it is recommended that the couple take a week off from work. It is possible that attempting penetration at home may take time or may not always be sexually exciting, and thus Viagra (sildenafil) or Cialis (tadalafil) may be prescribed to facilitate easy maintenance of her partner's erection. Following exposure, there are 2–4 follow-up sessions (over 10 weeks). A detailed treatment manual is available [78, 79].

A recent uncontrolled study in Iran [12] successfully replicated this approach, although the mean number of in vivo therapy sessions was 5.71 ($SD = 2.47$, range 2–11) as compared with a mean of 1.88 therapy sessions ($SD = 0.77$; range 1–4 sessions) reported in ter Kuile et al.'s study from the Netherlands [78]. Overall, this treatment approach seems highly promising, and the RCT should be independently replicated. It should be noted that the sole focus of this treatment intervention is on penetration success, and it does not deal with pleasure or pain during intercourse. In fact, for about half the participants in the Netherlands, outcome measures for sexual satisfaction and pain were still not within the healthy range of sexually well-functioning women, suggesting that some women were reporting discomfort or pain during intercourse after the therapist-aided exposure therapy [78]. This is not surprising, since some of these women had previously avoided most sexual contact and pleasure in addition to penetration. If sexual satisfaction, sexual functioning, or pain remains problematic after successful treatment for penetration, then follow-up treatment with other professionals (e.g., a psychologist, sex therapist, or pelvic floor physiotherapist) may be beneficial. If dyspareunia still persists, a further evaluation for organic causes of introital allodynia must be explored. Organic etiologies may not be obvious to practitioners not experienced in the evaluation of vulvodynia and dyspareunia, and, therefore, this may warrant a referral, if possible, to a specialist in vulvar pain disorders (e.g., www.ISSVD.org, www.ISSWSH.org).

24.6 Case Study

This case study used an approach similar to ter Kuile et al.'s therapist-aided exposure [78, 79]. Although the ter Kuile et al.'s treatment approach is typically implemented by a psychologist who coaches women on how to do insertion on her own without physically assisting the woman, our case illustrates an interdisciplinary team approach including both a psychologist and physiotherapist. This format allows the physiotherapist to be "hands on" by utilizing manual techniques, physical modalities, and exercise, complemented by the psychologist who addressed the woman's psychological needs.

[3] A combination of fear, anxiety, and tension, subsequently referred to as fear.

Fatima[4] consulted at a university hospital Sex and Couples Therapy Service, where a doctoral-level psychology intern (SP) began weekly 1-hour psychotherapy sessions. After four sessions, and with knowledge of the efficacy of therapist-aided exposure, the psychology intern consulted with a physiotherapist (CB) with over 20 years experience in pelvic floor physical therapy and who had recently been trained by the ter Kuile team in Holland. They offered Fatima the therapist-aided exposure treatment, and she agreed to this treatment course. A convenient week of treatment was scheduled during which the couple could be absent from work. Psychotherapy with Fatima alone continued for seven sessions until the scheduled week of intensive therapist-aided exposure treatment.

24.6.1 Identification

Fatima was a 39-year-old Middle Eastern French-speaking woman referred by a medical practitioner from a nearby fertility clinic. The physician told Fatima that fertility treatment would not be possible until the couple was able to have vaginal penetrative sexual intercourse.

24.6.2 Motive for Consultation

Fatima had been married for 12 years but was had never had penetrative sex despite many attempts at penetration. Motivation was high because of her approaching 40th birthday and the desire to have children.

24.6.3 History of Presenting Problem

Fatima had never been able to tolerate tampon or finger insertion or a gynecological examination. Fatima reported symptoms of panic in response to attempted penetration, described as an intense fear and "blacking out." She said that she has improved slightly in recent months as she and her husband could now touch her labia externally without her panicking. She reported desire and pleasure when the couple was intimate during other non-penetrative sexual activities. She had never masturbated and grimaced during the interview when asked why. Fatima reported no premarital partners or attempts at vaginal intercourse. There was no history of abuse or trauma.

[4] Name has been altered to preserve confidentiality.

24.6.4 Past Psychiatric/Medical History

Fatima reported animal phobias (e.g., snakes, dogs) and a fear of dark voids, but denied being generally anxious. Fatima had never visited a mental health professional prior to her evaluation by the Sex and Couple Therapy Service nor had she been diagnosed with a psychiatric disorder. She reported no recurrent illness and had never used any contraception.

24.6.5 Mental Status

During the assessment, Fatima was quite personable, talkative, and socially appropriate.

24.6.6 DSM-5 Diagnosis

Fatima met DSM-5 criteria for GPPPD, lifelong and generalized.

24.6.7 Hypothesized Origin of Presenting Problem

Within the context of psychotherapy, Fatima explained that most women in her country of origin practice abstinence until marriage. She mentioned that she had been told that if a bride is unable to have intercourse on her wedding night, the elderly women of the town insert an oil candle in the vagina the following day. Fatima referred to her inability to have sex as a "blockage."

24.6.8 Content of Psychotherapy Sessions

Fatima was extremely unfamiliar with her vaginal anatomy, and asked how many holes women had. The psychology intern (SP) provided psychoeducation about female anatomy (e.g., pictures, diagrams) and opportunities to respond to questions about the female body/sexuality. She was also asked to purchase a women's sexual health book. One of her first homework assignments was to look at her genitals using a mirror. Fatima was extremely reluctant at first, although was able to examine her genitals and found them to be pretty. She was often tearful in session and mad at herself for having this problem for so long. Psychotherapy provided a safe place for her to discuss her disappointment and frustrations. The psychology intern explained how her sexuality was dormant for many years and praised Fatima for opening up her sexual self. On subsequent sessions, the therapist encouraged Fatima to go home and take a cotton swab or her pinky finger and to touch the outer vaginal labia and around the vaginal opening, which she was successfully able to do. The therapist explained the interplay between emotions, thoughts, and behaviors, as Fatima had high anxiety about not being able to get pregnant. The therapist also did some deep breathing and relaxation exercises with Fatima. The psychology intern developed a strong therapeutic alliance with Fatima. The psychology intern introduced and prepared Fatima for the plan of therapist-aided exposure. Fatima's husband attended the eleventh session to discuss the treatment plan and how the couple could work together to navigate this process.

The therapist-aided exposure was led by a physiotherapist (CB). The psychology intern, Fatima, and Fatima's husband were all present for the following five sessions:

24.6.9 Session 1 (1 h, Day 1)

There was a team introduction, followed by a psychosocial history intake by the physiotherapist. The physiotherapist then educated and informed Fatima about the female anatomy using diagrams and a three-dimensional model of the pelvis with removable organs, which made it easy for the couple to visualize and understand the anatomy. Fatima's husband explained that she physically blocks vaginal penetration by closing her legs. Fatima explained past symptoms of phobic reactions to penetration, such as feeling that there is a hole in her heart, having sweaty palms, and feeling "cut" at the throat. The team discussed the physical signs that she exhibits when she is beginning to have anxiety and fear-based reactions so that she could act upon them early should they present during treatment. Fatima was fully briefed on the therapist-aided exposure program and provided with an information package to take home (adapted and translated version of ter Kuile et al. treatment manual) [78, 79].

24.6.10 Session 2 (1 h, Day 6)

Fatima was taught deep breathing (20 min), followed by global stretching exercises (adductors and hamstrings, hip rotators). The physiotherapist identified genital anatomical structures as Fatima held a hand mirror. The physiotherapist applied external pressures on the surface of vulva and instructed Fatima on how to engage in pelvic floor contraction and relaxation. Fatima purchased a kit of graduated insertion devices. She was also given a fear ladder to complete at home (see Fig. 24.1) with instructions on listing items in a hierarchy of increasing fear/anxiety in relation to insertion. The ladder was to include physiotherapist's finger, two fingers, a silicon penis, and intercourse. Glaxal Base cream was suggested for daily application because of Fatima's dry skin and history of fissures.

24.6.11 Session 3 (3 h, Day 7)

This was the first therapist-aided exposure therapy session. The physiotherapist reviewed anatomical structures and answered the couple's questions. Next, the team reviewed, in detail,

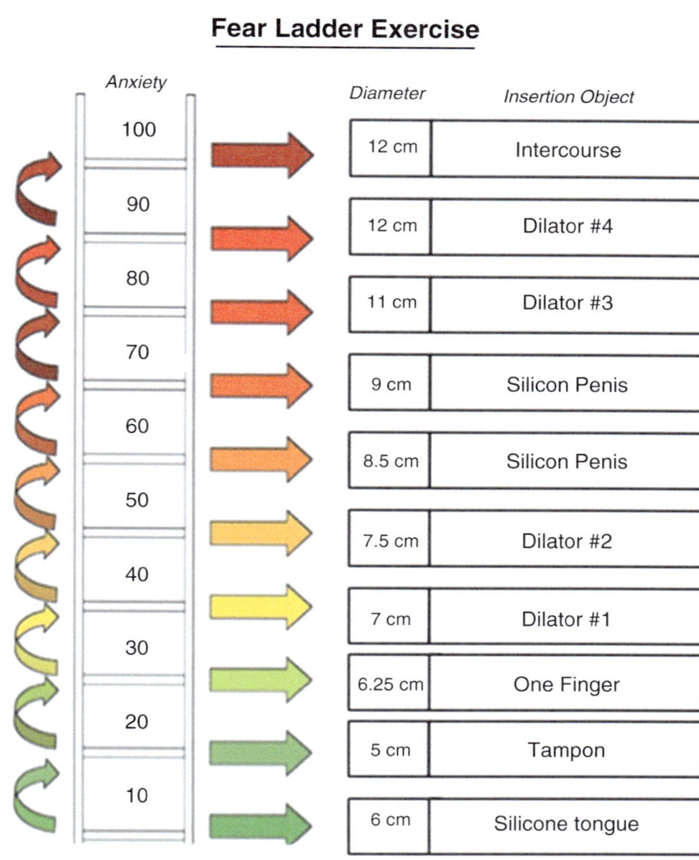

Fig. 24.1 Fear ladder exercise. With permission from ter Kuile MM, Reissing ED. Lifelong Vaginismus. In: Binik YM, Hall KSK, editors. Principles and Practice of Sex Therapy, Fifth Edition 2014© Guilford Publications 2004 [1]

Fatima's hierarchical fear ladder. In this session, she was able to successfully climb the 8th rung on her ladder (see Fig. 24.1). To begin the gradual exposure therapy, Fatima started by inserting a 0 fear-inducing object, a silicone tongue-shaped object. During each insertion, the psychology intern asked Fatima to rate her anxiety and pain level. Next, a tampon applicator was inserted by Fatima. The physiotherapist then inserted one finger and performed muscle identification techniques including stretching and techniques where Fatima learned to actively contract and relax her muscles. Subsequently, dilator number one was inserted by Fatima, followed by dilator number two, and then a silicone penis that Fatima had previously purchased. Next, the physiotherapist inserted two fingers and performed additional manual techniques. Fatima then partially inserted dilator number three, which was the first insertion device that produced great anxiety, recognized via her emotional and physical reactions (e.g., she mentioned that her heart was racing and that she had sweaty palms). The exposure session ended with guided mindfulness techniques by the psychology intern, who congratulated and reinforced Fatima's progress and indicated that the team and her husband were supporting her. Fatima was emotional and tearful, but left comforted, happy with her progress, and proud of herself.

24.6.12 Session 4 (2 h, Day 9)

This was the second therapist-aided exposure therapy session. Fatima and her husband had worked on her fear ladder at home and arrived at the same point that had been reached during session 3. Session 4 began at the bottom of the ladder using device 0 on the fear ladder and progressed gradually: silicone tongue, dilator number one, dilator number two, physiotherapist's two fingers, and manual techniques. The physiotherapist then showed Fatima's husband how to insert his finger into her vagina. Fatima reported some discomfort, and the physiotherapist applied xylocaine cream, which helped significantly. Fatima then inserted dilator three, followed by partial insertion of dilator four. At this point, Fatima reported an anxiety level of 7/10 and a pain level of 5/10. The physiotherapist demonstrated a counterpressure technique to decrease pain during dilator removal. Fatima requested information on ideal positions for intercourse, which the physiotherapist explained.

24.6.13 Session 5 (2 h, Day 15)

The couple was happy to report that they were able to have intercourse on day 9. Fatima was able to insert devices at the top of the fear ladder on Day 10 and had intercourse again on day 11. The psychology intern and physiotherapist debriefed and received feedback from couple for the potential treatment of future women suffering from vaginismus.

24.6.14 Two Months Post-treatment

Fatima remains in psychotherapy to discuss non-related sexual issues (e.g., work-related anxieties). The couple continues to have satisfying vaginal penetrative sex 2–3 times/week and is trying to conceive naturally.

In summary, our treatment is diverged from ter Kuile et al.'s protocol [78, 79], as there were two therapists present from different disciplines working together, complementing and keeping each other on track during the therapist-aided exposure, which proved to be helpful for both therapists. A similar approach using a physiotherapist and psychotherapist is currently being carried out [10]. Moreover, the physiotherapist was able to use physical exercise instruction, physical guidance for the insertion, and manual techniques. It remains unclear whether the 11 sessions of psychotherapy were needed. However, post hoc, Fatima informed the therapists that she did not believe that she would have consulted or been prepared to begin the therapist in vivo gradual exposure immediately. She appreciated the time in psychotherapy to discuss her sexuality, her frustrations, and to feel confident enough to see the physiotherapist with her psychologist and husband present.

24.7 Conclusion

The therapist-aided exposure treatment appears to be highly effective for women with lifelong vaginismus and could also be considered for women presenting with acquired vaginismus. It remains to be seen who would be the ideal professional to deliver this treatment and act as therapist, be it a gynecologist, a pelvic floor physiotherapist, a psychologist, or perhaps all who are capable to be trained in the therapist-aided exposure approach. One practical problem with a psychologist as the therapist is whether a psychologist is ethically allowed to treat a woman who is undressed and is exposed from the waist down, although this was approved by the Dutch Society of Psychologist ethics boards in Holland [80]. Ethical professional considerations, gender of the treatment provider (e.g., thus far only female), and location of treatment (e.g., cultural context [25]) should all be evaluated in future research and clinical practice.

It is our opinion that an integrated, interdisciplinary treatment with a gynecologist, psychologist, and pelvic floor physiotherapist could provide comprehensive care for women suffering from vaginismus [10, 68, 71]. This would further address any additional symptoms of vaginismus including pain, generalized anxiety, sexual satisfaction, desire, and relationship/couple issues. Independent of the therapist's profession and the method of delivery, there is currently a highly effective, evidence-based treatment for women with vaginismus, which makes sexual intercourse possible.

References

1. ter Kuile MM, Reissing ED. Lifelong vaginismus. In: Binik YM, Hall KSK, editors. Principles and practice of sex therapy. 5th ed. New York: Guilford Press; 2014.
2. Reissing ED, Binik YM, Khalifé S, Cohen D, Amsel R. Vaginal spasm, pain, and behavior: an empirical investigation of the diagnosis of vaginismus. Arch Sex Behav. 2004;33(1):5–17.
3. Rosenbaum T. Addressing anxiety in vivo in physiotherapy treatment of women with severe vaginismus: a clinical approach. J Sex Marital Ther. 2011;37(2):89–93.
4. Melles RJ, ter Kuile MM, Dewitte M, van Lankveld JJ, Brauer M, de Jong PJ. Automatic and deliberate affective associations with sexual stimuli in women with lifelong vaginismus before and after therapist-aided exposure treatment. J Sex Med. 2014;11(3):786–99.
5. Watts G, Nettle D. The role of anxiety in vaginismus: a case-control study. J Sex Med. 2010;7(1pt1):143–8.
6. De Kruiff M, Ter Kuile M, Weijenborg PTM, van Larikveld J. Vaginismus and dyspareunia: is there a difference in clinical presentation? J Psychosom Obstet Gynecol. 2000;21(3):149–55.
7. Reissing ED, Armstrong HL, Allen C. Pelvic floor physical therapy for lifelong vaginismus: a retrospective chart review and interview study. J Sex Marital Ther. 2013;39(4):306–20.
8. Lahaie M-A, Boyer SC, Amsel R, Khalifé S, Binik YM. Vaginismus: a review of the literature on the classification/diagnosis, etiology and treatment. Womens Health. 2010;6(5):705–19.
9. Lahaie MA, Amsel R, Khalife S, Boyer S, Faaborg-Andersen M, Binik YM. Can fear, pain, and muscle tension discriminate vaginismus from dyspareunia/provoked vestibulodynia? Implications for the new DSM-5 diagnosis of genito-pelvic pain/penetration disorder. Arch Sex Behav. 2014.
10. Katz D, Tabisel RL. Private pain. It's about life, not just sex... Understanding Vaginismus and Dyspareunia. 2nd ed. Plainview, NY: Katz-Tabi Publications; 2005.
11. Silverstein JL. Origins of psychogenic vaginismus. Psychother Psychosom. 1989;52(4):197–204.
12. Molaeinezhad M, Salehi M, Borg C, Yousefy A, Latifnejad Roudsari R, Salehi P, et al. Marriage consummated for 32 Iranian women using therapist-aided exposure therapy: a brief report. Sex Relat Ther. 2014;29(3):293–306.
13. Borg C, Georgiadis JR, Renken RJ, Spoelstra SK, Weijmar Schultz W, de Jong PJ. Brain processing of visual stimuli representing sexual penetration versus core and animal-reminder disgust in women with lifelong vaginismus. PLoS One. 2014;9(1), e84882.
14. Cherner RA, Reissing ED. A psychophysiological investigation of sexual arousal in women with lifelong vaginismus. J Sex Med. 2013;10(5):1291–303.
15. de Jong PJ, van Overveld M, Schultz WW, Peters ML, Buwalda FM. Disgust and contamination sensitivity in vaginismus and dyspareunia. Arch Sex Behav. 2009;38(2):244–52.
16. Engman M. Long-term coital behaviour in women treated with cognitive behaviour therapy for superficial coital pain and vaginismus. Cogn Behav Ther. 2010;39(3):193.
17. American Psychiatric Association. Diagnostic and statistical manual of mental disorders: DSM-5. Washington, D.C.: American Psychiatric Association; 2013.
18. Binik YM. The DSM, diagnostic criteria for vaginismus. Arch Sex Behav. 2010;39(2):278–91.
19. Peer Commentaries on Binik (2005). Arch Sex Behav. 2005;34(1):23–61.
20. Binik YM, Brotto LA, Graham CA, Segraves RT. Response of the DSM-V sexual dysfunctions subworkgroup to commentaries published in JSM. J Sex Med. 2010;7(7):2382–7.
21. Reissing ED, Borg C, Spoelstra SK, ter Kuile MM, Both S, de Jong PJ, et al. Throwing the baby out with the bathwater: the demise of vaginismus in favor of genito-pelvic pain/penetration disorder. Arch Sex Behav. 2014;43(7):1209–13.
22. Segraves R, Balon R, Clayton A. Proposal for changes in diagnostic criteria for sexual dysfunctions. J Sex Med. 2007;4(3):567–80.
23. Binik Y. Should dyspareunia be retained as a sexual dysfunction in DSM-V? A painful classification decision. Arch Sex Behav. 2005;34(1):11–21.
24. Hiller J. Defining vaginismus. Sex Relat Ther. 2000;15(1):87–90.
25. Ng M-L. Vaginismus – a disease, symptom or culture-bound syndrome? Sex Marital Ther. 1999;14(1):9–13.
26. Simonelli C, Eleuteri S, Petruccelli F, Rossi R. Female sexual pain disorders: dyspareunia and vaginismus. Curr Opin Psychiatry. 2014;27(6):406–12.
27. Reissing ED, Binik YM, KhalifÈ S. Does vaginismus exist? A critical review of the literature. J Nerv Ment Dis. 1999;187(5):261–74.
28. American Psychiatric Association. Diagnostic and statistical manual of mental disorders. Washington, D.C.: American Psychiatric Association; 1980.
29. American Psychiatric Association. Diagnostic and statistical manual of mental disorders: DSM-III-R. Washington, DC: American Psychiatric Association; 1987.
30. World Health O. ICD-10 international statistical classification of diseases and related health problems. Geneva: World Health Organization; 2005.
31. Reissing E, Brown C, Lord M, Binik Y, Khalifé S. Pelvic floor muscle functioning in women with vulvar vestibulitis syndrome. J Psychosom Obstet Gynecol. 2005;26(2):107–13.
32. Frasson E, Graziottin A, Priori A, Dall'Ora E, Didonè G, Garbin EL, et al. Central nervous system abnormalities in vaginismus. Clin Neurophysiol. 2009;120(1):117–22.

33. Huber JD, Pukall CF, Boyer SC, Reissing ED, Chamberlain SM. "Just Relax": physicians' experiences with women who are difficult or impossible to examine gynecologically. J Sex Med. 2009;6(3):791–9.
34. American Psychiatric Association. Diagnostic and statistical manual of mental disorders: DSM-IV-TR. Washington, DC: American Psychiatric Association; 2000.
35. Basson R, Althof S, Davis S, Fugl-Meyer K, Goldstein I, Leiblum S, et al. Summary of the recommendations on sexual dysfunctions in women. J Sex Med. 2004;1(1):24–34.
36. Ter Kuile MM, Van Lankveld JJ, Vlieland CV, Willekes C, Weijenborg PTM. Vulvar vestibulitis syndrome: an important factor in the evaluation of lifelong vaginismus? J Psychosom Obstet Gynecol. 2005;26(4):245–9.
37. Binik YM. Will vaginismus remain a "lifelong" baby? Response to Reissing et al. (2014). Arch Sex Behav. 2014;43(7):1215–7.
38. Ward E, Ogden J. Experiencing vaginismus – sufferers beliefs about causes and effects. Sex Marital Ther. 1994;9(1):33–45.
39. Ventegodt S. Sex and the quality of life in Denmark. Arch Sex Behav. 1998;27(3):295–307.
40. Fugl-Meyer KS, Fugl-Meyer AR. Sexual disabilities are not singularities. Int J Impot Res. 2002;14(6):487–93.
41. Peixoto MM, Nobre P. Prevalence and sociodemographic predictors of sexual problems in Portugal: a population-based study with women aged 18 to 79 years. J Sex Marital Ther. 2013;41(2):169–80.
42. Simonelli C, Tripodi F, Cosmi V, Rossi R, Fabrizi A, Silvaggi C, et al. What do men and women ask a helpline on sexual concerns? Results of an Italian telephone counselling service. Int J Clin Pract. 2010;64(3):360–70.
43. Amidu N, Owiredu W, Woode E, Addai-Mensah O, Quaye L, Alhassan A, et al. Incidence of sexual dysfunction: a prospective survey in Ghanaian females. Reprod Biol Endocrinol. 2010;8:106.
44. Oniz A. The prevalence and causes of sexual problems among premenopausal Turkish women. J Sex Med. 2007;4(6):1575.
45. Shokrollahi P, Mirmohamadi M, Mehrabi F, Babaei G. Prevalence of sexual dysfunction in women seeking services at family planning centers in Tehran. J Sex Marital Ther. 1999;25(3):211–5.
46. Dogan S. Vaginismus and accompanying sexual dysfunctions in a Turkish clinical sample. J Sex Med. 2009;6(1):184–92.
47. Rosen RC, Taylor JF, Leiblum SR, Bachmann GA. Prevalence of sexual dysfunction in women: results of a survey study of 329 women in an outpatient gynecological clinic. J Sex Marital Ther. 1993;19(3):171–88.
48. Simons JS, Carey MP. Prevalence of sexual dysfunctions: results from a decade of research. Arch Sex Behav. 2001;30(2):177–219.
49. Wijma B, Engman M, Wijma K. A model for critical review of literature-with vaginismus as an example. J Psychosom Obstet Gynecol. 2007;28(1):21–36.
50. Reissing ED, Binik YM, Samir K, Cohen D, Amsel R. Etiological correlates of vaginismus: sexual and physical abuse, sexual knowledge, sexual self-schema, and relationship adjustment. J Sex Marital Ther. 2003;29(1):47–59.
51. Basson R. Lifelong vaginismus: a clinical study of 60 consecutive cases. J Soc Gynecol Obstet Can. 1996;18:551–62.
52. Duddle M. Etiological factors in the unconsummated marriage. J Psychosom Res. 1977;21(2):157–60.
53. van Lankveld JJ, ter Kuile MM, de Groot HE, Melles R, Nefs J, Zandbergen M. Cognitive-behavioral therapy for women with lifelong vaginismus: a randomized waiting-list controlled trial of efficacy. J Consult Clin Psychol. 2006;74(1):168–78.
54. Spector IP, Carey MP. Incidence and prevalence of the sexual dysfunctions: a critical review of the empirical literature. Arch Sex Behav. 1990;19(4):389–408.
55. West SL, Vinikoor LC, Zolnoun D. A systematic review of the literature on female sexual dysfunction prevalence and predictors. Annu Rev Sex Res. 2004;15(1):40–172.
56. Graziottin A, Brotto LA. Vulvar vestibulitis syndrome: a clinical approach. J Sex Marital Ther. 2004;30(3):125–39.
57. Pacik PT. Understanding and treating vaginismus: a multimodal approach. Int Urogynecol J. 2014;25(12):1613–20.
58. Graziottin A. Sexual pain disorders: dyspareunia and vaginismus. In: Porst H, Buvat J, Medicine ISFS, editors. Standard practice in sexual medicine. Malden: Blackwell; 2006. p. 342–9.
59. Ogden J, Ward E. Help-seeking behaviour in sufferers of vaginismus. Sex Marital Ther. 1995;10(1):23–30.
60. Crowley T, Goldmeier D, Hiller J. Diagnosing and managing vaginismus. BMJ. 2009;338:b2284.
61. Basson R, Leiblum S, Brotto L, Derogatis L, Fourcroy J, Fugl-Meyer K, et al. Revised definitions of women's sexual dysfunction. J Sex Med. 2004;1(1):40–8.
62. Sims JM. On vaginismus. Transactions of the obstetrics. Soc Lond. 1861;3:356–67.
63. Cryle PM, Moore A. Frigidity: an intellectual history. Houndmills, Basingstoke, Hampshire. New York: Palgrave Macmillan; 2011.
64. Thorburn J. A practical treatise of the diseases of women. London, UK: Charles Griffin and Company; 1885.
65. Musaph H, Haspels A. Vaginisme. Ned Tijdschr Geneeskd. 1976;120:1589–92.
66. Fenichel L. The psychoanalytic theory of neurosis. NY, USA: Norton; 1945.
67. Masters WH, Johnson VE. Human sexual inadequacy. Boston: Little, Brown, and Company; 1970.
68. Rosenbaum TY. An integrated mindfulness-based approach to the treatment of women with sexual pain and anxiety: promoting autonomy and mind/body connection. Sex Relat Ther. 2013;28(1–2):20–8.

69. Rosenbaum TY. Physical therapy treatment of sexual pain disorders. In: Leiblum S, editor. Principles and practice of sex therapy. New York, NY: Guilford; 2007.
70. Rosenbaum T. Pelvic floor physiotherapy for women with urogenital dysfunction: indications and methods. Minerva Urol Nefrol. 2011;63(1):101.
71. Brown C. Recommendations for best-practice interdisciplinary management of women with vaginismus. Montreal, QC: McGill University; 2013.
72. Graziottin A. Evidence based physiotherapy for the pelvic floor. Bridging research and clinical practice. In: Bo K, Berghmans B, van Kampen M, Morkved S, editors. Treatment of sexual dysfunction. Oxford, UK: Elsevier; 2005.
73. McGuire H, Hawton KK. Interventions for vaginismus Cochrane Database of Systematic Reviews. 2001;2.
74. Melnik T, Hawton K, McGuire H. Interventions for vaginismus. Cochrane Database of Systematic Reviews. 2012;12.
75. Fuchs K, Hoch Z, Paldi E, Abramovici H, Brandes JM, Timor-Tritsch I, et al. Hypno-desensitization therapy of vaginismus. I. "In vitro" method. II. "In vivo" method. Int J Clin Exp Hypn. 1973;21(3):144–56.
76. Fertel NS. Vaginismus: a review. J Sex Marital Ther. 1977;3(2):113–21.
77. Reamy K. The treatment of vaginismus by the gynecologist: an eclectic approach. Obstet Gynecol. 1982;59(1):58–62.
78. ter Kuile MM, Melles R, de Groot HE, Tuijnman-Raasveld CC, van Lankveld JJ. Therapist-aided exposure for women with lifelong vaginismus: a randomized waiting-list control trial of efficacy. J Consult Clin Psychol. 2013;81(6):1127–36.
79. Ter Kuile MM, Bulte I, Weijenborg PT, Beekman A, Melles R, Onghena P. Therapist-aided exposure for women with lifelong vaginismus: a replicated single-case design. J Consult Clin Psychol. 2009;77(1): 149–59.
80. Ter Kuile MM. Personal communication about ethics procedure. [E-mail]. Message to: Irv Binik, Samara Perez, Claudia Brown. 2015 March 2. 2015.

Diagnosis and Management of Sexual Pain Disorders: Dyspareunia

25

Jill M. Krapf and Andrew T. Goldstein

25.1 Introduction

Pain with intercourse, or dyspareunia, may be one of the most common complaints in the gynecologic office setting. Despite this, it is one of the most difficult clinical problems to evaluate and treat, leading to understandable clinician discomfort. Based upon a systematic review by the World Health Organization (WHO), the incidence of painful intercourse ranges between 8 and 22 % [1]. In 2003, Basson et al. expanded the definition of dyspareunia to include women who experience pain with attempted vaginal entry, which is not included in the WHO definition and likely increases the true incidence of the condition [2].

To complicate these definitions further, the DSM-IV stipulates that dyspareunia should not include sexual pain resulting from a general medical condition or local pathology, but the recently released DSM-5 discarded the term vaginismus and introduced a combined definition: genito-pelvic pain/penetration disorder [3]. The decision that the two disorders could not be reliably differentiated was based on two primary considerations. First, the diagnostic formulation of vaginismus as "vaginal muscle spasm" was not supported by empiric evidence [4]. Second, fear of pain or fear of vaginal penetration is commonplace in clinical descriptions of vaginismus.

Pain with intercourse may also be a sign of vulvodynia, which is defined as chronic vulvar pain in the absence of infection, skin conditions, or neoplasia [5, 6]. Vulvodynia, and more specifically provoked vestibulodynia (pain at the vulvar vestibule), likely has a number of causes including inflammatory, hormonal, myofascial, and neurologic ones. Tight pelvic floor muscles (previously termed vaginismus, more appropriately termed hypertonic pelvic floor muscle dysfunction) may be a result, as well as a cause, of dyspareunia. This chapter will provide a general overview of diagnosis and management of dyspareunia, considering a broad differential diagnosis of painful intercourse. A comprehensive list of conditions associated with dyspareunia is summarized in Table 25.1.

25.2 Diagnosis

25.2.1 Approach to the Patient

A woman's experience of dyspareunia can be more complicated in presentation and evaluation than other medical conditions. Often, women do not

J.M. Krapf, M.D.
Department of Obstetrics and Gynecology,
George Washington University School of Medicine,
Washington, DC, USA

A.T. Goldstein, M.D., FACOG, IF (✉)
The George Washington University School
of Medicine, 3 Washington Circle NW, Suite 205,
Washington, DC 20027, USA
e-mail: obstetrics@yahoo.com

L.I. Lipshultz et al. (eds.), *Management of Sexual Dysfunction in Men and Women*, DOI 10.1007/978-1-4939-3100-2_25

Table 25.1 Conditions associated with dyspareunia

Hormonal:
Vulvovaginal atrophy
Hormonally mediated vestibulodynia
Inflammatory:
Skin allergy (semen allergy)
Lichen simplex chronicus
Vestibulodynia
Desquamative inflammatory vaginitis
Neurologic:
Pudendal neuralgia
Postherpetic neuralgia
Neuroproliferative vestibulodynia
Dermatologic:
Lichen sclerosus
Lichen planus
Vulvar granuloma fissuratum
Mucous membrane pemphigoid
Infectious:
Recurrent vulvovaginal candidiasis
Pelvic inflammatory disease
Sexually transmitted infection
Neoplastic:
Vulvar interepithelial neoplasm
Pelvic neoplasms (cervical, uterine, ovarian, colon)
Muscular:
Pelvic floor dysfunction
Vaginismus
Structural:
Endometriosis
Leiomyoma
Ovarian mass
Pelvic adhesions
Irritable bowel syndrome
Interstitial cystitis
Female genital cutting

disclose their symptoms to a health-care provider, and if they do, limitations of time and experience may hinder a comprehensive evaluation [7]. In addition to pain, an affected woman may experience embarrassment, shame, guilt, loss of self-esteem, frustration, depression, and anxiety related to her symptoms. It is not unusual for a woman with dyspareunia to have seen several health-care providers in an effort to evaluate and treat her condition [8]. It is important that the clinician promotes openness, comfort, trust, and confidence in the interaction with the patient. Assuring privacy and confidentiality is essential when conducting the medical interview. Although some patients may want their sexual partner present, this may also inhibit the patient from disclosing pertinent aspects of her medical or social history. Sensitivity to the patient's own initial preference is paramount in maintaining rapport. A partner may always be brought in subsequently if needed at a follow-up session. An overly intrusive partner can often be successfully managed and yet not offended.

Displaying understanding and empathy when appropriate and repeating the information back to the patient for confirmation further help to establish a positive interaction. Frequently, a patient will become emotional or there may be moments of silence, which can be cathartic for the patient. If there is not enough time to focus on the patient's concerns during a single visit, the patient should be reassured of the importance of her problem and scheduled for a follow-up visit to address the issue of sexual pain alone.

25.2.1.1 Medical History

After a chief complaint of painful intercourse is established, a history of the present illness should be obtained. Asking open-ended questions allows the patient to describe her experience of the condition. Encouraging the patient to give as much detailed information as possible and following a sequential timeline of her disease progression may facilitate this process. In regard to sexual pain, it is essential to determine timing, character, alleviating and aggravating factors, as well as associated symptoms.

The clinician should determine if the dyspareunia has been present since first attempt at intercourse (primary) or if the pain started after a period of pain-free intercourse (secondary). It is important to ask about first tampon use and experience with speculum examinations, as this may aid diagnosis. In cases of primary dyspareunia, it is more important to explore for a potential history of physical, sexual, and emotional abuse, as well as severe anxiety. If secondary, it is critical to ascertain whether or not the problem is partner-specific. In cases that are partner-specific, the following considerations should be explored: inadequate sexual technique, poor communication, incompatible sexual script, or no physical attraction. The provider may screen for severe difficulties in the couple's relationship through inquiry with a reassuring, "No one's relationship is perfect; are there any particularly difficult issues that exist at this time?" Monitor the degree of acrimony when the patient describes her complaints. For example, is the anger, hurt, or sadness a causative factor, or are these mild emotional frustrations of daily life? In practice, most providers lack the time for a thorough evaluation of all relationship issues, even if the partner joins the patient for the office visit. The goal is to pursue the diagnostic process sufficiently to determine if a referral for collaborative care with a sex or physical therapist is needed and/or identify an organic cause that may respond to a first-line treatment [9–11].

In a focused review, symptoms such as vaginal discharge, vulvar itching, irregular vaginal bleeding, and vulvar tearing can differentiate causes of dyspareunia. Changes in libido, decreased vaginal lubrication, and menopausal symptoms such as hot flushes and night sweats should be discussed. Use and effectiveness of artificial lubricant should be assessed. Urinary symptoms such as frequency, urgency, incomplete emptying, and leakage should be elucidated. It is also important to ask about bowel symptoms, including chronic constipation and rectal fissures.

After an accurate chief complaint, history of present illness, and review of symptoms have been established, additional information should be gathered to allow the clinician to narrow the differential diagnosis of dyspareunia. Depending on time, the sexual history can be expanded. It is of course important to obtain an obstetric and gynecologic history, as well as a past medical and surgical history. To the extent that time allows, additional elements of social history can be reviewed. Because certain medications may be associated with dyspareunia, it is essential to develop a timeline of medication use and compare this to the timeline of the patient's sexual pain history. The clinician should specifically inquire about herbal supplements, as well as over-the-counter topical preparations. Finally, there is always value in asking the patient what she thinks the cause of her problem is, if she has not already been forthcoming with an opinion. Most importantly, the collection of a detailed and specific history must be balanced by the need to maintain rapport, as a follow-up visit can always be scheduled if more information is needed prior to initiating treatment.

Hormonal contraceptives, antidepressants, and antibiotics are medications that can very commonly contribute to dyspareunia. In one case-control study, women who used oral contraceptives were 9.3 times more likely to develop vestibulodynia than controls [12]. In addition, women who used low-dose ethinyl estradiol oral contraceptives were more likely to develop vestibulodynia [13]. Oral contraceptives decrease free circulating testosterone, which may be harmful to the androgen-dependent mucin-secreting glands and endothelium of the vulvar vestibule, leading to pain symptoms and decreased lubrication [14]. Psychotropic medications are often implicated in hypoactive sexual desire disorder (HSDD) and female sexual arousal disorder (FSAD) and may decrease vaginal lubrication and lead to dyspareunia [15]. Although antibiotics do not cause sexual pain directly, long-term exposure may predispose to chronic yeast infections, which may lead to dyspareunia.

It is also important to recognize that some aspects of a patient's self-reported medical history may be inaccurate. For instance, a woman's self-diagnosis of a vulvovaginal yeast infection is inaccurate about half the time. In addition, studies surprisingly show that physician-aided diagnosis of candidiasis is frequently incorrect in the absence of microscopy and culture [16].

25.2.1.2 Physical Examination

All women with dyspareunia should undergo a thorough physical examination (Table 25.2). While this exam focuses mainly on the urogenital system, examination of other areas, such as the oral mucosa, may be warranted based upon a detailed history. Visual examination of the vulva involves noting any signs of inflammation, lichenification, changes in pigmentation, loss of architecture, scarring, fissures, or ulceration. While erythema is often a nonspecific finding, redness at

Table 25.2 Physical examination of dyspareunia

The vulva and vestibule
– Visual examination
– Vulvoscopy
– Sensory exam with cotton swab
– Consider biopsy
The vagina and cervix
– Visualization with speculum exam
– Wet mount with pH and KOH prep
– Vaginal culture
The uterus, ovaries, and bladder
– Bimanual exam to evaluate size, shape, and contour
– Rectovaginal exam
The pelvic floor
– Levator ani muscle trigger points
– Hypertonicity, weakness, tenderness
– Pudendal nerve tenderness

the ostia of the vestibular glands is suggestive of vestibulodynia. Vulvar skin abnormalities may indicate a dermatologic disease of the vulva and often warrant vulvar punch biopsy [17].

A moistened small cotton swab is used to perform a systematic sensory exam of the vulva. Women with sexual pain can exhibit allodynia, the perception of pain upon provocation by a normally non-painful stimulus, or hyperpathia, pain provoked by very light touch. Initially, the medial thigh, buttocks, and mons pubis are palpated to orient the patient to the examination. Then the labia majora, clitoral prepuce, perineum, and intralabial sulci should be palpated. Pain of the external vulva may indicate a vulvar dermatosis, vulvovaginal infection, or neuropathic process such as pudendal neuralgia. Attention is then turned to the labia minora, which are gently palpated first laterally and then medially to Hart's line (the lateral boundary of the vulvar vestibule). Within the vulvar vestibule, the clinician palpates five specific locations: the ostia of the Skene's glands (2 and 10 o'clock on the vulvar vestibule), the ostia of the Bartholin's glands (4 and 8 o'clock on the vulvar vestibule), as well as the fossa navicularis (6 o'clock on the vulvar vestibule) (Fig. 25.1).

Patients with vestibulodynia experience allodynia confined to the tissue of the vulvar vestibule, but have normal sensation of the external vulva, lateral to Hart's line. If the pain is localized to the vestibule, it is important to determine if the pain affects the entire vestibule or just the posterior vestibule. Pain with palpation anywhere on the vestibular tissue indicates an intrinsic pathology within the mucosa of the vestibular endoderm. Pain confined only to the posterior vestibule suggests an extrinsic cause, most commonly related to the underlying musculature, such as hypertonic pelvic floor muscle dysfunction [18].

A speculum exam of the vagina should be performed next to evaluate vaginal pathology and discharge. An appropriately sized speculum, such as a pediatric Graves speculum, and avoidance of touching the vulvar vestibule allow for a more tolerable examination. The clinician should note evidence of vaginal atrophy, erythema, erosions, ulcerations, scarring, and abnormal discharge. A cotton swab should be used to collect vaginal discharge for pH testing, wet mount, and potassium hydroxide (KOH) prep. The saline slide is examined for normal squamous epithelial cells, parabasal cells, an increased number of white blood cells (WBCs), budding hyphae indicating yeast, trichomonads, clue cells, and normal flora such as lactobacilli. As microscopic examination frequently misses candidiasis and trichomoniasis, a culture obtained at the time of vaginal inspection should be sent for speciation and sensitivity.

A manual exam is then performed with one finger, attempting to avoid the vestibule. The urethra and bladder trigone are gently palpated. Intrinsic tenderness of the urethra may be suggestive of a urethral diverticulum or interstitial cystitis, while tenderness of the bladder may be suggestive of either interstitial cystitis or endometriosis. The trigger points of the levator ani muscles are then palpated for hypertonicity, weakness, and tenderness, which can be evidence of hypertonic pelvic floor muscle dysfunction (also known as levator ani syndrome and previously vaginismus).

The ischial spine is then located and the pudendal nerve palpated as it enters Alcock's canal. Tenderness of the pudendal nerve is suggestive of pudendal neuralgia or pudendal nerve entrapment. Next, a bimanual examination is performed to assess the uterus and adnexa

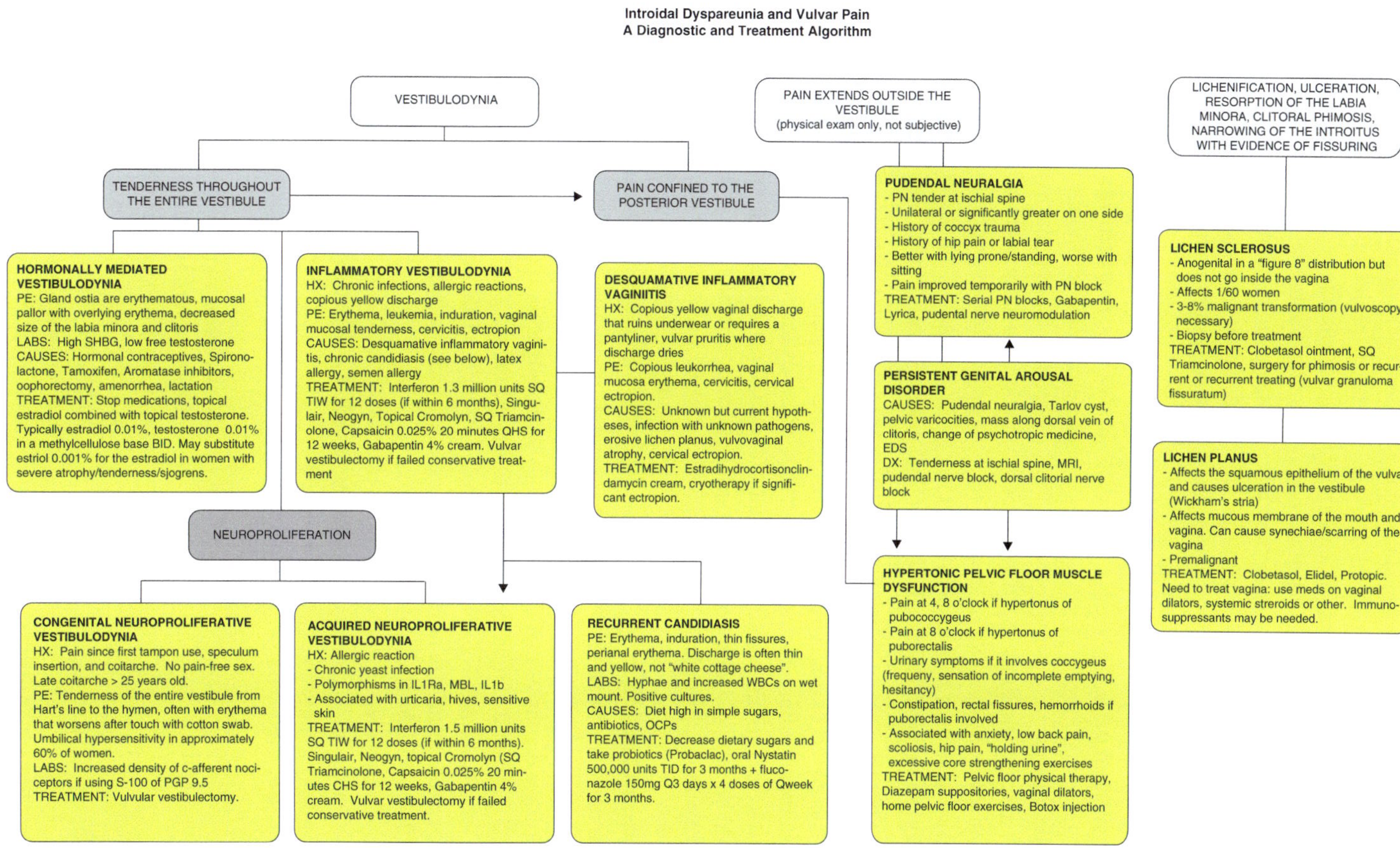

Fig. 25.1 A diagnostic and treatment algorithm for the treatment of dyspareunia and vulvar pain

(ovaries and fallopian tubes). Abnormalities in the size, shape, or contour may be indicative of a leiomyoma or adenomyosis. Enlargement or tenderness of the adnexa may represent an ovarian mass, pelvic inflammatory disease, or endometriosis. A rectovaginal examination is then performed to assess the rectovaginal septum and the posterior cul-de-sac for findings suggestive of endometriosis. Women who have undergone prior vaginal surgery or perineal laceration repair may have traumatic neuromas, which can also be a source of significant pain.

25.2.1.3 Histology

If there are specific findings on vulvar colposcopic examination suggestive of dermatoses, intraepithelial neoplasia, or neoplasia, a vulvar or vaginal biopsy should be obtained. A 4 mm punch biopsy may be used to obtain a sample at the edge of any ulcerations or erosions, if present. All biopsies should be closed with one or two stitches of absorbable suture such as 4-0 Vicryl-rapide (Ethicon, Inc., Somerville, NJ). Ideally, biopsies should be sent to a pathologist who specializes in dermatologic disorders.

25.2.1.4 Serum Testing

If a hormonal cause of sexual pain is suspected or if the cause is unknown, blood work may be helpful in determining a diagnosis and planning treatment (Table 25.3). Blood should be obtained for evaluation of serum estradiol, total testosterone, free testosterone, albumin, sex hormone-binding globulin (SHBG), follicle-stimulating hormone, and prolactin. A decreased serum estradiol level is frequently found in women with atrophic vaginitis or a hormonally mediated provoked vestibulodynia. Elevated SHBG and decreased free testosterone and estradiol are frequently found in women with provoked vestibulodynia caused by hormonal contraceptives [19–22]. An elevated prolactin level in reproductive-aged women can cause anovulation, which leads to atrophic vaginitis. Herpes serology should be obtained in women with symptoms of generalized vulvar burning or tingling or in those with pain concentrated in the clitoris (clitorodynia).

Table 25.3 Serum testing

Estradiol
Total testosterone
Free testosterone
Albumin
Sex hormone-binding globulin (SHBG)
Follicle-stimulating hormone (FSH)
Prolactin

25.2.1.5 Imaging and Diagnostic Procedures

Referrals for additional testing should be based on findings during the history and physical examination. Radiographic or ultrasonographic imaging may be appropriate to evaluate the uterus, ovaries, pelvis, or lower spine. Magnetic resonance imaging may help identify entrapment of the pudendal nerve.

Diagnostic laparoscopy may be necessary if there is significant evidence of endometriosis or utero-ovarian pathology that does not respond to initial conservative management. Colonoscopy, barium enema, and/or a CT scan with contrast may be used to rule out pathology of the lower gastrointestinal tract if deep thrusting dyspareunia is present along with dyschezia, hematochezia, or symptoms consistent with inflammatory bowel disease. Cystoscopy may be used to aid in the diagnosis of interstitial cystitis. An electromyelogram may be used to assess the tone and strength of the levator ani muscles when there is evidence of hypertonic pelvic floor dysfunction.

25.3 Management

25.3.1 Deep Dyspareunia

Dyspareunia may have a variety of causes. In order to determine the cause, the location of the pain must first be identified. Often, patients will describe pain with intercourse as deep and/or superficial. Deep dyspareunia may be attributed to a structural cause, including pathology of the genitourinary system, such as endometriosis, interstitial cystitis (painful bladder syndrome), or pelvic adhesions. Endometriosis is often difficult to manage, with treatment options ranging from a variety of hormonal preparations to surgical procedures including fulguration and excision of endometrial implants, as well as hysterectomy. Interstitial cystitis may be alleviated by dietary modification, although a referral to an urologist may be indicated for further workup or treatment. Treatment of pelvic adhesions is challenging, with management options involving both pain management as well as surgical lysis.

25.3.2 Vaginitis, Vulvovaginal Atrophy, and Vulvar Dermatoses

Pain with intercourse may occur with vaginal infection or cervicitis, vaginal atrophy, or vaginal scarring, such as that seen with intravaginal lichen planus. Vaginal infections such gonorrhea, chlamydia, and trichomonas should be treated per CDC guidelines [23]. Generally, treatment of bacterial vaginosis responds to a 5- to 7-day course of metronidazole, and uncomplicated vulvovaginal candidiasis is successfully treated using either a topical or oral azole medication. It should be noted that in the experience of the authors, recurrent bacterial vaginosis does not cause chronic dyspareunia.

Local estradiol preparations are the treatment of choice for vulvovaginal atrophy. These are available in many forms, including creams, tablets, and rings. A small amount of estradiol cream or gel applied to the vestibule may be necessary, in addition to vaginal or vulvar application, in cases of dyspareunia. Desquamative inflammatory vaginitis (DIV) is a poorly understood clinical condition involving diffuse exudative inflammation of the vagina leading to a profuse purulent discharge and dyspareunia. Although there are no controlled studies to inform management, intravaginal clindamycin and intravaginal hydrocortisone may alleviate symptoms [24]. Vulvar dermatoses, such as lichen planus and lichen sclerosus, are typically treated with a high-potency topical steroid, such as clobetasol [25].

25.3.3 Vulvodynia

Vulvar pain, which is usually more superficial, should be further characterized as generalized vulvar pain or specific pain isolated to the vulvar vestibule. Generalized vulvar pain may be related to an autoimmune dermatologic vulvar condition, such as lichen sclerosus, or may be a result of decreased estrogen levels, such as in vulvar atrophy. Generalized vulvar pain may also have a neurologic cause such as pudendal neuralgia, an infectious cause such as herpes simplex virus, or a neoplastic cause such as vulvar intraepithelial neoplasia. In the absence of defined neurologic, infectious, or neoplastic causes, vulvar pain is referred to as vulvodynia.

The term vulvar vestibulitis is often used in the literature to describe pain isolated to the vulvar vestibule; however, this condition may be more accurately called "provoked vestibulodynia." Emerging research supports possible hormonal, inflammatory, myofascial, and neurologic causes for provoked vestibulodynia [26]. A diagnostic and treatment algorithm for dyspareunia and vulvar pain was recently published and provides a systematic approach to management of women suffering from these symptoms. Figure 25.1 is an updated version of this algorithm.

Sexual pain due to hormonal causes includes vulvovaginal atrophy and hormonally mediated provoked vestibulodynia. The symptoms are often due to a decrease in estrogen and testosterone levels as a result of physiologic changes related to menopause or breastfeeding or due to the effects of a medication, such as combined oral contraceptives. Studies have shown that oral contraceptives may lower pain thresholds in the vestibular region and causes changes to the vaginal epithelium consistent with vulvovaginal atrophy [21, 22]. If oral contraceptive use is the main risk factor, the offending medication should be discontinued and alternative contraceptive methods may be considered, such as nonhormonal and progesterone-only options. In a non-placebo-controlled study, Burrows and Goldstein showed that a cream that combined estradiol

0.01 % and testosterone 0.1 % reduced visual analogue pain scores from 7.5 to 2.0 in 50 consecutive women who had developed provoked vestibulodynia from combined oral contraceptive pills [19]. In addition, an oral medication, ospemifene, was recently approved by the FDA for treatment of dyspareunia in postmenopausal women secondary to vulvovaginal atrophy [26].

Some research suggests a possible inflammatory cause of vestibulodynia. This may be the case in women with a history of chronic vulvovaginal infection or exposure-related sensitivities or allergic reactions in this area. To support this theory, Foster et al. [27] found that women with vestibulodynia exhibited increased levels of tumor necrosis factor beta and interleukin-1 alpha, which are inflammatory proteins. Several genetic defects have been identified that cause increased inflammation and increased susceptibility to vaginal infections [28]. Treatments using montelukast, submucosal betamethasone injections, and vestibular interferon injections have been tried with some success [29–31].

Several researchers have found that women with provoked vestibulodynia have up to ten times the density of c-afferent nociceptors nerve endings in their vestibular mucosa than normal women [32–34]. In addition, Bornstein et al. [35] found increased numbers of mast cells in vestibular tissue of women with vulvodynia. Persistently activated mast cells release nerve growth factor and heparinase that allow newly sprouted nerve endings to invade the superficial mucosa of the vestibule [36]. Topical lidocaine ointment has been used to treat "neuroproliferative vestibulodynia." Lidocaine may be applied using a 2 % jelly or 5 % ointment as needed prior to intercourse. In addition, long-term use of overnight topical lidocaine 5 % has been shown to significantly decrease pain with sexual activity, although long-term follow-up is not available [37].

Other topical medications have been investigated for provoked vestibulodynia including topical gabapentin, amitriptyline, and capsaicin. A retrospective, non-blinded, non-placebo-controlled study performed by Boardman et al. [38] revealed that topical gabapentin is an effective treatment for women with vulvodynia. Participants with both generalized (37 %) and localized (63 %) vulvodynia were treated with 2–6 % gabapentin for at least 8 weeks. The average pain score decreased 4.77 points, from 7.26 to 2.49 on a ten-point pain scale (mean pain score among the 35 evaluable women was significantly reduced from 7.26 to 2.49). Approximately 80 % of participants experienced at least a 50 % reduction in their pain. Furthermore, sexual function improved in the majority of participants, and all participants who had reported decreased participation in intercourse prior to treatment due to pain reported increased intercourse frequency after treatment [38, 39].

Pagano and Wong [40] performed a prospective study using topical amitriptyline 2 % cream that included 150 patients with provoked vestibulodynia and dyspareunia. One hundred and two participants exhibited purely provoked vestibulodynia, and 48 participants demonstrated both provoked and unprovoked vestibulodynia. Participants were encouraged to apply a pea-size amount of amitriptyline cream to the vulvar vestibule twice daily for 3 months. Of the 102 participants with purely provoked vestibulodynia, 84 (56 %) responded to the treatment (25 exhibited slight yet appreciable improvement, 44 exhibited moderate improvement, and 15 exhibited an excellent response defined as completely pain-free intercourse). The response rate was similar in the group of participants who experienced both provoked and unprovoked vestibulodynia; 48 % of them exhibited a positive response to treatment [40]. Lastly, in a retrospective chart review, topical capsaicin 0.025 % applied 20 min daily for 12 weeks decreased pain scores in patients with vulvodynia, but its use was limited by local irritation [38, 39].

In the past, oral medications have also been used for the treatment of vulvodynia and provoked vestibulodynia. Classes of oral medications used include tricyclic antidepressants (TCAs) (amitriptyline, desipramine), selective norepinephrine reuptake inhibitors (venlafaxine, duloxetine), and anticonvulsants (gabapentin, lamotrigine). Leo and Dewani [41] performed a literature review regarding the effectiveness of oral antidepressant medications in treating vulvodynia. The research included two randomized controlled trials, one quasi-experimental trial, seven nonexperimental studies, and three case reports; the majority of the 13 studies are TCA treatment. The authors concluded that there was a lack of sufficient evidence to support the use of antidepressant medication for treatment of vulvodynia [41].

In women who fail conservative treatments, vulvar vestibulectomy with vaginal advancement can be performed to remove the abnormal vestibular mucosa [42]. In 1983, Woodruff and Parmley were the first authors to describe vulvar vestibulectomy. Their procedure consisted of the excision of a semicircular segment of perineal skin, the mucosa of the posterior vulvar vestibule, and the posterior hymeneal ring. Three centimeters of the vaginal mucosa was then undermined and approximated to the perineum. Several variations of the procedure have been described to help decrease complications, such as dehiscence of the vaginal advancement flap, as well as to improve operative success. A complete vulvar vestibulectomy includes the excision of the mucosa of the entire vulvar vestibule including the mucosa adjacent to the urethra, while a modified vestibulectomy limits excision of the mucosa to the posterior vestibule [43].

In 2010, Tommola and colleagues did a systematic review of success and complication rates of the several variations of vulvar vestibulectomy and concluded, "There is no straightforward recommendation of the best technique. Certainly the surgeon's experience plays a critical role. As with all surgeries, the procedure should be extensive enough to remove all painful areas but also to avoid unnecessary risks." They examined 33 studies that addressed improvement in dyspareunia as a measure of surgical success for patients who had a partial or complete vulvar vestibulectomy. Seventeen of the 33 of those studies based improvement in dyspareunia solely on a patients' self-report on improvement of dyspareunia, alleviation of symptoms, or reduction in pain. Overall, these studies reveal that operative treatment provided significant relief in 78.5 % of patients, some relief in 88.8 % of patients, and no relief in 12.2 %. In nine studies that reported improvement in sexual function as a measure of success, all nine studies reported significant improvement in sexual function following vestibulectomy [44].

25.3.4 Hypertonic Pelvic Floor Muscle Dysfunction

It has been long acknowledged that tight pelvic floor muscles can contribute to provoked vestibulodynia. The muscles that compose the "floor of the pelvis" (levator ani muscles: the pubococcygeus, puborectalis, and transverse perineal muscles), which come together at the inferior aspect of the vestibule, can become tight and tender. Tight levator ani muscles cause a constriction of the arterioles, which leads to a decrease in blood flow to the muscles and the mucosa of the vestibule [45]. Decreased blood flow results in less oxygen delivery, leading to an increase in lactic acid in these tissues. This buildup of lactic acid causes the sensations of burning, rawness, throbbing, aching, and soreness. In response, the capillaries in the vestibule dilate to facilitate more blood to the area, causing an erythematous appearance of the vestibular mucosa [46].

Women with hypertonic pelvic floor dysfunction typically feel burning, rawness, and soreness. These symptoms can occur only with penetration or may be constant (non-provoked). In addition, there can be a sensation of ripping, tearing, or "hitting a wall" upon penetration. It is very important to understand that vestibulodynia caused by tight pelvic floor muscles only affects the back part of vestibule at 4, 6, and 8 o'clock because that is where the muscles attach directly under the mucosa of the vestibule. As there are no robust muscles in the vestibule around the urethra, tight pelvic floor muscles do not typically cause pain around the top part of the vestibule. Women with hypertonic pelvic floor dysfunction often have urinary symptoms such as frequency, urgency, and the sensation of incomplete emptying of the bladder. For this reason, women with hypertonic pelvic floor muscles are frequently misdiagnosed with a urinary tract infection or interstitial cystitis [45]. In addition, constipation, hemorrhoids, and rectal fissures are common. Women with hypertonic pelvic floor muscles frequently have low back pain and/or hip pain.

Women with other types of vestibulodynia (inflammatory, hormonally mediated, neuroproliferative) frequently will develop hypertonic pelvic floor dysfunction. In addition, women with more generalized vulvodynia almost always have some degree of hypertonic pelvic floor muscle dysfunction. The goal of treatment of hypertonic pelvic floor dysfunction is to relax and lengthen the pelvic floor muscles. As such, the mainstay of treatment is transvaginal pelvic floor physical therapy by a skilled women's health pelvic floor physical therapist [49]. Pelvic floor physical therapy can be augmented with biofeedback, vaginal dilators, home pelvic floor relaxation exercises, rectal or vaginal diazepam suppositories [47], oral muscle relaxants, trigger point injections, and botulinum toxin type A injections [48]. Pelvic floor physical therapists can be located using the following websites: www.womenshealthapta.org, www.hermanwallace.com, and www.isswsh.org.

25.4 Conclusion

Dyspareunia can be one of the most challenging complaints that providers encounter in the office setting. Ensuring adequate time and a comfortable setting to address a woman's concerns is essential in order to obtain an accurate and thorough history. Understanding the broad differential diagnosis of painful intercourse guides history taking. Certain medications and medical conditions may contribute to female sexual dysfunction. A thorough, yet focused, pelvic examination is necessary to determine the cause of the sexual pain.

Identifying the location of the pain is the first step in determining the diagnosis. Although specific conditions may be associated with dyspareunia, sexual pain often falls into the category of vulvodynia or more specifically provoked vestibulodynia. Vulvodynia has been historically considered a "diagnosis of exclusion," but with continued research and understanding of the condition, separate etiologies are becoming clear. Decreased estrogen and testosterone levels, as seen with oral contraceptive use or in menopause, may lead to sexual pain as well as other forms of female sexual dysfunction. Inflammatory and neurologic causes are being investigated with corresponding treatment options, including topical medications and vulvar vestibulectomy. Hypertonic pelvic floor muscle dysfunction may be a result, as well as a cause, of dyspareunia. This condition can be identified on physical examination, marked by pain in the posterior vestibule. Restoring blood flow and oxygen through relaxation of the pelvic floor muscles is the goal of therapy. Often, pelvic floor tightness and possible anxiety surrounding sexual intercourse must be addressed in addition to the primary cause of dyspareunia.

Sexual pain can significantly affect a woman's well-being and quality of life. Dyspareunia should be explored and addressed, either in the current or a separate medical visit. Restoration of lasting and satisfying sexual function often requires a multidimensional understanding of all of the forces that contribute to the condition. Each clinician should carefully evaluate his or her own competence and interest in treating female sexual pain, so that regardless of the treatment modality, the patient receives optimal care. Referral to a mental health profession and utilization of adjunctive consultation through sex therapists, psychologists, and physical therapists may help to alleviate physician time limitations and provide multimodal care.

References

1. Latthe P, Latthe M, Say L, Gulmezoglu M, Khan KS. WHO systematic review of prevalence of chronic pelvic pain: a neglected reproductive health morbidity. BMC Public Health. 2006;6:177–83.
2. Basson R, Leiblum S, Brotto L, et al. Definitions of women's sexual dysfunction reconsidered: advocating expansion and revision. J Psychosom Obstet Gynaecol. 2003;24:221–9.
3. APA. Diagnostic and statistical manual of mental disorders. 4th ed. Washington, DC: American Psychiatric Association; 2000.
4. Binik YM. The DSM diagnostic criteria for vaginismus. Arch Sex Behav. 2010;39:278–91.
5. Schultz WW, Basson R, Binik Y, et al. Women's sexual pain and its management. J Sex Med. 2005;2: 301–16.
6. Moyal-Barracco M, Lynch PJ. 2003 ISVVD terminology and classification of vulvodynia: a historical perspective. J Reprod Med. 2004;49(10):772–7.
7. Steege JF, Zolnoun DA. Evaluation and treatment of dyspareunia. Obstet Gynecol. 2009;113(5):1124–36.

8. Harlow BL, Stewart EG. A population-based assessment of chronic unexplained vulvar pain: have we underestimated the prevalence of vulvodynia? J Am Med Womens Assoc. 2003;58:82–8.
9. Perelman M. Psychosocial history. In: Goldstein I, Meston C, Davis S, Traish A, editors. Women's sexual function and dysfunction: study, diagnosis and treatment. Abingdon: Taylor and Francis; 2005.
10. Althof SE, Rosen RC, Perelman MA, Rubio-Aurioles E. Standard operating procedures for taking a sexual history. J Sex Med. 2012. doi:10.1111/j.1743-6109.2012.02823.x.
11. Perelman M. Combination therapy for sexual dysfunction: integrating sex therapy and pharmacotherapy. In: Balon R, Segraves R, editors. Handbook of sexual dysfunction. Boca Raton: Taylor and Francis; 2005. p. 13–41.
12. Bouchard C, Brisson J, Fortier M, et al. Use of oral contraceptive pills and vulvar vestibulitis: a case control study. Am J Epidemiol. 2002;156:254–61.
13. Greenstein A, Ben-Aroya Z, Fass O, et al. Vulvar vestibulitis syndrome and estrogen dose of oral contraceptive pills. J Sex Med. 2007;4:1679–83.
14. Panzer C, Wise S, Fantini G, Kang D, Munarriz R, Guay A, Goldstein I. Impact of oral contraceptives on sex hormone-binding globulin and androgen levels: a retrospective study in women with sexual dysfunction. J Sex Med. 2006;3(1):104.
15. Clayton AH, Campbell BJ, Favit A, et al. Symptoms of sexual dysfunction in patients treated for major depressive disorder: a meta-analysis comparing selegiline transdermal system and placebo using a patient-rated scale. J Clin Psychiatry. 2007;68:1860–6.
16. Ledger WJ, Monif GRG. A growing concern: inability to diagnose vulvovaginal infections correctly. Obstet Gynecol. 2004;130:782–4.
17. Goldstein AT, Goldstein GR. Vulvar punch biopsy. J Sex Med. 2009;6(5):1214–7.
18. King M, Rubin R, Goldstein A. Current uses of surgery for the treatment of genital pain. Curr Sex Health Rep. 2014;6(4):252–8.
19. Burrows LJ, Goldstein AT. The treatment of vestibulodynia with topical estradiol and testosterone. Sex Med. 2013;1:30–3.
20. Goldstein AT, Burrows L. Vulvodynia. J Sex med. 2008;5:5–15.
21. Bohm-Starke N, Johannesson U, Hilliges M, Rylander E, Torebjork E. Decreased mechanical pain threshold in the vestibular mucosa of women using oral contraceptives: a contributing factor in vulvar vestibulitis? J Reprod Med. 2004;49:888–92.
22. Harlow BL, Vitonis AF, Stewart EG. Influence of oral contraceptive use on the risk of adult-onset vulvodynia. J Reprod Med. 2008;53(2):102–10.
23. Centers for Disease Control and Prevention. Sexually transmitted diseases treatment guidelines, 2010. Ann Emerg Med. 2011;58(1):67–8.
24. Reichman O, Sobel J. Desquamative inflammatory vaginitis. Best Pract Res Clin Obstet Gynaecol. 2014;28(7):1042–50.
25. Krapf JM, Goldstein A. The vulvar dermatoses. Female Patient. 2012;37(4):1–5.
26. Goldstein SR, Bachmann GA, Koninckx PR, Lin VH, Portman DJ, Ylikorkala O. Ospemifene 12-month safety and efficacy in postmenopausal women with vulvar and vaginal atrophy. Climacteric. 2014;17(2):173–82.
27. Foster DC, Hasday JD. Elevated tissue levels of interleukin-1 beta and tumor necrosis factor-alpha in vulvar vestibulitis. Obstet Gynecol. 1997;89:291–6.
28. Gerber S, Witkin SS, Sucki D. Immunological and genetic characterization of women with vulvodynia. J Med Life. 2008;1:432–8.
29. Dede M, Yenen MC, Yilmaz A, Baser I. Successful treatment of persistent **vulvodynia** with submucous infiltration of betamethasone and lidocaine. Eur J Obstet Gynecol Reprod Biol. 2006;124(2):258–9.
30. Kamdar N, Fisher L, MacNeill C. Improvement in vulvar vestibulitis with montelukast. J Reprod Med. 2007;52(10):912–6.
31. Marinoff SC, Turner ML, Hirsch RP, Richard G. Intralesional alpha interferon: cost-effective therapy for vulvar vestibulitis syndrome. J Reprod Med. 1993;38(1):19–24.
32. Bohm-Starke N, Hilliges M, Falconer C, Rylander E. Increased intraepithelial innervations in women with vulvar vestibulitis syndrome. Gynecol Obstet Investig. 1998;46:256–60.
33. Westrom LV, Willen R. Vestibular nerve fiber proliferation in vulvar vestibulitis syndrome. Obstet Gynecol. 1998;91:572–6.
34. Bohm-Starke N, Hilliges M, Falconer C, Rylander E. Neurochemical characterization of the vestibular nerves in women with vulvar vestibulitis syndrome. Gynecol Obstet Investig. 1999;48:270–5.
35. Bornstein J, Goldschmid N, Sabo E. Hyperinnervation and mast cell activation may be used as histopathologic diagnostic criteria for vulvar vestibulitis. Gynecol Obstet Investig. 2004;58:171–8.
36. Bornstein J, Cohen Y, Zarfati D, Sela S, Ophir E. Involvement of heparanase in the pathogenesis of localized vulvodynia. Int J Gynecol Pathol. 2008;27:136–41.
37. Zolnoun DA, Hartmann KE, Steege JF. Overnight 5 % lidocaine ointment for treatment of vulvar vestibulitis. Obstet Gynecol. 2003;102(1):84–7.
38. Boardman LA, Cooper AS, Blais LR, Raker CA. Topical gabapentin in the treatment of localized and generalized vulvodynia. Obstet Gynecol. 2008;112(3):579–85.
39. Steinberg AC, Oyama IA, Rejba AE, Kellogg-Spadt S, Whitmore KE. Capsaicin for the treatment of vulvar vestibulitis. Am J Obstet Gynecol. 2005;192(5):1549–53.
40. Pagano R, Wong S. Use of amitriptyline cream in the management of entry dyspareunia due to provoked vestibulodynia. J Low Genit Tract Dis. 2012;16(4):394–7.
41. Leo RJ, Dewani S. A systematic review of the utility of antidepressant pharmacotherapy in the treatment of vulvodynia pain. J Sex Med. 2013;10:2497–505.

42. Goldstein AT, Klingman D, Christopher K, Johnson C, Marinoff SC. Outcome assessment of vulvar vestibulectomy with vaginal advancement for vulvar vestibulitis syndrome: results of a post-operative questionnaire survey. J Sex Med. 2006;3(5):923–31.
43. Goetsch MF. Simplified surgical revision of the vulvar vestibule for vulvar vestibulitis. Am J Obstet Gynecol. 1996;174(6):1701–7.
44. Tommola P, Unkila-Kallio L, Paavonen J. Surgical treatment of vulvar vestibulitis: a review. Acta Obstet Gynecol Scand. 2010;89(11):1385–95.
45. Rosenbaum TY, Owens A. The role of pelvic floor physical therapy in the treatment of pelvic and genital pain-related sexual dysfunction (CME). J Sex Med. 2008;5(3):513–23.
46. Hartmann D, Sarton J. Chronic pelvic floor dysfunction. Best Pract Res Clin Obstet Gynaecol. 2014;28(7):977–90.
47. Rogalski MJ, Kellogg-Spadt S, Hoffmann AR, Fariello JY, Whitmore KE. Retrospective chart review of vaginal diazepam suppository use in high-tone pelvic floor dysfunction. Int Urogynecol J. 2010;21(7):895–9.
48. Adelowo A, Hacker MR, Shapiro A, Modest AM, Elkadry E. Botulinum toxin type A (BOTOX) for refractory myofascial pelvic pain. Female Pelvic Med Reconstr Surg. 2013;19(5):288–92.
49. Rosenbaum TY. Pelvic floor involvement in male and female sexual dysfunction and the role of pelvic floor rehabilitation in treatment: a literature review. J Sex Med. 2007 Jan;4(1):4–13.

Commentary: Diagnosis and Management of Sexual Pain Disorder—Dyspareunia

Caroline F. Pukall and Emma Dargie

Dyspareunia remains a diagnosis with substantial discussion around causes and treatments. The recent modification of the fifth edition of the Diagnostic and Statistical Manual (DSM-5) diagnosis of dyspareunia to incorporate all genito-pelvic pain and penetration disorders into a single diagnosis has engendered significant debate in the community. Regardless, female genital pain remains a common condition that can be debilitating to the patient and a treatment challenge to the care team. In the preceding chapter, Krapf and Goldstein provide an overview of painful intercourse including etiologies, approach to the patient, and treatments focused on pharmacotherapy, surgery, and pelvic floor physical therapy. The chapter addresses both deep and more superficial dyspareunia, with an emphasis on how to more generally address these conditions in affected women.

In the following commentary, Pukall and Dargie also provide a perspective on genital pain, but dive more deeply into vulvodynia and even more specifically into provoked vestibulodynia (PVD). Complementing Krapf and Goldstein's chapter, the commentary hews more closely to a holistic approach integrating psychotherapy with physical therapy, and surgical intervention when appropriate, in the approach to PVD. By merging cognitive behavioral therapy (CBT) to alter thoughts and behaviors associated with pelvic pain with pelvic floor physical therapy to mitigate muscle tension, control, and awareness, significant gains can be made. In the absence of improvement, a surgical approach may be favored. Regardless of how dyspareunia is addressed, it is made clear in the chapter and accompanying commentary that a multidisciplinary approach tailored to the individual is likely to result in the most significant treatment benefit.

The Editors

Caroline F. Pukall, Ph.D. • Emma Dargie, M.Sc.
Department of Psychology, Queen's University,
Kingston, ON, Canada

Commentary

Introduction

Genital pain is a highly prevalent condition, with estimates ranging from 14 to 34 % in younger women and from 6.5 to 45 % in older women [1]. Genital pain conditions can affect women in mixed-sex and same-sex relationships [2], and they can have a negative impact on psychological and sexual relationship function and overall quality of life [3]. One of the most common characteristics associated with genital pain is dyspareunia (i.e., painful vaginal penetration in sexual situations). Pelvic floor muscle dysfunction, most commonly in the form of poor control and increased muscle tension, is also typically associated with pain in the genital area [4, 5]. The combination of intense genital pain and pelvic floor muscle dysfunction can result in significant issues with tolerating vaginal penetration, sometimes rendering penetration impossible (i.e., vaginismus).

Diagnosis

The International Society for the Study of Vulvovaginal Disease (ISSVD) proposed two main categories of chronic genital pain: *vulvar pain related to a specific disorder* (e.g., dermatologic, inflammatory, infectious) and *vulvodynia* [6]. When a medical cause is known, treatment is tailored to the presenting issue. Those patients who present with medically unexplained chronic vulvar pain would likely be diagnosed with vulvodynia. This diagnosis also applies in cases in which a condition that was believed to result in vulvar pain (e.g., bacterial vaginosis) was successfully treated without pain resolution. The ISSVD further defines subtypes of vulvodynia based on information such as location and temporal pattern, which is essential for diagnosis and treatment planning.

According to the ISSVD, vulvodynia is characterized as idiopathic burning pain with two main symptom presentations: *localized*, which involves only a portion of the vulva such as the clitoris or vulvar vestibule, or *generalized*, which involves the entire vulva [6]. The pain can be further specified according to its temporal pattern (i.e., when it occurs). If the pain is *provoked*, it occurs in response to contact; if it is *unprovoked*, it occurs spontaneously (i.e., independent of contact). The pattern of pain may also be *mixed* if the patient has a combination of both provoked and unprovoked pain. Provoked pain may occur in response to sexual, nonsexual (e.g., gynecological examinations), or both types of activities. In addition, research on a highly prevalent condition known as provoked vestibulodynia (PVD)—characterized as localized provoked pain upon the vaginal vestibule—has indicated that pain *onset* may also be an important factor to consider. The issue of whether the pain has been present since the patient's first episode of vaginal penetration (i.e., primary PVD) or after a period of pain-free activities (i.e., secondary PVD) can influence pain sensitivity [7] as well as treatment outcome [8].

When a patient reports experiencing dyspareunia or genital pain, a detailed pain history should follow [9]. Questions should cover, at a minimum, the following domains: pain location, descriptors, onset (e.g., gradual or sudden; primary or secondary), temporal pattern (e.g., when the pain occurs; how long the pain has been present), what factors change (increase or decrease) the pain, how severe is the pain (e.g., on a scale of 0–10), and any related symptoms (e.g., bladder pain). Furthermore, any previous treatment attempts and outcomes and the patient's personal explanation of the pain should be queried. Additionally, the impact of the pain should be thoroughly assessed in various domains, such as sexual functioning, body image, relationship adjustment, and psychological distress. A brief medical history should be ascertained, followed by a referral to knowledgeable medical professional for a complete medical history taking (including other pain conditions) and comprehensive gynecological examination. The gynecological examination should include a standard investigation (e.g., vaginal and cervical cultures) for routine infections and other issues, a full evaluation of potential causes of genital pain (e.g., dermatologic conditions, fissures), and the cotton swab test. This test consists of the palpation of various vulvar areas with a cotton swab while the patient rates her pain intensity; it is essential for determining the precise location and severity of the pain. Given the presence of sensory abnormalities and the contribution of the pelvic floor muscle dysfunction in the maintenance of PVD, referral to a pelvic health physical therapist for an in-depth pelvic floor assessment is also recommended.

Throughout the assessment process, health-care professionals should take care to ensure that they validate the patient's pain experience. In many cases, women with vulvodynia have been indirectly or directly told that their pain may not be "real" given the lack of physical findings. Sending such messages may contribute to increased psychological distress and other symptoms, leading to a sense of hopelessness and worsening of psychological health. Instead, providing education about chronic pain and its usual lack of physical findings, the vicious cycle of pain (see Fig. 25.2), and genital anatomy can be helpful. Recommending appropriate resources to patients, such as the National Vulvodynia Association website (www.nva.org), can allow patients to learn about their condition and feel less "alone" in coming to terms with their diagnosis.

Proposed Etiologies

Countless etiological theories of genital pain exist, ranging from biomedical to psychosocial. It is likely that different combinations of factors lead to similar symptoms of genital pain and that discovering those factors does not always hold the key to successful treatment. As such, spending significant amounts of energy trying to find the "cause" may not be worthwhile. Indeed, what may start as an acute pain directly linked to a cause (e.g., infection) may—over time—evolve into chronic unexplained pain due to the involvement of other factors (e.g., psychological distress, muscular responses, central nervous system dysregulation; Fig. 25.2).

Two factors have been consistently identified as risk factors for the development of chronic vulvar pain. The first of these is the use of oral contraceptives and potentially other hormonal methods of contraception. In 1994, Bazin and colleagues [10] first reported the association between oral contraceptives and PVD in a small case-control study. This study was followed by Sjoberg et al.'s [11] investigation indicating that women with PVD used oral contraceptives for a longer period of time than did non-affected women. Other researchers have reported a similar pattern of findings [12–14]. It is possible that the use of oral contraceptives may increase vestibular sensitivity to the point of rendering touch to the area painful (i.e., allodynic), as has been demonstrated via quantitative sensory testing [15] and validated measures of sexual function [16]. However, these results may depend on the dose and composition of the oral contraceptives, given that a recent study demonstrated no significant differences in self-reported or vulvar sensitivity thresholds in women who used a low-dose oral contraceptive [17]. It is important to note that having ever used oral contraceptives is not a necessary and sufficient factor for the development of PVD or related genital pain conditions; not all affected women have used oral contraceptives, and many women use these medications for various periods of time without ever developing genital pain problems. It is possible that vulvodynia may be triggered by the use of oral contraceptives in women with certain predisposing factors.

The second factor that is consistently linked to PVD is a history of recurrent vulvovaginal candidiasis (i.e., three or more yeast infections annually; Farmer et al. [20]). Estimates indicate a strikingly higher prevalence of such infections in women with PVD (42–90 %) [17, 18] than in control women (5–8 %) [19]. Indeed, the vestibular hypersensitivity characteristic of PVD may be caused by previous inflammation from prolonged/repeated vaginal yeast colonization. Farmer and colleagues [20] investigated whether repeated, localized exposure of the vulva to *Candida albicans* could lead to the development of chronic pain in mice. A subset of the mice that had been infected developed prolonged vulvar mechanical allodynia (i.e., painful response to touch) and hyperinnervation (i.e., an increase in

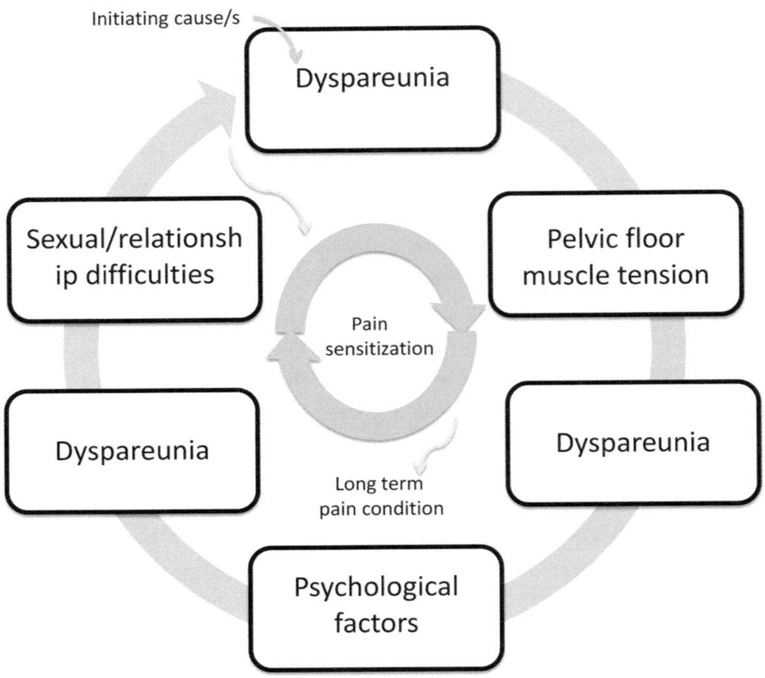

Fig. 25.2 The vicious cycle of pain. Once the experience of pain is initiated and continues for a prolonged period of time, the pain begins to influence and is influenced by many different factors (e.g., muscular, psychological, sexual). The involvement of these different factors can lead to increased pain and distress and can explain pain maintenance in the absence of physical findings. This cycle can start at any point or at multiple points simultaneously

the number of nerve fibers). This pattern echoes research on women with PVD, with evidence pointing to vestibular allodynia (see [21] for a review) and hyperinnervation [22–24], lending credence to the possibility that repeated yeast infections can render the vestibule hypersensitive in some affected women.

Other factors are likely involved in the etiology and maintenance of chronic vulvar pain, and these influences may be less evident at a local (vulvar) level. Research increasingly suggests that both peripheral (i.e., vulvar) and central (e.g., spinal, neural, psychological) factors are involved in the expression of chronic genital pain conditions (Fig. 25.2) [21]. Although just beginning to be studied, there appears to be evidence of heightened sensitivity to stimulation outside of the genital region [25, 26], indications of increased neural response to stimulation [27–29], and suggestions of an increased number of functional pain and other conditions (e.g., fibromyalgia, irritable bowel syndrome, depression) [30, 31] in women with vulvodynia. For some women, the pain may start locally and, over time, involve more central mechanisms. For other women, there may be a central dysregulation associated with having a chronic pain condition that, with repeated local (vulvar) injury, develops into a genital pain condition. Still others may develop the local and more generalized pain simultaneously.

Treatment

Treatment algorithms for vulvodynia exist [32]; however, most of the evidence for these algorithms is based on nonempirical sources (e.g., clinical experience, descriptive/observational studies, committee reports). Although highly important for informing research, the use of such algorithms may not accurately guide treatment. For example, oral medications (e.g., tricyclic antidepressants) are commonly recommended for pain control in vulvodynia, yet a recently published review [33] indicates that there is currently no empirical evidence for such practices. Looking at the evidence-based literature, three major treatment avenues have shown the most promise for PVD: psychological approaches, pelvic floor physical therapy, and surgical intervention.

Oftentimes, the first line of treatment recommended within these three is either psychological or pelvic floor physical therapy; they are sometimes recommended concurrently. If either or both of these treatments do not result in pain reduction, then surgical intervention (i.e., vestibulectomy) is recommended. Indeed, many patients must try different combinations of treatments before satisfactory results occur.

Cognitive behavioral therapy (CBT) is often recommended for women with vulvodynia. Similar to approaches taken with other pain conditions, CBT typically targets specific cognitive, emotional, relational, and behavioral goals related to the pain experience. For PVD, psychoeducation would be the first step, with an emphasis on the patient viewing her pain in relation to her thoughts, feelings, and behaviors as well as the interactions among these factors. Maladaptive patterns would be identified, with steps taken to modify them; positive coping strategies (e.g., relaxation, mindfulness, distraction) would be utilized. The maintenance of therapeutic gains would also be a focus of treatment. CBT can be particularly useful when patients with vulvodynia report unwanted cognitions or behaviors, difficulties with emotions, and/or issues with sexual/relationship function [9]. CBT for PVD has been shown to be more effective than other forms of therapy [34] and equally as effective as surgery in both a prospective randomized study [35] and a randomized treatment outcome study [36].

Pelvic floor physical therapy (PFPT) has also been shown to effectively treat PVD. PFPT targets muscle tension, control, and awareness through a variety of techniques (e.g., education, exercises, manual therapy, biofeedback). In a retrospective PFPT study, Bergeron and colleagues [37] found that self-reported pain during intercourse and gynecological examinations was reduced from pre- to posttreatment; in addition, significant increases in intercourse frequency, sexual desire, and sexual arousal were reported. A prospective study [5, 38] demonstrated reductions in pain during vaginal palpation, self-reported pain during intercourse, and self-reported pain during a gynecological examination from pre- to posttreatment. Furthermore, significant improvements in sexual function and a normalization of pelvic floor function were reported at posttreatment.

Vestibulectomy typically involves the surgical removal of parts or all (which leads to more successful outcomes) of the vaginal mucosa surrounding the opening to a depth of 1–2 mm. The success rates for vestibulectomy range between 60 and 90 % [32], and removal of all parts of the vaginal mucosa is more successful than removal of just the painful parts. However, given its invasiveness, the lack of a standardized definition of "successful" outcome, the relative lack of randomized comparisons, and the insufficient data on complication rates, it is not typically recommended as a first-line treatment [32].

Conclusions

Vulvodynia is a highly prevalent and distressing condition. Although the specific etiology or etiologies may never be uncovered for each patient, effective treatments exist. Empirically validated therapeutic interventions that focus on reducing pain intensity, coping with the presence of pain, enhancing muscular control, and potentially reestablishing sexual feelings and connections can be beneficial for many women. Validation of the pain as a chronic pain condition and education about pain processes and correlates should be provided to all patients presenting with vulvodynia and related conditions. Given the numerous factors involved in vulvar pain, treatment should ideally involve a variety of health-care professionals that work together in a collaborative manner.

References

1. van Lankveld JJ, Granot M, Weijmar Schultz WC, Binik YM, Wesselmann U, Pukall CF, et al. Women's sexual pain disorders. J Sex Med. 2010;7(1 Pt 2):615–31.
2. Blair K, Pukall CF, Smith KB, Cappell J. The differential associations of communication and love in heterosexual, bisexual and lesbian women's perceptions and experiences of chronic vulvar and pelvic pain. J Sex Marital Ther; in press.

3. Meana M, Binik YM, Khalife S, Cohen DR. Biopsychosocial profile of women with dyspareunia. Obstet Gynecol. 1997;90(4):583–9.
4. Reissing ED, Laliberte GM, Davis HJ. Young women's sexual adjustment: the role of sexual self-schema, sexual self-efficacy, sexual aversion and body attitudes. Can J Hum Sex. 2005;14(3):77–85.
5. Gentilcore-Saulnier E, McLean L, Goldfinger C, Pukall CF, Chamberlain S. Pelvic floor muscle assessment outcomes in women with and without provoked vestibulodynia and the impact of a physical therapy program. J Sex Med. 2010;7(2 Pt 2):1003–22.
6. Moyal-Barracco M, Lynch PJ. 2003 ISSVD terminology and classification of vulvodynia: a historical perspective. J Reprod Med. 2004;49(10):772–7.
7. Sutton KS, Pukall CF, Chamberlain S. Pain, psychosocial, psychosexual, and psychophysical characteristics in women with primary versus secondary vestibulodynia. J Sex Med. 2009;6(1): 205–14.
8. Heddini U, Bohm-Starke N, Nilsson KW, Johannesson U. Provoked vestibulodynia—medical factors and comorbidity associated with treatment outcome. J Sex Med. 2012;9(5):1400–6.
9. Dargie E, Pukall CF. Chronic genital pain. In: Porst H, Reisman Y, Kirana E, Tripodi F, editors. ESSM syllabus of sexual medicine for psychologists. 1st ed. Amsterdam: Medix; in press.
10. Bazin S, Bouchard C, Brisson J, Morin C, Meisels A, Fortier M. Vulvar vestibulitis syndrome: an exploratory case-control study. Obstet Gynecol. 1994;83(1): 47–50.
11. Sjoberg I, Nylander Lundqvist EN. Vulvar vestibulitis in the north of Sweden. An epidemiologic case-control study. J Reprod Med. 1997;42(3):166–8.
12. Berglund AL, Nigaard L, Rylander E. Vulvar pain, sexual behavior and genital infections in a young population: a pilot study. Acta Obstet Gynecol Scand. 2002;81(8):738–42.
13. Bouchard C, Brisson J, Fortier M, Morin C, Blanchette C. Use of oral contraceptive pills and vulvar vestibulitis: a case-control study. Am J Epidemiol. 2002; 156(3):254–61.
14. Harlow BL, Vitonis AE, Stewart EG. Influence of oral contraceptive use on the risk of adult-onset vulvodynia. J Reprod Med. 2008;53(2):102–10.
15. Bohm-Starke N, Johannesson U, Hilliges M, Rylander E, Torebjork E. Decreased mechanical pain threshold in the vestibular mucosa of women using oral contraceptives—a contributing factor in vulvar vestibulitis? J Reprod Med. 2004;49(11):888–92.
16. Battaglia C, Battaglia B, Mancini F, Busacchi P, Paganotto MC, Morotti E, et al. Sexual behavior and oral contraception: a pilot study. J Sex Med. 2012; 9(2):550–7.
17. Lee M, Morgan M, Rapkin A. Clitoral and vulvar vestibular sensation in women taking 20 mcg ethinyl estradiol combined oral contraceptives: a preliminary study. J Sex Med. 2011;8(1):213–8.
18. Bohm-Starke N, Hilliges M, Blomgren B, Falconer C, Rylander E. Increased blood flow and erythema in the posterior vestibular mucosa in vulvar vestibulitis. Obstet Gynecol. 2001;98(6):1067–74.
19. Witkin SS, Gerber S, Ledger WJ. Differential characterization of women with vulvar vestibulitis syndrome. Am J Obstet Gynecol. 2002;187(3):589–94.
20. Sobel JD. Vulvovaginal candidosis. The Lancet. 2007;369(9577):1961–71.
21. Farmer MA, Taylor AM, Bailey AL, Tuttle AH, MacIntyre LC, Milagrosa ZE, et al. Repeated vulvovaginal fungal infections cause persistent pain in a mouse model of vulvodynia. Sci Transl Med. 2011;3(101):101ra91.
22. Pukall CF, Cahill CM. New developments in the pathophysiology of genital pain: role of central sensitization. Curr Sex Health Rep. 2014;6(1):11–9.
23. Bohm-Starke N, Hilliges M, Falconer C, Rylander E. Increased intraepithelial innervation in women with vulvar vestibulitis syndrome. Gynecol Obstet Invest. 1998;46(4):256–60.
24. Chadha S, Gianotten WL, Drogendijk AC, Weijmar Schultz WC, Blindeman LA, van der Meijden WI. Histopathologic features of vulvar vestibulitis. Int J Gynecol Pathol. 1998;17(1):7–11.
25. Pukall CF, Binik YM, Khalife S, Amsel R, Abbott FV. Vestibular tactile and pain thresholds in women with vulvar vestibulitis syndrome. Pain. 2002; 96(1–2):163–75.
26. Pukall CF, Baron M, Amsel R, Khalife S, Binik YM. Tender point examination in women with vulvar vestibulitis syndrome. Clin J Pain. 2006;22(7):601–9.
27. Pukall CF, Strigo IA, Binik YM, Amsel R, Khalife S, Bushnell MC. Neural correlates of painful genital touch in women with vulvar vestibulitis syndrome. Pain. 2005;115(1–2):118–27.
28. Schweinhardt P, Kuchinad A, Pukall CF, Bushnell MC. Increased gray matter density in young women with chronic vulvar pain. Pain. 2008;140(3):411–9.
29. Hampson JP, Reed BD, Clauw DJ, Bhavsar R, Gracely RH, Haefner HK, et al. Augmented central pain processing in vulvodynia. J Pain. 2013;14(6):579–89.
30. Arnold LD, Bachmann GA, Rosen R, Kelly S, Rhoads GG. Vulvodynia: characteristics and associations with comorbidities and quality of life. Obstet Gynecol. 2006;107(3):617–24.
31. Arnold LD, Bachmann GA, Rosen R, Rhoads GG. Assessment of vulvodynia symptoms in a sample of US women: a prevalence survey with a nested case control study. Am J Obstet Gynecol. 2007;196(2): 128.e1–6.
32. Stockdale CK, Lawson HW. 2013 vulvodynia guideline update. J Low Genit Tract Dis. 2014;18(2):93.
33. Leo RJ, Dewani S. A systematic review of the utility of antidepressant pharmacotherapy in the treatment of vulvodynia pain. J Sex Med. 2013;10(10):2497–505.
34. Masheb RM, Kerns RD, Lozano C, Minkin MJ, Richman S. A randomized clinical trial for women

with vulvodynia: cognitive-behavioral therapy vs. supportive psychotherapy. J Pain. 2009;141(1): 31–40.
35. Weijmar Schultz WC, Gianotten WL, vanderMeijden WI, vandeWiel HBM, Blindeman L, Chadha S, et al. Behavioral approach with or without surgical intervention to the vulvar vestibulitis syndrome: a prospective randomized and non randomized study. J Psychosom Obstet Gynecol. 1996;17(3):143–8.
36. Bergeron S, Khalife S, Glazer HI, Binik YM. Surgical and behavioral treatments for vestibulodynia: two-and-one-half year follow-up and predictors of outcome. Obstet Gynecol. 2008;111(1):159–66.
37. Bergeron S, Brown C, Lord MJ, Oala M, Binik YM, Khalife S. Physical therapy for vulvar vestibulitis syndrome: a retrospective study. J Sex Marital Ther. 2002;28(3):183–92.
38. Goldfinger C, Pukall CF, Gentilcore-Saulnier E, McLean L, Chamberlain S. A prospective study of pelvic floor physical therapy: pain and psychosexual outcomes in provoked vestibulodynia. J Sex Med. 2009;6(7):1955–68.

26 New Concepts in the Understanding of Female Sexual Dysfunction

Marita P. McCabe

26.1 Points of Focus

- Need for an understanding of etiology in order to develop treatments for FSD.
- Biological, psychological, and relationship factors are likely to contribute to FSD.
- New treatment approaches involve mindful-based therapy and Internet therapy.

26.2 Introduction

Female sexual dysfunction (FSD) including female orgasmic disorder, female sexual interest arousal disorder, and genito-pelvic pain (APA, 2013) [1] causes significant concerns for women and has an impact on their relationships as well as their overall quality of life. This chapter discusses the factors that contribute to FSD, as well as models of how these various factors interact with one another to exacerbate these conditions. Recent advances in the treatment of FSD will also be considered, with a particular focus on mindfulness-based therapy and therapy in an online format.

26.3 New Information on the Etiology of FSD

Current understandings of the causes of sexual dysfunction acknowledge the contribution of biological, psychological, and social factors consistent with a biopsychosocial approach. For example, a study by Kontula and Haavio-Mannila [2] found evidence for the role of biological and psychosocial factors in sexual functioning in that, among both men and women, positive sexual functioning was associated with good health, positive sexual self-esteem, and a sexually skillful partner.

There has been limited research on the biological causes of sexual dysfunction in women. The biological causes of sexual dysfunction in men, in particular erectile dysfunction (ED), have received a great deal of research attention in recent years. This literature has established the role of several variables including age, disease, and drug use in the development of male sexual dysfunction. Similar research studies need to be conducted among women with FSD.

Numerous drugs have been implicated in the development of sexual dysfunction. Pharmacological agents used for treating nonsexual disorders, such as antidepressant medication, have been found to be associated with sexual dysfunction [3, 4]. In addition, recreational drugs, cigarette smoking, and alcohol have been found to negatively affect sexual functioning [5, 6].

M.P. McCabe, Ph.D. (✉)
Institute for Health and Ageing, Australian Catholic University, Melbourne, Australia
e-mail: marita.mccabe@deakin.edu.au

L.I. Lipshultz et al. (eds.), *Management of Sexual Dysfunction in Men and Women*, DOI 10.1007/978-1-4939-3100-2_26

A comprehensive review of the psychological and interpersonal factors that contribute to sexual dysfunction has been published by McCabe et al. [7]. This review evaluates the role of each developmental, individual, and relationship factor, and the interactions between them, in the etiology of sexual dysfunction. The model that includes these broad categories of etiological factors (see Fig. 26.1) was initially developed by McCabe [8]. The model begins with the premise that both individuals in a relationship bring a range of personal characteristics into their relationship. These characteristics may stem from a variety of sources, including developmental experiences (i.e., past experiences in the individual's life, especially experiences relevant to sexual activity such as a history of sexual abuse) and current aspects of the individual's functioning (e.g., depression, body image, and stress). These factors influence what each individual brings to the relationship generally and the sexual relationship specifically. For example, an individual may experience depression, which has a negative impact on the relationship, and this, in turn, may reduce the individual's sexual desire for his/her partner. As a result of this withdrawal, the partner may feel rejected from both the relationship and from sexual interaction, which exacerbates both the relationship and sexual problems. Once this occurs, treatment focused on one individual may not be successful in resolving the sexual problems, as both individuals in the relationship are now affected. As a result, therapy is most likely to be effective if it involves both partners in the relationship.

In this interactional model of sexual dysfunction, developmental, individual, and relationship factors influence one another. In addition, cognitions—that is, the interpretations that individuals place on events in the relationship—are crucial [9]. The meaning individuals give to sexual events (e.g., interpreting a partner's ED as rejection) is seen to be more important in predicting sexual dysfunction than the event itself. Also important is the meaning individuals give to nonsexual aspects of the relationship (e.g., interpreting a partner's depression-related withdrawal as rejection). Most importantly, if these evaluations are negative and are not expressed to the partner directly, the model proposes that they might be expressed indirectly in the form of a sexual dysfunction (e.g., a loss of sexual desire for the partner).

26.4 Female Sexual Dysfunction and Relationships

As noted above, biological, psychological, and interpersonal factors may all affect a woman's normal sexual functioning/response and consequently

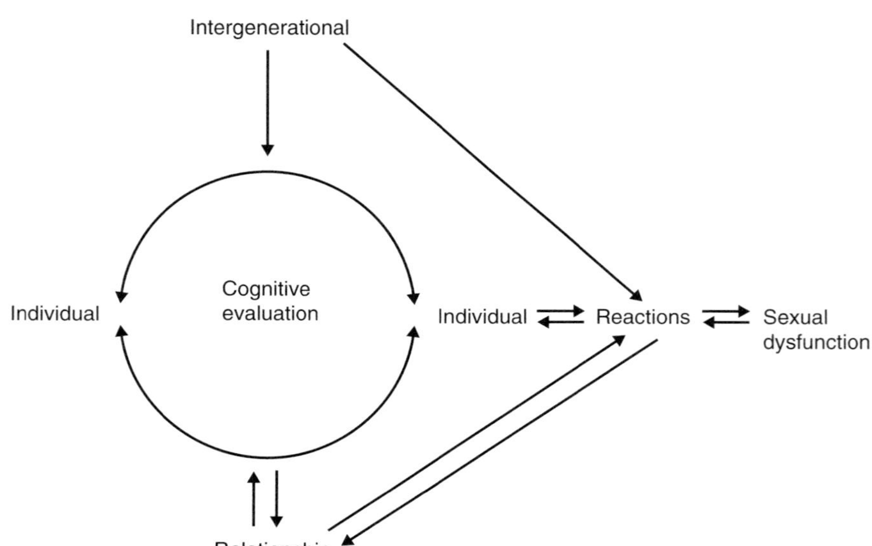

Fig. 26.1 Model to explain the development of sexual dysfunction within a relationship [8]

contribute to the development and maintenance of FSD. A recent Australian study found that interpersonal factors were more important to women's experience of sexual desire, whereas biological and individual (psychological) characteristics were more strongly associated with genital arousal and orgasmic function [10]. In a recent study conducted by King, Holt, and Nazareth [11], the most commonly perceived causes of sexual difficulties cited by women, regardless of whether they were assigned a diagnosis of FSD, were relationship difficulties. Research has furthermore indicated that women diagnosed with HSDD are more likely to have negative feelings about the quality of their relationship, particularly related to poor interpersonal communication and a lack of intimacy within their relationship in general [12].

It has been shown that, in general, women place greater emphasis on relationships as a context for sexual feelings and behaviors than do men [13]. This emphasis may be a result of differences in socialization between genders; women are socialized to place an emphasis on emotional connection (with a partner) as a prerequisite for sexual expression [14].

The causal association between FSD and relationship satisfaction remains elusive at present. For example, whereas desire problems can lead to interpersonal conflict [15], a poor relationship with a partner predicts low levels of sexual desire [16]. Research findings often suggest a bidirectional association between interpersonal factors such as relationship and sexual satisfaction, intimacy, communication, unresolved conflict, and partner sexual dysfunction and a woman's sexual desire [17]. Clearly then, there is a need to acknowledge and address such factors when assessing this aspect of women's sexuality.

Emotional intimacy between partners serves as a foundation for healthy sexual functioning and may be one of the primary interpersonal factors contributing to a woman's sexual response [18]. Higher levels of intimacy have been associated with greater levels of sexual satisfaction and orgasm among heterosexual couples in long-term relationships [19, 20]. A critical task in the treatment of sexual dysfunction is to promote a change in the couple's sexual style that focuses on emotional intimacy as a core process [18]. Some authors have suggested that the relatively poor treatment success for problems in sexual desire is due to an inadequate recognition of, and attention to, the relational aspects of these problems [21]. Research findings demonstrating that the quality of the relationship between partners improves following successful treatment of the disorder in sexual desire support this assertion [12].

26.5 New Treatment Approaches to FSD

Developments in the area of sexual pharmacology, particularly following the introduction of Viagra™ by Pfizer onto the market for the treatment of ED in 1998, have arguably resulted an increased biological reductionism of FSD, with an emphasis on physiological processes and a focus on women's genital performance [22]. Sex therapists warn that taking a purely medical approach to the treatment of female sexual problems is unlikely to be successful, if psychosocial and interpersonal contributors remain unexamined [23].

A major barrier to the development of clinical research and practice has been the absence of a well-defined, broadly accepted diagnostic framework and classification for FSD [24], and this problem is also reflected in the fact that fewer treatment options are currently available for women than for men [25]. It has been suggested that including an assessment of a woman's emotional experience within her sexual context is necessary to facilitate a complete understanding of sexual dysfunction [2]. An evaluation of the context in which sexual interactions occur (or do not currently occur) is necessary in order to tailor an effective treatment intervention that addresses the multitude of factors associated with the woman's sexual dysfunction.

26.6 Mindfulness

A recent and promising addition to the cognitive behavior therapy (CBT) approach for FSD involves the inclusion of mindfulness—a Buddhist meditation practice [26–32]. Mindfulness techniques facilitate nonjudgmental observation and present-moment awareness and, in the context of FSD, help to decrease cognitive and affective distractions and performance anxiety during sexual activity and increase women's attention and awareness of pleasurable sensations [33, 34].

To date, five studies have evaluated the incorporation of mindfulness training into group interventions for women with FSDs. In the first study [28], a mindfulness-based CBT intervention was delivered to a group of 26 women seeking treatment for acquired sexual desire and/or arousal difficulties. This treatment group reported significant improvements in sexual desire and sexual distress at posttest, as well as improvements in perception of genital arousal despite a lack of change in objective sexual arousal. The second study [29] involved the delivery of a mindfulness-based CBT intervention to a group of 22 women with early-stage gynecological cancer seeking treatment for acquired sexual arousal difficulties. This treatment group reported significant improvements in sexual desire, arousal, orgasm, satisfaction, and sexual distress. Trends toward improvement were also reported for both objective and perceived genital arousal, and women reported a significant improvement in overall well-being.

The third study [30] evaluated the effectiveness of a mindfulness-based CBT intervention for a group of 31 female survivors of endometrial or cervical cancer who reported sexual desire and/or sexual arousal difficulties. This study involved a waitlist control group, and results demonstrated that the women in the treatment group reported significant improvements in all areas of sexual response, as well as a trend toward improvement on scores of sexual distress, as compared to the control group. Women's ability to perceive genital arousal during an erotic film also increased significantly in the treatment group, despite no change in objective sexual arousal, and improvements were maintained at 6-month follow-up [30].

Upon further inspection of Brotto and colleagues' [28] results from the mindfulness-based CBT intervention, it was found that women with a history of sexual abuse had greater levels of improvement on various measures of sexual function and distress as compared to those without a history of sexual abuse. To further explore these results, the fourth study [31] compared the effectiveness of a mindfulness-based intervention to a CBT intervention for 22 partnered women with sexual difficulties, associated distress, and a history of childhood sexual abuse. Results suggested that women in the mindfulness-based treatment group reported significantly greater levels of subjective sexual arousal at posttest as compared to the CBT group and that both treatment groups experienced significant decreases in sexual distress [31].

It has also been theorized that mindfulness training may benefit women with sexual pain disorders [35, 36]. There are currently no quantitative data to support this hypothesis, but qualitative findings from a pilot study assessing the use of mindfulness-based approaches for women with provoked vestibulodynia, a chronic pelvic pain condition, suggest that participants benefited from the intervention and experienced a greater sense of control over pain management [30].

The fifth study implemented the *Pursuing Pleasure* (*PP*) program which was an Internet-based intervention for FSD [37]. The *PP* program introduced mindfulness in a nonsexual context first and then made the exercises more sensually and sexually oriented. This gradual introduction of mindfulness gave women the opportunity to learn basic mindfulness skills and troubleshoot any problems that arose, before incorporating mindfulness into sexual activity. Mindfulness training for FSDs slotted well into sensate focus, which also begins with a focus on nonsexual aspects of the practice and then gradually becomes more sexually oriented. From the experiences of women in the *PP* studies, it appears that mindfulness offers the following unique additions to traditional sensate focus: (1) Mindfulness training teaches women how to cultivate greater present-moment awareness and focus during sensate focus exercises. (2) Mindfulness exercises teach women new skills for managing cognitive and affective distractions during sexual activity. (3) Mindfulness training helps women develop the ability to manage distressing thoughts or emotions triggered before, during, or after sex. (4) Mindfulness practice can lead to a heightened awareness of genital arousal during sexual activity. (5) A mindful stance during sensate focus encourages a less judgmental stance toward self and partner. (6) Mindful awareness allows for a greater focus on letting go of expectations and predictions about sex and the outcome of sexual activity (e.g., orgasm, lubrication). Therefore, mindfulness training appears to offer women benefits above and beyond those offered by traditional sensate focus alone, and mindfulness can easily be incorporated into sensate focus exercises after basic mindfulness skills are acquired.

26.7 Internet-Based Treatments

Online CBT and Female Sexual Dysfunction In comparison to the number of studies investigating face-to-face treatment effects of FSD, only two studies were located that have used the Internet as a treatment modality for women. Jones and McCabe [38] conducted a study evaluating the effectiveness of an Internet-based CBT program titled *Revive*, for women experiencing various FSDs within a heterosexual relationship. A total of 39 women participated in the study (17 in the treatment group and 19 in the control group). *Revive* consisted of sensate focus, communication exercises, and unlimited e-mail contact with a therapist. The main aim of the e-mail contact was to address maladaptive cognitions as well as individual and relationship problems impacting sexual functioning [38]. The program consisted of five modules, with each module expected to take approximately 2 weeks to complete. Partners were expected to participate in the sensate focus and communication exercises.

Female sexual functioning and relationship functioning were assessed pretest, posttest, and at a 3-month follow-up. It was found that the women who completed the *Revive* program improved significantly on measures of sexual desire, arousal, lubrication, orgasm, sexual satisfaction, and pain compared to those in the control group, although 33 % of participants were still experiencing sexual problems more than 50 % of the time after treatment completion [38]. The treatment group also reported significantly greater improvements in sexual intimacy, emotional intimacy, and communication, but not for overall relationship satisfaction. Gains remained stable over the 3-month follow-up period and some participants reported further gains in sexual functioning. These results provide preliminary support for the use of Internet-based psychological therapy for mixed female sexual dysfunctions as an alternative to face-to-face sex therapy.

The second study was conducted by Hucker and McCabe [37] and evaluated the *PP* program discussed above. It was an online, mindfulness-based, CBT program for FSD. The program contained sensate focus, communication exercises, and unlimited e-mail contact with a therapist. *PP* also utilized online chat groups as a platform for cognitive therapy and social support. As well as being designed to improve women's sexual functioning, the program targeted relationship factors involved in FSD. Women who completed the *PP* program demonstrated significantly greater improvements in all aspects of sexual functioning as well as sexual intimacy, emotional intimacy, and communication as compared to the control group. This is consistent with past evaluations of the online treatment for female sexual dysfunction [38] and is not surprising given that the program consisted of communication- and intimacy-based exercises. Despite these improvements, the treatment group did not report significantly greater improvements in overall relationship satisfaction as compared to the control group, and this is also consistent with prior research [38].

26.8 Medical Treatments

In recent years, the focus of treatment for FSD has shifted from predominantly psychologically based techniques toward a more medical approach [25, 39–41]. For instance, a recent review of behavioral and CBT treatments for FSD indicated that there have been some recent studies, but that most treatment outcome studies have focused on medical interventions [42].

The discovery of effective pharmacological agents for male erectile dysfunction has led researchers to attempt to develop similar agents for females [43].

An extensive review of the literature on the effectiveness of pharmacological treatments for women found mixed results, although in the majority of cases, these approaches were found to be largely unsuccessful [25, 44, 45]. The female sexual response is vastly different from that of males, and unlike their male counterparts, the potential role of hormonal factors and various medical treatments on the sexual interest and activity of women remains unclear [40]. A medical approach to the treatment of sexual disorders in women fails to take into account the many individual factors and the quality of the relationship described by women as being related to the development of their dysfunction [39, 44, 46].

Only one published clinical trial supports the use of sildenafil for the treatment of female sexual arousal disorder in a sample of 51 young premenopausal women [47]. In contrast, a well-controlled clinical trial involving 583 women showed no difference in levels of sexual arousal between those who received drug sildenafil and a placebo group. Chives and Rosen [48] conducted a review of 16 studies that examined the effectiveness of PDE5i on female sexual functioning and found a general lack of efficacy of these agents. The authors attributed this lack of efficacy to gender differences in the concordance between physiological and psychological arousal in men and women. In regard to other medical interventions, a number of studies have found the use of a transdermal testosterone patch to be effective in the treatment of low sexual desire among naturally menopausal women [49, 50], as well as those who experience either an oophorectomy or hysterectomy [51]. Flibanserin has also been shown to be effective for the treatment of low sexual desire among premenopausal women through a series of a number of randomized controlled trials [52–54] as well as an open-label extension study over a period of 52 weeks [55]. In relation of women with major depressive disorder (MDD), gepirone-ER has been shown to be effective for low sexual desire [56]. Further, since women with these disorders are frequently taking SSRIs, Moll and Brown [57] conducted a review of the literature that found that the use of monoaminergic agents (e.g., bupropion, buspirone, and ropinirole) was effective in treating the sexual dysfunction associated with both MDDs as well as the use of these SSRIs.

The medical model of FSD tends to emphasize quantity, performance, and objective measures (e.g., frequency of orgasm and adequate lubrication) over the quality of sex and measures of subjective experience (e.g., pleasure, satisfaction, and intimacy) which women describe as being particularly relevant in their motivation to engage in sexual activity [38, 39]. As noted by Al-Azzawi et al. [58], there are both pharmacological and non-pharmacological treatments available for women with female sexual dysfunction. Based on this literature, their recommendation was that non-pharmacological treatment that focuses on lifestyle and psychosexual therapy should be trialled first. Undoubtedly, pharmacotherapy may play a role in the treatment of a limited number of sexual disorders, but the use of these treatments for women requires further development.

26.9 Conclusion

In order to treat FSD effectively, it is important to have a clear understanding of the nature of the problem(s) as well as the etiology of the various disorders. There have been recent promising developments in both mindfulness-based therapy and Internet therapy. As for sexual dysfunctions in men, it is likely that the most effective approach for FSD will be shown to be a combination of a medical and psychological intervention. Substantially more research is required for us to be confident in the development of such a treatment program.

References

1. American Psychiatric Association. Diagnostic and statistical manual of mental disorders. 5th ed. Arlington, VA: APA; 2013.
2. Kontula O, Haavio-Mannila E. The impact of aging on human sexual activity and sexual desire. J Sex Res. 2009;46:46–56.

3. Kennedy SH, Eisfeld BS, Dickens SE, Bacchiochi JR, Bagby RM. Antidepressant induced sexual dysfunction during treatment with moclobemide, paroxetine, sertraline, and venlafaxine. J Clin Psychiatry. 2000;61:276–81.
4. Wincze JP, Carey MP. Sexual dysfunction: a guide for assessment and treatment. 2nd ed. New York: Guildford Press; 2001.
5. McVary KT, Carrier S, Wessells H. Smoking and erectile dysfunction: evidence based analysis. J Urol. 2001;166:1624–32.
6. Miri SM, Meyer RE, Mendelson JH, Ellingboe J. Opiate use and sexual function. Am J Psychiatry. 1980;137:909–15.
7. McCabe MP. Sexual and relationship problems. In: Rieger E, editor. Abnormal psychology: leading researcher perspectives. 2nd ed. Melbourne: McGraw-Hill; 2011. p. 312–54.
8. McCabe MP. The development and maintenance of sexual dysfunction: an explanation based on cognitive theory. Sex Marital Ther. 1991;6:245–60.
9. Nobre PJ. Determinants of sexual desire problems in women: testing a cognitive-emotional model. J Sex Marital Ther. 2009;35:360–77.
10. Hayes RD, Dennerstein L, Bennett CM, Fairley CK. What is the "true" prevalence of female sexual dysfunctions and does the way we assess these conditions have an impact? J Sex Med. 2008;5:777–87.
11. King M, Holt V, Nazareth I. Women's views of their sexual difficulties: agreement and disagreement with clinical diagnoses. Arch Sex Behav. 2007;36:281–8.
12. Trudel G, Marchand A, Ravart M, Aubin S, Turgeon L, Fortier P. The effect of a cognitive-behavioral group treatment program on hypoactive sexual desire in women. Sex Relat Ther. 2001;16:145–64.
13. Peplau LA. Human sexuality: how do men and women differ? Curr Dir Psychol Sci. 2003;12:37–40.
14. Baumeister RF, Vohs KD. Sexual economics: sex as female resource for social exchange in heterosexual interactions. Pers Soc Psychol Rev. 2004;8:339–63.
15. Althof SE, Dean J, Derogatis LR, Rosen RC, Sisson M. Current perspectives on the clinical assessment and diagnosis of female sexual dysfunction and clinical studies of potential therapies: a statement of concern. J Sex Med. 2005;2:146–53.
16. Stuart FM, Hammond DC, Pett MA. Inhibited sexual desire in women. Arch Sex Behav. 1987;16:91–106.
17. Metz ME, Epstein N. Assessing the role of relationship conflict in sexual dysfunction. J Sex Marital Ther. 2002;28:139–64.
18. McCarthy BW, Thestrup M. Integrating sex therapy interventions with couple therapy. J Contemp Psychother. 2008;38:139–49.
19. Costa RM, Brod S. Women's relationship quality is associated with specifically penile-vaginal intercourse orgasm and frequency. J Sex Marital Ther. 2007;33:319–27.
20. Haning RV, O'Keefe SL, Randall EJ, Kommor MJ, Baker E, Wilson R. Intimacy, orgasm likelihood, and conflict predict sexual satisfaction in heterosexual male and female respondents. J Sex Marital Ther. 2007;33:93–113.
21. Talmadge LD, Talmadge WC. Relational sexuality: an understanding of low sexual desire. In: The Hatherleigh guide to marriage and family therapy. New York: Hatherleigh Press; 1996. p. 191–218.
22. Balon R, Segraves RT. Handbook of sexual dysfunction. Boca Raton: Taylor and Francis; 2005.
23. Goldberg DC, Pervin LA. Progress in the treatment of sexual desire disorders. PsycCRITIQUES. 2006;35:786–7.
24. Basson R, Berman J, Burnett A, Deogatis L, Ferguson D, Fourcroy J, et al. Report of the international consensus development conference on female sexual dysfunction: definitions and classification. J Urol. 2000;163:888–93.
25. Segraves RT, Balon R. Introduction: treatment of sexual disorders in the 21st century. In: Balon R, Segraves RT, editors. Handbook of sexual dysfunction. Boca Raton: Taylor and Francis; 2005. p. 1–11.
26. Everaerd W, Both S, Laan E. The experience of sexual emotions. Annu Rev Sex Res. 2006;17:183–99.
27. Althof SE. What's new in sex therapy (CME). J Sex Med. 2010;7:5–13.
28. Brotto LA, Basson R, Luria M. A mindfulness-based group psychoeducational intervention targeting sexual arousal disorder in women. J Sex Med. 2008;5:1646–59.
29. Brotto LA, Heiman J, Goff B, Greer B, Lentz GM, Swisher E, et al. A psychoeducation intervention for sexual dysfunction in women with gynecologic cancer. Arch Sex Behav. 2008;37:317–29.
30. Brotto LA, Erskine Y, Carey M, Ehlen T, Fionalyson S, Heywood M, et al. A brief mindfulness-based cognitive behavioral intervention improves sexual functioning versus wait-list control in women treated for gynecologic cancer. Gynecol Oncol. 2012;125:320–5.
31. Brotto LA, Seal BN, Rellini A. Pilot study of a brief cognitive behavioral versus mindfulness-based intervention for women with sexual distress and a history of childhood sexual abuse. J Sex Marital Ther. 2012;38:1–27.
32. Haln TN. The miracle of mindfulness: a manual on meditation. Boston, MA: Beacon; 1975.
33. Brotto LA, Heiman JR. Mindfulness in sex therapy: applications for women with sexual difficulties following gynecologic cancer. Sex Relat Ther. 2007;22:3–11.
34. Brotto LA, Krychman M, Jocabson P. Eastern approaches for enhancing women' sexuality: mindfulness, acupuncture, and yoga. J Sex Med. 2008;6:2741–8.
35. Basson R. The recurrent pain and sexual sequelae of provoked vestibulodynia: a perpetuating cycle. J Sex Med. 2012;9:2077–92.
36. Brotto LA, Basson R, Carlson M, Zhu C. Impact of an integrated mindfulness and cognitive behavioural treatment for provoked vestibulodynia (IMPROVED): a qualitative study. Sex Relat Ther. 2013;28(1):3–19.

37. Hucker A, McCabe MP. Incorporating mindfulness and chat groups in online cognitive-behavioral therapy for mixed female sexual problems. J Sex Res. 2015; 52(6) 627–639.
38. Jones L, McCabe MP. The effectiveness of an internet-based psychological treatment program for female sexual dysfunction. J Sex Med. 2011;8:2781–92.
39. Kleinplatz PJ. What's new in sex therapy? From stagnation to fragmentation. Sex Relat Ther. 2003;18: 95–106.
40. McCarthy BW. An integrative cognitive-behavioral approach to understanding, assessing and treating female sexual dysfunctions. J Fam Psychother. 2004;15:19–35.
41. Tiefer L. Beyond the medical model of women's sexual problems: a campaign to resist the promotion of 'female sexual dysfunction'. Sex Relat Ther. 2002;17: 127–35.
42. Stinson RD. The behavioral and cognitive-behavioral treatment of female sexual dysfunction: how far we have come and the path left to go. Sex Relat Ther. 2009;24:271–85.
43. Segraves RT. Female sexual disorders: psychiatric aspects. Can J Psychiatry. 2006;47:419–25.
44. Basson R, Brotto LA. Sexual psychophysiology and effects of sildenafil citrate in oestrogenised women with acquired genital arousal disorder and impaired orgasm: a randomized controlled trial. Int J Obstet Gynaecol. 2003;110:1014–24.
45. Heiman JR. Sexual dysfunction: overview of prevalence, etiological factors, and treatments. J Sex Res. 2002;39:73–8.
46. Basson R. The female sexual response: a different model. J Sex Marital Ther. 2000;26:51–65.
47. Caruso S, Intelisano G, Lup L, Agnello C. Premenopausal women affected by sexual arousal disorder treated with sildenafil: a double-blind, crossover, placebo-controlled study. Br J Obstet Gynecol. 2001;108:623–8.
48. Chives ML, Rosen RC. Phosphodiesterase type 5 inhibitors and female sexual response: faculty protocols or paradigms? J Sex Med. 2010;7:858–72.
49. Davis SR, Braunstein GD. Efficacy and safety of testosterone in the management of hypoactive sexual desire disorder in postmenopausal women. J Sex Med. 2012;9:1134–48.
50. Panay N, Al-Azzawai F, Bouchard C, Davis SR, Eden J, Lodhi I, et al. Testosterone treatment of HSDD in natural menopausal women: the ADORE study. Climacteric. 2010;13:121–31.
51. Shifren JL, Braunstein GD, Simon JA, Casson PR, Buster JE, Redmond GP, et al. Transdermal testosterone treatment in women with impaired sexual function after oophorectomy. N Engl Med. 2000;343: 682–8.
52. Goldfischer ER, Breaux J, Katz M, Kaufman J, Smith WB, Kimura T, et al. Continued efficacy and safety of flibanserin in premenopausal women with hypoactive sexual desire disorder (HSDD): results from a randomized withdrawal trial. J Sex Med. 2011;8: 3160–72.
53. Derogatis LR, Komer L, Moreau M, Kimura T, Garcia Jr M, Wunderlich G, Pyke R, VIOLET Trial Investigators. Treatment of hypoactive sexual desire disorders in premenopausal women: efficacy of flibanserin in the VIOLET study. J Sex Med. 2012;9:1074–85.
54. Thorp J, Simon J, Dattani D, Taylor L, Kimura T, Garcia Jr M, et al. Treatment of hypoactive sexual desire disorder in premenopausal women: efficacy of flibanserin in the DAISY study. J Sex Med. 2012;9:793–804.
55. Jayne C, Simon JA, Taylor LV, Kimura T, Lesko LM, SUNFLOWER study investigators. Open-label extension study of flibanserin in women with hypoactive sexual desire disorder. J Sex Med. 2012;9: 3180–8.
56. Fabre LF, Brown CS, Smith LC, Derogatis LR. Gepirone-ER treatment of hypoactive sexual desire disorder (HSDD) associated with depression in women. J Sex Med. 2011;8:1411–19.
57. Moll JL, Brown CS. The use of monoamine pharmacological agents in the treatment of sexual dysfunction: evidence in the literature. J Sex Med. 2011;8: 956–70.
58. Al-Azzawi F, Bitzer J, Brandernbury U, et al. Therapeutic options for postmenopausal female sexual dysfunction. Clumacteric. 2010;13:103–20.

Female Sexual Dysfunction and Cancer

27

Alyssa Dweck and Michael Krychman

27.1 Introduction

The American Cancer Society cites almost 800,000 new cancer diagnoses in 2012 with 5-year survival rates on the rise [1]. Survivorship and quality of life issues, including sexual function, are gaining more popular attention. It should come as no surprise that sexual dysfunction affects the majority of women treated for cancer, with some reports suggesting that nearly all women with breast cancer have treatment-related sexual complaints [2]. Female sexual dysfunction (FSD) includes a broad range of psychological, physical, and interpersonal issues. Common complaints include loss of libido, difficulty with arousal, dyspareunia, and anorgasmia. Despite these reports, sexual function is often a neglected part of the survivor experience. Practitioners cite time constraints and lack of training in sexual health as barriers to treatment. This chapter will discuss not only the broad issues regarding female sexuality faced universally by cancer patient/survivors, but also elucidate on nuances specific to specific cancers.

A. Dweck, M.S., M.D., F.A.C.O.G., C.S.T.
Mount Kisco Medical Group, Northern Westchester Hospital, Mt. Kisco, NY, USA

Mt. Sinai School of Medicine, New York, NY, USA

M. Krychman, M.D., C.M. (✉)
Southern California Center for Sexual Health and Survivorship Medicine, Newport Beach, CA, USA

University of California Irvine, Irvine, CA, USA
e-mail: mkrychman@aol.com

27.2 Patient History

When addressing sexual problems in the cancer patient, it is critical to consider what predates the cancer diagnosis. Is chronic disease or mental illness an issue? Are current medications and doses impacting the sexual response cycle? Is the patient happily partnered or not? Are other life stressors present that may be contributing to sexual complaints? Are age-related changes in sexuality an issue? What was the sexual repertoire prior to diagnosis? This demographic and historical background is essential and should be elicited through a focused sexual history with inquiry about the least intrusive topics first, followed by the more intimate ones. Open-ended questions are most effective to retrieve important history. Patients want their healthcare professional to initiate discussions of sexuality at diagnosis, prior to, during, and after treatment. Women want to know whether and when sex is permissible during and after treatment and appreciate detailed and candid advice regarding sexual intimacy. However, women may find it embarrassing, awkward, inappropriate, or taboo to bring up the subject of sexuality themselves, especially in

L.I. Lipshultz et al. (eds.), *Management of Sexual Dysfunction in Men and Women*, DOI 10.1007/978-1-4939-3100-2_27

light of a life-threatening illness. Some may feel guilt contemplating sex in that they should just be "happy to be alive." Patients may be overwhelmed with medical information and fail to ask.

An important educational resource for both healthcare professionals and patients is the American Cancer Society pamphlet (2013): *Sexuality for the Woman with Cancer* (http://www.cancer.org/acs/groups/cid/documents/webcontent/002912-pdf.pdf).

27.3 Common Complaints Affecting Sexuality in Cancer Patients and Survivors

27.3.1 Fatigue

Fatigue is ubiquitous in cancer patients and can present at the time of diagnosis, after medical or surgical therapy, or persist after treatment. Cancer-related fatigue is often a complex phenomenon since it can be due to separate medical issues, treatment related, or due to the cancer itself. A productive counseling point can be to encourage patients to time sexual relations around their most energetic time of day. Patients should be given permission to consider sex a priority in the morning, for example, when energy levels may be highest and fatigue at its lowest. Resuming exercise, which increases energy and improves mood, is another important clinical suggestion. The clinician must also address other causes of fatigue including cancer-related anemia, hypothyroidism, depression, poor nutrition, and poor sleep habits.

27.3.2 Fertility

Many women will be diagnosed with cancer in their reproductive years, including up to 25 % of women with breast cancer [3]. Patients interested in fertility preservation should undergo pretreatment counseling regarding options such as embryo or oocyte cryopreservation, egg donation, gestational surrogacy, and adoption. It is crucial to have this conversation and engage a reproductive endocrinologist in a timely fashion. By the same token, contraception may be needed or need to be altered in light of new cancer diagnosis. Hormonal contraception is contraindicated for those with breast or uterine cancers or other hormonally sensitive tumors. The nonhormonal IUD, barrier methods, and permanent sterilization may be the only viable options in these cases. Some women may become amenorrheic and seemingly menopausal without the need for contraception, particularly in their 40s during chemotherapy, only to see the return of menses months after chemotherapy cessation. Contraception should be reconsidered in these patients if menses resume and menopause is not definitive. Some women who experience a permanent and irreversible loss of fertility may experience mood changes, including depression and anxiety. Since many view reproduction as the primary goal of sexuality, the loss of fertility may impact a woman's perception of sexuality and she may report sexual disinterest.

27.3.3 Pain

Pain is an often a universal symptom for the cancer patient/survivor. Surgical site pain, chronic bone and muscle pain, and pain or heightened sensitivity due to radiation injury are common. As a result, analgesia may be necessary before sexual intercourse. Premedication with narcotics, acetaminophen, or nonsteroidal anti-inflammatory medication appropriately administered before sex may be beneficial. Topical anesthetics such as xylocaine jelly applied to painful areas may also be helpful. Open communication between partners is essential. Sexual repertoires may need to be altered since what may have previously been stimulating may now be uncomfortable. For example breast skin that was once sensual when touched may be painful after radiation. Abdominal scars might be sensitive or numb. In contrast, scars may be sensual and erotic for some. Finally, some patients experience phantom pain or chronic pain, which may impair sexual function. A pain management consultation may be valuable in these cases.

27.3.4 Menopausal Symptoms

Vasomotor symptoms, sleeplessness, and genitourinary syndrome of menopause (GSM) (which was previously called vulvovaginal atrophy) are common, particularly for those with estrogen-sensitive cancers – especially in those women who are taking aromatase inhibitors or selective estrogen receptor modulators. Conservative treatment options include dressing in layers with moisture-wicking fabrics, dietary manipulation to avoid caffeine, alcohol, and spicy or large meals. Cooling sheets and pillows, fans, lowered thermostat settings, and over-the-counter or prescription sleeping aids may also help, although definitive data from randomized clinical trials may be lacking. Mindfulness exercises, meditation, yoga, and regular exercise are also considered beneficial. Antidepressants, in particular selective serotonin reuptake inhibitors (SSRIs), serotonin norepinephrine reuptake inhibitors (SNRIs), and dopamine agonists, are commonly used. Anxiolytics, clonidine, and gabapentin are also medical options for vasomotor symptoms in those patients who cannot or will not take estrogen therapy. Low-dose paroxetine was recently FDA approved as the first nonhormonal medication with efficacy for reducing frequency and severity of moderate to severe vasomotor symptoms due to menopause. This novel medication may be appropriate for some cancer patients with vasomotor symptomatology. Nutraceuticals, vitamins, and herbal supplements remain controversial in the cancer patient and should be considered with extreme caution. In fact, the American College of Obstetricians and Gynecologists (ACOG) claims soy, over-the-counter phytoestrogens, dong quai, and ginseng are ineffective for vasomotor symptoms [4].

27.3.5 Dyspareunia and VVA

Dyspareunia and GSM can directly result from chemical or surgical castration. Estrogen depletion diminishes blood flow and natural lubrication to the genito-pelvic organs. Subsequent abstinence due to avoidance may worsen the situation. For those without estrogen-dependent cancers, this conundrum can be treated effectively with minimally absorbed local vaginal estrogen in the form of a local cream, ring, or tablet. In addition, there is a recently approved oral medication, ospemifene, a selective estrogen receptor modulator for the treatment of moderate to severe dyspareunia, a symptom of GSM due to menopause; safety of use in cancer patients is based on individual malignancies. Although in some oncological populations the use of local intravaginal estrogen products has gained popularity, long-term safety trials on the use of minimally absorptive local estrogens in cancer patients, especially those with hormonally sensitive tumors, are lacking [5]. All patients can benefit from nonhormonal vaginal moisturizers used regularly and long term. Replens™, for example, used regularly 2–3 times weekly, is over the counter, may restore vaginal pH, is generally well tolerated, and typically provides relief. Compounded hyaluronic acid used vaginally twice weekly or vitamin E capsules are effective moisturizers as well. Water-based, silicone-based, or oil-based lubricants are encouraged during sexual relations. Common products include KY Jelly™, Astroglide™, Wet Platinum™, Good Clean Love, and coconut oil. Paraben, glycerin, fragrance, bactericide, and spermicidal and dye-free options are gaining popularity, and these additives should be avoided in the menopausal cancer survivor. Vulvar soothing creams like Neogyn™ are effective for vulvar pain.

27.3.6 Psychological and Relationship Issues

Emotional consequences due to or in spite of physical changes from cancer treatments include feeling unattractive, changes in sexual self-esteem, lacking femininity, and direct impact on partner or relationship. Sexual well-being is central to psychological well-being and quality of life. Sexual intimacy assists in the cancer recovery process [6]. The transition from lover and marital partner to caretaker or housemate can disrupt the relationship creating excessive tension and impact effective communication. Concerns about infidelity due to discrepancy in sexual interest cannot be ignored and sexually transmitted infection screening may be appropriate. Negative consequences experienced by *partners* of breast cancer patient/survivors include fear of causing pain during sex, lack of interest in sex, difficulties in communication, and change in roles. These concerns do not differ according to age, relationship status, sexual orientation, or current stage of cancer treatment [6].

In those studied seeking new relationships, "not feeling desirable" and "fear of rejection" were most commonly reported and more so by women seeking new heterosexual relationships compared with those seeking same sex ones [6]. Perhaps this discrepancy speaks to the importance of penetrative vaginal intercourse in heterosexual couples. Exploration of noncoital sexual practices should be emphasized when counseling these patients.

Some feel a true sense of loss when vaginal intercourse, the "ideal expression of marital intimacy," is lost. Others report lack of intercourse not distressing with satisfaction from oral sex, self-stimulation, or alternative sexual expression. This is clearly dependent on the importance placed on intercourse prior to cancer diagnosis. Some are so grateful to have "survived" cancer and alive intercourse is secondary. Other survivors feel the lack of intercourse is age and not cancer related and that intercourse is not needed to maintain a harmonious marital relationship and that intimacy is more emotional/mental than physical. For some couples, a platonic nonsexual or celibate relationship becomes acceptable and less complicated than dealing with a reconfigured body and a partner [7].

In regard to couples' fate after cancer diagnosis, some report communication problems or increased conflict and attribute this relationship breakdown to cancer [6]. Other couples living with cancer are no more likely to separate than those in the general community [8]. In some instances, cancer may have a positive relationship effect by creating greater intimacy [9].

Rarely, women with cancer report an increased sexual pleasure or desire and that sex is a way of feeling alive during treatment. These cases are in the minority but suggest that detrimental sexual effects cannot be assumed for all women [9].

27.4 Medical Sex Therapy

Sexual function after cancer diagnosis and treatment may not return to baseline and realistic expectations should be discussed. Sexual medicine focuses on a "new normal." First, it is imperative to manage underlying chronic medical conditions. Address medications particularly antidepressants and antihypertensives which have direct effects on arousal, libido, and orgasm. Nutrition and exercise optimization are crucial. Stress reduction and fatigue management are paramount. Specific sexual assignments may be given including bibliotherapy or erotic/instructional book reading or video exploration, self-stimulation exercises, and relaxation techniques. Mindfulness training and sensate focus exercises including non-genital touching, solo or mutual masturbation, and if and when ready genital and coital activity can follow. Partners need to agree not to proceed to intercourse unless both are adequately prepared.

Vaginal moisturizers and lubricants remain the mainstay treatments for moderate to severe dyspareunia due to GSM. Books such as *The Joy of Sex* by Dr. Alex Comfort [10] illustrate alternate sexual positioning and additions to the sexual repertoire in cases where intercourse is not possible. Alternate sexual pleasuring techniques can be introduced, including manual, digital, or oral stimulation. Formal graduated dilator programs in combination with moisturizers and lubricants are essential for those with pelvic floor hypertonus, vaginal stenosis, narrowing, and scarring; and subsequent dyspareunia. Specialty trained pelvic floor physical therapists employ manipulative techniques and intravaginal diazepam or trigger point injections to treat hypertonic pelvic muscles to alleviate sexual pain. Vibrators/self-stimulators give additional stimulation to the clitoris and vagina and provide novelty to the sexual experience. Another handheld sexual device, the Eros Clitoral Stimulator®, provides suction to increase clitoral vasocongestion and stimulation which has been shown to be effective in small clinical trials in certain subpopulations including those who have cervical cancer [11].

Hypoactive Sexual Desire Disorder (HSDD) The antidepressant bupropion has been used off-label to treat lowered sexual desire complaints, and one study suggests a positive effect on arousal and orgasm in women [12]. Testosterone therapy has often been used off-label for HSDD in women and is not FDA approved. In fact, a randomized crossover trial in 150 women with cancer showed no differences in sexual function using testosterone cream over placebo during a 4-week treatment period [13]. The efficacy and safety of androgen therapy in cancer patients are unknown. Phosphodiesterase inhibitors used to treat erectile dysfunction in men have not proven efficacious in trials with women and remain unstudied in the cancer population [14]. Zestra®, an over-the-counter arousal botanical oil used topically prior to sex, has shown increased arousal and sexual satisfaction in women [15]. A small case series presentation suggests a positive sexual response to Zestra in breast cancer patients [16]. Flibanserin, a 5-HT1A agonist and 5-HT2A antagonist, and bremelanotide, a melanocortin agonist, are two medications that are in clinical development. They show excellent promise for the treatment of female sexual dysfunction and may be considered for use in the oncological patients given the fact that they are nonhormonal.

27.5 Specific Cancer Considerations

27.5.1 Breast Cancer

Breast cancer survivors make up a large proportion of cancer survivors in the US; in fact the American Cancer Society estimates a staggering 232,670 new diagnoses in 2014 [17]. Disfiguring surgery is not uncommon and tends to be more significant in younger women [18]. Breast cancer survivors may hide their bodies from their partners with lingerie, dim lights, or blatant avoidant behavior. Scars and skin fibrosis of the breast and axilla can limit range of motion. Lymphedema may present. During intimacy, position changes and liberal use of pillows for comfort may be helpful. Radiation can lead to skin changes including rash, burning, decreased sensation, skin thickening, and discoloration. Of particular concern is numbness or discomfort in the previously erogenous breast and chest. Chemotherapy may cause nausea, vomiting, diarrhea, and alopecia on the head, eyelashes and eyebrows, and genitals. Weight gain is common, particularly in those receiving chemotherapy and endocrine therapies. All of these medical issues have a negative effect on sexual self-esteem and feelings of attractiveness. Tamoxifen can cause hot flashes, vaginal discharge and itching, dysfunctional uterine bleeding, and uterine cancer. Severe atrophic changes in the genitals, bone loss, and fracture risk exist for those on aromatase inhibitors. Immediate premature menopause may occur and existing menopausal symptoms may worsen due to chemotherapy or endocrine treatment.

The psychological ramifications of breast cancer are significant. Research shows that the strongest predictor of sexual problems after breast cancer is lower perceived sexual attractiveness [18]. In addition women who have a poor body image after breast cancer have lower rates of sexual satisfaction and are more dissatisfied with their sexual relationship than those with a positive body image [19]. While the physical pain associated with mastectomy diminishes with time, the emotional pain may persist and women grieve the loss of their breast(s) and feel mastectomy is associated with being "half a woman" [20]. In fact, the quality of a woman's relationship is a stronger predictor of sexual satisfaction, sexual functioning, and sexual desire after breast cancer than the physical or chemical damage to the body after treatment [21–23].

27.5.2 Endometrial Cancer

The American Cancer Society estimates about 52,630 new cases of uterine cancer for 2014 [17]. Surgical staging remains the standard of care and includes total hysterectomy, removal of ovaries and tubes, and possible lymph node dissection. Laparoscopy is both safe and feasible and associated with quality of life advantage over laparotomy [24]. Endometrial cancer is often diagnosed at an early stage and the overall prognosis is excellent. Postoperative external beam radiation to the pelvis and/or intracavitary vaginal brachytherapy may be used for later-stage disease. In general, sexual function and fear of sex declined after surgery for uterine cancer but recovered to preoperative levels by 6 months [25]. Laparoscopy patients indicated physical appearance as more important and had higher scores of satisfaction with stomach appearance, overall appearance, and in feeling like a women although improvement over time was noted in both groups [25]. In other words, minimally invasive surgery did not differ from laparotomy regarding resumption of or improvements in sexual function postoperatively, but laparoscopic patients were more satisfied with their overall feminine appearance [25]. One study suggested that while uterine cancer patients treated with either surgery alone or surgery and intravaginal brachytherapy reported symptoms of dry, short, and tight vaginas, there was no significant difference in sexual functioning, sexual worry, or sexual enjoyment between the two [26]. It should be noted that since endometrial cancer is usually a diagnosis in older ages, baseline sexual function might be lower due to a variety of factors including relationship duration, age, and hormone status.

27.5.3 Cervical Cancer

Cervical cancer is usually diagnosed in reproductive-aged women so fertility or potential lack thereof may be an issue. A majority of patients are sexually active at the time of diagnosis in part due to younger age. Treatment of early-stage cervical cancer consists of cervical conization, radical trachelectomy, or radical hysterectomy with pelvic lymphadenectomy. As such, shortening of the vagina and disruption in neurovascular supply can result in dyspareunia, arousal, orgasm, and sexual positioning difficulties. Changes in position during intercourse to avoid deeper thrusting are advised. Alternatives to missionary position, such as female superior, side by side, or rear entry, are helpful. The Come Close® device, available in the United Kingdom, may be placed around the base of the penis to prevent deep thrusting and collision dyspareunia. Decreased libido and diminished vaginal lubrication seem to be the only side effects that persisted in a two-year study period [27]. If adjuvant radiotherapy is needed, treatments can cause bloody and foul smelling vaginal discharge, vaginal stenosis, polyuria, and bleeding. Lymphedema in the lower extremities can occur and can be managed with compression stockings, physical therapy, and lymph massage locally.

In one study, the ability to achieve orgasm was unimpaired in cervical cancer survivors; however, dyspareunia was more common than in healthy controls [28]. This was more frequently reported and lasted longer in patients treated with radiotherapy compared to surgery [28]. Lack of lubrication was more frequent in cervical cancer survivors than in healthy controls. In general, in the cervical cancer population, impaired sexual function seems to be accompanied by pain during vaginal intercourse, and decreased desire and arousal are, at least in part, a result of pain [28]. As such, if treatment focuses on avoidance of pain, arousal and desire will improve. The vast majority of cervical cancer is caused by human papilloma virus (HPV) infection. Since this is sexually transmitted, it may be associated with complex psychological ramifications.

Unique to cervical cancer is the media impact achieved with advertisements related to HPV. Women question their own or their partners' past relations or feel embarrassed discussing their cancers because of the potential blame on sexual conduct [29].

27.5.4 Colorectal Cancer

The American Cancer Society estimates 66,000 new colorectal cancer diagnoses for 2014 [17]. An overwhelming patient concern in the treatment colorectal cancer is the potential ostomy. Women are frightened and concerned for potential odor, gas, soiling, and fecal or fatal accidents. Patients should be educated to carefully orchestrate ostomy management techniques when engaging in sexual activity. The various techniques employed to manage a stoma and appliance before, during, and after sex are numerous and creative. Women may apply a new bag so it is empty during relations. Cover the pouch with towels and fixate its position with tube tops or nightgowns to keep the pouch stable, insure accident prevention, and keep the pouch hidden [30]. Others may place special tablets within the ostomy bag to mask potential odors, while others may opt for sexy coverings for their ostomy appliance.

27.5.5 Anal Carcinoma

Anal cancer is distinct from colorectal cancer. Risk factors include smoking, history of multiple sexual partners and anal intercourse, impaired immunity including HIV, HPV infection, and age over 50. Anal carcinoma is treated with surgical resection with or without chemoradiation, and in some cases permanent colostomy is needed. Issues with ostomy care and rituals regarding sexuality are discussed above. Acute effects of treatment include skin reaction including desquamation, pain, nausea, vomiting, diarrhea, and hair loss. Later effects include vaginal stenosis, changes in rectal or anal function, flatus and fecal incontinence, pain, and acceleration of menopausal symptoms. Psychosocial effects include depression, embarrassment, and, specific to anal cancer, anxiety over the relationship of anal carcinoma to sexual practices, HIV or HPV infection, and the possibility of needing a colostomy. The skin is a sensual organ so prevention of skin changes and early treatment for radiation induced skin damage are essential. Extreme sensitivity to touch can occur due to radiation. Guidance may be needed to avoid "touch" that is experienced as discomfort [31].

27.5.6 Ovarian Cancer

Ovarian cancer is unique since early detection is limited. Typical treatment is surgical debulking with adjuvant chemotherapy depending on stage. Total hysterectomy with removal of ovaries and tubes has profound emotional and psychological impact at the core of femininity and fertility. First-line chemotherapy usually involves a platinum or taxane compounds known to cause fatigue, nausea, vomiting, weight change, changes in cognition, alopecia, peripheral neuropathy, and symptoms of menopause. In addition, preexisting sexually transmitted diseases often flare as a result of induced immune suppression. Oral antiviral therapy for genital or oral herpes and antifungal treatment for yeast vaginitis may be required. Long-term sexual consequences of taxane and platinum chemotherapy regimens may include clitoral neuropathy, affecting sensation and pain tolerance. Since the majority of women diagnosed with ovarian cancer are older than 60, sexual activity may already have declined due to age, hormonal decline, and partner and relationship status. In fact, predictive of greater levels of sexual activity after ovarian cancer were satisfaction with the appearance of one's body, being younger than age 56, not being actively treated, and being married [32].

27.5.7 Vulvar Cancer

Vulvar cancer accounts for only 3–5 % of gynecologic malignancies [33]. Uniquely, many of these patients may have avoided sex prior to diagnosis due to symptoms of their cancer including vulvar pain, itching, burning, soreness, bleeding, ulcers, or the existence of multifocal lesions. Surgical treatments including wide local excision, simple or radical vulvectomy with lymphadenectomy, and adjuvant radiation therapy have further negative sexual consequences. Depending on the location of the vulvar lesion, in order to obtain adequate surgical margins, clitorodectomy may be necessary, causing obvious sexual dysfunction. Inability to have intercourse due to vaginal stenosis can occur and even aggressive vaginal rehabilitation with dilators and physical therapy may be warranted. Women feel "lopsided" after hemivulvectomy; complain of loss of sexual sensation, due to fibrosis and lymphedema; and have concern about loss of control over bodily functions. In addition, since so much publicity surrounds the more common breast or colon cancers, lack of public awareness may contribute to the vulvar cancer patient's sense of aloneness [34]. Lastly, as the majority of vulvar carcinomas occur secondary to vulvar dermatoses such as lichen sclerosus, preexisting scarring and sexual dysfunction from these conditions may contribute to sexual dysfunction and need to be addressed.

27.6 Conclusion

As more women survive cancer due to medical and treatment advances, the need for optimal strategies that address quality of life facets including sexual function are critical. While cancer and its treatments directly contribute to sexual dysfunction, many confounding medical issues also influence post-cancer sexual functioning. Medications, partner status, depression and anxiety, personal self-esteem, premorbid sexual status, and cultural and religious influences are paramount etiological factors which must be addressed in tandem with the physiological and psychological ramification of cancer and its treatments. As such, addressing sexual dysfunction in the cancer patient requires education, open communication, lifestyle modifications, therapy, and support from a multidisciplinary team of healthcare professionals. Specialized cancer centers with survivorship programs are ideally suited to provide comprehensive care since they offer a multifaceted approach to sexual health and involve gynecology, internal medicine, sex therapy, social work, pharmacology, psychology, nutrition support, physical therapy, and spiritual healing.

27.7 Patient and Provider Resources

The American Cancer Society (ACS): http://www.cancer.org/

North American Menopause Society (NAMS): http://www.menopause.org/

International Society for the Study of Women's Sexual Health (ISSWSH): http://www.isswsh.org

International Society for Sexual Medicine (ISSM): www.issm.info

European Society for Sexual Medicine (ESSM): www.essm.net

American Congress of Obstetricians and Gynecologists (ACOG): http://www.acog.org/

References

1. American Cancer Society. Cancer facts and figures. Atlanta, GA: American Cancer Society; 2012.
2. Krychman ML. Sexual rehabilitation medicine in a female oncology setting. Gynecol Oncol. 2006;101:380–4.
3. Dizon DS. Quality of life after breast cancer: survivorship and sexuality. Breast J. 2009;15(5):500–4.
4. American College of Obstetricians and Gynecologist Task Force on Hormone Therapy. Sexual Dysfunction. Obstet Gynecol. 2004;104:85S–91.
5. Memorial Sloan-Kettering Cancer Center Clinical Trial. Serum estradiol levels in post menopausal women with breast cancer receiving adjuvant aromatase inhibitors and vaginal estrogen. NCT00984300. 2009. Available at http://www.ClinicalTrials.gov. Accessed 26 Sept 2010.
6. Wsshe JM, Perz J, Gilbert E. Changes to sexual wellbeing and intimacy after breast cancer. Cancer Nurs. 2012;35(6):456–65.
7. Ramirez M, McMullen C, Grant M, Altschuler A, Hornbrook MC, Krouse RS. Figuring out sex in a reconfigured body: experiences of female colorectal cancer survivors with ostomies. Women Health. 2009;49(8):608–24.
8. Schover LR. Myth-busters: telling the true story of breast cancer survivorship. J Natl Cancer Inst. 2004;96:1800–1.
9. Manne S, Ostroff J, Rini C, et al. The interpersonal process model of intimacy: the role of self-disclosure, partner disclosure, and partner responsiveness in interactions between breast cancer patients and their partners. J Fam Psychol. 2004;18(4):589–99.
10. Comfort A. The joy of sex the timeless guide to lovemaking. New York: Octopus Publishing Group Ltd.; 2008.

11. Schroder MA, et al. Clitoral therapy device for treatment of sexual dysfunction in irradiated cervical cancer patients. Int J Radiat Oncol Biol Phys. 2005; 61(4):1075.
12. Seagraves R, Clayton A, Croft H, Wolf A. Warnock Jl Bupropion sustained release for the treatment of hypoactive desire disorder. J Clin Psychopharmacol. 2004;24:339–42.
13. Barton DL, Wender DB, Sloan JA, et al. Randomized controlled trial to evaluate transdermal testosterone in female cancer survivors with decreased libido; North Central Cancer Treatment Group protocol N02C3. J Natl Cancer Inst. 2007;99:672–9.
14. Derzko C, Elliott S, Lam W. Management of sexual dysfunction in postmenopausal breast cancer patients taking adjuvant aromatase inhibitor therapy. Curr Oncol. 2007;14 suppl 1:S20–40.
15. Ferguson D, Hosmane B, Heiman JR. Randomized, placebo-controlled, double blind, parallel design trial of the efficacy and safety of Zestra R in women with mixed desire/interest/arousal/orgasm disorders. J Sex Marital Ther. 2010;36:66–86.
16. Krychman ML, Kellogg S. A case series of female orgasmic complaints in cancer survivors treated with a topical applied blend of botanical oils and extracts. In: ISSM/SMSNA Cancer survivorship and sexuality annual meeting. Unmoderated Poster. Annual Meeting. Washington, DC. 2011.
17. American Cancer Society. Facts and figures. Atlanta, GA: American Cancer Society; 2014.
18. Burwell SR, Case DL, Kaelin D, et al. Sexual problems in younger women after breast cancer surgery. J Clin Oncol. 2006;24(18):2815–21.
19. Speer JJ, Hillenberg B, Sugrue DP, et al. Study of sexual functioning determinants in breast cancer survivors. Breast J. 2005;11(6):440–7.
20. Manderson L, Stirling L. The absent breast: speaking of the mastectomized body. Feminism Psychol. 2007;17(1):75–92.
21. Alder J, Zanetti R, Wight E, et al. Sexual dysfunction after premenopausal stage 1 and 11 breast cancer: do androgens play a role? J Sex Med. 2008;5: 1898–906.
22. Alicikus ZA, Gorken IB, Sen RC, Kentli S, Kinay M, Alanyali H, Harmancioglu O. Psychosexual and body image aspects of quality of life in Turkish breast cancer patients: a comparison of breast conserving treatment and mastectomy. Tumori. 2009;95(2):212–18.
23. Engel J, Kerr J, Schlesinger-Raab A, Sauer H, Hölzel D. Quality of life following breast-conserving therapy or mastectomy: results of a 5-year prospective study. Breast J. 2004;10(3):223–31.
24. Walker JL, Piedmonte MR, Spirtos NM, et al. Recurrence and survival after random assignment to laparoscopy versus laparotomy for comprehensive surgical staging of uterine cancer Gynecologic Oncology Group LAP2 Study. J Clin Oncol. 2012; 30:695–700.
25. Carter J, Huang H, Chase DM, Walker JL, Cella D, Wenzel L. Sexual function of patients with endometrial cancer enrolled in the Gynecologic Oncology Group LAP2 Study. Int J Gynecol Cancer. 2012;22(9):1624–33.
26. Quick AM, Seamon LG, Abdel-Rasoul M, Salani R, Martin D. Sexual function after intracavitary vaginal brachytherapy for early-stage endometrial carcinoma. Int J Gynecol Cancer. 2012;22(4):703–8.
27. Jensen PT, Groenvold M, Klee MC, Thranov I, Peterson MA, Machin D. Early stage cervical carcinoma, radical hysterectomy and sexual function. A longitudinal study. Cancer. 2004;100:97–106.
28. Lammerink EA, de Bock GH, Pras E, Reyners AK, Mouris MJ. Sexual functioning of cervical cancer survivors: a review with a female perspective. Maturitas. 2012;72(4):296–304.
29. Bilodeau K, Bouchard L. The sexuality of Quebec women with cervical cancer: looking for love despite radiotherapy's trauma to their sexual body. Can Oncol Nurs J. 2011;21(4):233–7.
30. Ramirez M, McMullen C, Grant M, Altschuler A, Hornbrook MC, Krouse RS. Figuring out sex in a reconfigured body: experiences of female colorectal cancer survivors with ostomies. Women Health. 2009;49(8):608–24.
31. Wood GA, Sauder BL. Sexual side effects in women with anal carcinoma. Oncol Nurs Forum. 2009;36(3): 275–8.
32. Wilmoth MC, Hatmaker-Flanigan E, LaLoggia V, Nixon T. Ovarian cancer survivors: qualitative analysis of the symptom of sexuality. Oncol Nurs Forum. 2011;38(6):699–708.
33. Coleman R, Santosa J. Vulvar carcinoma. Curr Treat Options Oncol. 2000;1:177–90.
34. Jefferies H, Clifford C. Aloneness: the lived experience of women with cancer of the vulva. Eur J Cancer Care (Engl). 2011;20(6):738–46.

Female Sexual Dysfunction and Premature Menopause with Focus on Women's Wording

28

Alessandra Graziottin
and Monika Ewa Lukasiewicz

28.1 Introduction

Women are never too young to become menopausal, as a result of either a spontaneous or iatrogenic process of premature ovarian failure (POF) or insufficiency (POI). Here the POF acronym will be preferred, while premature menopause (PM) will be used when issues are shared both in spontaneous and iatrogenic menopause. The earlier the menopause, the more severe and complex the impact on women's sexuality can be [1–3]. Women report changes on their sexual identity, sexual function, and sexual relationships, the major contributors of women's sexual well-being, which is modulated by life events, reproduction-related events, health, relationships, and sociocultural variables [1, 4, 5]. According to the POF etiology, body image [6–8] and body feelings may change dramatically.

The younger the woman, the less she realizes the different key goals of her life cycle (feeling sexy, seductive and attractive, falling in love, having a satisfying sexual life, forming a stable couple/getting married, having children) and, consequently, the more pervasive the impact on her sexual identity, sexual function, and sexual relationship can be [1–3].

Female sexual dysfunction (FSD) can occur at any age but it tends to increase with age, with an accelerated impairment after the menopause and beyond [8, 9]. Three important overlapping factors that affect female sexuality in women with PM are indeed the aging process, menopause, and the systemic inflammation. The latter being a critical component of the former two [10].

The number of women complaining of PM is increasing, mainly as a result of prolonged survival after cancer treatment. The paper will focus on key sexual issues at menopause with this special perspective and a prominent attention on biologically based sexual issues, maintaining the key areas of sexual identity, sexual function, and sexual relationships [1–19] while psychosocial variables will be only briefly addressed [2]. The goal is to empower physicians' competence in addressing the many sexual issues triggered by PM.

A. Graziottin, M.D. (✉)
Center of Gynecology and Medical Sexology, H. San Raffaele Resnati, Via Enrico Panzacchi 6, 20123 Milan, Italy

Graziottin Foundation for the cure and care of pain in women, Milan, Italy
e-mail: a.graziottin@studiograziottin.it; segreteria@studiograziottin.it
http://www.alessandragraziottin.it; http://www.fondazionegraziottin.org

M.E. Lukasiewicz, M.D.
Department of Obstetrics and Gynecology, The Medical Center of Postgraduate Education, Bielanski Hospital, Warsaw, Poland

L.I. Lipshultz et al. (eds.), *Management of Sexual Dysfunction in Men and Women*, DOI 10.1007/978-1-4939-3100-2_28

28.2 Prevalence of PM

Spontaneous POF affects on average 1 % of women under 40 years of age [12–14, 20, 21]. Ethnicity is a contributor: the highest figure of spontaneous POF is reported among African American and Hispanic (both 1 and 4 %) and the lowest in Japanese (0 and 1 %) [20]. Iatrogenic menopause, for benign and malignant conditions, secondary to pelvic or gynecologic surgery, systemic chemotherapy, and pelvic or total body radiotherapy, affects 3.4–4.5 % [1–3, 22]. The latter figure is increasing worldwide due to the increased effectiveness of treatments and survival.

28.3 Etiology of PM

Heterogeneity is the hallmark of the PM etiology, which can be genetic, autoimmune, associated with chronic diseases, or iatrogenic in the context of benign or malignant diseases [1–3, 11–14, 21]. Leading etiologies of PM are summarized in Table 28.1.

PM impact on health and sexuality varies accordingly [23]. It may be limited in women affected by POF, who already have a family and are on optimal HRT or HT, as it is currently defined. It may be dramatic when the consequences of PM are superimposed to a serious medical condition which currently contraindicates HT, such as breast cancer and/or uterine adenocarcinoma in a childless younger woman and couple [1, 24, 25]. Multiple pathologies (and associated treatments) further increase the risk of systemic inflammation and accelerated aging, as exemplified when PM is associated to cancer or autoimmune diseases [12, 13, 21]. Neuroinflammation, a still neglected component of systemic inflammation associated with diseases, menopause, and aging, may contribute to sexual dysfunction through the associated physical and emotional depression, pain, loss of energy, and pervading fatigue [10, 26].

Key Point Surgical menopause *suddenly* deprives the woman of total ovarian hormone production, with a rapid impact on her well-being and sexuality. POF, either spontaneous or iatrogenic, has a gradual, *insidious* evolution over 2 or more years.

Table 28.1 Etiology of premature menopause

• Premature ovarian failure (POF):
Idiopathic
Genetic: Turner's syndrome
Fragile X syndrome
Mosaicism
Deletion/inversion
Galactosemia
BRCA1 mutation
Autoimmune, associated with: Celiac disease
Lupus erythematosus
Rheumatoid arthritis
Associated with chronic disease:
Chronic renal insufficiency
Primary biliary cirrhosis
• Iatrogenic for benign conditions:
Endometriosis
Bilateral dysgerminoma
Ovariectomy concomitant to hysterectomy
• Iatrogenic in women at risk of breast and/or ovarian cancer:
BRCA1 and/or BRCA2 carrier
• Iatrogenic for established malignant conditions:
Bilateral oophorectomy
Chemotherapy
Pelvic radiotherapy
Total body irradiation

Modified from Graziottin and Basson (2004) [1]

Occasional ovulation, due to the last recruitment of primordial oocytes, is possible for 2–3 years and pregnancy may occur in up to 10 % of women after POF diagnosis [12, 21]. This opportunity must not be missed by "masking" the first menstrual irregularities with a pill, without thinking about diagnosing or excluding PM before!

28.4 Prevalence of FSD in PM

Systematic studies on prevalence of female sexual disorders (FSD) in women affected by PM are limited. The prevalence of low desire for younger surgically menopause (SM) women is significantly higher (32 %) than that found for premenopausal women of the same age (19 %) ([4, 27]). The probability of hypoactive sexual desire disorder (HSDD) increases with age, while the *distress* associated with the loss of desire is inversely correlated with age [27]. SM is associated with low sexual desire and distress in 35 % of women in the United Kingdom, 44 % in Italy, 16 % in Germany, and 56 % in France [4].

The majority of the papers on the subject focus on qualitative aspects of PM impact on women's sexual function [1, 2, 8].

28.5 Women's Wording of Sexual Feelings and Concerns at PM

Women's wording is essential, to set the scenario, understand the key vulnerabilities in their sexuality, and perceive the overall sense of sexual loss they feel when PM occurs (Box 28.1). This is more important here as the paucity of studies specifically focused on sexual problems after PM may otherwise make this issue underappreciated.

Box 28.1 Women's Wording on Sexual Issues at PM

- *Sexual identity*

  "With all those hot flushes and sweating I feel like an old lady. And I'm only 35!"

  "I do not sleep well any more, since my (early) menopause. And when I get up in the morning I feel more tired than the night before. I have no energy at all…"

  "My skin is drier, I see more and more wrinkles every day. I cannot look at myself in the mirror."

  "My pubic hairs are getting white so early! I feel so ashamed!"

  "I'm getting fatter, without having changed anything in my diet! And I have this horrible 'menopausal look' with all the fat going on my belly."

  "I have pain in all my joints. I feel stiff and rigid in the morning as if I were trapped in an armor of rust. I feel so old."

  "Without my ovaries (or my uterus) I do not feel I'm a woman anymore."

  "After my early menopause, nobody looks at me, nobody dates me! I feel sexually invisible."

  "I feel asexual."

  "I feel no more feminine since chemo caused the loss of my beautiful hair. They were my pride, and now I feel so ugly…."

- *Sexual function*

  "I do not have any more sexual drive, for anybody."

  "Since I became menopausal too early, I had a worsening vaginal dryness. Sex is no longer a pleasure."

  "I had an early menopause at 32. Now, at 40, it takes ages to get aroused, my orgasm is fading and weak. I'm too young to feel so old!"

  "My clitoris is dead."

  "My vagina is so tied and dry, I cannot make love any more. It hurts too much!

  "Having sex is a nightmare now: I have a cystitis every time I have intercourse!"

- *Sexual relationship*

  "My husband has lost interest in making sex with me, since I lost my periods."

  "My partner says that I have lost my scent of woman. He does not like to do oral sex with me anymore, while we both loved it before!"

  "I feel so hurt. Since I got menopausal so early, he became interested only in looking at other women! But it denies and this gets me crazy of jealousy."

  "Why should I make love, if I cannot have children anymore?"

  "We were looking for our first child with no success. My periods were delayed. The results of the hormonal exams were shocking: I was getting menopausal! My husband had always longed for a child and said he cannot accept remaining childless. I've lost him because he wants a natural pregnancy."

  "Please give me all the info on how I can get pregnant. Do I have a last chance with my ovary? Is ovum donation safe? Which problems would I or my child have?"

Women's reported feelings explain why *sexual identity*, the sense of femininity and sexual attractiveness, as well as the potential for pregnancy, is perceived as definitely wounded or lost. Their wording about how they see themselves in the mirror and in their cognitive mind-set (*body image*) and how they perceive the changes in their physical and emotional feelings (*body feelings*) well indicates why PM may affect so dramatically their sexual identity. Body image concerns, such as skin and hair changes, changes in body shape, and tendency for weight gain and central adiposity, may impair the sense of personal attractiveness, contributing to loss of self-confidence and self-esteem, and a general sense of "feeling and looking older" [1, 3, 5, 6, 24, 25]. Sexual identity is more vulnerable when PM disrupts the process of psychosexual maturity, after peripubertal spontaneous POF or after iatrogenic POF, for childhood or adolescent cancers, for example, lymphoma [4, 5]. Body image issues may become prominent in women who underwent breast or gynecologic oncology surgery and associated treatments causing PM. POF after brain cancer surgery and chemo may cause even worse sexual damages. Chemotherapy may have a pervading impact on sexual identity when hair loss and skin, nail, and genital mucosal changes become prominent. The woman's health, coping attitude, and quality of sexuality *before* PM may all affect the sexual outcome after PM. Women at higher risk of negative sexual outcome after PM are younger, single or in conflicting relationships, and childless, with lower education and socioeconomic status [1, 6, 24, 25].

Women's wording on the impairment of their *sexual function* is more clear-cut and informative than pure statistics. Different etiologies of PM may independently contribute to FSD. For example, dysmetabolic diseases, such as diabetes, are at higher risk in overweight PM women and generally in obese menopausal subjects, and this further contributes to FSD. Corticosteroids, when needed to treat the leading autoimmune pathology, such as systemic lupus erythematosus (SLE) or rheumatoid arthritis (RA), affect sexuality as well [28–30].

The report on the impact of PM on relationships suggests facts and nuances that are more frequently told to a physician with training in sexual medicine. Stage in life cycle may contribute to FSD, fertility being a major issue in childless women and couples [1–3, 15]. The partner's reaction to the associated infertility and the quality of the relationships before and after PM modulate the individual and couple's coping attitudes. Contextual factors—both relational and sociocultural, such as ethnicity—further contribute [15].

Women's words well express the need for complex sexual help. They indicate how pervasive the discovery of PM can be for the three dimensions of women sexuality and how we must keep in mind the complexity, without limiting the listening and intervention to the sexual function. A multidisciplinary approach, medical, rehabilitative, and psychosexual, may offer the most comprehensive and satisfying outcomes for the woman and the couple (either hetero- or homosexual). However, no specific papers on the impact of PM on homosexual couples have been published in the author's knowledge.

28.6 How to Diagnose PM

Impending PM should be considered when menstrual irregularities are complained of, more so if menopausal symptoms appear in women younger than 40 years of age. Predictors of PM include: raised basal FSH when the sample is performed in the third or fourth day after the beginning of period, low anti-Mullerian hormone (AMH) and inhibin B, and/or a poor response to ovarian stimulation. Definite diagnosis is based on FSH levels above 40 IU/L in two consecutive samples at 1-month distance. Echography may show small ovaries for the age, with no or a few residual oocytes. PM is implicit when bilateral oophorectomy is performed in women younger than 40 years of age [12, 13, 21, 31].

28.7 Premature Menopause: A Challenge for Sexuality

Progress in oncology has significantly increased the number of survivors of childhood and adolescent cancers. Unfortunately, the impact of chemotherapy and radiotherapy, pelvic or total body radiotherapy, on oocytes may precipitate a PM [1, 3]. The complexity of the clinical picture, the increased vulnerability to accelerated aging for the combined effect of PM and side effects of chemotherapy and/or radiotherapy, and the survivor's expectations for a better quality of life (QoL), both in general and sexual terms, challenge the physician's ability to tailor the more appropriate medical and psychosexual treatment [1, 3].

Receptors for sexual hormones are present in virtually all organs and tissues. *Estrogen receptor alpha* is mainly located in the breast, genitals, and hypothalamus ("the reproductive system"). They modulate the *proliferative actions of estrogens. Estrogen receptor beta* is present in all the organs (brain, lung, bowels, bone, joints): they mediate *antiproliferative and reparative actions.* PM causes a dramatic loss of sexual hormones: distribution of receptors explains why it is associated with an increased risk of accelerated aging—the younger the woman, the higher the risk, unless appropriate HT, when feasible, is initiated and adequately maintained at appropriate doses [1, 11, 14, 32, 33]. Morbidity and mortality from cardiovascular disease, stroke, accelerated brain aging, and osteoporosis present a greater risk in PM women compared to controls [34–37]. Some observational studies indicate that effects of estrogens on the brain (neuroprotective or harmful) depend on age of onset of the menopause [36, 38, 39]. In a recent study Bove et al. showed that an earlier age of surgical menopause is associated with decline in global condition and increase burden of Alzheimer's disease [39]. Rocca et al.'s study on the effect of mono- or bilateral oophorectomy, without subsequent HT, indicates an odds ratio of 1.46 of accelerated brain aging and an odds ratio of 1.68 of Parkinsonism (with borderline significance for Parkinson disease) in women who underwent this surgery in the fertile age. The data strongly indicate that the younger the woman, the more vulnerable the brain [14]. The dramatic vulnerability of both the cognitive and motor systems well indicates how pervasive the brain damage and the associated neuroinflammation are, when the consequences of PM are neglected.

Sexual dysfunctions are reported with higher frequency and more significant personal distress after surgical menopause [4]. Overall sense of well-being and achievements of life goals are variably affected.

28.8 Hormones and the Pathophysiology of Sexual Dysfunction After PM

Estrogens and androgens modulate the neurobiology of brain aging. Their trophic role in neuronal membrane repair, in promoting neuronal sprouting and interneuronal connectivity as well as the levels of neurotransmitters, is gaining increasing evidence [1, 4, 40]. They also modulate sexual desire and mental arousal and the neurovascular cascade of events leading to genital arousal, lubrication, and orgasm. Estrogens are modulators of sexual response and "permissive" factors for the vasoactive intestinal polypeptide (VIP), which "translates" desire and central arousal into vaginal congestion and lubrication (reference).

Testosterone has an initiating role on desire and central arousal, acting on the dopaminergic appetitive-seeking pathway, and a modulator role of the peripheral response, as a permissive factor for nitric oxide (NO), the main mediator of clitoral and cavernosal body congestion [1, 4, 40].

Loss of estrogens and androgens contributes to impaired brain aging, as exemplified by increased and anticipated neurovegetative, affective, cognitive, and motor disorders in PM women (reference). It reduces sexual desire, central and peripheral arousal, with vaginal dryness, and causes/worsens orgasmic difficulties and dyspareunia, causing loss of self-confidence and self-esteem, and increases anxiety and concerns (reference). Loss of estrogens and androgens (particularly of testosterone and DHEA) increases the vulnerability to neuroinflammation, a still underappreciated aspect of brain aging (reference). Sexual hormone loss may as well contribute to the neurobiological etiology of depressed mood that coexists so often with acquired loss of desire and potentiates the depressive feelings (reference) consequent to the many losses that PM—and menopause in general—implies [5]. Comorbidity of FSD is frequent. The issue of FSD cannot be separated from the impact on sexuality of concomitant medical comorbidities associated with or consequent to different etiologies of PM [1].

28.9 Clinical Features Contribute to FSD After PM

Premature menopause is strongly connected with vasomotor symptoms (more severe after surgical menopause), sleep disturbances, insomnia, depression, anxiety, lack of concentration, and fatigue, more prominent when HH is not feasible, not offered, or inadequate in terms of quality and duration.

Vaginal symptoms, urinary symptoms, and comorbid disorder further contribute to the sense of accelerated sexual aging [12, 13, 21, 23]. They include vaginal atrophy, reduced vaginal secretion, delayed time of vaginal lubrication during sexual intercourse, vaginal dryness, and loss of vaginal rugae, elasticity, and transudate. Urinary symptoms as dysuria, urge or stress incontinence, and recurrent postcoital cystitis can have a further detrimental effect on QoL and sexual health.

Joint pain, sarcopenia, and accelerated osteopenia further impair women's general health and sense of vital energy and strongly influence QoL [12, 13, 21, 23].

Last but not least, severity of vasomotor symptoms predicts and increases the vulnerability to depression and Alzheimer's and Parkinson diseases [32, 36, 38, 39]. They gradually undermine the sense of self-confidence and self-esteem, when the feeling of a progressively incompetent memory threatens the basis of the social and professional role (reference).

28.10 Diagnosis of FSD After PM

FSD may be antecedent to PM, concomitant to PM, and/or specifically caused and/or maintained by PM. Diagnosis should consider the multifactorial etiology of FSD (with special attention to predisposing, precipitating, and maintaining factors, biological and psychosexual), the disorder being generalized or situational, lifelong, or acquired, as well as the level of distress it causes.

In stable relationships, counseling to *both* partners is a crucial part of the diagnosis and management. Accurate physical examination is mandatory, given the importance of biological factors associated to PM, with focus on trophism and appearance of external genitalia, vagina and vaginal pH, pelvic floor tonicity, and "pain map," in case of dyspareunia [1, 41]. A poor quality of genital sexual feedback is usually an underevaluated contributor of loss of sexual desire/interest in all women, more so in PM and menopausal women for the additional aging and hormone-deprivation contributing role.

Key Point Hormone samples should be included in diagnosis of POF as well as vaginal pH. Specific exams should be considered according to the clinical history and etiology of PM.

28.11 Medical Management of FSD Associated with PM

The first-line intervention should be focused on improving lifestyles as major contributors of health, body image, and body shape, of a better sense of femininity, and of a (still) fulfilling sexual life [8]. Daily physical exercise to feel fitter; appropriate food choice and intake; avoidance of smoking, alcohol, and leisure drugs; and better care of hairs, nails, skin, all are subtle and substantial changes that should be encouraged. The woman should fully understand her sense of loss after PM and then be positively encouraged to move across the mourning and the sense of having lost something essential to get a "reconquered" life. Empowering her feeling of being an even more aware protagonist of her own life is a key step in the counseling pathway. Specifically, treatment of POF should be etiologically based on hormonal (replacement) therapy (HT), when medically/oncologically feasible, in order to avoid the consequences of estrogen and androgen insufficiency [1, 2, 5, 8, 16–19, 33]. HT may minimize the impact of PM on general health, menopausal symptoms and signs, and couple dynamics. Interdisciplinary approach is sometimes indicated to offer the best opportunity to tailor treatment according to the woman's clinical situation and to optimize the treatment choices to her and her partner's sexual needs [42, 43].

Options include bioidentical estradiol and progesterone at individualized doses: 25, 50, or 75 pg/mL of plasmatic estradiol should be obtained according to age and individual vulnerabilities, particularly in younger patients, when specific somatic concerns (early onset osteopenia and sarcopenia, among others) are in play [1, 2, 8, 37]. Estrogens' and testosterones' anti-inflammatory properties on the brain are of increasing interest [26]. Route of administration can be oral, vaginal, and transdermal, according to the woman's preferences. When the uterus is present, 12 days of progesterone or progestins/month should be prescribed [1, 8, 33]. Women without uterus can use estradiol alone, with the good news that it does significantly *decrease* the risk of breast cancer. Topical testosterone cream, compounded by the pharmacist with the medical prescription, may improve the clitoral and genital responsiveness to sexual stimulation. Systemic testosterone, previously available with the transdermal patch [16–19], is now administered through bioidentical compounds, but no study on these treatments have been performed in the authors' knowledge, in spite of their increasing use. DHEA (10 or 25 mg/day, orally) is increasingly considered as a critical and yet underevaluated part of a well-tailored HT.

However, no guidelines are available on the optimal dose and schedule treatment for PM patients in the authors' knowledge. The sentence "lowest hormone dose for the shortest period of time," currently used for the HT after natural menopause around 50 years of age is a biological nonsense for women who have to face 20, 30, or more years hormoneless at a very young age. Consensus exists that they should be offered treatment at least until the age of 51, in absence of major contraindications [1, 8].

Management of FSD due to POF differentiates according to the most important sexual issues: (1) age, physical and psychological impact of PM or natural menopause; (2) effects of estrogen and androgen loss on general and sexual health; (3) severity of menopausal symptoms; and (4) loss of fertility and its meaning to both partners [1].

The focus here will be on treatment of FSD associated to PM or natural menopause. An updated critical review of available treatment for menopausal FSD has been published by Al-Azzawi et al. [33].

28.12 Desire/Interest and Central Arousal Disorders

Reduced libido is observed in about 7–22 % of women with POF [4]. Desire and central arousal overlap. Although some clinical studies have failed to demonstrate a direct correlation between testosterone level and FSD [44], there is evidence that women with POF demonstrate reduced total and free testosterone level compared to control group [45, 46]. Randomized controlled trials (RCT) indicate the positive effect of testosterone in estrogen-repleted women after surgical menopause, when etiology of FSD appears to be hormone dependent. RCT have shown that treatment with 300-μg/day testosterone patches on estrogen-repleted women significantly increased sexual desire, frequency of satisfying sexual activity, and reduced sexual distress and was well tolerated [16–19]. Two systematic reviews of RCT indicate a positive effect of testosterone on all dimensions of sexual function and some psychological benefits as well [24, 29]. According to a Cochrane Review and a high-quality RCT, sexual function of postmenopausal women given testosterone therapy in addition to standard hormone therapy was improved [47, 48].

Secondary outcomes indicate a significant improvement of arousal and orgasm and of self-image and self-esteem and a significant reduction in anxiety and concerns. The testosterone patch treatment has been approved by the European Agency for the Evaluation of Medicinal Products (EMEA) in July 2006. However, controversy still exists on the indication of androgen therapy in women [49].

In spite of its clear-cut efficacy on all dimensions of sexual function, the testosterone patch has been withdrawn from the market by Warner Chilcott, the company that held the rights to market *Intrinsa*, in October 2012. The real truth being it proved to be an economic failure as only a small percentage of physicians did prescribe it.

Tibolone and HT with estradiol and norethisterone are other options to improve sexual desire [50]. Bupropion is a nonhormonal drug that may as well improve it when HT is not feasible [51].

28.13 Genital Arousal Disorders

Vaginal estrogenic treatment is indicated when the genital arousal disorder causes and/or is associated with vaginal dryness, dyspareunia, postcoital cystitis, urogenital atrophy, and/or urinary incontinence, mostly of the urge type. Accelerated urogynecological comorbidity will be delayed with appropriate HT [1, 8, 33, 41, 52, 53]. Safety of vaginal estrogen therapy has been documented in RCT and in observational studies; however, controversy about using vaginal estrogens in breast cancer patients still exists [6, 7, 25].

To minimize the impact of radiotherapy on vaginal tissue, it is crucial to start vaginal estrogenic treatment, pelvic floor stretching, and vaginal molds as early as possible. The proper, early treatment may maintain vaginal elasticity, optimal length, and "habitability" during pelvic or vaginal radiotherapy for cervical cancer [54, 55].

In 2013 ospemifene (an estrogen agonist/antagonist) was approved by the US Food and Drug Administration (FDA) for the treatment of moderate-to-severe dyspareunia associated with vulvovaginal atrophy [56].

Intravaginally administered dehydroepiandrosterone (DHEA) on daily basis improves symptoms of vaginal atrophy in postmenopausal women and reduces burning, itching, and dryness [57].

Testosterone applied daily on the vulva and vaginal introitus may anecdotally improve vulvovaginal trophism, clitoral sensitivity, genital arousal, and erotic response. It may therefore improve the genital feedbacks that may contribute to maintain sexual desire/interest and central arousal. However, more studies are needed [58, 59].

28.14 Orgasmic Disorder

True orgasmic disorder acquired subsequent to PM may benefit from HT. Increasing evidence supports a positive role of testosterone in restoring orgasmic potential [5, 16–19, 47]. Pelvic floor rehabilitation is indicated when (a) hypotonia is diagnosed as contributing to reduced orgasmic sensations and (b) hyperactive pelvic floor causes introital dyspareunia and vaginal dryness, preventing the genital engorgement ("orgasmic platform," according to Masters and Johnson [60], thus impairing the coital component of orgasm). Comorbid stress or urge incontinence with fear of leakage, respectively, with thrusting or with orgasm is to be appropriately addressed [1].

28.15 Sexual Pain Disorders (Dyspareunia)

Dyspareunia, introital and/or deep, requires a careful pathophysiologic understanding of its complex biological etiology (cutaneous, muscular, endocrine, vascular, nervous, immune, iatrogenic) and meaning to design an effective treatment [41]. Friction introital dyspareunia, secondary to vaginal dryness, may benefit from vaginal ET. Reflexive pelvic muscle tightening ("hyperactivity of the levator ani," secondary to pain) may benefit from self-massage and stretching, electromyographic biofeedback, and/or physiotherapy [1, 8, 61].

28.16 Treatment of PM and Associated Fertility Issues

Prevention of infertility in women facing impending POF is critical in childless women. Three lines of *research* are currently raising new hopes in the pursuit of fertility protection in young women [1, 8, 62]: (a) Cryopreservation of oocytes or ovarian tissue before cancer therapy is an option in women with impending POF. (b) Cryopreservation of embryos is feasible in women with a partner, when both are committed to have a baby, but requires a cycle of in vitro fertilization (IVF): time before cancer treatment may be a key limiting factor. (c) Cryopreservation of ovarian tissue is very promising, also in the prepubertal years [1, 8, 62]. Ovarian suppression with GnRHa during chemotherapy can be also an option [7]. However, with an impending PM, the current possibility of having a child is very rare. An honest disclosure of current limits of all these techniques should be clearly acknowledged in counseling with patients and their partner. Referral to a reproductive specialist should be offered to patients who are interested in fertility preservation. Ovodonation can be considered, if accepted by the woman and the couple, in countries where it is legal or abroad [62].

28.17 Couple Issues After PM

In women with either POF or natural menopause, appropriate listening to the sexual concerns and to the real personal motivation to treatment is essential for treatment planning and psychosexual management of FSD (Box 28.2). Specific concerns triggered by body image issues, loss of fertility, or menopausal symptoms that cannot be hormonally treated (i.e., in breast cancer patients) should be considered also with the couple perspective, when indicated [7, 63]. After the natural menopause, 48 % of women [4] report low desire, but only a minority feel distressed because of it and motivated to seek for treatment. Moreover, the older the woman, the higher the probability that the partner himself may have concomitant personal sexual problems, i.e., male sexual disorders (MSD), that may preexist to menopause, be concomitant to it, or consequent to the many FSD menopausal women may complain about [2]. The partner can be the *symptom inducer*, when, for example, his persistent or worsening erectile deficit may cause or contribute to her loss of desire or when his inadequate personal care or hygiene precipitates her loss of sexual interest; or he can be the *symptom carrier*, when his loss of desire is consequent to her avoidant behavior toward any form of sexual intimacy; when her vaginal atrophy, with dyspareunia and introital narrowing, "precipitates" his erectile deficit, while erection could have been still acceptable, although not perfect, with a well-lubricated vagina; or when the many physical changes induced by PM, including the reduction of sexual pheromones, may precipitate a loss of desire and interest in the partner.

Box 28.2 Psychosexual Management in Case of FSD

- Individual behavioral therapy
  - In case of dyspareunia:
    Behavioral therapy with vaginal inserts/molds and progressive rehabilitation of the pelvic floor
    Pharmacological treatment for any associated intense phobic avoidance.
- Psychotherapy to cope with the many losses PM and its e tiology have caused on health and sexuality
- Couple therapy to address sexual and/or nonsexual couple issues, such as conflicts, poor erotic skills, or communication inadequacies

Key Point Evaluate and treat, when indicated, both partners, to have a comprehensive diagnosis of his/her contribution to the current sexual complaint after PM

28.18 Conclusions

PM accelerates general health and sexual aging, unless appropriate HT, when non-contraindicated, is initiated and maintained over time, at least until the age of 51. FSD reporting after PM increases. Women with PM are at higher risk for distressing sexual disorders. RCT indicate that HT, with estrogen and testosterone, may have positive effects on all domains of sexual function, especially after surgical PM. Attention to sexuality may be essential and welcomed for POF women in spite of the difficulty to raise sexual issues. Simple and open question may ease the dialogue between patient and gynecologist.

The questions "How's your sexual life?," "Is there any sexual concern you'd like to discuss?," or "Would you like to improve your sexual life, if you are not currently satisfied?" show the women that the health-care provider is at ease with this issue. She will be listened to and counseled would she be willing to raise her concerns to get a proper diagnosis and treatment. In sexual medicine a well-tailored, integrated medical and psychosexual approach may offer POF women and couples a long-lasting satisfying sexual season. The best outcome is obtained when a well-tailored HT, when feasible and oncologically appropriate, is combined with healthy lifestyles. Psychotherapy, of either the woman or couples, may prove useful when specific issues are not addressed by simply restoring the hormonal equilibrium.

References

1. Graziottin A, Basson R. Sexual dysfunctions in women with premature menopause. Menopause. 2004;11(6):766–77.
2. Graziottin A, Leiblum SR. Biological and psychosocial pathophysiology of female sexual dysfunction during the menopausal transition. J Sex Med. 2005;2 Suppl 3:133–45.
3. Madanat LMS, Malila N, Dyba T, Hakulinen T, Sankila R, Boice Jr JD, Lähteenmäki PM. Probability of parenthood after early onset cancer: a population-based study. Int J Cancer. 2008;123(12):2891–8.
4. Graziottin A, Koochaki PE, Rodenberg CA, Dennerstein L. The prevalence of hypoactive sexual desire disorder in surgically menopausal women: an epidemiological study of women in four European countries. J Sex Med. 2009;6(8):2143–53.
5. Alexander JL, Dennerstein L, Burger H, Graziottin A. Testosterone and libido in surgically and naturally menopausal women. Womens Health (Lond Engl). 2006;2(3):459–77.
6. Graziottin A. Breast cancer and its effects on women's self-image and sexual function. In: Goldstein I, Meston C, Davis S, Traish A, editors. Women's sexual function and dysfunction: study, diagnosis and treatment. London: Taylor and Francis; 2006. p. 276–81.
7. Cardoso F, Loibl S, Pagani O, Graziottin A, Panizza P, Martincich L, Gentilini O, Peccatori F, Fourquet A, Delaloge S, Marotti L, Penault-Llorca F, Kotti-Kitromilidou AM, Rodger A, Harbeck N. The European Society of Breast Cancer Specialists recommendations for the management of young women with breast cancer. Eur J Cancer. 2012;48(18):3355–77.
8. Graziottin A. Menopause and sexuality: key issues in premature menopause and beyond. Ann N Y Acad Sci. 2010;1205:254–61.
9. Nicolosi A, Laumann EO, Glasser DB, Moreira Jr ED, Paik A, Gingell C, Global Study of Sexual Attitudes and Behaviors Investigators' Group. Sexual behavior and sexual dysfunctions after age 40: the global study of sexual attitudes and behaviors. Urology. 2004;64(5):991–7.
10. Graziottin A, Skaper S, Fusco M. Mast cells in chronic inflammation, pelvic pain and depression in women. Gynecol Endocrinol. 2014;30(7):472–7.
11. Fassnacht W, Mempel A, Strowitzki T, Vogt PH. Premature ovarian failure (POF) syndrome: towards the molecular clinical analysis of its genetic complexity. Curr Med Chem. 2006;13(12):1397–410.
12. Meskhi A, Seif MW. Premature ovarian failure. Curr Opin Obstet Gynecol. 2006;18(4):418–26.
13. Anasti JN. Premature ovarian failure: an update. Fertil Steril. 2006;70:1–15.
14. Rocca WA, Bower JH, Maraganore DM, Ahlskog JE, Grossardt BR, de Andrade M, Melton 3rd LJ. Increased risk of cognitive impairment or dementia in women who underwent oophorectomy before menopause. Neurology. 2007;69(11):1074–83.
15. Rauck A, Green DM, Yasui Y, Mertens A, Robinson LL. Marriage in the survivors of childhood cancer: a preliminary study description from the Childhood Cancer Survivor Study. Med Pediatr Oncol. 1999;33:60–3.
16. Shifren JL, Braunstein J, Simon JA, et al. Transdermal testosterone treatment in women with impaired sexual function after oophorectomy. N Engl J Med. 2000;343:682–8.
17. Buster JE, Kingsberg SA, Aguirre O, et al. Testosterone patch for low sexual desire in surgically menopausal women: a randomized trial. Obstet Gynecol. 2005;105(5 Pt 1):944–52.
18. Simon J, Braunstein G, Nachtigall L, et al. Testosterone patch increases sexual activity and desire in surgically menopausal women with hypoactive sexual desire disorder. J Clin Endocrinol Metab. 2005;90(9):5226–33.
19. Davis SR, van der Mooren MJ, van Lunsen RH, et al. Efficacy and safety of a testosterone patch for the treatment of hypoactive sexual desire disorder in surgically menopausal women: a randomized, placebo-controlled trial. Menopause. 2006;13(3):387–96.
20. Luborsky JL, Meyer P, Sowers MF, Gold EB, Santoro N. Premature menopause in a multi-ethnic population study of the menopause transition. Hum Reprod. 2003;8(1):199–206.
21. De Vos M, Devroey P, Fauser BC. Primary ovarian insufficiency. Lancet. 2010;376(9744):911–21.
22. Puukko LMR, Hirvonen E, Aalberg V, Hovi L, Rautonen J, Siimes MA. Sexuality in young women surviving leukemia. Arch Dis Child. 1997;76:197–202.

23. Shuster LT, Rhodes DJ, Gostout BS, Grossardt BR, Rocca WA. Premature menopause or early menopause: long-term health consequences. Maturitas. 2010;65(2):161–6.
24. Schover LR. Sexuality and body image in younger women with breast cancer. J Natl Cancer Inst Monogr. 1994;16:177–82.
25. Graziottin A, Castoldi E. Sexuality and breast cancer: a review. In: Studd J, editor. The management of the menopause. The millennium review. London: Parthenon Publishing; 2000. p. 211–20.
26. Vegeto E, Benedusi V, Maggi A. Estrogen anti-inflammatory activity in brain: a therapeutic opportunity for menopause and neurodegenerative diseases. Front Neuroendocrinol. 2008;29(4):507–19.
27. Graziottin A. Prevalence and evaluation of sexual health problems – HSDD in Europe. J Sex Med. 2007;4 Suppl 3:211–9.
28. Poggiogalle E, Di Lazzaro L, Pinto A, Migliaccio S, Lenzi A, Donini LM. Health-related quality of life and quality of sexual life in obese subjects. Int J Endocrinol. 2014;2014:847871.
29. Yilmaz H, Polat HA, Yilmaz SD, Erkin G, Kucuksen S, Salli A, Ugurlu H. Evaluation of sexual dysfunction in women with rheumatoid arthritis: a controlled study. J Sex Med. 2012;9(10):2664–70.
30. García Morales M, Callejas Rubio JI, Peralta-Ramírez MI, Henares Romero LJ, Ríos Fernández R, Camps García MT, Navarrete Navarrete N, Ortego Centeno N. Impaired sexual function in women with systemic lupus erythematosus: a cross-sectional study. Lupus. 2013;22(10):987–95.
31. Leader B, Baker VL. Maximizing the clinical utility of antimüllerian hormone testing in women's health. Curr Opin Obstet Gynecol. 2014;26(4):226–36.
32. Soni M, Hogervorst E. Premature ovarian insufficiency and neurological function. Minerva Endocrinol. 2014;39(3):189–99. Epub 2014 June 19.
33. Al-Azzawi F, Bitzer J, Brandenburg U, Castelo-Branco C, Graziottin A, Kenemans P, Lachowsky M, Mimoun S, Nappi RE, Palacios S, Schwenkhagen A, Studd J, Wylie K, Zahradnik HP. Therapeutic options for postmenopausal female sexual dysfunction. Climacteric. 2010;13(2):103–20.
34. Wu X, Cai H, Kallianpur A, Li H, Yang G, Gao J, Xiang YB, Ji BT, Yu-Tang, Zheng W, Shu XO. Impact of premature ovarian failure on mortality and morbidity among Chinese women. PLoS One. 2014;9(3):e89597.
35. Rocca WA, Grossardt BR, Miller VM, Shuster LT, Brown Jr RD. Premature menopause or early menopause and risk of ischemic stroke. Menopause. 2012;19(3):272–7.
36. Rocca WA, Grossardt BR, Shuster LT. Oophorectomy, estrogen, and dementia: a 2014 update. Mol Cell Endocrinol. 2014;389(1–2):7–12.
37. Kurtoglu-Aksoy N, Akhan SE, Bastu E, Gungor-Ugurlucan F, Telci A, Iyibozkurt AC, Topuz S. Implications of premature ovarian failure on bone turnover markers and bone mineral density. Clin Exp Obstet Gynecol. 2014;41(2):149–53.
38. Phung TK, Waltoft BL, Laursen TM, Settnes A, Kessing LV, Mortensen PB, Waldemar G. Hysterectomy, oophorectomy and risk of dementia: a nationwide historical cohort study. Dement Geriatr Cogn Disord. 2010;30(1):43–50.
39. Bove R, Secor E, Chibnik LB, Barnes LL, Schneider JA, Bennett DA, De Jager PL. Age at surgical menopause influences cognitive decline and Alzheimer pathology in older women. Neurology. 2014;82(3):222–9.
40. Bachmann G, Bancroft J, Braunstein G, et al. FAI: the Princeton consensus statement on definition, classification, and assessment. Fertil Steril. 2002;77:660–5.
41. Graziottin A. Sexual pain disorders (Dyspareunia and vaginismus). In: Porst H, Buvat J, editors. ISSM (International Society of Sexual Medicine) Standard Committee Book, standard practice in sexual medicine. Oxford: Blackwell; 2006. p. 342–50 (available at: www.alessandragraziottin.it)
42. King J, Wynne CH, Assersohn L, Jones A. Hormone replacement therapy and women with premature menopause—a cancer survivorship issue. Eur J Cancer. 2011;47(11):1623–32.
43. Luisi S, Orlandini C, Biliotti G, Scolaro V, De Felice G, Regini C, Petraglia F. Hormone replacement therapy in menopause and in premature ovarian insufficiency. Minerva Ginecol. 2013;65(6):607–20.
44. Davis SR, Davison SL, Donath S, Bell RJ. Circulating androgen levels and self-reported sexual function in women. JAMA. 2005;294(1):91–6.
45. Kalantaridou SN, Calis KA, Vanderhoof VH, Bakalov VK, Corrigan EC, Troendle JF, Nelson LM. Testosterone deficiency in young women with 46, XX spontaneous premature ovarian failure. Fertil Steril. 2006;86(5):1475–82.
46. Guerrieri GM, Martinez PE, Klug SP, Haq NA, Vanderhoof VH, Koziol DE, Popat VB, Kalantaridou SN, Calis KA, Rubinow DR, Schmidt PJ, Nelson LM. Effects of physiologic testosterone therapy on quality of life, self-esteem, and mood in women with primary ovarian insufficiency. Menopause. 2014;21(9):952–6.
47. Somboonporn W, Davis S, Seif MW, Bell R. Testosterone for peri- and postmenopausal women. Cochrane Database Syst Rev. 2005;4, CD004509.
48. Davis SR, Worsley R. Androgen treatment of postmenopausal women. J Steroid Biochem Mol Biol. 2014;142:107–14.
49. Wierman ME, Basson R, Davis SR, Khosla S, Miller KK, Rosner W, Santoro N. Androgen therapy in women: an endocrine society clinical practice guideline. J Clin Endocrinol Metab. 2006;91(10):3697–710.
50. Ziaei S, Moghasemi M, Faghihzadeh S. Comparative effects of conventional hormone replacement therapy and tibolone on climacteric symptoms and sexual dysfunction in postmenopausal women. Climacteric. 2010;13(2):147–56.

51. Clayton AH, Croft HA, Handiwala L. Antidepressants and sexual dysfunction: mechanisms and clinical implications. Postgrad Med. 2014;126(2):91–9.
52. Goldstein I, Alexander JL. Practical aspects in the management of vaginal atrophy and sexual dysfunction in perimenopausal and postmenopausal women: review. J Sex Med. 2005;2 Suppl 3:154–65.
53. Tan O, Bradshaw K, Carr BR. Management of vulvovaginal atrophy-related sexual dysfunction in postmenopausal women: an up-to-date review. Menopause. 2012;19(1):109–17.
54. Mariani L, Gadducci A, Vizza E, Tomao S, Vici P. Vaginal atrophy in breast cancer survivors: role of vaginal estrogen therapy. Gynecol Endocrinol. 2013;29(1):25–9.
55. Incrocci L, Jensen PT. Pelvic radiotherapy and sexual function in men and women. J Sex Med. 2013;10 Suppl 1:53–64.
56. McLendon AN, Clinard VB, Woodis CB. Ospemifene for the treatment of vulvovaginal atrophy and dyspareunia in postmenopausal women. Pharmacotherapy. 2014;34:1050–60.
57. Archer DF. Dehydroepiandrosterone intra vaginal administration for the management of postmenopausal vulvovaginal atrophy. J Steroid Biochem Mol Biol. 2014;145:139–43.
58. Witherby S, Johnson J, Demers L, Mount S, Littenberg B, Maclean CD, Wood M, Muss H. Topical testosterone for breast cancer patients with vaginal atrophy related to aromatase inhibitors: a phase I/II study. Oncologist. 2011;16(4):424–31. Epub 2011 March 8.
59. Fernandes T, Costa-Paiva LH, Pinto-Neto AM. Efficacy of vaginally applied estrogen, testosterone, or polyacrylic acid on sexual function in postmenopausal women: a randomized controlled trial. J Sex Med. 2014;11(5):1262–70. Epub 2014 Feb 25.
60. Morrow R. Sex research and sex therapy: a sociological analysis of Masters and Johnson. New York: Routledge; 2008. p. 105.
61. Capobianco G, Donolo E, Borghero G, Dessole F, Cherchi PL, Dessole S. Effects of intravaginal estriol and pelvic floor rehabilitation on urogenital aging in postmenopausal women. Arch Gynecol Obstet. 2012;285(2):397–403.
62. Tomasi-Cont N, Lambertini M, Hulsbosch S, Peccatori AF, Amant F. Strategies for fertility preservation in young early breast cancer patients. Breast. 2014;23(5):503–10. 2014 June 13 Epub ahead of print.
63. Gilbert E, Ussher JM, Perz J. Sexuality after breast cancer: a review. Maturitas. 2010;66(4):397–407.

Female Sexual Dysfunction and Infertility

29

Elizabeth Grill and Glenn L. Schattman

Infertility is defined as the failure to achieve pregnancy after 12 months or more of appropriate, timed unprotected intercourse or donor insemination [1]. Women who are over age 35 are encouraged to initiate an evaluation after only 6 months of trying to become pregnant due to the lower probability of achieving pregnancy each month compared to younger women. This recommendation stems from the shorter window of remaining reproductive potential when compared with younger women. In couples in whom known or suspected infertility risk factors may be present, i.e., history of irregular periods, severe endometriosis, factors that predispose to tubal occlusion such as pelvic inflammatory disease, or a known or suspected male factor like undescended testicles or prior chemotherapy, an evaluation may be initiated after only 3 months of trying.

While initial attempts to conceive often start as "let's just see what happens when we stop using contraception" and possibly an increased frequency of sex, the frustration and anxiety of failed conceptions quickly escalate after each menstrual period, resulting to a methodical and planned scheduling of one's sex life around anticipation of ovulation and the "fertile window." The myth that a couple will have sex once and get pregnant or that pregnancy should happen the first month you try despite advancing age of the female partner is unfortunately a widely held belief. The most important factor in determining a woman's eventual chances for conception is her age. A German study evaluating time to pregnancy in couples stopping natural family planning methods documented a cumulative probability of pregnancy of 38 %, 68 %, 81 %, and 92 % at one, three, six, and 12 cycles, respectively, [2]. Most couples conceived within 6 months of trying. In women undergoing donor insemination due to a severe male factor such as azoospermia, pregnancy rates after up to 12 cycles of insemination with donor sperm were 74 % in women <31 years of age. The negative impact of age on fertility was clearly evident as women >35 years of age had a pregnancy rate of only 54 % after 12 months of appropriately timed donor insemination.

29.1 Evaluation

In couples who fail to conceive, a thorough evaluation of identifiable and potentially correctable causes of infertility should be initiated. This starts with a history and physical examination. Most couples are referred to an OB/GYN or reproductive endocrinologist, a physician trained to focus

E. Grill, Psy.D. (✉) • G.L. Schattman, M.D.
The Ronald O. Perelman and Claudia Cohen Center for Reproductive Medicine, Weill Cornell Medical College, New York, NY, USA
e-mail: eag2001@med.cornell.edu

L.I. Lipshultz et al. (eds.), *Management of Sexual Dysfunction in Men and Women*, DOI 10.1007/978-1-4939-3100-2_29

on abnormalities of the female reproductive tract, and the conversation usually starts with a complete menstrual and gynecologic history of the female partner. Questions regarding the woman's menstrual cycles and symptoms may provide information about ovulation, while questions pertaining to prior gynecologic problems including abnormal PAP smears, sexually transmitted infections, surgeries, and even prior pregnancies with other partners may reveal anatomic conditions reducing chances of pregnancy. Questions to both partners then focus on other risk factors including medications, exposures to reproductive toxicants like smoking or chemotherapy, as well as family history. Men are asked to provide a semen sample for analysis. If normal, other than the initial semen analysis and providing sperm when needed (which can even be cryopreserved for future use), the remainder of the evaluation and treatments falls on the female partners' shoulders to endure.

The examination of the woman includes, but is not limited, to an examination of her thyroid gland and breasts for secretions or masses, pelvic examination, cervical cultures, and transvaginal sonogram to assess ovarian "reserve," a measure of the relative quality and quantity of follicles remaining (albeit not a very accurate marker). If an identifiable etiology of infertility can be determined, directed measures to correct the abnormality may be undertaken depending on the chances of success. For example, if tubal pathology is identified in a 38-year-old nulligravid woman and surgical correction yields a 20 % probability of conception after 12 months with 25 % of all conceptions being tubal ectopic pregnancies, the decision to forgo surgery and proceed to IVF or remove the fallopian tubes to improve the odds of IVF being successful would be reasonable.

Testing for identifiable and correctable causes of female factor infertility is relatively straightforward and should not take more than a single cycle to complete. The testing falls into three main buckets: hormonal (ovulation and luteal function post-ovulation), anatomic factors (cervical abnormalities, endometrial defects, and tubal/peritoneal factors), and egg factors (advanced age with diminished egg quantity and anticipated high rate of oocyte aneuploidy). Testing for these factors includes documentation of ovulatory cycles, which can be obtained from the history and is supported by the patient having regular menstrual cycles with molimina. Infertility in up to 15 % of all infertile couples and up to 40 % of infertile women is due to ovulatory disturbances [3]. In the presence of regular cycles, a serum progesterone level, basal body temperatures, urine LH testing, and especially endometrial biopsy are unnecessary.

Anatomic abnormalities are detected with a hysterosalpingogram (HSG), during which radiopaque contrast is injected into the uterine cavity and fluoroscopy confirms the shape of the uterine cavity and identifies any anatomic defects as well as spillage of dye from the fallopian tubes into the peritoneal cavity, consistent with tubal patency. If performed properly, rarely will there be false-positive or false-negative interpretations which would require surgery to confirm. In the presence of a normal HSG, laparoscopy is not indicated. Cervical factors, including abnormalities of cervical mucus, have traditionally been evaluated with a "post-coital" test where a sample of the peri-ovulatory cervical mucus is looked at under a microscope within 12 h post-coitum. The presence of motile sperm in the setting of thin, watery "egg white"-like mucus is considered a normal result. However because the findings correlate poorly to the ability to conceive a pregnancy, this test is no longer recommended [4].

Ovarian "reserve," a measure of the quantity and quality of remaining eggs, is also difficult to determine. The most predictive variable in a couple's ability to achieve pregnancy is chronologic age of the female partner. Advanced age of the female partner, independent of oocyte quantity, is the best predictor of artificial reproductive technology (ART) outcome. Surrogate markers for ovarian function include cycle day 3 follicle-stimulating hormone (FSH) and estradiol levels as well as anti-Müllerian hormone (AMH) levels. High-frequency ultrasound can also provide an objective measure of quantity of antral follicles in the ovary and a close correlation with total number of retrievable oocytes. High levels of AMH indicate a larger number of potentially recruitable eggs similar to a higher antral follicle count (AFC). High levels of FSH, on the other hand, indicate diminished ovarian reserve and fewer potential oocytes. However, the threshold for FSH as a marker of ovarian reserve has not been determined, and there is high intra-cycle variability in FSH levels, limiting its utility in fertility evaluation in women. At this time, none of the ovarian reserve markers, unless a very high threshold is used, have a strong correlation with pregnancy outcome.

29.2 Treatment

When a specific abnormality can be identified, treatment can be directed at correcting the abnormality, i.e., tubal pathology can be surgically corrected or bypassed with in vitro fertilization. Having a diagnosis, however, even if not correctable, makes treatment easier to undergo. An etiology of infertility is not identified in up to 30 % of couples and even more if considering those couples in whom a diagnosis is made, but treatment remains ineffective [5]. In some, the diagnosis is merely reduced cycle fecundity due to advanced age of the female partner and pregnancy rates are expected to be low. A common but ineffective treatment for infertility is intrauterine insemination, where washed and concentrated sperm are placed high into the uterus, bypassing the need for the sperm to travel through the vagina and cervix. Pregnancy rates using IUI and those from timed intercourse are low: 4.8 % with IUI and 2.1 % with timed intercourse or intracervical insemination [6].

Because the chances for pregnancy with a single egg developing each month are low, most infertility treatments are aimed at stimulating multiple follicles to develop and mature in the hopes of increasing the chances that at least one will fertilize and implant; this process is termed ovulation induction. First-line therapy is often in the form of oral medications that antagonize the production of, or response to, estrogen. Clomiphene citrate (CC), a weak estrogen, stimulates FSH secretion and follicle development by blocking the estrogen receptor, while letrozole, an aromatase inhibitor, blocks the production of estrogen. Neither agent has proven superior over the other, but pregnancy rates remain quite low per cycle for both drugs. With CC alone, cycle fecundity rates were 5.6 %, and the combination of CC/IUI increased cycle fecundity rates slightly to 8.3 % [6]. Cycle fecundity rates with daily injections of FSH (gonadotropin) for 2 weeks to facilitate egg maturation were 8 % per cycle and 18 % per cycle when IUI was performed in addition to the use of ovulation-inducing medications [7]. It should be considered that the anticipated success of each subsequent treatment declines with each failed cycle, so the above success rates per cycle do not continue indefinitely.

While ovulation induction seems to be a reasonable approach to enhancing fertility, there are risks associated with this process, with the greatest risk involving the possibility of multiple gestations. In fact, this approach is responsible for many more twins and triplets than IVF [8]. Clomiphene citrate treatment results in a twin pregnancy rate of ~8 to 10 % and gonadotropin treatment increases this to ~33 % [7, 9]. IVF is an effective treatment for infertility due to all causes of infertility except for uncorrectable uterine factors and advanced female age. Success rates per cycle are 40.1 % at <35 years of age and decrease to 21.2 % between 38 and 40 years of age and 4.5 % in women over 42 years old [10]. Given unlimited resources and time, cumulative success rates would be rather good with the majority of younger couples achieving their goal of having one or more children. Unfortunately this is often not the reality. Each cycle of ovulation induction involves multiple, almost daily blood tests, transvaginal ultrasound examinations, and hormone injections. If that does not reduce the desire for intimacy with your partner, knowing that until the developing eggs are ready there is no reproductive purpose to having sex usually significantly decreases sexual desire. For this reason, FSD is common in women experiencing infertility.

Studies have linked the physical, psychological, and financial challenges of assisted reproduction to increased marital conflict, decreased sexual self-esteem, feelings of inadequacy, and decreased frequency of sexual intercourse [11, 12]. Women struggling with infertility experience greater levels of psychosocial distress than men with respect to grief, guilt, denial, anxiety, cognitive disturbance, depression, and hostility [13]. More often women initiate medical treatment for infertility and are more invested in having a child. Typically, women are more aware of the limits of their reproductive potential and are more willing to consider extreme or alternative measures to achieve parenthood than their partners. For women, reproduction and sexuality may be more intrinsically intertwined than they are for men, so that disturbances in one area reverberate in other areas [14].

Sexual dysfunction is high in all infertile women, and women with secondary infertility suffer more from impaired sexual function than those with primary infertility [15]. Various studies have detected increased sexual dysfunction in 40–62 % of infertile women and reported loss of desire and arousal as the leading cause of dysfunction [14, 16–19]. Overall, infertility is associated with decreased sexual activity and appears to become worse as the number of childless years increases [20].

It has been speculated that three factors operate together in driving women's distress level higher than their spouses' [21]. First, the social responsibility of conceiving and pregnancy is still attributed mainly to the female partner [22]. Women often feel failure with regard to sexual and reproductive functions (further reinforced by medical terminology such as premature ovarian "failure" or "incompetent" cervix). Women view the role of mother as an integral part of their femininity, gender identity, and sexuality. Consequently, anything that threatens this role has the potential for negative social pressure and internal conflict.

Second, fertility treatment is more intrusive, time consuming, and often painful for women than it is for men [21, 22]. Infertility-related stress for women can be associated with not only the diagnosis but also treatment procedures, many of which are physically, psychologically, or pharmacologically invasive. Sexual intercourse can lose its spontaneity and erotic value as the goal becomes pregnancy, and sex becomes restricted to fertile times of the month [23]. This distortion of a sexual relationship can be long lasting and even cause disruptions to a couple's sexual life long after treatment [24].

Finally, coping strategies differ between men and women: men tend to deny and remain active, while women cannot imagine life without children and develop depressive reactions [21, 22]. Researchers found that positive reinterpretation and active coping strategies had a positive impact on sexual functioning, while planning and self-restraint coping had an adverse effect on sexual functioning [25].

The link between infertility and sexuality is complex. Sexual dysfunction may have an etiological role in infertility, or it may be a consequence of the disorder secondary to psychological stress in either or both partners. Regardless of the cause of infertility, research has consistently shown that in response to infertility and its treatment, women experience greater emotional distress than men and often assume more personal responsibility while enduring a disproportionate share of medical treatment [14]. In short, infertility clearly impacts the sexual functioning and sexual health of women in numerous ways.

29.3 Infertility Leading to Sexual Dysfunction

Women undergoing fertility treatment characterize infertility as the most stressful experience of their lives [26–28] likely contributing to higher reported rates of depression and sexual dysfunction [29, 30]. Sexual impairment in infertile couples is often due to the performance pressure experienced in response to planned sex, pressure to perform on demand, extensive and painful tests, intense feelings of anxiety, and the highly personal matter of sexuality being turned over to the external control of a physician and the psychological feeling of the medical team in the bedroom [31, 32]. As infertility drags on, feelings of sexual inadequacy and depression can occur due to the close association between sexuality and fertility [33].

Couples in infertility treatment report avoiding sexual intimacy during non-fertile times. Men and women lose pleasure from non-procreative sexual activity and develop an apathetic attitude about sex [34]. Similarly, women with tendencies to hypoactive sexual desire may find themselves avoiding sex except when they are ovulating or avoiding foreplay in order to facilitate a more rapid ejaculation from their partner. Regrettably and all too frequently, relationship building and recreational aspects of sexual activity are abandoned especially when large sums of money and sometimes invasive procedures are employed to induce ovulation. Sex on demand and providing an erection and ejaculation that is timely and efficient become the goals of sex [14, 35]. These tensions frequently lead to a reduction in nonsexual affection, resulting in feelings of disconnection and exacerbating relationship tension [36].

29.4 The Evaluation and Treatment of FSD and Infertility

It is clear that the stress, psychological demands, and physically intrusive procedures associated with infertility treatment can affect sexual self-image, desire, and performance. Whether sexual dysfunction is a preexisting condition or an unwelcome side effect of infertility treatment, it can be a devastating and discouraging blow, compounding the disappointment of childlessness and the distress of medical treatment.

Most infertile couples are reluctant to discuss the private sexual aspects of their relationship, but even more so when they fear it will interrupt medical treatment [37]. Consequently, the sexual problems of infertile couples are ignored or minimized in a belief that they will dissipate on their own or will have few long-term consequences. Unfortunately, although some sexual problems may disappear when the pressures of infertility treatment end, sexual difficulties may linger or become more problematic after treatment ends or parenthood is achieved [21, 22].

Even couples who never encounter major or disrupting sexual problems often experience episodic or situational diminished sexual desire and satisfaction in response to the emotional distress or physical strains of infertility or a specific treatment. Episodic loss of desire in one or both partners can usually be addressed with minimal education and reassurance. However, consistent and extensive diminished sexual desire in infertile men and women is more problematic and usually multifactorial.

Numerous partner-related psychosexual issues may adversely affect outcome. Contextual factors, including difficulties with the current interpersonal relationship, should be clarified, and previous sexual scripts should be assessed [14]. Preexisting psychiatric conditions as well as psychological issues that develop as a result of an infertility diagnosis and/or treatment should also be evaluated and addressed.

Ideally, if the sexual problems reflect more fundamental relationship problems, it may be more important that those issues take precedence over further infertility treatment. However, questions about whether treatment should be denied or postponed often pose very real dilemmas for medical caregivers and for infertile couples, especially if couple's fixation on parenthood clouds their judgment about the health and well-being of their marriage, family, their potential children, and themselves [14].

Sex therapists can assist fertility specialists and can intervene on several different therapeutic levels by providing patient education and helping patients with treatment decisions. Although some patients may proceed with infertility treatment in the presence of some sexual dysfunctions, medical treatment should be in conjunction with psychotherapy and/or sex therapy, emphasizing the importance of sexual health and well-being in infertile couples.

References

1. ASRM. Definitions of infertility and recurrent pregnancy loss: a committee opinion. Fertil Steril. 2013;99:63.

2. Gnoth C, Godehardt D, Godehardt E, Frank-Herrmann P, Freundl G. Time to pregnancy: results of the German prospective study and impact on the management of infertility. Hum Reprod. 2003;18:1959–66.
3. Mosher WD, Pratt WF. Fecundity and infertility in the United States: incidence and trends. Fertil Steril. 1991;56:192–3.
4. Oei SG, Helmerhorst FM, Bloemenkamp KWM, et al. Effectiveness of the postcoital test: randomised controlled trial. BMJ. 1998;317:502–5.
5. Dodson WC, Whitesides DB, Hughes Jr CL, Easley 3rd HA, Haney AF. Superovulation with intrauterine insemination in the treatment of infertility: a possible alternative to gamete intrafallopian transfer and in vitro fertilization. Fertil Steril. 1987;48:441–5.
6. ASRM. Effectiveness and treatment for unexplained infertility. Fertil Steril. 2006;86:S111–14.
7. Guzick D, Sullivan M, Adamson GD, et al. Efficacy of treatment for unexplained infertility. Fertil Steril. 1998;70:207–13.
8. ASRM. Multiple gestation associated with infertility therapy: an American Society for Reproductive Medicine Practice Committee opinion. Fertil Steril. 2012;97:825–34.
9. Tarlatzis BC, Grimbizis G. Future use of clomiphene in ovarian stimulation. Will clomiphene persist in the 21st century? Hum Reprod. 1998;13:2356–8.
10. SART. Clinic summary report: all member clinics. Retrieved Accessed 9 April 2015, from https://www.sartcorsonline.com/rptCSR_PublicMultYear.aspx?ClinicPKID=0
11. Andrews F, Abbey A, Halman L. Is fertility-problem stress different? Fertil Steril. 1992;57:1247–53.
12. Whiteford LM, Gonzalez L. Stigma: the hidden burden of infertility. Soc Sci Med. 1995;40:27–36.
13. Dunkel-Schetter C, Lobel M. Psychological reactions to infertility. New York: Plenum; 1991.
14. Burns LH. Sexual counseling and infertility. New York: Parthenon Publishing; 2006.
15. Keskin U, Coksuer H, Gungor S, et al. Differences in prevalence of sexual dysfunction between primary and secondary infertile women. Fertil Steril. 2011;96:1213–17.
16. Hurwitz MB. Sexual dysfunction associated with infertility. A comparison of sexual function during the fertile and the non-fertile phase of the menstrual cycle. S Afr Med J. 1989;76:58–61.
17. Oskay UY, Beji NK, Serdaroglu H. The issue of infertility and sexual function in Turkish women. Sex Disabil. 2010;28:71–9.
18. Millheiser LS, Helmer AE, Quintero RB, et al. Is infertility a risk factor for female sexual dysfunction? A case-control study. Fertil Steril. 2010;94:2022–5.
19. Boivin J, Takefman JE, Brender W, Tulandi T. The effects of female sexual response in coitus on early reproductive processes. J Behav Med. 1992;15:509–18.
20. Nene UA, Coyaji K, Apte H. Infertility: a label of choice in the case of sexually dysfunctional couples. Patient Educ Couns. 2005;59:234–8.
21. Wright J, Duchesne C, Sabourin S, et al. Psychosocial distress and infertility: men and women respond differently. Fertil Steril. 1991;55:100–8.
22. Benazon N, Wright J, Sabourin S. Stress, sexual satisfaction, and marital adjustment in infertile couples. J Sex Marital Ther. 1992;18:273–84.
23. Cousineau TM, Domar AD. Psychological impact of infertility. Best Pract Res Clin Obstet Gynaecol. 2007;21:293–308.
24. Wirtberg I, Moller A, Hogstrom L, Tronstad SE, Lalos A. Life 20 years after unsuccessful infertility treatment. Hum Reprod. 2007;22:598–604.
25. Bar-Hava M, Azam F, Yovel I, et al. The interrelationship between coping strategies and sexual functioning in in vitro fertilization patients. J Sex Marital Ther. 2001;27:389–94.
26. Kaplan HS. The evaluation of sexual disorders: psychological and medical aspects. New York: Brunner/Mazel; 1995.
27. Meana M, Binik YM, Khalife S, et al. Dyspareunia: more than bad sex. Pain. 1997;71:211–12.
28. Freeman EW, Boxer AS, Rickels K, Tureck R, Mastroianni Jr L. Psychological evaluation and support in a program of in vitro fertilization and embryo transfer. Fertil Steril. 1985;43:48–53.
29. Nelson CJ, Shindel AW, Naughton CK, Ohebshalom M, Mulhall JP. Prevalence and predictors of sexual problems, relationship stress, and depression in female partners of infertile couples. J Sex Med. 2008;5:1907–14.
30. Lukse MP, Vacc NA. Grief, depression, and coping in women undergoing infertility treatment. Obstet Gynecol. 1999;93:245–51.
31. Applegarth LD, Grill EA. Psychological issues in reproductive disorders. Philadelphia: Hanley and Belfus; 2004.
32. Daniluk J. Women's sexuality across the life span: challenging myths, creating meanings. New York: Guilford; 1998.
33. Kedem P, Mikulincer M, Nathanson YE, Bartoov B. Psychological aspects of male infertility. Br J Med Psychol. 1990;63(Pt 1):73–80.
34. Leiblum SR, editor. Love, sex and infertility: the impact of infertility on the couple. New York: Wiley; 1997.
35. Keye WR. The impact of infertility on psychosexual function. Fertil Steril. 1980;34:308–9.
36. Perelman MA. The impact of relationship variables on the etiology, diagnosis and treatment of erectile dysfunction. Adv Primary Care Med Clin Updat. 2007;3:3–6.
37. Bachmann GA, Leiblum SR, Grill J. Brief sexual inquiry in gynecologic practice. Obstet Gynecol. 1989;73:425–7.

Female Sexual Dysfunction: Impact of the Life Cycle (Pregnancy, Children, and Aging)

30

William D. Petok

While the hope of most women is that sexual function will remain consistent throughout their life span, certain normal events can play a role in sexual function and dysfunction, most notably, pregnancy, children, and aging. Traversing these events without significant problem will be the course for most women. However, some will develop sexual problems that require intervention. Health-care providers who are prepared for these events in their patients' lives will be able to assist them with these important transition experiences and help them to reduce the psychological impact these disorders can cause.

30.1 Pregnancy

Casey, a 25-year-old married to Robert for 2 years, was 2½ months pregnant with her first child when she sought therapy. She was anxious about the pregnancy, concerned that her desire was waning and equally worried that her husband was rapidly losing interest in her. He had declined to have intercourse with her several times over the past 2 weeks, saying he was tired. She certainly was tired but couldn't understand why he would use fatigue as a reason to avoid something they had enjoyed so much for the past several years. A meeting with both of them revealed that he was worried about harming the baby growing inside her uterus. This, he said, was why he had avoided intercourse. He was embarrassed to tell her the truth and created the story.

For most women pregnancy is an expected consequence of their sexual lives. A number will experience the lack of pregnancy as a significant impediment to satisfying sex. The impact of infertility on sexual experience is discussed in Chap. 28.

One of the more common sexual problems during pregnancy is not a diagnostic entity at all. It involves a male's reaction to the fact that his partner is carrying a child. A frequent comment notes his concern that intercourse will in some way harm the developing fetus. Treatment can be as simple as explaining that the fetus is well protected and he has nothing to worry about or more complicated and require significant education and assessment of potential anxiety issues that could underlie his concern.

It is significant to note that review articles conclude that female sexual function declines steadily during the course of pregnancy with the greatest decrements taking place during the third trimester [1]. These same authors highlight the complex interplay of psychological, cultural, ethical, and sexological factors along with organic and neurologic components that contribute to this end result.

W.D. Petok, Ph.D. (✉)
Independent Practice, 479 Jumpers Hole Road, Suite 304 B, Severna Park, MD 21146, USA
e-mail: bpetok@comcast.net

L.I. Lipshultz et al. (eds.), *Management of Sexual Dysfunction in Men and Women*, DOI 10.1007/978-1-4939-3100-2_30

Changes in desire are common during pregnancy. Depending on the incidence of morning sickness and fatigue, some women will find that desire declines during the first trimester and rebounds into the second and third [2]. One would hardly consider this decrement in desire a dysfunction, but it should be acknowledged as a normal occurrence. Similar symptoms at other times of the day will certainly create an impediment to desire that is understandable. Many health-care providers hear reports from pregnant women that they are unusually tired during the first trimester. Given that sex when tired is less desirable, some women will experience reduced sexual activity for this reason. Hormonal changes that can lead to decreased desire are also implicated in breast tenderness and anxiety that can further reduce desire and arousal [1]. Usually, reassurance that this will diminish with time is sufficient for the woman who is concerned about the situation.

As her abdomen increases in size and other physical effects of pregnancy are felt, desire may not be the issue. Rather, comfort during intercourse is the focal point. Women report difficulty with intercourse in the missionary position for a variety of reasons. Having a partner on top pushes the baby into her other organs and creates discomfort. A natural outgrowth of this situation can be a decline in desire. Experimentation with alternate positions for coitus as well as other forms of sexual stimulation can relieve the discomfort and maintain desire and sexual satisfaction. However, there is evidence that libido, clitoral sensitivity, and orgasm are all reduced during pregnancy [3, 4].

Women report fears that intercourse during pregnancy will cause abnormal bleeding, fetal damage, vaginal or urinary infections, and vaginal pain [3]. Research indicates that these events occur with relatively low frequency. More importantly, it appears that women are not very likely to discuss these concerns with their physician, suggesting that good practice anticipates questions about sexual function and associated problems early in pregnancy care to allay fears and prevent reduced sexual satisfaction during this time. Simply raising the issue by saying "Many people are concerned about sexual activity during pregnancy. Do you have concerns about this," can open the door for a fruitful and prophylactic conversation. This approach is consistent with the observation that patients want to talk about sexual function and prefer their health-care providers to raise the issue because they may be embarrassed to do so themselves.

Most women are advised to refrain from intercourse for 6 weeks postpartum to allow for vaginal healing. This recess from sexual activity also takes into account the very real fatigue that women (and most likely their spouses) experience caring for a newborn. Problems with sexual function have been noted at 3 months postpartum that include coital pain, lack of vaginal lubrication, difficulty with orgasm, changes in vaginal "fit," bleeding or irritation after sex, and loss of sexual desire [5]. Significant improvements in many of these symptoms were noted at 6 months postpartum. Several other studies have confirmed these findings. Elevated prolactin levels, which occur during lactation, suppress gonadotropin secretion and result in persistently reduced estrogen levels, thereby mimicking menopausal symptoms. Once again, preemptive counseling is recommended to help couples traverse what can be a sexually difficult period [1].

Clinical experience indicates that couples are often misinformed about how pregnancy will impact their sexual experience and are reluctant to bring the topic up with care providers. They may become anxious or depressed if they encounter problems. Having established that sexual function is part of overall health care can provide entry to this area [6], affording an opportunity to prevent the psychological impact if problems do arise.

30.2 Parenthood

Anna, 34, and Juan, 35, have 3 children who are 7, 4, and 2 years old. Anna works part time as a nurse, and Juan is a mechanical engineer. She entered therapy at the advice of her gynecologist after she reported a total loss of desire for sex. She was upset and worried that Juan would lose interest in her and even more so that she no longer wanted to engage in sex.

Raising children has its challenges and rewards. The opportunity to nurture new lives into productive people is something many women look forward to. While they may understand that the time invested in rearing children must come from somewhere, they may not appreciate how it can impact sexual activity and function. Popular culture complicates matters. Shoppers are inundated with sexual images and pronouncements from every grocery store checkout counter magazine section. Their overwhelming message is that phenomenal sexual experiences are what every woman wants and has. Reality is typically different. Such was the case with Anna and Juan.

Women's intimate relationships necessarily change with parenthood. Some do report enhanced sexual intimacy, but a more frequent experience is dissatisfaction due to less time, energy, and opportunity for sexual activity with their partners. The physical and social demands of parenting are significant and include increased financial pressures as well as the tasks that raising children requires. Some find themselves "sandwiched" between children and aging parents that require attention of their own. For newer parents, the introduction of other members to a family can interrupt the rhythm that the couple has established prior to the arrival of children. A consequence is that couples must readjust their expectations of what is reasonable sexually. If one partner takes on a disproportionate responsibility for child-rearing, the other can feel abandoned or sexually undesirable. This can lead to discord about what is the optimal level of sexual closeness.

In some cases, a resolution is as simple as helping the couple define what the problem is and how they can set aside time for intimacy that is comfortable for both. In other cases, it will be more complex. Sexual dysfunctions can develop during child-rearing years that are more significant. The biological bases of these problems and their treatment are discussed in the preceding chapters in this section.

Declines in desire that are the result of unsatisfying sexual relations do take place. Changes in sexual patterns that worked well for the couple in the early stages of their relationship can suffer when fatigue prevents either the length of time available or the energy for similar kinds of activity that were satisfying before. For example, a woman may take more time to relax enough to achieve an orgasm and her partner may tire before she climaxes, or she may have grown accustomed to time snuggling after sex and her partner now falls asleep quickly afterwards, leaving her less satisfied by the encounter. As a result, desire for sexual activity wanes.

Pain problems can also occur. Women who have had episiotomies and do not heal properly can find intercourse painful. Similarly, changes in lubrication can also cause discomfort. Some women will develop pain related to vulvodynia or other related problems. While not associated with parenting, if these conditions develop during child-rearing years, they will influence the trajectory of the couple's sexual interactions.

Partners can also have pressures, financially and otherwise, that render them less desirous of sexual activity. In some cases, longer work hours to compensate for lost income because a spouse is now home with children rather than earning produce less interest. Similarly, anxiety about insuring a family's financial stability can result in decreased sexual desire.

Remarkably, little research exists on the impact of parenthood on sexual function and satisfaction. Twenge et al. [7] reviewed the research on the impact of parenthood on marital satisfaction and noted that having children actually causes small declines in marital satisfaction. They postulated that some of the dissatisfaction is caused by men's greater desire for sex producing frustration due to the demands that childbearing and child-rearing place on sexual availability of partners. As children grew older, the dissatisfaction of women with their marriages declined. In other words, women with older children had greater marital satisfaction.

Ahlborg et al. [8] reported that average sexual frequency declined from prior to pregnancy and childbirth and remained low between 6 months postpartum and the first child's fourth birthday. Tiredness as a hindrance to having sex was the primary factor for this decline. Another study of 2081 women 33–43 years old found that multiparous women had fewer orgasm problems compared to nulliparous women. The authors also determined that nulliparous women had more pain problems and had less sexual satisfaction than women with children, irrespective of the number of children, providing a positive perspective on the impact of children on partner sexual relations [9].

Finally, and quite interestingly, a study evaluated the impact of stress on sexual relationships in couples [10]. The majority of partners were 31 or more years old. While the number of children was not specifically studied, it is reasonable to assume that many of the couples had children. Sexual desire problems were the most frequently reported issue for both men and women. The second most common problem for women was orgasmic difficulties. Premature ejaculation was second most reported problem for men. The authors concluded that stress arising from issues between the partners played a significant role in understanding sexual dysfunctions in the women in the study. Stress from life events outside of the partner relationship played a lesser and statistically insignificant role. Several recommendations are offered including the application of stress management and improved partner problem resolution and communication skills.

Anna and Juan benefited from adjusting to the idea that sex would be more likely to take place when they could create time in their schedule for it. Many couples object to the loss of spontaneity that they believe "should" accompany sexual activity. However, once they see that busy lives with complicated schedules leave little "spontaneous" opportunity, they can see the value of a somewhat more plan-full approach. This isn't to suggest that sex becomes scheduled like a carpool. It does mean that some thought put into "when and how" will make for a more satisfying outcome. Some even find that anticipation of these events leads to greater arousal and closeness.

30.3 Aging

Sharon, 75, and her husband, Robert, 79, hadn't made love in 8 years. She'd developed arthritic hips and had gained weight over the years, making intercourse difficult. Add to that the discomfort that thrusting caused, and it seemed obvious why they had been sexually inactive. But that wasn't the full story. Robert had melanomas on both legs, and the treatment was painful. In addition, his erectile dysfunction hadn't responded to medication interventions. However, the most significant issue was that they never talked about their lack of sex.

Joan and Gary were married 40 years as she was turning 70. Both were retired and engaged in activities together and separately. Fortunately, their health was good and they were mobile. She noticed that while they continued to share an intimate relationship that included sex, it was different than it had been in their 30s. It took both of them longer to become aroused, and they enjoyed a different kind of sensuality that included less frequent intercourse. Instead, they had more manual and oral stimulation which they found satisfying. She continued to be orgasmic and still found their sexual experience very pleasurable.

Both of the vignettes above describe possible outcomes for women as they age. The first describes a woman who has dealt with significant issues of her own. Her sexual experience has been compounded by the physical constraints of her partner. Most importantly, the manner in which she and her husband relate with one another has a substantial impact on her satisfaction. In the second vignette, normal and predictable changes in sexual response seem to have minimal impact on the outcome of the woman's sexual experience. She and her partner have accommodated to these changes and probably improved what was a good sexual relationship prior to menopause. Could it be that the best predictor of the present is the past?

Women who have regular reproductive health care can be prepared for the inevitable changes that menopause and later life can bring to sexual function. They can be aware that many processes which contribute to a positive sexual experience will slow down or diminish. Thinning of the vaginal epithelium, reduced pelvic blood flow and vaginal lubrication can lead to discomfort with intercourse. Muscles that aren't as strong, joints that aren't as flexible, and changes in the nervous system can make some activities less satisfying.

All of these normal occurrences can require adaptations to sexual activities in order to ensure a pleasurable outcome. And of course, a partner who is capable and willing to adapt is essential.

The Rancho Bernardo Study highlights the understanding that older women can have satisfying sexual lives [11]. A cohort of women with a median age of 67 and a mean number of years postmenopause of 24.6 years was studied. The researchers note that, as one would expect, sexual activity, frequency, and desire declined with age. At the same time, despite partner status or sexual activity, 61 % of the cohort reported being moderately or very satisfied with their overall sexual life.

The same study also reported that a very small fraction of the women reported sexual desire "almost always" or "always," and they were in the younger portion of the sample. Interestingly, current hormone use, sexual activity, and frequency of arousal, lubrication and orgasm were positively associated with sexual desire. This suggests that older women who "use it" don't lose it! In the group of sexually active women over 80 years old, 23 % reported arousal almost always or always, and 28 % of women who were aroused reported lubrication at the same level as arousal. There was no significant relationship between hormone use and lubrication, and 37.5 % of the oldest age group reached orgasm always or almost always. Pain or discomfort with intercourse was reported as low, very low, or nonexistent by 71 % of the oldest cohort. The authors note that there are limitations to their research including the homogeneity of the population studied and response bias that could exist from only those with the best emotional and physical health participating. Nevertheless, the research indicates that sexual function in older age can be satisfying and active [11].

However, there are some women who will not have such a good outcome and will have an experience more like Sharon in the first vignette. For those women who wish to have more satisfying encounters, modifications to their sexual activity will be necessary and can require psychological as well as sexological counseling that involves both them and their partners. Intercourse may not be possible for a variety of reasons. Pain, both from intromission or other physical constraints, may make intercourse very uncomfortable. They may benefit from interventions that increase physical touch along the lines of sensate focus exercises [12]. While a variety of medical interventions such as lubricants, vaginal moisturizers, and hormonal therapies can be useful, communication skills to improve how a woman discusses sexual interaction with her partner can also help. Creating expectations for sexual experience that are in line with their physical realities is also essential. Women may have been led to believe that aging and sexual activity are diametrically opposed. On the other hand, they may have come to believe that sexual activity and satisfaction are invariant throughout the life span. The former group will benefit from an improved awareness of the possibilities and the latter from a recalibration in a different direction. At a minimum, counseling that offers hope and provides direction on how to achieve greater satisfaction is useful.

For example, Sharon and Robert benefited from directed discussion about what each of them found comfortable with regard to physical activity during sex. She was thrilled to have him touch her gently and not necessarily on her genitals. He was pleased that his erection wasn't the most important thing to her. Sensate focus helped them with this. Separate work with Robert to help him deal with the loss of sexual function was necessary. A therapist competent in dealing with aging issues and the losses inherent in them is essential in these cases.

30.4 Summary

Various normally occurring events in the life cycle can and do have an impact on sexual function and satisfaction. Health-care providers who are aware of these events and can predict some of the possibilities for their patients will serve to limit the potential negative impact of these events. Normalizing changes in sexual function throughout the life span is an essential first step. Providing good resources and referrals is a close second.

References

1. Serati M, Salvatore S, et al. Female sexual function during pregnancy and after childbirth. J Sex Med. 2010;7:2782–90.
2. Gokyildiz S, Beji NK. The effects of pregnancy on sexual life. J Sex Marital Ther. 2005;31: 201–15.
3. Fok WY, Chan LY, Yuem PM. Sexual behavior and activity in Chinese pregnant women. Acta Obstet Gynecol Scand. 2005;84:934–8.
4. Erol B, Sanli O, Korkmaz D, Seyhan A, Akman T, Kadioglu A. A cross-sectional study of female sexual function and dysfunction during pregnancy. J Sex Med. 2007;4:1381–7.
5. Barrett G, Pendry E, Peacick J, Victor C, Thakar R, Manyonda I. Women's sexual health after childbirth. BJOG. 2000;107:186–95.
6. Maurice WL. Sexual medicine in primary care. St. Louis: Mosby; 1999.
7. Twenge JM, Campbell WK, Foster CA. Parenthood and marital satisfaction: a meta-analytic review. J Marriage Fam. 2003;65:574–83.
8. Ahlborg T, Rudeblad K, Linner S, Linton S. Sensual and sexual marital contentment in parents of small children – a follow-up study when the first child is four years old. J Sex Res. 2008;45:295–304.
9. Witting K, Santtila P, Alanko K, Harlaar N, Jern P, Johansson A, Von Der Pahlen B, Varjonen M, Sandnabba NK. Female sexual function and its association with number of children, pregnancy and relationship satisfaction. J Sex Marital Ther. 2008;34:89–106.
10. Bodenmann G, Ledermann T, Blattner D, Galluzzo C. Associations among everyday stress, critical life events and sexual problems. J Nerv Ment Dis. 2006; 194:494–501.
11. Trompeter SE, Bettencourt R, Barrett-Connor E. Sexual activity and satisfaction in healthy community-dwelling older women. Am J Med. 2012;125:37–43.
12. Masters WH, Johnson VE. Human sexual inadequacy. New York: Little-Brown; 1970.

Part III

Sexual Dysfunction and the Couple

It Takes Two to Tango: Evaluation and Treatment of Sexual Dysfunction in the Couple

31

Stanley E. Althof and Rachel Needle

31.1 Introduction

Sexual dysfunctions do not occur in a vacuum; they impact the symptom bearer and his/her partner—sexually, emotionally, and interpersonally. This chapter will focus on the evaluation and treatment of sexual dysfunction(s) in the couple with an emphasis on the construct of the sexual equilibrium.

31.2 Sexual Equilibrium

The construct of couples having a sexual equilibrium is the foundation for understanding the impact that one partner's sexual dysfunction has upon the other and the resistances that may be encountered in treating such couples. We have always thought of the sexual equilibrium akin to Newton's second law of motion implying that any change in one partner will produce a change in the other [1]. It is not difficult to appreciate that a man's erectile dysfunction (ED) could impact the female partner's sexual arousal/interest/desire (FSAID) or that her genital pain disorder might affect the man's ejaculatory function. Conversely, when treating couples, as one partner's sexual dysfunction appears to be improving, it is always surprising when the other partner develops a new and seemingly unexplained sexual problem. The concept of sexual equilibrium needs to be broadened to include alterations in the interpersonal and emotional realms as well as the sexual. For instance, rather than developing a new and seemingly unexplained sexual problem, the partner may become depressed.

The construct of the sexual equilibrium needs to remain front and center when evaluating and treating couples for a sexual problem. The partner's role as a precipitating or maintaining factor has often been overshadowed by focusing on the initial symptom bearer's medical, psychological, or interpersonal issues. There is a dynamic and reciprocal relationship between each partner's sexual function, sexual satisfaction, and physical and mental health [2, 3].

31.3 Vignette

The sexual life of a young professional couple that had been married for 1 year was marred by Joe's psychogenic ED. His difficulties began

S.E. Althof, Ph.D. (✉)
Case Western Reserve University School of Medicine, Cleveland, OH, USA

Center for Marital and Sexual Health of South Florida, West Palm Beach, FL, USA
e-mail: Stanley.althof@case.edu

R. Needle, Psy.D.
Center for Marital and Sexual Health of South Florida, West Palm Beach, FL, USA

Advanced Mental Health Training Institute, West Palm Beach, FL, USA

Nova Southeastern University, West Palm Beach, FL, USA

L.I. Lipshultz et al. (eds.), *Management of Sexual Dysfunction in Men and Women*, DOI 10.1007/978-1-4939-3100-2_31

shortly after they were married. His wife Laura felt entitled to a satisfying sexual life and was distressed by Joe's lack of concern about his continued problem and avoidance of any form of sexual play. They had not touched one another for 6 months prior to their seeking consultation.

Both Joe and Laura had attended parochial schools; however, he was currently more invested in Catholicism than she. Prior to marriage, they had dated for 2 years and had engaged in premarital intercourse. While dating, Laura became pregnant and chose to terminate the pregnancy.

During the evaluation, Joe said, "It was like dragging her down the sewer. I forced her to have sex with me, and look what happened!" Laura responded that he didn't force her, that she very much wanted to be sexual and had enjoyed it. She regretted the abortion but thought it was the right decision given the circumstances.

I (SA) suggested that treatment should focus on their premarital sexual life and resolving the feelings about the pregnancy termination. They agreed, and Joe's potency returned the following week. Joe seemed pleased, but Laura had suddenly lost her sexual desire. As Joe was talking about "robbing Laura of her virginity," she seemed increasingly uncomfortable. When I asked what was troubling her, she "confessed" that Joe had not been the first. We then shifted the focus as to why she had allowed Joe to believe she was a virgin. She explained that she felt very guilty about her past behavior and feared Joe would not love her if she told him about the others. Although Joe felt angry and betrayed by Laura's "secret," he also felt relieved that he was not the only one who had done something they both perceived as wrong sexually prior to their marriage. The couple began to appreciate their need for some sexual symptom to alleviate their collective guilt. Over the next two sessions, Laura's desire returned and Joe's potency remained intact. At a 2-month follow-up, the sexual gains were maintained.

31.4 Commentary

This vignette dramatically illustrates how sexual symptoms can impact the other partner (Laura's disappointment with not having a satisfying sexual life) and that symptoms can shift between partners during treatment (Joe regaining his potency and Laura losing sexual interest). This was a resilient and loving couple who were able to integrate revelations about the other. They understood that their symptoms had meaning relating to their shared history, and they sought to forgive one another and move forward positively. While this case is atypical in terms of how quickly the symptoms shifted and resolved, it is offered to the reader to illustrate the importance of the sexual equilibrium construct.

31.5 The Biopsychosocial Model and Assessment

We strongly recommend that clinicians employ a biopsychosocial perspective when evaluating and treating couples who present with sexual dysfunction [4, 5]. The biopsychosocial model is an integrative and dynamic model that is always changing and helps to elucidate the multiple influences on the patient's sexual dysfunction. It assesses the potential medical problems associated with the dysfunction—vascular, hormonal, neurologic, disease, and surgery related and potential problems with medication(s). It also takes into account lifestyle issues that may impact sexual function, such as obesity, smoking, drugs, alcohol, and exercise.

It is vital that the patient, partner, and clinician are mutually involved in the assessment process. Taking a collaborative approach, the clinician collects the sexual, medical, relational, contextual, and psychological information that he/she synthesizes into a cohesive treatment plan. When questions are asked in a logical and empathic manner, the patient and partner often gain a fresh perspective on the multiple issues related to his/her sexual problem. Not every partner will be present at the initial consultation; nonetheless, the partner should be invited to participate when able, as his/her perspective often proves helpful in understanding the context of the current situation (e.g., did he tell you he's a drinker). The partner often has important insights regarding the relationship dynamics and is an important ally in the success of any treatment intervention [6].

The clinician should begin with a complete description of the presenting sexual problem, as well as other areas of sexual function, since there is often an overlap between dysfunctions. Other chapters in this volume will focus on the specifics of taking an individual's sexual history; we are more focused on the partner and his/her response to the problem. If the partner is not present at the initial consultation, we suggest you begin by asking the patient if the partner knows that they have sought treatment. Ask whether the partner misses sexual intimacy and how he/she has responded to the sexual dysfunction. Is the partner angry, hurt, sad, or frustrated that the patient has delayed seeking treatment or pleased that because of the dysfunction sexual life is behind them? Is he/she likely to be a willing and supportive partner in the patient's treatment or are there interpersonal obstacles that need to be overcome? Does he/she have any sexual problems and what have they done, if anything, to overcome their own difficulties?

Psychological factors are also assessed in the partner. Suggested questions include the following: Has the sexual dysfunction caused a loss of confidence? Has the patient or partner suffered from depression? Is the patient or partner now avoidant of sexual behavior or is there a relevant historical event that significantly influences the development and maintenance of the dysfunction? For instance, is there a history of sexual/physical/psychological abuse, an invasive traumatic surgery, or parental divorce or abandonment?

What is the quality of the interpersonal relationship? Is the couple's attachment secure, anxious, or chaotic? What impact does the development of the dysfunction have on the partner? Does his/her response to the symptom bearer make matters better or worse? Also, how do previous relationship experiences such as abandonment, power and control struggles, infidelity, alcohol/drug abuse, etc. impact upon the present relationship?

Lastly, what are the cultural/social issues that are relevant to the dysfunction? How does the couple's ethnic/religious background intersect with the couple's sexual problems? Is there sufficient privacy? Do they work different shifts? Are there current economic or vocational concerns?

The answers to these questions help us to understand the forces that came together to give birth to and maintain a sexual symptom. Such a comprehensive biopsychosocial assessment allows for thoughtful stepwise treatment planning whether it is for individual, for couples, pharmacotherapy, or combined medical and psychological treatment.

31.6 Empirical Support for the Notion of the Sexual Equilibrium

In the late 1980s, the Case Western Reserve group began a research study of men who presented with erectile dysfunction and received either intracavernosal injection (ICI) or vacuum tumescence therapy (VTT). Those were the days that preceded the introduction of Viagra™, Cialis™, or Levitra™, and ICI and VTT were the most innovative treatments available at the time. All couples (except when medically contraindicated) were given the choice of which treatment they wished to receive. Couples were seen at baseline, 1 month after treatment was initiated, and then at 3, 6, and 12 months. At each visit, the men and women completed questionnaires that assessed sexual function, mental health (SCL-90R), relationship satisfaction (Dyadic Adjustment Scale), anxiety (Spielberger State-Trait Anxiety Inventory), self-esteem (personal evaluation questionnaire), and depression (Beck Depression Inventory).

After 12 months, men were injecting themselves 4.3 times per month with 83 % of the erections labeled as satisfactory, while the men in the vacuum group were using the device 3.5 times per month with 74 % of the erections labeled as satisfactory. Additionally, significant positive changes were observed in quality of the men's erection, frequency of lovemaking (intercourse), sexual satisfaction, all 12 scales of the SCL-90R, Beck Depression Inventory, and Spielberger trait anxiety score [7, 8].

Women responded equally well to both interventions. In both the injection and vacuum groups, women demonstrated significant positive changes in sexual satisfaction, sexual arousal, frequency of lovemaking (intercourse), and frequency of coital orgasm. Women reported feeling more at ease in their relationships and attributed this to how the men felt about themselves. They emphasized how stressful intercourse had been before their partner initiated ED treatment—because the men fostered hurried and anxious attempts at lovemaking. Improving the men's erectile difficulties led to measurable positive changes in the women and overall couple. The positive effects reported by the women seem to be the result of changes within the couple's equilibrium. Any change in one partner produced a change in the other and in the dyadic system [9].

Fifteen years later, Fisher and colleagues published the results of their study entitled, "Sexual Experience of Female Partners of Men with Erectile Dysfunction: The Female Experience of Men's Attitudes to Life Events and Sexuality (FEMALES) Study" [10]. They reported on the partners of 293 men with ED who received vardenafil (Levitra™) and responded to questionnaires assessing frequency of sexual activity, nature of their sexual experience, both before and after the development of their partner's ED, and the nature of the partner's sexual experience after her partner began using vardenafil.

ED had a significant negative effect on the female partners' sexual experience. The women reported a reduced frequency of sexual activity after their partner developed ED and described declines in their sexual desire, arousal, orgasm, and satisfaction. Following the man's treatment with vardenafil, the women's desire, arousal, orgasm, and satisfaction almost returned to their pre-ED levels. The man's use of vardenafil improved the woman's sexual function.

There is also evidence of the negative impact of premature ejaculation (PE) on the female partner's sexuality. This has been confirmed in several epidemiological studies where PE has been found to be correlated to overall female sexual dysfunction, sex not being pleasurable, and problems with desire, arousal and orgasmic problems, as well as low sexual satisfaction and sexual distress [11–14]. Graziottin described the impact of PE on female partners and the emotional process they experience [15]. Most women begin by not addressing the sexual problem for fear of hurting the man's feelings and/or of increasing his feeling of inadequacy. They enter into a collusion of silence hoping that with time things will magically improve. When they don't, she may raise the issue of her frustration with their sexual life but often the man is reluctant to discuss the problem. As the PE continues unabated, she becomes increasingly frustrated, angry, and contemptuous of the man's problem. Finally, Hobbs describes the negative impact that PE has on the female partner's sexual life [16]. Comparing the female partners of men with and without PE, Hobbs reported that the female partners of men with PE experienced half as much sexual desire, arousal, and orgasm.

Unfortunately, there is not a great deal of empirical research on the impact of female sexual dysfunction on male partners. Additionally, there has been very little research on the impact of male or female sexual dysfunction with men who have sex with men or with women who have sex with women.

Reporting on the male partners of women with vaginismus, Dogan and Dogan reported that 50 % of the partners of women with vaginismus had PE [17]. We believe that partners of women with female sexual interest/arousal disorder (FSIAD) are puzzled as to why the women have lost their desire or arousal. They may miss the intimacy, blame themselves for her dysfunction, and wonder if she is having an affair, or question whether she still loves him. Often times a vicious cycle develops where the male partner of a woman with low desire may become exasperated and demand lovemaking, causing her desire to diminish further—resulting in an increase in the man's sexual demands.

31.7 Treatment Concerns

The first consideration, from the therapist's perspective, is whether the presenting problem is best treated in an individual, conjoint, or a combined medical/psychological format. In the USA, there are currently no approved medications for female sexual dysfunction except for the treatment of dyspareunia. For men, there is an assortment of medical treatments for ED and testosterone therapy for hypogonadal men, but no approved treatment for premature ejaculation.

We generally see individuals with lifelong sexual problems in individual therapy because we consider such individuals as having failed to surmount some developmental hurdles that predated the relationship. We see acquired disorders more often in conjoint treatment with the exception of extremely chaotic relationships, or severe individual psychopathology, such as substance abuse, bipolar disorder, or profound character pathology. When there are no serious psychosocial obstacles and there is an approved medication available, we tend to favor a combination of medical and psychological treatment since it offers the best of both worlds.

Interventions that specifically address relationship issues are usually more successful than treatments focused only on the presenting sexual symptoms [18, 19]. Having a better pretreatment relationship has been associated with successful sex therapy treatment outcomes [20].

Much work still needs to be done in terms of empirically demonstrating the efficacy of individual and conjoint psychosocial interventions for sexual problems. Studies generally have small samples, consist of exclusively heterosexual couples, and have little to no follow-up.

31.8 Conclusion

The sexual equilibrium is a powerful construct when working with couples who present for treatment of a sexual dysfunction. Keeping this construct "front and center" allows the therapist to better understand and properly consider the partner's responses to the sexual problem and help the couple to work through the sexual, psychological, and interpersonal issues related to the dysfunction.

References

1. Althof S. Psychogenic impotence: treatment of men and couples. In: Leiblum S, Rosen R, editors. Principles and practice of sex therapy. New York: Guilford Press; 1989. p. 237–68.
2. McCabe M. Intimacy and quality of life among sexually dysfunctional men and women. J Sex Marital Ther. 1997;23:276–90.
3. McCabe MP, Cobain M. The impact of individual and relationship factors on sexual dysfunction among males and females. J Sex Marital Ther. 1998;13(2):131–43.
4. Althof SE, Leiblum SR, Chevret-Measson M, et al. Psychological and interpersonal dimensions of sexual function and dysfunction. J Sex Med. 2005;2:793–800.
5. Rosen RC, Barsky JL. Normal sexual response in women. Obstet Gynecol Clin N Am. 2006;33:515–26.
6. Pollets D, Ducharme S, Pauporte J. Psychological considerations in the assessment of erectile dysfunction. Sex Disabil. 1999;17:129–45.
7. Althof S, Turner L, Levine S, et al. Intracavernosal injection in the treatment of impotence: a prospective study of sexual, psychological and marital functioning. J Sex Marital Ther. 1987;13:155–67.
8. Turner L, Althof S, Levine S, Kursh E, Bodner D, Resnick M. Treating erectile dysfunction with external vacuum devices: impact upon sexual, psychological and marital functioning. J Urol. 1990;141:79–82.
9. Althof S, Turner L, Levine S, Bodner D, Kursh E, Resnick M. Through the eyes of women: the sexual and psychological responses of women to their partners' treatment with self-injection or vacuum constriction therapy. J Urol. 1992;147:1024–7.
10. Fisher WA, Rosen RC, Eardley I, Sand M, Goldstein I. Sexual experience of female partners of men with erectile dysfunction: the female experience of men's attitudes to life events and sexuality (FEMALES) study. J Sex Med. 2005;2:675–84.
11. Giuliano F, Patrick DL, Porst H, et al. Premature ejaculation: results from a five-country European observational study. Eur Urol. 2008;53:1048–57.
12. Patrick DL, Althof SE, Pryor JL, et al. Premature ejaculation: an observational study of men and their partners. J Sex Med. 2005;2:358–67.
13. Riley A, Riley E. Premature ejaculation: presentation and associations. An audit of patients attending a sexual problems clinic. Int J Clin Pract. 2005;59:1482–7.
14. Rosen R, Althof S. Impact of premature ejaculation: the psychological quality of life and sexual relationship consequences. J Sex Med. 2008;5:1296–307.
15. Graziottin A, Althof S. What does premature ejaculation mean to the man, the woman and the couple? J Sex Med. 2011;8:304–9.
16. Hobbs K, Symonds T, Abraham L, May K, Morris MF. Sexual dysfunction in partners of men with premature ejaculation. Int J Impot Res. 2008;20:512–7.

17. Dogan S, Dogan M. The frequency of sexual dysfunctions in male partners of women with vaginismus in a Turkish sample. Int J Impot Res. 2008;20:218–21.
18. Althof S, Leiblum S, Chevret M, et al. Psychological and interpersonal dimensions of sexual function and dysfunction. In: Lue T, Basson R, Rosen R, Giuliano F, Khoury S, Montorsi F, editors. Sexual medicine: sexual dysfunctions in men and women. Paris: Edition 2004
19. Zimmer D. Does marital therapy enhance the effectiveness of treatment for sexual dysfunction? J Sex Marital Ther. 1987;13:193–209.
20. Hawton K, Catalan J. Prognostic factors in sex therapy. Behav Res Ther. 1986;24:377–85.

Infertility and Sexual Dysfunction (SD) in the Couple

32

Elizabeth Grill, Rose Khavari, Jonathan Zurawin, Juan Ramon Flores Gonzalez, and Alexander W. Pastuszak

32.1 Introduction

Sexual dysfunction can significantly affect both partners in a relationship as well as the couple as a whole. Thus, a couple's sexuality should be considered as a dyadic unit encompassing a reciprocal exchange of positive and negative feedback. One partner's libido and climax positively influences the other's sexual desire, helping to affirm sexual identity. Conversely, if one partner perceives a lack of sexual response from the other, his or her self-image may be undermined. For instance, women whose partners have erectile dysfunction (ED) report a decline in their own sexual desire, arousal, orgasm, and satisfaction [1, 2]. Accordingly, optimal dyadic sexual function is an important element for a couple's bonding.

Contemporary population-based studies assessing the prevalence and incidence of sexual dysfunction are not available and a paucity of data exists. Previous analysis of the National Health and Social Life Survey data from 1992 observed sexual dysfunction in the United States in 43 % of women and 31 % of men [3]. However, only approximately 12 % of 31,581 women endorsed the combined presence of sexual problems and distress associated with those problems, a more valid indicator of the impact of sexual dysfunction in women [4]. While there are numerous causes of sexual dysfunction, in this chapter we focus on the impact of infertility on sexual dysfunction in the man, woman, and couple, with special consideration of the couple as a unit. Given the growing body of knowledge relating organic and psychological causes of sexual dysfunction, as well as the growing rate of fertility evaluation, providing a perspective on the interplay between infertility and sexual dysfunction and appropriate management is necessary. Here, we dissect the relationships between infertility and sexual dysfunction in men and women individually, as well as in the couple.

E. Grill, Psy.D.
The Ronald O. Perelman and Claudia Cohen Center for Reproductive Medicine, Weill Cornell Medical College, New York, NY, USA

R. Khavari, M.D.
Houston Methodist Center for Restorative Pelvic Medicine, Houston Methodist Hospital Department of Urology, Houston, TX, USA

J. Zurawin, M.D.
Baylor College of Medicine, Houston, TX, USA

J.R.F. Gonzalez, M.D.
Department of Surgery, University of Texas Medical School at Houston, Houston, TX, USA

A.W. Pastuszak, M.D., Ph.D. (✉)
Baylor College of Medicine, Division of Male Reproductive Medicine and Surgery, Center for Reproductive Medicine, Scott Department of Urology, Houston, TX, USA
e-mail: pastusza@bcm.edu

L.I. Lipshultz et al. (eds.), *Management of Sexual Dysfunction in Men and Women*, DOI 10.1007/978-1-4939-3100-2_32

32.2 Infertility and Sexual Dysfunction in the Man, Woman, and Couple

Infertility is defined as "the inability to conceive after 1 year of unprotected sex" [5] and may affect up to 15 % of couples [5, 6]. Importantly, male and female factors each can contribute independently to fertility difficulties in up to 50 % of cases [7–9]. Sexual function and childbearing are considered important aspects of most partnerships and deeply impact quality of life. For many couples, the inability to conceive or give birth to a healthy child often forces partners to reevaluate their sense of femininity and masculinity, gender identity, and ultimately the meaning of their relationship. Furthermore, couples with fertility difficulties confront many challenges including societal and parental pressures for propagation, physical and psychological burdens, and potential financial burdens if considering assisted reproductive technologies. Such stressors can lead to poor marital adjustment and decreased quality of life, as well as to sexual dysfunction. Common feelings in the setting of infertility, such as loss, anger, guilt, despair, depression, shame, and anxiety, often overshadow the usual feelings of warmth, affection, and emotional connection that are the natural prerequisites of sexual intimacy [10, 11]. Sex lives are quickly taken from the intimacy of the bedroom to the control of the healthcare establishment [12]. Sex is altered and becomes methodical, predictable, and unexciting for many couples struggling with infertility, and couples begin to associate sex with failure to conceive and may avoid it.

Infertility, with its direct link to procreative sexual behavior, is thus experienced as a stressful life crisis that has been compared to that of cancer, AIDS, and other devastating illnesses as well as the loss of a loved one [13–15]. Infertile couples have reported sexual problems ranging from lack of desire, pleasure, or spontaneity to sexual dysfunction. Keye [16] determined that the three areas of sexual difficulty in infertile couples were (1) the actual physical condition causing infertility or resulting from treatment, (2) sexual intercourse becoming only a means of reproduction rather than intimacy or pleasure, and (3) the global psychological impact of the infertility experience.

Organic sexual dysfunctions are regarded as a minor cause of infertility, impacting approximately 5 % of all infertility cases [17]. Overall, sexual dysfunction alone is common, with 40–45 % of adult women and 20–30 % of adult men with at least one manifestation of sexual dysfunction [18]. Male sexual disorders such as chronic ED and anejaculation make natural conception impossible, whereas in women, severe presentation of genito-pelvic pain/penetration disorders such as vaginismus and apareunia prevent natural pregnancy [19]. However, sexual problems are common in infertile couples, with women more affected than men [20]. As the focus of sexual activity continues to emphasize procreation, infertile men and women may feel depressed, lose interest in "sex-on-demand," or find it difficult to feel sexual when they are chronically frustrated and unhappy due to childlessness. Loss of libido may be the result of chronic health problems or the invasiveness of medical treatment for infertility. It may be due to the medications and hormones that can interfere with sexual response and/or interest or to the stresses and demands that infertility places on the marriage, social relationships, work life, or financial resources [21].

Studies have linked the physical, psychological, and financial challenges of assisted reproduction to increased marital conflict, decreased sexual self-esteem, feelings of inadequacy, and frequency of sexual intercourse [13, 22]. Overall, infertility is associated with decreased sexual activity and appears to become worse as the number of childless years increases [19]. The interplay between the infertility and sexual dysfunction can affect one's reproductive potential and impact interpersonal relationships and self-image.

32.3 Infertility and Sexual Dysfunction in Men: A Medical Perspective

The male sexual dysfunctions most likely to affect male fertility are those that cause ED and affect sexual desire, arousal (reviewed in Chap. 16

"Hypoactive Sexual Desire in Men"), and ejaculation (reviewed in Chap. 14, "Evaluation and Treatment of Disorders of Ejaculation" and Chap. 15 "Evaluation and Treatment of Orgasmic Disorders"), limiting the ability to effectively inseminate the female partner [23]. In 1999, Laumann et al. reported on sexual dysfunction in a modern young US population, observing ED in 7–9 % of men 18–39 years old [24]. In this population, ED was associated with emotional stress, low physical satisfaction, and low general happiness.

The causes of ED are often multifactorial, comprising a mix of organic and psychogenic factors, although a psychogenic factor is a contributor in almost all cases, particularly in younger men (reviewed in Chap. 6 "Urologic and Clinical Evaluation of the Male with Erectile Dysfunction") [25]. Importantly, depression and other psychological factors are also linked to ED. The Massachusetts Male Aging Study (MMAS) observed an increased risk of ED (OR 1.82) in men with depressive symptoms [26], and other studies have supported this relationship [27]. When considering psychogenic ED, the link with sexual confidence and performance anxiety should not be overlooked, and numerous studies have reinforced a clear association between ED and sexual confidence [28, 29].

Medications can result in male sexual dysfunction and can negatively impact fertility. Some common medications affecting the male sexual response include thiazide diuretics and beta-blockers (i.e., propranolol) that can decrease blood flow to the penis and cause decreased libido and ED [30]. Decreased sexual desire, ejaculatory difficulties, and ED can also occur with the use of spironolactone, antipsychotics, SSRIs, SNRIs, and tricyclic antidepressants [30].

When considering male factor infertility, 6 % of men who are evaluated for infertility have coexisting significant pathologies, including genetic abnormalities, malignancy, and endocrinopathy, and as a result a diagnosis of infertility is directly linked to general male health [31]. Cancer and its treatment using radiation, surgery, and/or chemotherapy is well known to negatively impact male fertility, either via direct effects on the gonads (chemotherapy, radiation) or on structures required for male sexual function (surgery) [32, 33]. Most commonly in younger men, metastatic testicular cancer requiring retroperitoneal lymph node dissection (RPLND) may disrupt the lumbar sympathetic and hypogastric plexuses causing anejaculation or retrograde ejaculation, as well as ED [34–36]. Retroperitoneal procedures may also cause obstruction of the vas deferens or ejaculatory ducts [37]. Radical prostatectomy and cystoprostatectomy carry with them a risk of ED from neurovascular injury and infertility due to transection of the vas deferens, removal of the seminal vesicles, and injury to lumbar and hypogastric plexuses [37]. Iatrogenic disturbance of the bladder neck with resultant urinary incontinence during transurethral resection of the prostate, and less so following bladder neck incision, can result in retrograde ejaculation in up to 75 % of men who undergo those procedures for benign causes as well [38, 39].

Whether the cause is vascular, neurogenic, hormonal, drug induced, anatomic, or psychogenic, the end result is the same, with decreased sexual desire, an inability to achieve and maintain an adequate erection, or the inability to deliver sperm to the optimal location for fertilization. This sexual dysfunction not only limits the man's fertility but can also have a profound negative impact on self-esteem, quality of life, psychosocial health, and relationships.

32.4 Infertility and Sexual Dysfunction in Men: Psychosocial Implications

Having a diagnosis of infertility or subfertility is a psychological and relationship stressor and is associated with sexual dysfunction [15, 40]. Some studies suggest that infertile men experience less distress than women using various indices of emotional state [41, 42]. However, over time, male partners of infertile couples report significantly less desire, more stressful marital relationships, and worse sexual function and satisfaction compared to fertile control couples [43, 44]. Having a diagnosis of male factor infertility lasting 3–6 years contributes to decreased relationship stability, sexual activity, and lower sexual satisfaction in both male and female partners from infertile couples, with the decrease in sexual activity increasing as the amount of fruitless years accrue [19, 45]. Men also report less ability to control ejaculation and less satisfaction with their sexual performance in general [5, 46, 47], and men who are the sole contributors to infertility in the relationship have a higher incidence of depression compared with men who were either fertile or shared the problem with their partners [48].

The emotional ramifications of a diagnosis of infertility, no matter the etiology, can further impact procreative potential through alteration of physical function, and a vicious cycle can develop where one condition can potentiate the other. Men in infertile relationships have a higher than expected incidence of ED and depressive symptoms, lower self-esteem, higher anxiety, more somatic symptoms, and more dysfunctional sexual relationships [49]. During infertility, many men develop performance anxiety, sexual avoidance, or even aversion to sex, especially if sex is for "procreation purposes only" and their partner is sexually unresponsive. Regimenting intercourse can decrease libido in 10 % of patients, and ED may occur in up to 20 % of men engaging in timed intercourse [50]. Frequently, infertile men complain of feeling "used" like "stud service" (that all his partner wants from him is his sperm) or of the "queen bee syndrome" (his sole importance is to fertilize his partner) [51, 52]. In a study of infertile men in Germany, a short-lasting partnership and high sexual dissatisfaction prior to the diagnosis of infertility caused more distress in infertile men, whereas being in a longer-lasting and sexually satisfying partnership seemed to have a buffering effect with regard to sexual distress and infertility [53].

32.5 Infertility and Sexual Dysfunction in Women: A Medical Perspective

Although the term "infertility" is generally used to indicate a couple with challenges in conceiving pregnancy naturally, as compared to the general population (20 % per cycle), the more appropriate term should be "subfertility," suggesting a decreased capacity for conceiving naturally. The National Survey of Family Growth reports 10.9 % (6.7 million) of women 15–44 years of age with impaired fecundity between 2006 and 2010 in the United States. Of these women, 11.9 % (7.4 million) have ever received any fertility services [54]. The incidence of etiologies causing infertility varies between different populations. However, among 14,141 couples in 21 publications, abnormal semen factors contributed to 25 % of infertility cases and female factors 54 %, with ovulatory disorders implicated in 27 % of cases, tubal disorders in 22 %, and endometriosis in 5 % [55].

Ovulatory disorders represent a major cause for subfertility and infertility, and polycystic ovary syndrome (PCOS) is the primary disorder in this category that leads to anovulation or oligoovulation. While PCOS can significantly affect a woman's health-related quality of life including fertility, body image, self-esteem, and menstrual cycles, it can also negatively affect the sexual desire and arousal that directly contributes to the couple's sexual health [56]. Medical management and hormonal developments in the recent decades have improved management of PCOS [57].

Tubal abnormalities and obstruction can contribute to 22 % of infertility causes in couples and can be evaluated using hysterosalpingogram and managed accordingly. Uterine causes of female subfertility include intrauterine adhesions and leiomyomas. Intrauterine adhesions can be lysed using hysteroscopic intervention, which can increase the rate and success of pregnancies in this patient population [58]. In general leiomyomas do not interfere with pregnancy unless they are large and result in uterine distortion or are located in the cervical area, distorting the endocervix and interfering with sperm transport.

Endometriosis, the presence and growth of uterine glands and stroma in aberrant locations, can contribute significantly to infertility, pain, and detriments to sexual health. Endometriosis symptoms vary widely from mild to severe. The significant pelvic adhesions and inflammation caused by endometriosis are the main factors leading to challenges in conceiving normally, which can further burden the relationship and sexual health in a couple. In addition, the pain that is present in many patients with endometriosis contributes to sexual pain disorders and can play a significant role in the couple's sexual dynamic [59]. Montanari and colleagues evaluated 182 women with deep infiltrating endometriosis and showed significantly lower satisfaction scores in Sexual Health Questionnaire (SHOW-Q) that correlated with decrements in quality of life [60]. Other conditions included in the genito-pelvic pain and penetration disorder (formerly known as dyspareunia and vaginismus) that may limit vaginal penetration during intercourse are atrophic vaginitis, vulvodynia, and painful bladder syndrome (interstitial cystitis).

Other gynecological disorders that may be indirectly related to female fertility that may negatively affect sexual function in a female, and thus in the couple, include pelvic organ prolapse, urinary and fecal incontinence, and anal, bladder, colorectal, and gynecological malignancies.

Despite the high prevalence of sexual dysfunction in couples dealing with fertility difficulties, sexual dysfunctions more commonly result *from* fertility difficulties rather than cause infertility. Sexual dysfunction and infertility have emotional and psychological ramifications within a couple's relationship, and data suggest that patients with secondary infertility may have higher prevalence of sexual dysfunction [60, 61].

32.6 Infertility and Sexual Dysfunction in Women: Psychosocial Implications

Evaluation and treatment of infertility in the female and couple, beginning with semen analysis and the female evaluation, can result in emotional stress and affect the couple's sexual relationship. This is exacerbated with timing of intercourse and postcoital testing performed at some centers, interfering with the spontaneity of a couple's intimacy. However, these stresses appear to manifest more prominently in the female partner, as shown by Oddens et al. while surveying 281 women prior to starting treatment for infertility. The authors showed lower scores for coital frequency, sexual interest, and pleasure in non-mothers when compared to an age and relationship duration matched group of mothers [62]. In contrast, in a study by Müller et al., 68 men surveyed at an andrology clinic before and after fertility treatment revealed no change in their sexual satisfaction [63]. Emotional stress within couples resulting from fertility treatments, particularly in the female partner, was evaluated by Hammarberg et al., who observed that 2–3 years after infertility treatment, 59 % of 116 women reported treatment as having a negative impact on their sexual relationship [64]. In addition, when used in women for ovulatory stimulation, hormonal therapy alone can cause weight gain, breast tenderness, and mood imbalances that can negatively affect a couple's sexual health.

Sexual dysfunction is high in all infertile women, and women with secondary infertility suffer more from impaired sexual function compared with those with primary infertility [61]. Hurwitz et al. [65] detected increased sexual dysfunction in 50 % of females and reported loss of sexual desire as the leading cause of dysfunction. Oskay et al. [66] found sexual dysfunction in 61.7 % of infertile women and in 42.9 % of fertile women, and Millheiser et al. [67] detected sexual dysfunction in 25 % of fertile and 40 % of infertile women. Both research groups found lower scores of desire and arousal parameters in the infertile group as compared to the fertile group. Women reported severe marital strain, as well as sexual inhibitions, anorgasmia, and reduced interest in sex [68]. Andrews and associates found that infertility-specific stress had a stronger negative impact on women's sense of sexual identity and self-efficacy than it did on men [69].

32.7 Treatment of Sexual Dysfunction in the Couple

Even couples that never encounter major or disrupting sexual problems often experience episodic or situational diminished sexual desire and satisfaction in response to the emotional distress or physical strains of infertility or a specific treatment. Episodic loss of sexual desire in one or both partners can usually be addressed with minimal education and reassurance. However, consistent and extensive diminished sexual desire in infertile men and women is more problematic and usually multifactorial.

Infertile couples are reluctant to discuss sexual dysfunction if they fear that it will interrupt medical treatment. Even so, no clinician working with infertile couples should assume that a couple is having regular sexual intercourse sufficient for reproduction or ignore the possibility of unusual sexual practices that interfere with conception and/or medical treatment plans [21]. Clinicians treating sexual problems can intervene on several different therapeutic levels and are encouraged to provide patient education to patients and their partners in treatment decisions whenever possible [70].

Overall, the management of sexual dysfunction is best provided by a combination approach, which successfully integrates both physical and psychosocial factors [71]. Combination therapy integrating sex therapy and oftentimes sexual pharmaceuticals is frequently the best treatment approach for sexual dysfunction. Contextual factors, including difficulties with a current interpersonal relationship, should also be clarified and previous sexual scripts should be assessed [72]. In some couples, partners blame themselves or each other for infertility or medical diagnosis, resulting in anger that interferes with sexual desire and functioning. Several questions should be asked, including whether sexual relations were ever good with the current partner, what changed, and what the patient's view of causation is. Other questions to consider when assessing infertility patients are whether anything changed in their emotional or sexual relationship since they have been trying to conceive and how often they engage in sexually intimate acts and/or have penetrative sex [21]. Numerous partner-related psychosexual issues may also adversely affect outcome. If the sexual problems reflect more fundamental relationship problems, it may be that marital issues must take precedence over further infertility treatment.

32.8 Referral, Consultation, and Collaboration

It is clear that the stress, psychological demands, and physically intrusive procedures associated with infertility treatment can affect sexual self-image, desire, and performance. Whether sexual dysfunction is a preexisting condition or an unwelcome side effect of infertility treatment, it can be a devastating and discouraging blow, compounding the disappointment of childlessness and the distress of medical treatment. All too often, the sexual problems of infertile couples are ignored or minimized in a belief that they will dissipate on their own or will have few long-term consequences. Unfortunately, although some sexual problems may disappear when the pressures of infertility treatment end, sexual difficulties typically linger or become more problematic after treatment ends or parenthood is achieved [10, 73]. Depending on the comfort level, preference, resources, and availability, the physician may choose to treat the couple or refer them to a sex therapist and/or infertility counselor [21, 74].

32.9 Conclusions

Infertility in the man, woman, and couple can result in significant distress and sexual dysfunction. In both men and women, infertility can result in sexual dysfunction, and vice versa, as a function of frequently coexisting organic and psychological factors. Importantly, the interplay between the organic and psychosocial factors leading to infertility-related sexual dysfunction cannot be overlooked, and appropriate treatment should be targeted to both individual and the couple to address the organic and psychosocial issues.

References

1. Jiann BP, Su CC, Tsai JY. Is female sexual function related to the male partners' erectile function? J Sex Med. 2013;10(2):420–9.
2. Boddi V, Corona G, Fisher AD, Mannucci E, Ricca V, Sforza A, et al. "It takes two to tango": the relational

domain in a cohort of subjects with erectile dysfunction (ED). J Sex Med. 2012;9(12):3126–36.
3. Latif EZ, Diamond MP. Arriving at the diagnosis of female sexual dysfunction. Fertil Steril. 2013;100(4):898–904.
4. Shifren JL, Monz BU, Russo PA, Segreti A, Johannes CB. Sexual problems and distress in United States women: prevalence and correlates. Obstet Gynecol. 2008;112(5):970–8.
5. Monga M, Alexandrescu B, Katz SE, Stein M, Ganiats T. Impact of infertility on quality of life, marital adjustment, and sexual function. Urology. 2004;63(1):126–30.
6. Mosher WD. Infertility trends among U.S. couples: 1965–1976. Fam Plan Perspect. 1982;14(1):22–7.
7. Thonneau P, Marchand S, Tallec A, Ferial ML, Ducot B, Lansac J, et al. Incidence and main causes of infertility in a resident population (1,850,000) of three French regions (1988–1989). Hum Reprod. 1991; 6(6):811–16.
8. Eisenberg ML, Lathi RB, Baker VL, Westphal LM, Milki AA, Nangia AK. Frequency of the male infertility evaluation: data from the national survey of family growth. J Urol. 2013;189(3):1030–4.
9. Wong WY, Thomas CM, Merkus JM, Zielhuis GA, Steegers-Theunissen RP. Male factor subfertility: possible causes and the impact of nutritional factors. Fertil Steril. 2000;73(3):435–42.
10. Burns L. An overview of sexual dysfunction in the infertile couple. J Fam Psychother. 1995;6:25–46.
11. Irvine S. Male infertility and its effect on male sexuality. Sex Relat Ther. 1996;11:273–80.
12. Applegarth L, Grill E. Psychological issues in reproductive disorders. In: Chan P, Goldstein M, Rosenwaks Z, editors. Reproductive medicine secrets. Philadelphia: Hanley and Belfus; 2004. p. 391–402.
13. Andrews FM, Abbey A, Halman LJ. Is fertility-problem stress different? The dynamics of stress in fertile and infertile couples. Fertil Steril. 1992;57(6):1247–53.
14. Domar AD, Zuttermeister PC, Friedman R. The psychological impact of infertility: a comparison with patients with other medical conditions. J Psychosom Obstet Gynaecol. 1993;14(Suppl):45–52.
15. Lenzi A, Lombardo F, Salacone P, Gandini L, Jannini EA. Stress, sexual dysfunctions, and male infertility. J Endocrinol Investig. 2003;26(3 Suppl):72–6.
16. Keye W. The impact of infertility on psychosexual function. Fertil Steril. 1980;34:308–9.
17. Wischmann TH. Psychogenic infertility—myths and facts. J Assist Reprod Genet. 2003;20(12):485–94.
18. Lewis RW, Fugl-Meyer KS, Corona G, Hayes RD, Laumann EO, Moreira Jr ED, et al. Definitions/epidemiology/risk factors for sexual dysfunction. J Sex Med. 2010;7(4 Pt 2):1598–607.
19. Nene UA, Coyaji K, Apte H. Infertility: a label of choice in the case of sexually dysfunctional couples. Patient Educ Couns. 2005;59(3):234–8.
20. Wischmann TH. Sexual disorders in infertile couples. J Sex Med. 2010;7(5):1868–76.
21. Burns L. Sexual counseling and infertility. In: Burns LH, Covington SN, editors. Infertility counseling: a comprehensive handbook for clinicians. New York: Parthenon Publishing; 2006. p. 212–35.
22. Whiteford LM, Gonzalez L. Stigma: the hidden burden of infertility. Soc Sci Med. 1995;40(1):27–36.
23. Lewis RW, Fugl-Meyer KS, Bosch R, Fugl-Meyer AR, Laumann EO, Lizza E, et al. Epidemiology/risk factors of sexual dysfunction. J Sex Med. 2004;1(1):35–9.
24. Laumann EO, Paik A, Rosen RC. Sexual dysfunction in the United States: prevalence and predictors. JAMA. 1999;281(6):537–44.
25. Ralph D, McNicholas T. UK management guidelines for erectile dysfunction. BMJ. 2000;321(7259): 499–503.
26. Araujo AB, Durante R, Feldman HA, Goldstein I, McKinlay JB. The relationship between depressive symptoms and male erectile dysfunction: cross-sectional results from the Massachusetts male aging study. Psychosom Med. 1998;60(4):458–65.
27. Perelman MA. Erectile dysfunction and depression: screening and treatment. Urol Clin N Am. 2011; 38(2):125–39.
28. Althof SE, Wieder M. Psychotherapy for erectile dysfunction: now more relevant than ever. Endocrine. 2004;23(2–3):131–4.
29. Morse WI, Morse JM. Erectile impotence precipitated by organic factors and perpetuated by performance anxiety. Can Med Assoc J. 1982;127(7):599–601.
30. Nudell DM, Monoski MM, Lipshultz LI. Common medications and drugs: how they affect male fertility. Urol Clin N Am. 2002;29(4):965–73.
31. Kolettis PN, Sabanegh ES. Significant medical pathology discovered during a male infertility evaluation. J Urol. 2001;166(1):178–80.
32. Howell SJ, Shalet SM. Spermatogenesis after cancer treatment: damage and recovery. J Natl Cancer Inst Monogr. 2005;34:12–7.
33. Osterberg EC, Ramasamy R, Masson P, Brannigan RE. Current practices in fertility preservation in male cancer patients. Urol Ann. 2014;6(1):13–7.
34. Stahl PJ, Stember DS, Mulhall JP. Options for fertility preservation in men and boys with cancer. Adv Exp Med Biol. 2012;732:29–39.
35. Kedia KR, Markland C, Fraley EE. Sexual function after high retroperitoneal lymphadenectomy. Urol Clin N Am. 1977;4(3):523–8.
36. Nijman JM, Schraffordt Koops H, Oldhoff J, Kremer J, Sleijfer DT. Sexual function after surgery and combination chemotherapy in men with disseminated nonseminomatous testicular cancer. J Surg Oncol. 1988;38(3):182–6.
37. Hendry WF. Iatrogenic damage to male reproductive function. J R Soc Med. 1995;88(10):579P–84P.
38. Bettocchi C, Verze P, Palumbo F, Arcaniolo D, Mirone V. Ejaculatory disorders: pathophysiology and management. Nat Clin Pract Urol. 2008;5(2):93–103.
39. Wein AJ, Kavoussi LR, Campbell MF. In: Wein AJ (editor-in-chief), Kavoussi LR, et al., editors.

Campbell-Walsh urology. 10th ed. Philadelphia, PA: Elsevier Saunders; 2012.
40. Link PW, Darling CA. Couples undergoing treatment for infertility: dimensions of life satisfaction. J Sex Marital Ther. 1986;12(1):46–59.
41. Wright J, Duchesne C, Sabourin S, Bissonnette F, Benoit J, Girard Y. Psychosocial distress and infertility: men and women respond differently. Fertil Steril. 1991;55(1):100–8.
42. Stanton AL, Tennen H, Affleck G, Mendola R. Cognitive appraisal and adjustment to infertility. Women Health. 1991;17(3):1–15.
43. Berg BJ, Wilson JF. Psychological functioning across stages of treatment for infertility. J Behav Med. 1991;14(1):11–26.
44. Khademi A, Alleyassin A, Amini M, Ghaemi M. Evaluation of sexual dysfunction prevalence in infertile couples. J Sex Med. 2008;5(6):1402–10.
45. Drosdzol A, Skrzypulec V. Evaluation of marital and sexual interactions of Polish infertile couples. J Sex Med. 2009;6(12):3335–46.
46. Abbey A, Andrews FM, Halman LJ. Provision and receipt of social support and disregard: what is their impact on the marital life quality of infertile and fertile couples? J Pers Soc Psychol. 1995;68(3):455–69.
47. O'Brien JH, Lazarou S, Deane L, Jarvi K, Zini A. Erectile dysfunction and andropause symptoms in infertile men. J Urol. 2005;174(5):1932–4; discussion 4.
48. Slade P, Raval H, Buck P, Lieberman BE. A 3-year follow-up of emotional, marital, and sexual functioning in couples who were infertile. J Reprod Infant Psychol. 1992;10:233–43.
49. Shindel AW, Nelson CJ, Naughton CK, Ohebshalom M, Mulhall JP. Sexual function and quality of life in the male partner of infertile couples: prevalence and correlates of dysfunction. J Urol. 2008;179(3):1056–9.
50. Sigg C. Sexuality and sterility. Therapeutische Umschau Revue therapeutique. 1994;51(2):115–19.
51. Zoldbrod A. Men, women, and infertility: intervention and treatment strategies. New York: Lexington Books; 1993.
52. Mazor M. Emotional reactions to infertility. In: Mazor M, Simons H, editors. Infertility: medical, emotional and social considerations. New York: Human Science Press; 1984. p. 23–35.
53. Schilling G, Muller MJ, Haidl G. Sexual dissatisfaction and somatic complaints in male infertility. Psychother Psychosom Med Psychol. 1999;49(8):256–63.
54. Impaired Fecundity: CDC [cited 2015 May 1]. Available from http://www.cdc.gov/nchs/nsfg/key_statistics/i.htm-impaired
55. Collins HA. Unexplained infertility. In: Key WR, Chang RJ, Rebar RW, Soules MR, editors. Infertility: evaluation and teatment. Philadelphia, PA: Saunders; 1995.
56. Bazarganipour F, Ziaei S, Montazeri A, Foroozanfard F, Kazemnejad A, Faghihzadeh S. Health-related quality of life in patients with polycystic ovary syndrome (PCOS): a model-based study of predictive factors. J Sex Med. 2014;11(4):1023–32.
57. Mahan ME. Ovulatory disorders and infertility. J Reprod Med. 2008;53(4):311; author reply.
58. March CM, Israel R. Gestational outcome following hysteroscopic lysis of adhesions. Fertil Steril. 1981;36(4):455–9.
59. Buster JE. Managing female sexual dysfunction. Fertil Steril. 2013;100(4):905–15.
60. Montanari G, Di Donato N, Benfenati A, Giovanardi G, Zannoni L, Vicenzi C, et al. Women with deep infiltrating endometriosis: sexual satisfaction, desire, orgasm, and pelvic problem interference with sex. J Sex Med. 2013;10(6):1559–66.
61. Keskin U, Coksuer H, Gungor S, Ercan CM, Karasahin KE, Baser I. Differences in prevalence of sexual dysfunction between primary and secondary infertile women. Fertil Steril. 2011;96(5):1213–17.
62. Oddens BJ, den Tonkelaar I, Nieuwenhuyse H. Psychosocial experiences in women facing fertility problems—a comparative survey. Hum Reprod. 1999;14(1):255–61.
63. Muller MJ, Schilling G, Haidl G. Sexual satisfaction in male infertility. Arch Androl. 1999;42(3):137–43.
64. Hammarberg K, Astbury J, Baker H. Women's experience of IVF: a follow-up study. Hum Reprod. 2001;16(2):374–83.
65. Hurwitz MB. Sexual dysfunction associated with infertility. A comparison of sexual function during the fertile and the non-fertile phase of the menstrual cycle. S Afr Med J. 1989;76(2):58–61.
66. Oskay U, Beji N, Serdaroglu H. The issue of infertility and sexual function in Turkish women. Sex Disabil. 2010;28:71–9.
67. Millheiser LS, Helmer AE, Quintero RB, Westphal LM, Milki AA, Lathi RB. Is infertility a risk factor for female sexual dysfunction? A case-control study. Fertil Steril. 2010;94(6):2022–5.
68. Boivin J, Takefman JE, Brender W, Tulandi T. The effects of female sexual response in coitus on early reproductive processes. J Behav Med. 1992;15(5):509–18.
69. Andrews FM, Abbey A, Halman LJ. Stress from infertility, marriage factors, and subjective well-being of wives and husbands. J Health Soc Behav. 1991;32(3):238–53.
70. Dunn ME, Althof SE, Perelman MA. Phosphodiesterase type 5 inhibitors' extended duration of response as a variable in the treatment of erectile dysfunction. Int J Impot Res. 2007;19(2):119–23.
71. Perelman M. Combination therapy for sexual dysfunction: integrating sex therapy and pharmacotherapy. In: Balon R, Segraves R, editors. Handbook of sexual dysfunction. Boca Raton: Taylor and Francis; 2005. p. 13–41.
72. Gagnon JH, Rosen RC, Leiblum SR. Cognitive and social aspects of sexual dysfunction: sexual scripts in sex therapy. J Sex Marital Ther. 1982;8(1):44–56.
73. Boxer A. Infertility and sexual dysfunction. Infertil Reprod Med Clin N Am. 1996;7:565–75.
74. Perelman MA. Sex coaching for physicians: combination treatment for patient and partner. Int J Impot Res. 2003;15 Suppl 5:S67–74.

Couples Therapy and Counseling

33

Barry McCarthy and Lana M. Wald

33.1 Introduction

Traditionally, physicians in sexual medicine (e.g., urologists, gynecologists, sexual medicine specialists, and psychiatrists) focused on biomedical factors that caused sexual dysfunction. The first-line intervention was medication (pro-erection medications or hormonal enhancement); the second-line intervention included injections, external pumps, or the MUSE® system; and the third-line intervention was surgical (penile prosthesis). Although there is literature on female dysfunction, especially the newly named diagnosis of sexual interest arousal disorder (SIAD), the great majority of the work in sexual medicine focused on male dysfunction. Since the introduction of sildenafil [1], the biomedical model has been the predominant approach to the study and treatment of sexual function and dysfunction. Rowland [2] raised concerns that psychological and relational assessments and interventions were being ignored both in clinical practice and research. Although the dramatic increase in understanding of vascular, neurological, and hormonal components of sexual function and dysfunction was extremely welcomed, in reality, the biomedical model as a stand-alone intervention has not delivered the promised results. The best example is the treatment of erectile dysfunction (ED). Contrary to advertisements and media hype, the man taking a pro-erection medication rarely returns to having easy, predictable erections and intercourse 100 % reliably. The most important understanding is that the woman's role is much more than encouraging the man to ask his physician for medication [3]. In the Good-Enough Sex (GES) approach to male and couple sexuality, the best predictor of maintaining satisfying couple sexuality is the woman's active role in treatment and her investment in their sexual relationship [4]. Although the standard biopsychosocial model gives "lip service" to psychological and social/relational factors, these are usually not addressed unless the medical intervention has been unsuccessful [5].

The new mantra in couple sexuality is desire, pleasure, eroticism, and satisfaction [6]. From this perspective, the most important factor is desire. The couple approach is not an optional resource, but is the optimal intervention.

Traditionally, in assessment and treatment of male sexual dysfunction, the woman usually had no therapeutic role. The biomedical model for premature ejaculation (PE) emphasizes PE as a biophysiological dysfunction involving treating solely the man using a stand-alone medication intervention [7]. This approach is also true for ED, whether

B. McCarthy, Ph.D. (✉) • L.M. Wald, M.A.
Department of Psychology, American University, 4400 Massachusetts Avenue, NW, Washington, DC 20016, USA
e-mail: bmccar@american.edu; mccarthy160@comcast.net

L.I. Lipshultz et al. (eds.), *Management of Sexual Dysfunction in Men and Women*, DOI 10.1007/978-1-4939-3100-2_33

treated by a primary care physician or urologist. The man is seen alone, assessed for any comorbid illness, and prescribed a PDE5 inhibitor with little or no counseling about psychosexual factors to optimize results. This is a major factor leading to disappointing outcomes and a high treatment dropout rate [8]. When he stops medication, the man reverts to a pattern of anticipatory anxiety, performance anxiety about erection and intercourse as a pass-fail sex test, frustration, embarrassment, and eventually sexual avoidance. The decision to stop trying to be sexual and to avoid any sexual touch is often made unilaterally and conveyed nonverbally. The woman is usually confused and distressed, unsure whether to blame herself, the medication, or her partner [9].

McCarthy and Fucito [10] suggest a couple approach to the assessment, treatment, and relapse prevention of ED. This is also relevant to PE, ejaculatory inhibition (delayed ejaculation), and male hypoactive sexual desire disorder (HSDD). In the comprehensive, integrative biopsychosocial approach, the couple is the prime patient. The urologist or primary care physician sees the man for assessment and gives a prescription for a PDE5 inhibitor or other medical intervention. Ideally, the couple therapist and physician work together in a synergistic manner, which is in the best interest of the man and couple. This is the special challenge of a mental health-medical team approach. Rather than the physician being the team leader, the physician and therapist cooperate as trusting colleagues working in a coordinated manner for the man, woman, and couple.

The couple therapist is working in the context of the biopsychosocial model and educates the partners to take personal responsibility for sexuality while recognizing that, in essence, sexuality is a "team sport." This combination of personal responsibility/intimate sexual team is at the core of this approach to sexual function and dysfunction [11]. In the four-session assessment model, the clinician seeks to identify the biological, psychological, and socio-relational factors which subvert healthy sexuality, especially sexual desire [12].

If at all possible, the initial session is conducted with the couple. This emphasizes the powerful therapeutic message that, at its core, intimacy and sexuality are a couple issue. In the initial session, we seek to identify when sexuality was most positive and what they valued about each other and as a couple. It is important to assess the sexual problems the couple has tried to address on their own so that mistakes are not repeated. The clinician does not overpromise or set unrealistic expectations, but it is therapeutic to be positive and realistic about changing intimacy and sexuality.

If the psychological/relational/sexual history is done with the partner present, it is likely the clinician will receive a "sanitized" version rather than a genuine narrative, which includes a careful exploration of emotional and sexual vulnerabilities. Appropriate therapeutic intervention (medically, psychologically, and relationally) requires a genuine understanding of personal strengths and vulnerabilities, especially motivational factors. Ideally, the couple would share the value of a satisfying, secure, and sexual relationship. However, the clinician should not assume this, but recognize the need to assess motivational factors. Common causes for failure of medical interventions include lack of motivation on the part of one or both partners, negative emotions such as resentment or shame, sex as a manipulation rather than a sharing of pleasure, a secret sexual life of variant arousal or greater confidence with masturbation than couple sex, a question of sexual orientation, an extramarital affair, a focus on fertility but not value of sexuality, a history of sexual trauma which is a shameful secret, or a hidden health issue such as an eating disorder or bipolar disorder. Understanding each partner's psychological, relational, and sexual strengths and vulnerabilities is crucial for treatment planning and a successful outcome.

The fourth session in the assessment model is a 90-minute couple feedback session where the clinician has three areas of focus:

1. Sharing a genuine individual narrative with each partner, with the other present, involving processing past and present psychological, relational, and sexual issues.
2. Discussing couple sexual strengths and vulnerabilities. Establishing a therapeutic plan with mutually acceptable goals.

3. Assigning the first psychosexual skill exercise to be completed in the privacy of the couple's home. The message is that half of the therapy occurs in the therapist's office (including when to implement the medical intervention), and the other half of the change process occurs in the reality of the couple's home [13]. There is neither nudity nor touching in the clinician's office, but it is crucial to implement a new couple sexual style in the couple's home.

The issue of integrating medical interventions into the couple's sexual style of intimacy, pleasuring, and eroticism is discussed in the couple feedback session and is a focus for discussion and implementation in therapy. The danger of the biomedical model, where the physician sees the patient alone and asks the yes-no question "Is sex ok?" or "Are there any problems?" is that the patient, especially the man, will give the easy, socially desirable response that everything is ok. However, if the therapist or physician has both partners in the office and asks an open-ended question such as "At this time, how are desire, pleasure, eroticism, and satisfaction progressing? What is going best and what is most problematic?" This encourages the couple to be forthcoming and specific about individual and couple sexuality so that the intervention can be modified and tailored for the couple's needs.

Sex therapy is more focused, time-limited, and change-oriented than most couple therapy. Although there is a range of interventions from a single couple consultation to therapy lasting years, the most typical format is therapy involving 6–25 sessions over a 3-month to 1-year period. Typically, couple therapy begins on a weekly basis, but sessions usually transition to biweekly within 4–6 weeks.

A special feature is an individualized relapse prevention program to ensure gains are maintained and couple sexuality continues to have a 15–20 % role in relationship vitality and satisfaction. Ideally, the couple can call for a booster session to ensure a lapse does not turn into a relapse. Hopefully, the couple would schedule follow-up sessions every 6 months over a 2-year period. The follow-up sessions involve discussing the couple's sexual style to reinforce the desire, pleasure, eroticism, and satisfaction mantra as well as establish a new goal for the next 6 months to facilitate continued sexual growth. The core focus is on strong, resilient sexual desire.

33.2 Case Study: Alexis and Alexander

Forty-four year-old Alexis and 52-year-old Alexander were an alienated, demoralized couple when they appeared for sex therapy. This was a second marriage for both. They married 4 years ago, but the marriage was clearly headed toward divorce due to being nonsexual as a result of Alexander's struggles with ED. The referral for therapy came from the third urologist Alexander had consulted. He was afraid that Alexander's tearfulness in the individual consultation could indicate a suicide risk. This urologist had recommended a third-level intervention—a penile prosthesis. Over the past 3 years, Alexander had tried Viagra, Cialis, MUSE, and penile injections, but found only fleeting improvement and then a regression. Over the 3 years, Alexander had consulted three urologists, an internist, an endocrinologist, a cardiologist, and a psychiatrist. Only the psychiatrist had asked to see Alexis for one individual consultation.

When Alexander called the sex therapist, he was seeking an individual appointment, but the therapist suggested the four-session assessment approach, with the first session being with the couple.

In the first couple session, the therapist asked whether desire, pleasure, eroticism, and satisfaction had ever been a part of Alexander and Alexis's relationship. Sexuality had been a major strength and a factor in taking the risk to commit to a second marriage. Alexis felt left out of the medical consultations and interventions, and it was she who was threatening to leave the marriage. Her feeling was that no matter what Alexander said, he no longer found her attractive nor did he love her. She did not think surgery was a good idea nor would it resolve the core issue of lack of love and desire. Alexander felt blamed and shamed. He did not want to be divorced a second time, but felt besieged by Alexis's negativity. She had become his worst critic and blamed him for anything that was wrong. The destructive sexual power struggle dominated their relationship.

In the first session, each person is asked to sign release of information form(s) so the therapist can contact past or present, individual or couple, and medical or mental health providers. The perspective of other clinicians and their treatment suggestions can be of value. Rather than wait for a written report, the clinician calls the medical and/or mental health professionals.

A second suggestion for the initial session is to provide the couple with reading not to exceed 20 pages. Reading does not cure a dysfunction, but it serves to destigmatize the problem. For example, it was helpful for Alexis to learn that one in five married couples have a nonsexual marriage (i.e., sex less than ten times a year), most commonly occurring within the first 2 years of the marriage. In addition, learning that few men experience the dramatic turnaround with Viagra illustrated in the television advertisements served to reassure the couple that they were not alone.

The individual psychological/relational/sexual history (sessions two and three) begins with the therapist saying, "I appreciate you being as honest and forthcoming as possible about your life both before this marriage and since you became a couple. At the end, you can red flag anything you do not want shared with your spouse. I will not share this without your permission. I do need to know as much as possible to help you understand and change this difficult sexual situation." Like 85 % of couples, both Alexis and Alexander had sensitive/secret material.

In conducting the history, it is crucial to ask open-ended questions and to elicit the genuine stories, including confusing, sad, or traumatic experiences. For example, rather than asking, "Have you ever had an affair?" the question is, "The majority of people have thoughts, feelings, fantasies, or experiences of being sexual outside their marriage. Tell me about your experiences." Another example is, "Before leaving home, what was the most confusing, negative, guilt-inducing, or traumatic experience that happened to you sexually or emotionally?"

A core issue in Alexander's history was the humiliation he endured during his first intercourse attempt (ejaculation prior to intromission). His first marriage ended because his ex-wife found marital sex dull and routine and had an affair. Alexander now frequented massage parlors twice a month and paid extra for manual stimulation to orgasm (he had an erection). He loved her, but resented her criticalness, especially sexually.

Alexis had a very different set of vulnerabilities. As an adolescent, she had two abortions, which she had never discussed with her first husband or Alexander. She had used an affair (in her first marriage) as a reason to leave a fatally flawed marriage. Alexander's sexual enthusiasm and desire were a major motivator for Alexis to take the risk of a second marriage. Although she loved Alexander, she felt the ED was a sign the marriage was doomed. She was confused that Alexander could become erect but quickly lost his erection when she touched him. She was very hurt that he was unwilling to pleasure her to orgasm, although she had never asked.

The clinician lobbied each partner to share sensitive and vulnerable issues to help motivate them to work together in changing the nonsexual state of their marriage. Both Alexander and Alexis agreed to share sensitive/secret material at the couple feedback session.

The challenge for Alexis and Alexander was to rebuild sexual desire and address ED as an intimate sexual team. In the couple feedback session (session four), we processed each partner's sexual narrative in order to understand and change the pattern of sexual avoidance. This involved Alexis understanding that Alexander's ED was caused by a combination of physiological vulnerability, anticipatory anxiety, and approaching intercourse as a pass-fail performance test. Alexis had a vital role in helping them develop a new couple sexual style focused on sharing pleasure and adopting the GES approach in order to confront performance anxiety.

For Alexander, the challenge was to turn toward Alexis as his intimate and erotic ally and accept the GES approach that 85 % of sexual encounters will flow to intercourse and orgasm. When sexuality does not flow to intercourse, he is open to sensual or erotic alternative scenarios, rather than panicking or apologizing. A core challenge for Alexander was to rebuild sexual desire based on being present and sharing pleasure-oriented touching.

In the ongoing therapy sessions, mostly conducted with the couple (although the therapist recommended that Alexander and Alexis ask for an individual session as needed), the focus was on revitalizing sexual desire, developing the complementary couple sexual style which balanced each partner's sexual autonomy with being an intimate sexual team, and learning to value both synchronous sexual encounters (both Alexander and Alexis experience desire, pleasure, eroticism, and satisfaction) with asynchronous scenarios (the experience was better for one partner than the other). A major breakthrough for Alexander was experiencing that Alexis could enjoy an erotic scenario to orgasm with manual and/or oral stimulation. He learned to "piggyback" his arousal on her arousal.

The change process was neither easy nor straightforward. There were emotional and sexual successes intermixed with frustration and disappointment. At the therapist's urging, Alexander, accompanied by Alexis, was referred to a new urologist who recommended they utilize a daily low dose of Cialis for a 3-month trial period. This urologist reinforced positive, realistic GES expectations rather than overpromising a return to 100 % predictable erections and intercourse. Alexis made the point to Alexander that even when couple sex was at its best early in their relationship, she was not orgasmic 100 % of the time. In addition, Alexis was similar to a great many women, although she valued orgasm during intercourse, her orgasmic response was easier, both in frequency and intensity, through erotic stimulation.

In the 3-month follow-up session with the urologist, Alexis and Alexander queried about the option of using regular dose Cialis on an as-needed basis. The urologist was willing to try that regimen, but since the present regimen was working so well, he recommended maintaining the daily dose.

A particularly valuable component of the couple integrative biopsychosocial model is the individualized relapse prevention plan. In most health and mental health treatment programs, relapse prevention is ignored or the problem is dealt with by focusing on medications and dosage. Developing an individualized relapse prevention program is an integral component of the couple biopsychosocial model. Sexuality, especially ED and desire problems, cannot be treated with benign neglect. Healthy couple sexuality requires thought, energy, and communication. Alexis and Alexander agreed to three dimensions in their relapse prevention plan: (1) quarterly, they would have a sensual date with a prohibition on intercourse and orgasm to reinforce sensuality as a shared pleasure; (2) if they went 3 weeks without a positive sexual experience, they would schedule a "booster" session to ensure a lapse did not become a relapse; and (3) they would schedule a follow-up session every 6 months for 2 years in order to ensure they maintain gains and set new sexual goals aimed at reinforcing their commitment to a vital, resilient, sexual desire.

33.3 Summary

The comprehensive integrated couple biopsychosocial model for sexual dysfunction includes couple sex therapy as the core dimension. The physician, couple therapist, and other professionals work as a respectful, collaborative team as they engage in a comprehensive assessment, treatment, and relapse prevention program for sexual problems. The prime client is the couple rather than the individual. The focus is not on individual sex dysfunction, but building desire, pleasure, eroticism, and satisfaction. In assessment and treatment, the biological, psychological, and relational factors that subvert sexuality are confronted, and the biological, psychological, and relational factors that promote healthy couple sexuality are reinforced. Rather than hoping for a "cure" and a return to "normal" sexual performance with totally predictable erections and intercourse for the man and totally predictable orgasms, ideally during intercourse, for the woman, there is an acceptance of the inherent variability and flexibility of couple sexuality. The GES approach and expectations are a key to maintaining sexual desire and satisfaction while accepting the complexity of roles and meanings for couple sexuality.

References

1. Goldstein I, Lue T, Padma-Nathan H, Rosen R, Steers W, Wicker P. Oral sildenafil in the treatment of erectile dysfunction. N Engl J Med. 1998;338:1397–404.
2. Rowland D. Will medical solutions to sexual problems make sexological care and science obsolete? J Sex Marital Ther. 2007;33:385–97.
3. Leiblum S. After sildenafil: bridging the gap between pharmacological treatment and satisfying sexual relationships. J Clin Psychiatry. 2002;63:17–22.
4. Metz M, McCarthy B. The "Good Enough Sex" (GES) model. In: Kleinplatz P, editor. New directions in sex therapy. 2nd ed. New York: Routledge; 2012.
5. Berry M. Historical revolutions in sex therapy. J Sex Marital Ther. 2013;39:21–39.
6. Foley S, Kope S, Sugrue D. Sex matters for women. 2nd ed. New York: Guildford; 2012.
7. Waldinger M. Lifelong premature ejaculation. World J Urol. 2005;23:102–8.
8. Rosen R, McKenna K. PDE-5 inhibition and sexual response: pharmacological mechanisms and clinical outcomes. Annu Rev Sex Res. 2002;13:36–88.
9. McCarthy B, McDonald D. Assessment, treatment, and relapse prevention: male hypoactive sexual desire disorder. J Sex Marital Ther. 2009;35:58–67.
10. McCarthy B, Fucito L. Integrating medication, realistic expectations, and therapeutic interventions in the treatment of male sexual dysfunction. J Sex Marital Ther. 2005;31:319–28.
11. McCarthy B, Wald LM. Sexual desire and satisfaction: the balance between individual and couple factors. Sex Relat Ther. 2012;27(4):310–21.
12. McCarthy B, Thestrup M. Couple therapy and the treatment of sexual dysfunction. In: Gurman A, editor. Clinical handbook of couple therapy. 4th ed. New York: Guilford; 2008.
13. McCarthy B, McCarthy E. Sexual awareness. 5th ed. New York: Routledge; 2012.

The Intersection of Sexually Transmitted Infection and Sexual Disorders in the Couple

34

William Fisher

> *Sex therapists are in the business of restoring sexual function and enabling sexual behavior. Sexual behavior, however, may take place in the context of the risk of contracting a sexually transmitted infection (STI), the subjective fear of contracting an STI, the acute acquisition of an STI, or the chronic carriage of an STI, each of which may result in a cascade of negative effects on the couple's sexual and relationship health.*
>
> Fisher and Holzapfel (2014)

Sexually transmitted infection (STI) concerns may profoundly influence the sexual and relationship health of the individual and the couple. This chapter reviews clinical scenarios in which STI issues may play an important role in the etiology, maintenance, and exacerbation of sexual and relationship dysfunction in the couple context. We explore the psychological and relationship impacts of STIs on individuals and their partners and consider counseling principles that may prove useful in working with men and women who are dealing with STI-related sexual and relationship problems.

34.1 Case Study

Cindy and Eric are in their late 30s and have been married for 5 years. They wish to have a child and have attempted to conceive for 6 months without result. Frustrated, the couple underwent fertility investigation and was advised that they will have difficulty conceiving due to tubal factor problems. They have been referred for IVF but are unsure about the invasive procedures, expense, and uncertain outcome. Cindy's level of sexual desire, never strong, has waned, provoking conflict with Eric, further downward spiral in Cindy's sexual interest, and her eventual complete withdrawal from sexual contact. Miserable, Cindy and Eric present at the sexual medicine clinic to seek help for what they conceive to be her problem with absent desire. As a routine part of Cindy's individual interview, her physician asks, "Is there anything else I should know that might help me understand the issues you two are dealing with?" Cindy reports that when she was in college, she was diagnosed with chlamydia and treated for pelvic inflammatory disease. She adds that she has had deep pelvic pain since this episode, making intercourse uncomfortable, and that now, with tubal factor infertility, she feels she is "paying for past behavior." Her husband is not aware of this history. As a routine part of Eric's individual interview, the physician asks, "Is there anything else I should know that might help me understand the issues that you and your partner are dealing with?" Eric informs the physician that, since Cindy's withdrawal from sex, he has had a one-time affair with a coworker. "I'm terrified I caught something. I'm terrified I'll give her something! I want you to test me for *everything*. Now!"

W. Fisher, Ph.D. (✉)
Department of Psychology, University of Western Ontario, London, Ontario, Canada

Department of Obstetrics and Gynaecology, University of Western Ontario, London, Ontario, Canada
e-mail: fisher@uwo.ca

L.I. Lipshultz et al. (eds.), *Management of Sexual Dysfunction in Men and Women*, DOI 10.1007/978-1-4939-3100-2_34

As this case study illustrates, STI issues, individual, partner, or both and historical, concurrent, or both, may be of pivotal importance in the management of sexual and relationship dysfunction. Beyond case illustrations, systematic evidence concerning the impact of STI on sexual and relationship health has been reported, and relevant findings are considered in the section that follows.

34.2 Impact of STI on Sexual Function and Relationship Health

A number of general reviews of the impact of STI on sexual function have appeared in recent years [1–4]. Perusal of this work leads to a number of conclusions concerning the impact of STI on the couple. First, nearly all research concerning STI and sexual function focuses on the individual, not the couple, though there are very clear implications of STI impact on the individual that may reasonably be assumed to affect the sexual and relationship health of the couple. Second, there is very little population-based research concerning the association of STI and sexual dysfunction in representative national samples, although when such research is conducted, associations between STI and sexual function have been observed. Third, it appears that the sexual and relationship implications of infection with bacterial STI, which may readily be cured, may differ considerably from the implications of infection with viral STIs, which are not curable and which may result in chronic carriage and couple discordance of infection. Finally, it is often the case that clinicians who manage sexual dysfunction in men, women, and couples require "…a foundation of knowledge concerning STI prevention, prevalence, natural history, testing, treatment, and sexual and medical sequelae in order to be able to provide competent care in relevant situations" although this has not consistently been the standard of training or care in sex therapy or sexual medicine [1].

With respect to bacterial STI, a number of clinical issues are relevant. First, bacterial STIs, including chlamydia and gonorrhea, are often asymptomatic, and may be detected, to the potential shock and surprise of the individual, in the context of screening as opposed to symptomatic presentation [5]. Given asymptomatic carriage over varying periods of time, issues of the source of infection and transmission to sexual partners may be ambiguous [6, 7], and caution is warranted in relation to false-positive screening results in low prevalence populations [4, 7]. What is not in doubt, however, is occurrence of the negative impact of bacterial STI on the individual and often by extension on the couple. Gottleib et al. [7] enrolled 1807 women who were undergoing routine chlamydia testing as part of family planning clinic appointments, some 8.8 % of who tested positive for infection. At 4- to 6-week follow-up, chlamydia-positive women showed a 75 % increase from baseline in anxiety about sexual aspects of their life on a validated survey instrument. Nearly all of the women (99 %) who tested positive for chlamydia were worried that they could have been exposed to other STIs, 87 % felt it would be difficult to trust future partners, more than 75 % stated that they were "not very proud of their actions," more than two-thirds felt betrayed by their partner, and substantial numbers of chlamydia-positive women were angry, afraid to tell their partner, and concerned about future fertility. At follow-up, three times as many chlamydia-positive women as chlamydia negative had broken up with their relationship partner. Duncan et al. [6] report similar findings for self-disgust and anxiety about the male partner and concern about future fertility in qualitative research with a smaller sample of women who tested positive for chlamydia. We note that a history of chlamydia or other bacterial STI may serve as a predisposing factor in future development of sexual and relationship dysfunction precipitated by contemporaneous events. We note as well that diagnosis of chlamydia or other bacterial STI, whether as the result of screening and identification of past infection or acute symptomatic presentation of current infection as a result of extra-relationship sexual contact, may precipitate relationship crisis [1].

With respect to the impact of viral—and therefore manageable, but not curable—STI, research concerning the impact of herpes simplex virus (HSV), human papillomavirus (HPV), and human immunodeficiency virus (HIV) on sexual and relationship health is informative. Sexual and relationship impact of viral STI infection may stem from the infection and its clinical symptoms; anxiety about chronic carriage of the virus; concerns about transmission of the virus to or from a sexual partner or during childbirth; extended, painful, and sometimes ineffective treatment of symptoms; and direct iatrogenic impact of pharmacotherapy of the infection [4, 8–10].

Mindel and Marks [3] have reviewed the literature concerning the psychosexual impact of HSV infection, noting that genital herpes is a common, chronic, and recurrent challenge. Within the limitations of existing research—which include focus on clinical samples and lack of controls—it appears to be the case that individuals with herpes may experience depression, anger, diminished self-esteem, hostility toward the partner perceived to be the source of infection, and fear of transmission to others. Research suggests that individuals experiencing a first episode may be particularly affected, while individuals who have lived with HSV for a length of time may have learned to cope with it better, but at the same time, those with recurrent HSV outbreaks may continue to experience psychosexual challenge at significant levels. Mindel and Marks [3] review directs special attention to the availability of serological testing for HSV and to the potential for psychosexual morbidity among those testing positive who have no history of herpes infection. In this connection, Melville et al. [11] conducted qualitative research with 24 individuals who tested positive for HSV-2 and who had no clinical history of disease. Short-term emotional responses to the herpes diagnosis included surprise, distress, and self-blame, and importantly, long-term concerns included worries about partner acceptance, concern about transmitting HSV infection to the partner, feeling sexually undesirable, feeling like damaged goods, avoidance of sex, and relationship problems after diagnosis. Mindel and Marks [3] suggest that management of psychosocial consequences of HSV infection can include rapid diagnosis, accurate information about the infection and its consequences, strategies for reducing the risk of transmission to others, advice about antiviral suppressive treatments to limit recurrence, and psychological support, including cognitive behavioral therapy to alter affected individuals' way of thinking about herpes and means of coping with the infection. Online support and community-based support groups are also available [12].

Studies of the psychosexual impact of HPV infection have appeared both before [9, 13] and after [14–18] availability of HPV vaccine protection and movement toward routine HPV DNA screening as a cervical cancer screening approach [5, 19]. From the perspective of challenge to couple sexual and relationship health, it is important to note that HPV infection is exceedingly prevalent, it may spontaneously clear or remain chronic, and it may be asymptomatic or result in the appearance of genital warts (low-risk HPV types), cervical dysplasia and cervical, vulvar, oropharyngeal, penile, and anal cancer (high-risk HPV types) [5]. HPV infection may also be transmitted from mother to infant, though rarely, resulting in recurrent pharyngeal papillomatosis [20].

The occurrence of each of the pathological sequelae of HPV infection—as well as worry about the possible future occurrence of these outcomes—may predispose, maintain, or exacerbate sexual and relationship problems. Graziottin and Serafini's [15] review of psychosexual consequences of HPV infection highlights challenges that include depression, anxiety, and anger, feeling worse about one's sexual relationship, concern over "who infected who," and sexual problems specifically associated with HPV-related genital warts and their repeated and painful treatment. Individual studies of psychosexual impact of HPV diagnosis may be particularly informative. For example, Daley and colleagues [14] examined the effect of HPV infection in a sample of HPV-positive women who attended routine gynecological examinations that included Pap tests that, if abnormal, were followed up with HPV DNA testing. Findings revealed impacts of HPV infection that have significant implications for couples' sexual function and relationship health, including stigma (70 % of HPV-positive women worried that people would judge them), shame (68 %), feeling that they are paying for past behavior (68 %), feeling "unclean" (59 %), and reporting that "having HPV in my body is disgusting to me" (55 %). Drolet et al. [21] evaluated the psychological status of a large group of women who received abnormal cervical smear results indicative of HPV infection compared to a control group of women with normal cervical smears. Findings indicated both immediate and sustained impact of abnormal cervical smear results on women's anxiety level and on each measured dimension of an HPV Impact Profile [22] including emotional impact, self-image, sexual impact, and concern about partner and transmission issues. In related research, Drolet et al. [17] examined the psychosexual reactions of men and women who were undergoing treatment for HPV-related genital warts. Findings indicated significant elevations in anxiety and depression, pain and discomfort, and multiple dimensions on the HPV Impact Profile [22] including sexual activity, worries about partner and transmission of infection, and self-image. Negative impacts of HPV-related genital warts persisted for as long as the warts persisted. Notably, at 6-month follow-up, 51 % of participants—all of whom had received treatment—still had genital warts and elevated psychosexual challenge. Findings indicated similar negative psychological and sexual impact on men and women and similar impact from initial compared to recurrent episodes of genital warts. Also of relevance to sexual and relationship health of the couple are findings concerning disclosure and nondisclosure of HPV infection to a partner, although the efficacy of partner disclosure for prevention of transmission has not been demonstrated [23]. Some 66 % of HPV-positive women in Daley et al.'s [14] research indicated that they would disclose their HPV status to a future sex partner (though at the time of participation in this research, only 39 % had actually informed their partner) and 26 % were unsure about whether they would disclose their HPV infection to their partner. In an interesting parallel, Arima et al. [18] enrolled university student men in a longitudinal study, testing periodically for incident HPV infection and assessing whether men with incident infection disclosed this to their partner. Men with incident HPV infections reported disclosing to their partner in 31 % of affected partnerships.

As cervical cancer screening moves toward routine reliance on HPV DNA testing [19], it is critical to note that a substantial proportion of midlife women will test positive for HPV infection at midlife as the result of chronic carriage of much earlier infection [1, 5]. HPV diagnoses may thus be expected to increase substantially in future years with a corresponding increase in negative sexual and relationship impact on the couple. Specific illustration of sexual and relationship impact of an HPV diagnosis is provided in a venerable study by Campion and colleagues [13]. These investigators evaluated women who had HPV infection, with or without cervical intraepithelial neoplasia (CIN). Compared to controls, women with HPV infection or HPV and CIN reported substantial declines in spontaneous sexual interest, frequency of intercourse, adequacy of vaginal lubrication and sexual arousal, frequency of orgasm, and a substantial increase in painful intercourse. Critically, with respect to relationship health, women with HPV infection or HPV and CIN reported a substantial increase in negative feelings about sexual intercourse with their current partner or (if there was no current partner, toward intercourse in general), compared to controls. McCaffery and colleagues [16] report similar negative impact of HPV infection on feelings about sexual partners: "… HPV+ women demonstrated significantly greater concerns about their sexual relationships than women who tested HPV−…These findings are suggestive of a marked negative impact on feelings about sexual relationships among women who were HPV+" [16].

To provide some balance to this litany of negative effects of STIs on sexual and relationship health, we note that close reading of the literature suggests there may also be reasons for some degree of optimism. Clinical case reports of the management of HPV infection [9] indicate that specific clinical care steps—including crisis management upon diagnosis, if necessary; supportive counseling to empower the patient to take an active role in managing their infection and avoiding transmission; and clinical education concerning optimal medical follow-up—may represent a comprehensive approach to facilitating better outcomes over the longer term. Clearly, in relevant cases of affected couples, couple counseling could be added to this mix at each level of crisis management, empowerment, and education of patient and partner. Other reasons for a measure of optimum have surfaced as well [14]. Daley et al. [14] found that—in addition to multiple negative impacts of HPV diagnosis—some 52 % of women diagnosed with HPV reported feeling *closer* to their partner. Drolet et al.'s [17] report that within the broadly negative impact of an abnormal cervical smear on quality of life, anxiety, and sexual functioning and partner and transmission concerns, significant improvements were observed in each of these indicators at a 12-week follow-up interval, although each was still negatively impacted compared to controls. Drolet et al. [21] also report that the negative impact of anogenital warts resolved among the roughly 50 % of their affected sample of men and women whose warts were no longer present at follow-up. These findings for improvement with comprehensive and appropriate clinical care, time, and treatment progress may provide the basis for a measure of evidence-based optimism that can be conveyed to affected patients and partners.

HIV infection may represent an extreme version of the impact of chronic carriage of viral STI on couple sexual and relationship health. HIV infection is associated with sexual dysfunctions in men, including erectile dysfunction and low sexual desire [8, 24], as well as in women [25–27], for reasons that include the effects of HIV infection on sexual function; the effects of HIV antiretroviral (ARV) therapy on sexual function; the effects of HIV and ARV on body fat distribution, body image, and perceived attractiveness; HIV stigma; HIV-related depression; the HIV concordance or discordance of the couple; and the fear of transmission to others. As is the case with other STIs, individual and couple management may benefit from clinical education, treatment of HIV disease, and counseling concerning reduction of transmission risk, which in the case of HIV will involve adherence to ARV therapy, achievement of undetectable viral load, and consistent use of condoms. We note that meta-analytic evidence exists to support the effectiveness of cognitive behavioral therapy in improving the psychological health of HIV-infected individuals [28].

34.3 Counseling Principles at the Intersection of STI and Couple Sexual and Relationship Function

This review has considered a wide array of systematic evidence concerning the effect of STIs on an individual's sexual health and on the couple sexual relationship. We conclude with suggestions for management of couples whose sexual and relationship health is challenged by STI-related issues [1].

1. STI-related concerns may predispose, precipitate, maintain, or exacerbate couple sexual and relationship problems. It may prove valuable to routinely evaluate concurrent or historical STI issues and concerns of couple members.
2. STI screening and testing can indicate when an STI is present, but cannot always definitively state when and from whom the infection was contracted.
3. Clinicians may deal with couples in which an STI acquired historically, or sequelae of an STI acquired historically, surfaces within a relationship. The clinician can inform the couple that the infection is historical and does not represent relationship infidelity.
4. Clinicians may also deal with situations in which an acute STI acquired in extra-relationship sexual contact provokes a primary relationship crisis.
5. Clinicians managing acute or historical STI may systematically attend to crisis management, education concerning the infection to empower the patient and the partner to adapt to living with the infection, and medically relevant information concerning prevention of

transmission and self-care going forward, as may be relevant.

6. Clinicians may find that management of the sexual and relationship impact of STI on the couple benefits from comanagement with complementary clinical skills. Depending upon the clinician's training and experience, comanagement of the couple affected by STI issues may involve clinical teamwork with infectious disease specialists, couple therapists, and cognitive behavioral psychotherapists, among others.
7. The occurrence of negative impact of STIs on couple sexual and relationship function appears to be common. Accordingly, clinicians may seek foundational knowledge in STI prevention, prevalence, natural history, testing, treatment, and sexual and medical sequelae in order to be able to provide competent care for affected individuals and couples.
8. As a final point, we remind clinicians that effective sex therapy may facilitate sexual behavior in clients who will subsequently be exposed to STI risk. Clinicians should consider STI risk and provide STI prevention counseling in relevant situations.

References

1. Fisher WA, Holzapfel S. Suppose they gave an epidemic and sex therapy didn't attend? Sexually transmitted infection concerns in the sex therapy context. In: Binik YM, Hall KSK, editors. Principles and practice of sex therapy. 5th ed. New York: Guilford; 2014.
2. Mercer CH, Fenton KA, Johnson AM, Copas AJ, Macdowall W, Erens B, Wellings K. Who reports sexual function problems? Empirical evidence from Britain's 2000 National Survey of Sexual Attitudes and Lifestyles. Sex Transm Infect. 2005;81:394–9.
3. Mindel A, Marks C. Psychological symptoms associated with genital herpes virus infections. Epidemiology and approaches to management. CNS Drugs. 2005; 19(4):303–12.
4. Sadeghi-Nejad H, Wasserman M, Weidner W, Richardson D, Goldmeier D. Sexually transmitted diseases and sexual function. Journal of Sexual Medicine. 2010;7:389–413.
5. Fisher WA, Steben M. Sexually transmitted infection: at the junction of biology and behavior. In: Puckall C, editor. Human sexuality. Research and theory. Oxford: Oxford University Press; 2014.
6. Duncan B, Hart G, Scoular A, Bigrig A. Qualitative analysis of psychosocial impact of diagnosis of *Chlamydia trachomatis*: implications for screening. Br Med J. 2001;322:195–9.
7. Gottlieb SL, Stoner BP, Zaidi AA, Buckel C, Tran M, Leichliter JS, Berman SM, Markowitz LE. A prospective study of the psychosocial impact of a positive chlamydia trachomatis laboratory test. Sex Transm Dis. 2011;38(11):1004–11.
8. Asboe D, Catalan J, Mandalia S, Dedes N, Florence E, Schrooten W, et al. Sexual dysfunction in HIV-positive men is multi-factorial: a study of prevalence and associated factors. AIDS Care. 2007;19(8): 955–65.
9. Linnehan MJ, Groce E. Counseling and educational interventions for women with genital human papillomavirus infection. AIDS Patient Care STDs. 2000; 14(8):439–45.
10. Shindel AW, Horberg MA, Smith JF, Breyer BN. Sexual dysfunction, HIV, and AIDS in men who have sex with men. AIDS Patient Care STDS. 2011;6:341–9.
11. Melville J, Sniffen S, Crosby R, Salazar L, Whittington D, Dithmer-Schreck D, DiClemente R, Wald A. Psychosocial impact of serological diagnosis of herpes simplex virus type 2: a qualitative assessment. Sex Transm Infect. 2003;79:280–5.
12. Gupta R, Warren T, Wald A. Genital herpes. Lancet. 2007;370:2127–37.
13. Campion MJ, Brown JR, McCance DJ, Atia W, Edwards R, Cuzick J, Singer A. Psychosexual trauma of an abnormal cervical smear. Br J Obstet Gynaecol. 1988;95:175–81.
14. Daley EM, Perrin KM, McDermott RJ, Vamos CA, Rayko HL, Packing-Ebuen JL. The psychosocial burden of HPV. J Health Psychol. 2010;15(2):279–90.
15. Graziottin A, Serafini A. HPV infection in women: psychosexual impact of genital warts and intraepithelial lesions. J Sex Med. 2009;6:633–45.
16. McCaffery K, Waller J, Forrest S, Cadman L, Szarewski A, Wardle J. Testing positive for human papillomavirus in routine cervical screening: examination of psychosocial impact. Br J Obstet Gynaecol. 2004;111:1437–43.
17. Drolet M, Brisson M, Maunsell E, Franco EL, Coutlee F, Ferenczy E, Ratnam S, Fisher WA, Mansi JA. The impact of anogenital warts on health-related quality of life: a 6-month prospective study. Sex Transm Dis. 2011;38(10):949–56.
18. Arima T, Winer R, Kurth AE, Martin DP, Hughs JP, Stern ME, et al. Disclosure of genital human papillomavirus infection to sex partners by young men. Sex Transm Dis. 2012;39(8):583–7.
19. Cuzick J, Clavel C, Petry K-U, Meijer CJLM, Hoyer H, Ratnam S, et al. Overview of the European and North American studies on HPV testing in primary cervical cancer screening. Int J Cancer. 2006;119: 1095–101.
20. Derkay CS, Darrow DH. Recurrent respiratory papillomatosis. Ann Oncol Rhinol Laryngol. 2006;115(1): 1–11.

21. Drolet M, Brisson M, Maunsell E, Franco EL, Coutlee F, Ferenczy A, Fisher WA, Mansi JA. The psychosocial impact of an abnormal cervical smear result. Psycho-Oncology. 2012;21(10):1071–81.
22. Mast TC, Zhu X, Demuro-Mercon C, Cummings HW, Sings HL, Ferris DG. Development and psychometric properties of the HPV impact profile (HIP) to assess the psychosocial burden of HPV. Curr Med Res Opin. 2009;25(11):2609–19.
23. Canadian Guidelines on Sexually Transmitted Infections. 2014. Downloaded 19 Sept 2014 http://www.phac-aspc.gc.ca/std-mts/sti-its/
24. Lamba H, Goldmeier D, Mackie NE, Scullard G. Antiretroviral therapy is associated with sexual dysfunction and with increased serum oestradiol levels in men. Int J STD AIDS. 2010;15:234–7.
25. Florence F, Schrooten W, Dreezen C, Gordillo V, Schonnesson LN, Asboe D, The Eurosupport Study Group. Prevalence and factors associated with sexual dysfunction among HIV-positive women in Europe. AIDS Care. 2004;16(5):550–7.
26. Luzi K, Guaraldi G, Murri R, De Paola M, Orlando G, Squillace N, et al. Body image is a major determinant of sexual dysfunction in stable HIV-infected women. Antivir Ther. 2009;14:85–92.
27. Siegel K, Schrimshaw EE, Lekas H-M. Diminished sexual activity, interest, and feelings of attractiveness among HIV-infected women in two eras of the AIDS epidemic. Arch Sex Behav. 2006;35:437–49.
28. Crepaz N, Passin WF, Herbst JH, Rama SM, Mallow RM, Purcell DW, Wolistski RJ, The HIV/AIDS Prevention Research Synthesis (PRS) Team. Meta-analysis of cognitive-behavioral interventions on HIV-positive persons' mental health and immune functioning. Health Psychol. 2008;27(1):4–14.

Epilogue: Cautiously Optimistic for the Future of a Transdisciplinary Sexual Medicine

35

Michael A. Perelman

Sexuality, with its fundamental connection to reproduction, has been the subject of sustained and inordinate interest among all cultures since prehistoric ages. Sexual dysfunctions have been experienced as devastating problems to mankind since the beginning of recorded time, evidenced by Stone Age wall paintings and biblical references. The material contained in this volume's previous pages support sexual medicine as a postmodern, twenty-first-century solution to that prebiblical problem [1].

One cannot be anything but excited and extremely optimistic in the face of the huge progress made in the last two decades since the sildenafil clinical trials' success catalyzed a worldwide expansion of a sexual medicine subspecialty and simultaneously revitalized sex therapy[1] [2]. Given the advances in our knowledge about desire, arousal, ejaculation, and orgasm in women and men, there is no doubt that we will provide more optimal care for those suffering from the consequences of sexual disorders in the future by integrating appropriate use of medical and surgical techniques with adequate counseling.

The degree of advancement in our neurobiological, molecular, and genetic understanding of the mechanisms of sexual function and dysfunction at both the central and peripheral levels is extraordinary. There is no indication that this pace will slow down, and fortunately there is every indication that the rate at which we are accumulating such knowledge is accelerating. We are developing new pharmaceuticals for sexual indications at a speed unimaginable over 50 years ago when Masters and Johnson first published *Human Sexual Inadequacy* [3]. New technologies are in place as described in the Le and Burnett chapter to improve our treatments of erectile dysfunction. There is no drug approved for delayed ejaculation yet (nor is one in clinical trial at the time of this writing). However, there are a number of treatments for premature ejaculation that are being investigated and/or awaiting regulatory approval. The rapid advancement and use of novel, contemporary techniques in our ability to study animal models and patients with localized brain lesions provide much of our understanding about the neuroanatomical and biochemical pathways important for ejaculation and orgasm. With the emergence of

[1] While some referrals for ED were lost to mental health professionals, contrary to media hype, the introduction of sildenafil expanded opportunities for sex therapists. Sex therapy was reinvigorated with a new treatment tool, which expanded the number and range of individuals who could be restored to sexual health.

M.A. Perelman, Ph.D. (✉)
Psychiatry, Reproductive Medicine and Urology, Weill Medical College Cornell University, 70 East 77th Street, New York, NY 10075, USA

Co-Director, Human Sexuality Program, The New York Presbyterian Hospital, New York, NY, USA

Founder, MAP Education and Research Fund, New York, NY, USA
e-mail: michael@mapedfund.org

L.I. Lipshultz et al. (eds.), *Management of Sexual Dysfunction in Men and Women*, DOI 10.1007/978-1-4939-3100-2_35

noninvasive techniques including molecular-level resolution brain imaging and genetic analysis, there are opportunities to strengthen our current understanding and identify new central pathways that will lead to improved therapies for both men and women. Yet, there are potential downsides, which remain a source of concern for the professionalism and further maturation of our field.

35.1 Lack of a Sexual Health Formulary for Women

The lack of a robust sexual health formulary for women, particularly when juxtaposed against the number of products available for men, has been decried for years. In fact, the 2003 International Consultation held in Paris was a highly regarded professional milestone in the history of sexual medicine, in part because of the infamous debate on this topic between the English cardiologist Graham Jackson and the American psychologist Leonore Tiefer. Collaboration between major urology, sexual medicine, and sex therapy associations led to the assembly of more than 200 multidisciplinary experts (male and female) from five continents and 60 countries into 19 committees. The recommendations concerning state-of-the-art knowledge in the respective sexual medicine areas represented expert opinion developed over 2 years. This achievement reflected tremendous rebalancing of sexual medicine into a multidisciplinary movement [1]. Jackson and Tiefer debated whether "FSD was a construction of the pharmaceutical industry," the heart of public and professional concerns about the pharmaceuticalization and medicalization of sexual health in general and female sexual health specifically. The fine point was not whether women had sexual concerns and issues, but how they were defined, what gave rise to them, and what type of treatment (or not) they required. The US Food and Drug Administration's (FDA) failure to have approved a sex drug for women added much to the drama and legend.

Embedded for some was a "gender story" of a perceived overemphasis on male erection within the sexual medicine movement and a simultaneously held fear and concern regarding the commercialization of women's sexual complaints. Tiefer advocated a "new view of women's sexuality," [4] a collaborative grass roots effort of academic social scientists, therapists, and women's health activists. The audience declared Jackson the "winner," but Tiefer was ensconced as the iconic standard bearer of the "new view."

However, the situation for women is poised for improvement. In 2014, the FDA conducted a 2-day Patient-Focused Drug Development public meeting and scientific workshop on FSD. On day 1, the FDA was interested in obtaining patient input on the impact of the most common form of FSD, female sexual interest/arousal disorder (FSIAD) on daily life. In addition, the agency wanted to obtain patients' and some partners' views on currently available therapies to treat the condition. During the second day's workshop, the FDA facilitated discussions of the scientific challenges related to diagnosing the condition in both clinical trials and practice. There was further discussion about the importance of ensuring valid patient-reported outcome measures for the key efficacy end points used in clinical trials. Subsequent to that meeting, Sprout Pharmaceuticals resubmitted a new drug application (NDA) to the FDA for flibanserin, an investigational, once-daily, nonhormonal pill for hypoactive sexual desire disorder (HSDD) in premenopausal women. If approved, flibanserin would be the first and only FDA-approved treatment for any FSD.[2] Should that drug obtain regulatory approval, there is little doubt such success would be a watershed event that would trigger increased commercial funding for sex research and the next generation of sexual pharmaceuticals.

Whether one is for approval or not, the implications for sexual medicine and the public at

[2]On August 18, 2015 the U.S. Food and Drug Administration approved Addyi (flibanserin) to treat acquired, generalized hypoactive sexual desire disorder (HSDD) in premenopausal women, but with risk evaluation and mitigation strategies (REMS) required. "Today's approval provides women distressed by their low sexual desire with an approved treatment option," said Dr. Janet Woodcock, director of the FDA's Center for Drug Evaluation and Research (CDER) adding, "Because of a potentially serious interaction with alcohol, treatment with Addyi will only be available through certified health care professionals and certified pharmacies."

large will be profound. Yet, that meeting, like so many other issues in sexual medicine, was almost overwhelmed with controversy. Why?

35.2 Medicalization and Pharmaceuticalization

There are many reasons, but two are especially important, both the fear of medicalization and its related worry of pharmaceuticalization of normal variations of human sexual response. In part, this was a continuation of a century-old debate pitting reductionism against holism. The majority of professional societies concerned with the consequences of the FDA meeting supported the view that women should be offered the individual choice and opportunity to determine, with their healthcare professionals, what type of treatment would be best suited to help relieve their individual suffering. Other professionals and representatives of some women's organizations felt that flibanserin was insufficiently studied at that time to warrant approval, and they urged that the FDA should merely encourage the pursuit of more scientific knowledge about FSD. The debate about flibanserin is an important one in the history of sexual medicine, and the FDA meeting was a turning point regardless of the side one took. Yet, hidden within that conflict was another.

35.3 Who Are the Experts?

"Who are the experts" is one of the most important controversies dividing and perhaps defining the field of sexual medicine today. This important question determines who treats the problems, the nature of research, and how all is conceptualized. Throughout this book, those issues have been discussed both directly and at other times only tangentially and implicitly. Different healthcare specialists significantly and consistently reflect profession-of-origin bias. Some of those biases were offset in this book by the commentaries, allowing the readers to comprehend for themselves how to integrate the biological and psychosocial-behavioral and cultural components with sexual dysfunction diagnosis and treatment. Hopefully, this text laid the foundation for such integration, but inevitably a few oversimplifications appear within it. Yet, such lapses might be expected in a volume of this length, breadth, and depth. Generally, the mental health experts emphasized the importance of a biopsychosocial approach, often recognizing humanistic values. The urologists tended to emphasize better understanding of physiology, improved surgical techniques, new drugs to improve performance, and protocols for a variety of male-related illnesses and treatments with known sexual sequelae. Gynecologists emphasized the growing body of knowledge gained in understanding female sexual physiology, diagnosis, and treatments. All of the experts explicitly (or implicitly through citation) recognized the importance of the relatively recent emergence of sexual medicine professional societies (focused on men, women, or both) and the rise of learned journals devoted to this nascent specialization. So what is the problem, and what still remains a concern?

While the mission of this book is to advocate for a transdisciplinary approach where expertise is integrated for the benefit of the field and patients, not all stakeholders view sexual issues in the same light. Regrettably, many professionals continue to be unduly influenced by reports from some patients who previously had consulted with reportedly incompetent and judgmental sexual medicine practitioners, as well as sex therapists. Such experiences led them to seek interventions from practitioners of another discipline and to reject contact with members of the offending discipline. Moser [5] listed additional reasons for discord between disciplines: fears that another practitioner will "steal" their patients, mistrust of and/or disbelief in the other's approach, distrust of the other's motivation (e.g., beliefs that physicians are bought off by pharmaceutical companies and therapists are anti-physician), and fears that the other discipline will inordinately influence one's approach undesirably. It is to our field's detriment that few sex therapists attend conferences focusing on the latest advances in sexual medicine, and still fewer sexual medicine practitioners attend conferences focusing on the latest developments in sex therapy [1, 5].

Additionally, some mental health practitioners remain concerned whether or not sexual medicine as a profession will avoid falling again into the reductionist trap that characterized it from the 1980s through the beginning of the this new millennium. By 1984, our improved ability to diagnose organic pathology with sophisticated assessment devices led to a dramatic increase in the number of men undergoing surgical penile prosthesis placement. Why? Besides sex therapy, the primary treatment available to physicians at that time was surgery. There was substantial evidence that primary care physicians were becoming reluctant to refer cases for sex therapy, as the numbers of men with documented organic deficits increased. Yet, some of those deficits were minor and mirrored deficits found in the general population of men who were still able to function. Some men with ED experienced minor organic deficits escalating into very severe ED because of psychological and relational issues. Yet, frequently, the only solution offered by urologists in that presexual pharmaceutical era was surgery. Of course, the etiology of ED had not changed (it was always mental and physical), but the medical profession's and the lay public's outlook had shifted dramatically [1, 6].

Almost overnight, it seemed sexual disorders that were once considered a psychological problem were conceptualized as "purely a physical problem that required a medical solution." Initially, this was good for our field, as the 75-year emphasis from Freud through Masters and Johnson supporting a primarily psychological determination of sexual disorders had for too long overshadowed the biological factors that were proven to play such an important role. However, more rapidly than most mental health professionals could possibly imagine, that pendulum swung too far in the opposite direction. Was it really true, as many physicians then claimed in lectures and to the media, that "overwhelmingly 90 % of a sexual disorder's etiology was organic in origin?" Were there not alternative explanations and contributory factors, and if so, why were they not mentioned? The answer is an easy one: modern media and pharmaceutical marketing!

35.4 Modern Media and Marketing

Physician "thought leaders" who consulted to pharmaceutical companies were giving media interviews, arranged and facilitated by the public relations and marketing departments of the pharmaceutical companies who were manufacturing the most popularly prescribed vasoactive drugs and prostheses. Ironically, the very success of the medicalization of sexual concerns at that time also nurtured most of the public and professional controversies that surround the pharmaceutical treatment of sexual problems through today.

For a drug to receive FDA approval, there must be a "disease" that the drug addresses. For men in 1998, for instance, the branded disease du jour was "ED," and the drug was sildenafil. Furthermore, for a drug to receive acceptance in the medical community, an understandable narrative about its mechanism of action and evidence-based research supporting its efficacy and safety are all required. Tens of millions of dollars were spent proving that drugs do indeed successfully treat male erectile dysfunction. The vasoactive injectables were first, shortly followed by the same class of medication with a transurethral delivery system. Both were "safe and effective." However, they began to be abused and were later advertised as an easily available treatment for both ED and premature ejaculation (PE) often regardless of the actual etiology of the disorder [7]. These medical treatments and the PDE5 inhibitors (PDE5i's) that followed years later became the ubiquitous solution offered for any male sexual difficulty. Many found it cavalier and excessive that PDE5is were being overprescribed for every case of ED and other male sexual dysfunctions regardless of the diagnosis and the dysfunction's level of severity or its etiology.

Dismissed from public discourse and all but forgotten was the truism that every sexual disorder regardless of the severity of its organic etiology also has a psychosocial component: if not a causative one, certainly a consequence [6]. The media had a strong hand in this sea change, although those same promotions did usefully help open a dialogue between the public and the medical community about all aspects of human sexuality. However, nothing has changed the sexual landscape more than the anonymity and openness of the Internet [8]. Prior to the sildenafil launch, telecommunications and the Internet meaningfully amplified the controversy surrounding President Clinton's affair. In fact, the introduction of sildenafil, combined with the public investigation of President Clinton's extramarital behavior, changed the nature of polite discourse in the USA, if not the world [1]. What was once a private discussion between a man and his physician (or therapist) had become very public, replete with late-night television comedian commentary. The global media coverage of new techniques for restoring male sexual function was astounding, albeit often overly simplistic. The number of people reached was extraordinary. It became axiomatic in commercials and media interviews that "ED" was a disease you should discuss with your doctor. The exaggerated notion that psychological problems caused most sexual problems was replaced by the equally fallacious argument that sexual problems were the result almost exclusively of organic causes.

Many sex therapists were concerned that they would no longer have a viable role in the treatment of male ED. Many feared the medicalization of human sexuality that Tiefer had warned of years earlier would severely curtail their roles and access to patients [9]. McCarthy noted: "Some physicians and many in the media believe the introduction of sildenafil (Viagra™) is the death knell for sex therapy, at least with males [10]." The hyperbole was profound with some predicting that sex therapists would "soon become extinct, like dinosaurs" [1]. However, to paraphrase Mark Twain, early reports of our demise were greatly exaggerated [2].

All learned that men's desire for sex, the efficacy of PDE5i's, and men's interest in using them (also true for the vasoactive medications for penile injection therapy now used primarily for recalcitrant cases) could be adversely undermined by psychosocial-behavioral and cultural factors. Discontinuation rates as high as 50–60 % were reported in the literature, and greater emphasis and re-interest in relational and other psychological issues emerged within the sexual medicine and pharmaceutical communities [1, 11].

This all becomes particularly important in light of the transdisciplinary message articulated at the beginning of this book. It took the next 10 years for sex therapists and a few very knowledgeable urologists who specialized in sexual medicine to begin reshaping our understanding of etiology to one that had a better balance of both organic and psychogenic factors, e.g., "discontinuation issues" were not only caused by adverse events. These specialists brought to the understanding of sexual medicine the recognition that a binary, "is it organic or psychogenic?" is not the right question to be asked. Instead, one should be searching to identify the various underlying factors and try to determine their relative contributions. Etiology is almost always both mental and physical, but in varying proportions for every case of sexual dysfunction. Any other answer is usually a naive oversimplification.

Ironically though, it was the same pharmaceutical companies that had helped to exacerbate the problem that helped reverse the trend toward an overemphasis on the role of organicity. How? By the new millennium, Pharma had hired sex therapists as consultants to their advisory boards and put them on their speaker bureaus, in order to add a psychological balance to the sexual medicine equation. Funded by unrestricted educational grants, sex therapists spoke at medical meetings about sex coaching for physicians [12].[3] Pharmaceutical companies began looking at "partner issues" as relationship context emerged as a major factor in how successfully and

[3] Sex therapists have expanded their impact through public and colleague education. In terms of public education, media exposure broadened the scope, range, and size of the general audience who heard a sex therapy message integrated into open discussion. There was unprecedented opportunity with colleague education to reach non-sex therapy professionals with a psychological message. Primary care physicians and urologists learned that incorporating sex therapy techniques improved the effectiveness of sildenafil. Furthermore, sex therapists discovered that integrating adjunctive use of sildenafil with sex therapy accelerated the therapy process and improved outcome.

continuously their Pharma's drugs were used [13]. This led to the involvement of more female experts in sexual medicine who encouraged companies to also explore treatments for female sexual disorders. Pharma had initially funded ED epidemiological studies and later investigated the prevalence of other male sexual disorders. The sociologists, epidemiologists, and sexual medicine specialists who designed, ran, and analyzed those studies soon recognized and documented that women had as many, if not more, sexual problems than men [14]. This led to more research on women's sexual physiology, psychology, and treatments for their sexual dysfunctions as well as their inclusion in the leadership hierarchy of the 3rd International Consultation on Sexual Medicine (ICSM) mentioned earlier in this chapter, as well as the 2015 4th ICSM held in Madrid. By that time, the names and missions of the sexual medicine societies had expanded, including the International Society for Sexual Medicine (formerly the International Society for Impotence Research) and the 2001 formation of the International Society for the Study of Women's Sexual Health (ISSWSH). Journal mastheads brimmed with names of female sexual health experts, and journal content was expanded to focus on both male and female issues, as well as multiple treatment formats.

Whether Pharma's motivation was an altruistic search for a true understanding of sexual response across gender and culture for the benefit of mankind, or more cynically to identify and effectively secure and develop new markets, is a debate for others, although even that question is probably too binary and reflects the political and economic beliefs of those who choose to argue it. The result, however, was clear. Sexual medicine expanded and became more diverse and sophisticated. Urological and male hegemony was reduced. In fact, pharmaceutical companies again had a role as their drug "detail reps" (duplicating the marketing plan of SSRIs decades earlier) targeted primary care physicians and subsequently they, not urologists, became the largest prescribing cohort. So if journal editorships, reviewers, authors, presenters, and societies were now gender diverse and multidisciplinary, what is the concern?

35.5 We Are Once Again at a Crossroad

The aforementioned rebalancing took over two decades, but we are once again at a crossroad. Basic and early-stage clinical research using new investigative techniques including molecular imaging and genetic analysis will deepen our understanding of the biological underpinnings of sexual function and dysfunction. Such analysis uses sophisticated techniques that include, among others, whole-genome sequencing, neuroimaging with PET and fMRI studies, as well as better-quality plethysmography and thermography. Precision medicine and nanotechnology represent exciting trends and are some of the most interesting concepts of the day. But an influx of new biological discovery risks returns us to the unnecessary binary thinking that characterized the late twentieth century where many health professionals advocated an outdated, dichotomous, simplistic, etiological model of "organic versus psychological."

The increasingly contentious role of science and technology in modern society has given rise to controversies that often have profound social, political, and economic implications, and more and more often they feature public disagreements among scientific, technical, or medical experts [15]. What is the alternative to a back-to-the-future rush to overly reductionist thinking and an unnecessary binary view of the mental and physical? How can science advance and make the best use of the tremendous new opportunities that advanced technology makes available to creative and passionate investigators and clinicians? The answer lies in a transdisciplinary approach to sexual medicine.

We are on the cusp of being able to explain some of the varied findings that support and explain both the biological and psychological. We are actually coming closer to resolving the mind-body conundrum that has plagued philosophers for centuries.

For instance, there are new studies demonstrating that some elements of sexual response involve deactivation in areas throughout the prefrontal cortex, a region critical for higher-order functions that include, but are not limited to, both self-control and working memory [16]. Perhaps these data will identify biological correlates of the "spectatoring" phenomena described by Masters and Johnson as one of the most common causes of sexual dysfunction. Perhaps those with particular biological predispositions toward negative ruminative thinking could be identified. The Sexual Tipping Point® (STP) model could illustrate how minimizing such critical distraction with mindfulness or overriding it with erotic fantasy would offset the deleterious effect. In much the same way, the STP model could illustrate how a pharmaceutical could improve sexual response by lowering thresholds for excitement or increase the threshold that triggers sexual inhibition.[4] Greater enlightenment will be found within such integrated thinking.

35.6 Maintaining a Transdisciplinary Viewpoint Is a Critical Next Step

This book provides a springboard toward a transdisciplinary sexual medicine perspective for the reader wishing to integrate the lessons implicitly and explicitly offered. The future for sexual medicine does indeed seem bright. Yet, despite sexual medicine's impressive developments over the past 25 years, sexual worries, disorders, and dysfunctions not only remain with us but may also be increasing because of the problems caused by an ever-escalating saturation of society with sexual images and themes. The introduction of sildenafil foreshadowed a pharmaceutical and biotechnological revolution in the treatment of both male and female sexual dysfunction. As new drugs are developed and approved for men and women, opportunities for educating and assisting people in restoring sexual functioning will only increase. However, sex remains a highly emotionally charged act that always takes place within a psychological and cultural context. As such, sex therapists and physicians working together will continually have an opportunity and responsibility to participate in the restoration of their patients' sexual health. Yet, the goal of our work is not just to alleviate our patient's sexual symptom, but is also to improve their intimate relational lives. Our aspiration is for all healthcare practitioners to maintain a patient-centered holistic approach that integrates a variety of treatments as needed, whether for sexual concerns, disorders, or dysfunctions.

[4] The STP model is a registered trademark of the MAP Education and Research Fund, a 501(c)(3) public charity. STP illustrations are available free from mapedfund.org.

References

1. Perelman MA. The history of sexual medicine. In: Diamond L, Tolman D, editors. APA handbook of sexuality and psychology. Washington, DC: American Psychological Association; 2014.
2. Perelman MA. The impact of the new sexual pharmaceuticals on sex therapy. Curr Psychiatry Rep. 2001;3(3):195–201.
3. Masters W, Johnson V. Human sexual inadequacy. New York, NY: Little Brown; 1970.
4. Kaschak E, Tiefer L. A new view of women's sexual problems. New York, NY: Haworth Press; 2001.
5. Moser C. Sexual medicine, sex therapy, and sexual health care. In: Kleinplatz PJ, editor. New directions in sex therapy: innovations and alternatives. New York, NY: Routledge; 2012.
6. Perelman MA. Rehabilitative sex therapy for organic impotence. In: Segraves T, Haeberle E, editors. Emerging dimensions of sexology. New York: Praeger; 1984. p. 181–8.
7. Zarembo A. Clinic settles lawsuits but still faces scrutiny over erectile dysfunction injections. Los Angeles Times. 2 April 2011.
8. Kleinplatz PJ. New directions in sex therapy: innovations and alternatives. New York, NY: Routledge; 2012.
9. Tiefer L. Three crises facing sexology. Arch Sex Behav. 1994;23(4):361–74.
10. McCarthy BW, Fucito LM. Integrating medication, realistic expectations, and therapeutic interventions in the treatment of male sexual dysfunction. J Sex Marital Ther. 2005;31(4):319–28.
11. Althof S. Therapeutic weaving: the integration of treatment techniques. In: Levine S, editor. Handbook of clinical sexuality for mental health professionals. New York: Brunner-Routledge; 2003. p. 359–76.
12. Perelman MA. Sex coaching for physicians: combination treatment for patient and partner. Int J Impot Res. 2003;15 Suppl 5:S67–74.
13. Perelman MA. The impact of relationship variables on the etiology, diagnosis and treatment of erectile dysfunction. Adv Primary Care Med Clin Update. 2007;3:3–6.

14. Laumann EO, Paik A, Rosen RC. Sexual dysfunction in the United States: prevalence and predictors. JAMA. 1999;281(6):537–44.
15. Martin B, Richards E. Scientific knowledge, controversy, and public decision making. In: Jasanoff S, Markle GE, Petersen JC, Pinch TJ, editors. Handbook of science and technology studies. Thousand Oaks, CA: SAGE; 1995.
16. Huynh HK, Beers C, Willemsen A, Lont E, Laan E, Dierckx R, et al. High-intensity erotic visual stimuli de-activate the primary visual cortex in women. J Sex Med. 2012;9(6):1579–87.

Index

L.I. Lipshultz et al. (eds.), *Management of Sexual Dysfunction in Men and Women*, DOI 10.1007/978-1-4939-3100-2

G

H

M

N

O

P

MIX
Papier aus verantwortungsvollen Quellen
Paper from responsible sources
FSC® C105338

If you have any concerns about our products,
you can contact us on
ProductSafety@springernature.com

In case Publisher is established outside the EU,
the EU authorized representative is:
Springer Nature Customer Service Center GmbH
Europaplatz 3, 69115 Heidelberg, Germany

Printed by Libri Plureos GmbH
in Hamburg, Germany